Abdominal Pain: Clinical Assessment and Management

Abdominal Pain: Clinical Assessment and Management

Edited by Judy Landis

hayle
medical

New York

Hayle Medical,
750 Third Avenue, 9th Floor,
New York, NY 10017, USA

Visit us on the World Wide Web at:
www.haylemedical.com

ISBN: 978-1-63241-480-9

The publisher's policy is to use permanent paper from mills that operate a sustainable forestry policy. Furthermore, the publisher ensures that the text paper and cover boards used have met acceptable environmental accreditation standards.

Printed in China.

Cataloging-in-Publication Data

Abdominal pain : clinical assessment and management / edited by Judy Landis.
p. cm.
Includes bibliographical references and index.
ISBN 978-1-63241-480-9
1. Abdominal pain. 2. Abdominal pain--Diagnosis. 3. Abdominal pain--Treatment.
I. Landis, Judy.
RC809 .A23 2018
616.047 2--dc23

Table of Contents

Preface IX

Chapter 1 **Detection of Puumala Hantavirus Antigen in Human Intestine during Acute Hantavirus Infection** 1
Joerg Latus, Klara Tenner-Racz, Paul Racz, Daniel Kitterer, Daniel Cadar, German Ott, M. Dominik Alscher, Jonas Schmidt-Chanasit, Niko Braun

Chapter 2 **A School-Based Study with Rome III Criteria on the Prevalence of Functional Gastrointestinal Disorders in Chinese College and University Students** 8
Yan-Yan Dong, Fei-Xue Chen, Yan-Bo Yu, Chao Du, Qing-Qing Qi, Han Liu, Yan-Qing Li

Chapter 3 **Validation of the Fibromyalgia Survey Questionnaire within a Cross-Sectional Survey** 14
Winfried Häuser, Eva Jung, Brigitte Erbslöh-Möller, Mechthild Gesmann, Hedi Kühn-Becker, Franz Petermann, Jost Langhorst, Thomas Weiss, Andreas Winkelmann, Frederick Wolfe

Chapter 4 **Effects of Pregabalin on Central Sensitization in Patients with Chronic Pancreatitis in a Randomized, Controlled Trial** 20
Stefan A. W. Bouwense, Søren S. Olesen, Asbjørn M. Drewes, Jan-Werner Poley, Harry van Goor, Oliver H. G. Wilder-Smith

Chapter 5 **Non-Specific Abdominal Pain and Air Pollution: A Novel Association** 30
Gilaad G. Kaplan, Mieczyslaw Szyszkowicz, Jakub Fichna, Brian H. Rowe, Eugeniusz Porada, Renaud Vincent, Karen Madsen, Subrata Ghosh, Martin Storr

Chapter 6 **Preference for Different Anchor Descriptors on Visual Analogue Scales among Japanese Patients with Chronic Pain** 38
Junya Yokobe, Masaki Kitahara, Masato Matsushima, Shoichi Uezono

Chapter 7 **Influence of the Serotonin Transporter 5HTTLPR Polymorphism on Symptom Severity in Irritable Bowel Syndrome** 45
Rocchina Colucci, Dario Gambaccini, Narcisa Ghisu, Giuseppe Rossi, Francesco Costa, Marco Tuccori, Nicola De Bortoli, Matteo Fornai, Luca Antonioli, Angelo Ricchiuti, Maria Gloria Mumolo, Santino Marchi, Corrado Blandizzi, Massimo Bellini

Chapter 8 **Neurologic Manifestations Associated with an Outbreak of Typhoid Fever, Malawi - Mozambique, 2009: An Epidemiologic Investigation** 51
James Sejvar, Emily Lutterloh, Jeremias Naiene, Andrew Likaka, Robert Manda, Benjamin Nygren, Stephan Monroe, Tadala Khaila, Sara A. Lowther, Linda Capewell, Kashmira Date, David Townes, Yanique Redwood, Joshua Schier, Beth Tippett Barr, Austin Demby, Macpherson Mallewa, Sam Kampondeni, Ben Blount, Michael Humphrys, Deborah Talkington, Gregory L. Armstrong, Eric Mintz

Chapter 9 **Identification of a Novel Nonsense Mutation p.Tyr1957Ter of CACNA1A in a Chinese Family with Episodic Ataxia 2** 60
Yafang Hu, Haishan Jiang, Qun Wang, Zuoshan Xie, Suyue Pan

Chapter 10 **MicroRNA Profiling in Mucosal Biopsies of Eosinophilic Esophagitis Patients Pre and Post Treatment with Steroids and Relationship with mRNA Targets** 65
Shaolei Lu, Vincent A. Mukkada, Shamlal Mangray, Kelly Cleveland, Nick Shillingford, Christoph Schorl, Alexander S. Brodsky, Murray B. Resnick

Chapter 11 **Risk Factors for Development of Chronic Kidney Disease following Renal Infarction: Retrospective Evaluation of Emergency Room Patients from a Single Center** 76
Wen-Ling Lin, Chen-June Seak, Jiunn-Yih Wu, Yi-Ming Weng, Hang-Cheng Chen

Chapter 12 **Developmental Fluoxetine Exposure Normalizes the Long-Term Effects of Maternal Stress on Post-Operative Pain in Sprague-Dawley Rat Offspring** 84
Liesbeth Knaepen, Ine Rayen, Thierry D. Charlier, Marianne Fillet, Virginie Houbart, Maarten van Kleef, Harry W. Steinbusch, Jacob Patijn, Dick Tibboel, Elbert A. Joosten, Jodi L. Pawluski

Chapter 13 **Concordance of Sleep and Pain Outcomes of Diverse Interventions** 93
Anthony G. Doufas, Orestis A. Panagiotou, John P. A. Ioannidis

Chapter 14 **Enhanced Auditory Brainstem Response and Parental Bonding Style in Children with Gastrointestinal Symptoms** 100
Shizuka Seino, Satoshi Watanabe, Namiko Ito, Konosuke Sasaki, Kaori Shoji, Shoko Miura, Kanoko Kozawa, Kunihiko Nakai, Hiroshi Sato, Motoyori Kanazawa, Shin Fukudo

Chapter 15 **Catechol-O-Methyltransferase val158met Polymorphism Predicts Placebo Effect in Irritable Bowel Syndrome** 108
Kathryn T. Hall, Anthony J. Lembo, Irving Kirsch, Dimitrios C. Ziogas, Jeffrey Douaiher, Karin B. Jensen, Lisa A. Conboy, John M. Kelley, Efi Kokkotou, Ted J. Kaptchuk

Chapter 16 **Infant Safety during and after Maternal Valacyclovir Therapy in Conjunction with Antiretroviral HIV-1 Prophylaxis in a Randomized Clinical Trial** 114
Alison L. Drake, Alison C. Roxby, James Kiarie, Barbra A. Richardson, Anna Wald, Grace John-Stewart, Carey Farquhar

Chapter 17 **Regional Neuroplastic Brain Changes in Patients with Chronic Inflammatory and Non-Inflammatory Visceral Pain** 123
Jui-Yang Hong, Jennifer S. Labus, Zhiguo Jiang, Cody Ashe-Mcnalley, Ivo Dinov, Arpana Gupta, Yonggang Shi, Jean Stains, Nuwanthi Heendeniya, Suzanne R. Smith, Kirsten Tillisch, Emeran A. Mayer

Chapter 18 **Self-Reported Pain Intensity with the Numeric Reporting Scale in Adult Dengue** 131
Joshua G. X. Wong, Victor C. Gan, Ee-Ling Ng, Yee-Sin Leo, Siew-Pang Chan, Robin Choo, David C. Lye

Chapter 19 **Increased Diagnostic Yield of Capsule Endoscopy in Patients with Chronic Abdominal Pain** 137
Liping Yang, Yu Chen, Bingling Zhang, Chunxiao Chen, Min Yue, Juan Du, Chaohui Yu, Youming Li

Chapter 20 **The Analysis of Factors Associated with Progression of Isolated Terminal Ileal Lesions** 141
Zhang Fangbin, Hao Weiwei, Zhao Wugan, Zheng Cong, Chu Yanjun, Xu Feng

Chapter 21 **Gastro-Esophageal Reflux Disease Symptoms and Demographic Factors as a Pre-Screening Tool for Barrett's Esophagus** 148
Xinxue Liu, Angela Wong, Sudarshan R. Kadri, Andrej Corovic, Maria O'Donovan, Pierre Lao-Sirieix, Laurence B. Lovat, Rodney W. Burnham, Rebecca C. Fitzgerald

Chapter 22 **The Duration of Gastrointestinal and Joint Symptoms after a Large Waterborne Outbreak of Gastroenteritis in Finland in 2007 – A Questionnaire-Based 15-Month Follow-Up Study** 156
Janne Laine, Jukka Lumio, Salla Toikkanen, Mikko J. Virtanen, Terhi Uotila, Markku Korpela, Eila Kujansuu, Markku Kuusi

Chapter 23 **Excitability of the Motor Cortex in *De Novo* Patients with Celiac Disease** 162
Giovanni Pennisi, Giuseppe Lanza, Salvatore Giuffrida, Luisa Vinciguerra, Valentina Puglisi, Mariagiovanna Cantone, Manuela Pennisi, Carmela Cinzia D'Agate, Pietro Naso, Giuseppe Aprile, Giulia Malaguarnera, Raffaele Ferri, Rita Bella

Chapter 24 **How and when should NSAIDs be used for Preventing Post-ERCP Pancreatitis?** 169
Ignasi Puig, Xavier Calvet, Mireia Baylina, Álvaro Isava, Pau Sort, Jordina Llaó, Francesc Porta, Francesc Vida

Chapter 25 **The Association between GP Consultations for Non-Specific Physical Symptoms in Children and Parents** 177
Mujahed Shraim, Milisa Blagojevic-Bucknall, Christian D. Mallen, Kate M. Dunn

Chapter 26 **A School-Based Cross-Sectional Survey of Adverse Events following Co-Administration of Albendazole and Praziquantel for Preventive Chemotherapy against Urogenital Schistosomiasis and Soil-Transmitted Helminthiasis in Kwale County, Kenya** 187
Sammy M. Njenga, Paul M. Ng'ang'a, Mariam T. Mwanje, Fatuma S. Bendera, Moses J. Bockarie

Chapter 27 **The Impact of Sexual Abuse in Patients Undergoing Colonoscopy** 192
Melianthe P. J. Nicolai, Josbert J. Keller, Lieke de Vries, Andrea E. van der Meulen-de Jong, Jan J. Nicolai, James C. H. Hardwick, Hein Putter, Rob C. M. Pelger, Henk W. Elzevier

Chapter 28 **Typhoid Outbreak in Songkhla, Thailand 2009-2011: Clinical Outcomes, Susceptibility Patterns, and Reliability of Serology Tests** 200
Wannee Limpitikul, Narong Henpraserttae, Rachanee Saksawad, Kamolwish Laoprasopwattana

Chapter 29 **Revisiting Russell's Viper (*Daboia russelii*) Bite in Sri Lanka: Is Abdominal Pain an Early Feature of Systemic Envenoming?** 206
Senanayake A. M. Kularatne, Anjana Silva, Kosala Weerakoon, Kalana Maduwage, Chamara Walathara, Ranjith Paranagama, Suresh Mendis

Chapter 30 **Perceptions of Malaria in Pregnancy and Acceptability of Preventive Interventions among Mozambican Pregnant Women: Implications for Effectiveness of Malaria Control in Pregnancy** 214
Helena Boene, Raquel Gonzílez, Anifa Valá, Maria Rupérez, César Velasco, Sónia Machevo, Charfudin Sacoor, Esperança Sevene, Eusébio Macete, Clara Menéndez, Khátia Munguambe

Permissions

List of Contributors

Index

Preface

This book has been a concerted effort by a group of academicians, researchers and scientists, who have contributed their research works for the realization of the book. This book has materialized in the wake of emerging advancements and innovations in this field. Therefore, the need of the hour was to compile all the required researches and disseminate the knowledge to a broad spectrum of people comprising of students, researchers and specialists of the field.

Abdominal pain is the pain that occurs between the pelvis and the chest. The pain may vary from a mild stomach ache to severe pain. The cause can either be inflammation, trauma to stomach or bowel, peptic ulcer, etc. In order to diagnose the problem, tests such as colonoscopy, computed tomography and ultrasound can be performed. The book presents researches and studies performed by experts across the globe. Through this book, we attempt to further enlighten the readers about the new developments in this field.

At the end of the preface, I would like to thank the authors for their brilliant chapters and the publisher for guiding us all-through the making of the book till its final stage. Also, I would like to thank my family for providing the support and encouragement throughout my academic career and research projects.

Editor

Detection of Puumala Hantavirus Antigen in Human Intestine during Acute Hantavirus Infection

Joerg Latus[1], Klara Tenner-Racz[2], Paul Racz[2], Daniel Kitterer[1]*, Daniel Cadar[2], German Ott[3], M. Dominik Alscher[1], Jonas Schmidt-Chanasit[2,4], Niko Braun[1]

1 Department of Internal Medicine, Division of Nephrology, Robert-Bosch Hospital, Auerbachstrasse 110, Stuttgart, Germany, **2** Bernhard Nocht Institute for Tropical Medicine, WHO Collaborating Centre for Arbovirus and Haemmorrhagic Fever Reference and Research, Bernhard-Nocht-Strasse 74, Hamburg, Germany, **3** Department of Diagnostic Medicine, Division of Pathology, Robert-Bosch Hospital, Auerbachstrasse 110, Stuttgart, Germany, **4** German Centre for Infection Research (DZIF), partner site Hamburg-Luebeck-Borstel, Hamburg, Germany

Abstract

Background: Puumala virus (PUUV) is the most important hantavirus species in Central Europe. Nephropathia epidemica (NE), caused by PUUV, is characterized by acute renal injury (AKI) with thrombocytopenia and frequently gastrointestinal symptoms.

Methods: 456 patients with serologically and clinically confirmed NE were investigated at time of follow-up in a single clinic. The course of the NE was investigated using medical reports. We identified patients who had endoscopy with intestinal biopsy during acute phase of NE. Histopathological, immunohistochemical and molecular analyses of the biopsies were performed.

Results: Thirteen patients underwent colonoscopy or gastroscopy for abdominal pain, diarrhea, nausea and vomiting during acute phase of NE. Immunohistochemistry (IHC) revealed PUUV nucleocapsid antigen in 11 biopsies from 8 patients; 14 biopsies from 5 patients were negative for PUUV nucleocapsid antigen. IHC localized PUUV nucleocapsid antigen in endothelial cells of capillaries or larger vessels in the lamina propria. Rate of AKI was not higher and severity of AKI was not different in the PUUV-positive compared to the PUUV-negative group. All IHC positive biopsies were positive for PUUV RNA using RT-PCR. Phylogenetic reconstruction revealed clustering of all PUUV strains from this study with viruses previously detected from the South-West of Germany. Long-term outcome was favorable in both groups.

Conclusions: In patients with NE, PUUV nucleocapsid antigen and PUUV RNA was detected frequently in the intestine. This finding could explain frequent GI-symptoms in NE patients, thus demonstration of a more generalized PUUV infection. The RT-PCR was an effective and sensitive method to detect PUUV RNA in FFPE tissues. Therefore, it can be used as a diagnostic and phylogenetic approach also for archival materials. AKI was not more often present in patients with PUUV-positive IHC. This last finding should be investigated in larger numbers of patients with PUUV infection.

Editor: Niklas K. Björkström, Karolinska Institutet, Sweden

Funding: The authors have no support or funding to report.

Competing Interests: The authors have declared that no competing interests exist.

* E-mail: Daniel.Kitterer@rbk.de

Introduction

Hantaviruses are rodent-borne zoonotic viruses of the *Bunyaviridae* family [1] that can cause Hemorrhagic Fever with Renal Syndrome (HFRS) in Asia and Europe and Hantavirus Cardiopulmonary Syndrome in the Americas with reported case fatality rates up to 35% [2–5]. Puumala virus (PUUV) is the main hantavirus species in Central Europe and is known to cause a milder form of HFRS, which also is called nephropathia epidemica (NE) [6–11]. The clinical picture in NE includes acute kidney injury (AKI), thrombocytopenia, proteinuria and hematuria caused by tubular and glomerular involvement [12]. Both renal tubular and glomerular cells are affected by infection that leads to breakdown of cell-to cell contacts [13]. Therefore, the urinary sediment of patients with hantavirus infection contains tubular cells, with enlarged nucleoli, that are positive for hantavirus antigen [14–16]. At the level of histopathology, hantavirus infection leads to mild tubular interstitial changes and moderate interstitial infiltration with mononuclear cells [13,17]. Up to now, hantavirus antigen has been found only in the cytoplasm of tubular epithelial cells from kidney biopsies of infected patients [16,18–21]. In 1992, Nuutinen et al. [22] were the first who performed endoscopy (gastroscopy or colonoscopy) in 10 patients with acute NE (within 1–4 weeks after beginning of symptoms). In every case, hemorrhagic gastropathy was observed. Histopathological analysis of the intestinal biopsies showed that the hemorrhagic lesions were associated with edema in the lamina propria. No inflammatory changes could be detected within the biopsies [22].

A high percentage of patients with PUUV infection have severe gastrointestinal (GI) symptoms, e.g. abdominal pain, nausea and vomiting [12,23,24]. Recently we demonstrated PUUV antigen in the appendix of a NE patient with severe AKI, who underwent surgery due to severe abdominal pain. Immunohistochemistry (IHC) of the appendix from this patient showed PUUV antigen in capillary and large vessel endothelium. The capillaries with PUUV-positive, endothelial cells were located mainly in the lamina propria, including the gut associated lymphoid tissue (GALT). PUUV antigen in larger vessels was present mainly in the serosa and mesoappendix [25]. Rarely, viral antigen was found in lymphoreticular cells. In the present study, our aim was to investigate whether GI symptoms in some patients with NE is associated with PUUV infection of intestine. We have performed histopathological, immunohistochemical and molecular analyses of biopsies of the human intestine of 13 patients with NE and severe GI symptoms. The course of the disease and long- term outcome was investigated in these patients.

Materials and Methods

Patients

Since 2001, German laboratories report diagnosed PUUV infections to the local health authorities. All serologically and clinically confirmed NE patients from four selected local health authorities in southern Germany were contacted by mail. We identified 1.570 patients with NE between who became ill between 2001 and 2012. These patients were asked to attend the outpatient clinic between September 2012 and April 2013. Overall 456 NE patients could be followed at the outpatient department at the Robert-Bosch-Hospital Stuttgart, Germany. Three patients were excluded by age <18 years at the time of NE. All patients gave written informed consent before participating in the study, which was approved by the Ethics Committee of the Ethics Commission of the State Chamber of Medicine in Baden- Wuerttemberg (Stuttgart) (F-2012-046). Studies were conducted in concordance with the Declaration of Helsinki.

Data acquisition

Clinical and laboratory data during the acute phase of NE were obtained from medical reports and files from each patient or reported by the patient at time of follow-up. We identified patients who underwent colonoscopy or gastroscopy including biopsies during acute PUUV- infection. At time of follow-up at the outpatient department at the Robert-Bosch-Hospital Stuttgart, Germany detailed past and current medical histories were obtained, and a careful physical examination was done. AKI was classified on the basis of the RIFLE criteria [26]. Mild/ moderate AKI was defined in patients with no AKI and AKI Risk (R) and severe AKI was classified as RIFLE Injury (I) and RIFLE Failure (F). Information on pre-hospital baseline serum creatinine levels was available for all patients. Blood pressure was measured in all patients twice as recommended by the American Heart Association [27]. Hypertension stage 1 was defined by SBP of 140–159 mm Hg or DBP 90–99 mmHg and hypertension stage 2 by SBP >160 mm Hg or DBP >100 mmHg according to the classification of blood pressure for adults of the Seventh Report of the Joint National Committee on Prevention, Detection, Evaluation, and Treatment of High Blood Pressure [28].

All serum samples at time of follow-up were analyzed for PUUV-specific IgM and IgG in all patients using a strip-immunoblotassay (recomLine Bunyavirus IgG/IgM, Mikrogen, Germany) [29]. Hematuria was defined as a positive dipstick test for erythrocytes and over two erythrocytes per high-power field. Proteinuria was defined by an albumin/creatinine ratio (ACR)> 0.25 g/g creatinine in spot urine sample [30].

Biopsies and IHC

All patients had given their informed consent regarding a scientific work-up of tissues taken during routine procedures and eight different departments of pathology were involved in the routine pathological work-up of the biopsies. Twenty-five intestinal biopsies were fixed in 10% neutral-buffered formalin solution and embedded in paraffin. Five µm-thick sections were prepared and placed on slides coated with 3-amino-propyl-trethosilane. After deparaffinizing through xylene the sections were boiled in a domestic pressure cooker in citrate buffer pH 6 for 3 minutes and chilled down to room temperature. The sections were incubated with a PUUV monoclonal antibody raised against nucleocapsid protein (clone A1C5; dilution: 1:30; Progen Biotechnik, Heidelberg, Germany) for 30 min. Binding of antibody was visualized using the kit DCS Detection Line (DCS Innovative Diagnostik System, Hamburg, Germany) containing a secondary antibody coupled with biotin and a conjugate Streptavidin and horseradish peroxidase. The slides were developed using DAB (3,3′diaminobenzidine), counterstained with haematoxylin and mounted. To delineate the cells containing PUUV nucleocapsidantigen, immunohistochemical double labelling was applied. After developing the DAB step, the sections were then heat treated again for 2 min and incubated with the monoclonal antibody CD34 (dilution: 1:100; Dako) for overnight. The second antibody was visualized with alkaline phosphatase (Dako) Fast Blue salt. The sections were examined using an AxioIimager M1 microscope (Carl Zeiss, Jena, Germany). Vero E6 cells infected with PUUV strain Sotkamo served as positive control.

Molecular detection and phylogenetic characterization of PUUV from biopsies

A total of 8 biopsies from different patients (7 gastric and 1 colon), which were detected as positive by IHC, have been subjected to molecular investigation. In parallel, we used formalin fixed and paraffin embedded (FFPE) PUUV uninfected and infected Vero E6 cells as controls. Four 10-micron thickness sections from each FFPE biopsies were used for RNA extraction. Whole viral RNA was extracted from tissues by use of RNeasy FFPE Kit (Qiagen, Hilden, Germany) according to the manufacturer's instructions. RNA was then subjected to RT-PCR to recover partial S segment (144 bp) using a degenerate forward primer PUMAGJ1-F 5′-CAACMCGTGGGAGACARACTGT-3′ at position 429 and reverse primer PUMAGJ1-R 5′-CYTTCATRGTTGAYTGAGCAGT-3′ at position 572 both positions according to the complete nucleocapsid gene protein sequence of the Bavaria CG 33/04 strain (GenBank acc. no. DQ016430) designed based on all available European PUUV strains retrieved from the GenBank. Reverse transcription and PCR amplification (RT-PCR) of the 144 bp segment of the nucleocapsid gene was performed using the SuperScript III One-Step RT-PCR System with Platinum Taq High Fidelity (Invitrogen). The PCR was performed in a 50-ml volume containing 5 µl of sample RNA, 25 µl of 2x Reaction Mix, 2.5 µl of each primer (PUMAGJ1 and PUMAGJ2), 2 µl High Fidelity Enzym-Mix and ddH2O up to 50 µl. The reaction was then incubated in a thermocycler under the following conditions: 50°C for 50 minutes and 94°C as cDNA synthesis and pre-denaturation step; 45 cycles of 94°C for 20 seconds (denaturation), 55°C for 45 seconds (annealing), 72°C for 1 minute (extension) with a final elongation step at 72 °C for 10 min. The PCR product was visualized on a UV transilluminator following separation on 2.5% agarose gels containing ethidium bromide. Amplicons were sent to the company LGC Genomics for Sanger sequencing. Sequence data were analyzed using Geneious 7.4.1 program for multiple alignments. Phylogenetic analyses of the obtained sequences were performed in comparison to the strains belonging to different geographical regions as retrieved from GenBank. Evolutionary tree and distances (number of base substitutions per site) were generated by PhyML v3.1 [31]with the General-Time-Reversible model of sequence evolution with gamma-distributed rate variation among sites and proportion of invariable sites (GTR + Γ+I) found to be most appropriate model according to Akaike information criteria included in the jModelTest [32]. The PUUV sequences were shown in File S1.

Statistical analysis

Data are reported as median and range unless otherwise specified. All continuous variables were tested for normality using the Kolmogorov-Smirnov test. Comparisons between different groups were performed with the Mann-Whitney test or the Fisher's exact test, as appropriate. Analysis was performed using GraphPad statistical software package (San Diego, California, USA). A p value <0.05 was considered statistically significant.

Results

Overall, 456 patients were followed-up at our outpatient clinic with a median follow up time of 10 (7–29) months after acute NE. All patients lived in southern Germany and had laboratory and clinically confirmed NE between 2001 and 2012.Thirteen patients had colonoscopy or gastroscopy with biopsies during their acute PUUV- infection. Endoscopy was done 12 (9–15) days in the PUUV-positive group and 7 (4–9) days in the PUUV-negative group after beginning of symptoms associated with NE. The indications for endoscopy were severe abdominal pain, diarrhea, nausea and vomiting. Gastroscopy revealed gastritis with subepithelial hemorrhages and telangiectasia in all patients. The most prominent hemorrhagic findings were found in the antrum. In the PUUV-positive group, in two patients gastritis was associated with *Helicobater pylori* infection, whereas in the PUUV-negative group no *Helicobater pylori* infection could be found. In the PUUV-negative group, two patients had mild gastro-esophageal reflux disease and in one patient thrush esophagitis was present. Colonoscopy was done in 3 patients revealing spotty hemorrhage in all biopsies without any signs of inflammation.

IHC was done on 25 intestinal biopsies. Twenty-one of these were gastric; 1 was esophageal; and 3 were from colon. PUUV nucleocapsid antigen was detected in eleven biopsies from eight patients (9 gastric and 2 colon). Fourteen biopsies (12 gastric, 1 esophageal and 1 colon) from 5 patients were negative for PUUV nucleocapsid antigen. PUUV nucleocapsid antigen was mainly found in endothelial cell of capillaries or larger vessels in the lamina propria of biopsies from stomach or colon (see Figure 1 and 2). The intense immunohistochemical staining of cells expressing PUUV nucleocapsid antigen deposited in a granular pattern documents the involvement of the human intestine in PUUV infection. Biopsies from all patients, which were detected as positive by IHC, have been subjected to molecular investigation. All IHC positive biopsies were positive for PUUV RNA using RT-PCR.

Four out of eight patients in the PUUV-positive and three out of five patients in the PUUV-negative group presented with abdominal pain at time of diagnosis. Nausea and vomiting were present in five out of eight patients in the PUUV-positive and in three out of five patients in the PUUV negative group. In total, ten out of thirteen patients had AKI during PUUV infection. Neither higher rates of AKI, nor differences regarding severity of AKI could be detected in the PUUV-positive compared to the PUUV-negative group. At time of follow-up, kidney function was within the normal range in all patients. The prevalence of hypertension, proteinuria, hematuria and co-morbidities as long-term consequences after PUUV infection was not different between both groups. A detailed summary of study population including laboratory values during acute course of the disease and at time of follow-up is given in table 1 and table 2. Due to a possible selection bias, we compared baseline characteristics during acute course of the disease (e.g. laboratory values, severity of AKI, symptoms during acute course of the disease) and outcome data between the patients who underwent endoscopy with biopsies (n = 13) and the study population without endoscopy (n = 443 patients). No statistical significant differences could be observed between the groups (data not shown).

Phylogenetic reconstruction revealed clustering of all PUUV strains from this study with viruses previously detected from the South-West of Germany (Figure 3) [33].

Discussion

We investigated biopsies of the human intestine in patients with acute PUUV infection in order to understand why a majority of patients with NE have severe abdominal pain [23], for which there is no pathophysiologic explanation. We found 13 patients who had an endoscopy at time of acute Hantavirus infection due to severe gastrointestinal symptoms. Endoscopy was carried out during acute phase of NE and gastritis with hemorrhage could be observed in all patients. In line with the results from to the study of Nuutinen et al. [22], the hemorrhagic changes were more prominent in the proximal compared to the distal part of the stomach. In contrast, signs of inflammation could be detected in all intestinal biopsies in our study.

IHC demonstrated PUUV nucleocapsid antigen in 62% of the analyzed biopsies. PUUV nucleocapsid antigen was located mainly in endothelial cells of capillaries or larger vessels in the lamina propria. This finding accords with previous reports from patients with HCPS, with experimental PUUV infection in cynomolgus macaques and from our recent report [25,34,35]. Almost all hantavirus infections (especially southern Germany) are caused by PUUV [7,33], although Tula virus and Dobrava-Belgrade virus circulates in Germany and might cause symptomatic infections in humans [36–39].

Regarding clinical course of the disease, twelve out of thirteen patients had to be admitted to hospital. Duration of hospital stay was more than one week and ten out of thirteen patients had AKI, indicating that PUUV causes severe disease in most patients with NE. Although the number of patients is relatively small, a possible explanation could be an enhanced inflammatory response caused by a generalized PUUV infection. This systemic infection could be reflected by the presence of PUUV nucleocapsid antigen in human intestine and might explain the clinical phenotype of severe GI-symptoms. Further studies in larger numbers of NE patients are needed to investigate whether detection of PUUV nucleocapsid antigen in the human intestine might be a risk factor for severe course of the disease.

Remarkably, all IHC positive biopsies were positive for PUUV RNA using RT-PCR. Thus, the RT-PCR technique could be used to detect infection from archival or fixed materials. As an auxiliary advantage of RT-PCR, it is possible to sequence the amplicon, enabling more extensive molecular analyses. In this study, the nucleocapsid gene was chosen for amplification because it provides valuable information regarding the possible origin of the PUUV. The success of the development of this RT-PCR from FFPE biopsies enables work on PUUV in more flexible conditions

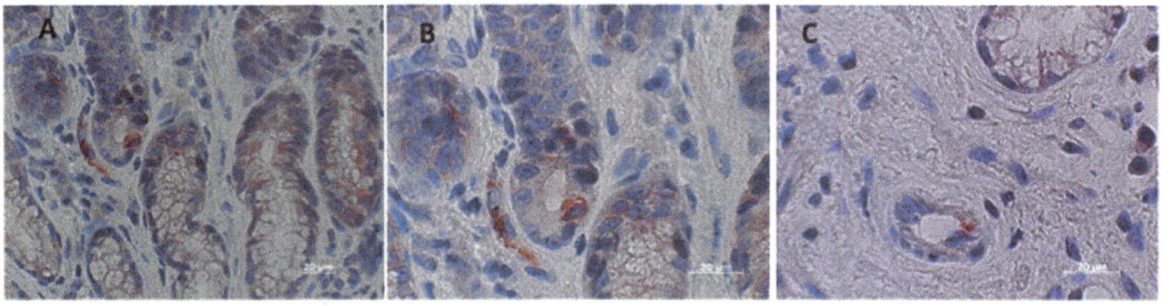

Figure 1. Detection of PUUV nucleocapsid antigen in the capillaries in the lamina propria of a gastric biopsy 8 days after beginning of symptoms associated with NE (fever, abdominal pain, nausea and vomiting) A Higher magnification demonstrates capillaries with positive endothelial cells in the lamina propria (same patient) B Endothelial cell with PUUV nucleocapsid antigen (same patient) C.

because FFPE could be handled without biosecurity concerns. In this study, phylogenetic reconstruction revealed clustering of all PUUV strains with viruses previously detected from South-West of Germany [33]. Based on Ettinger et al. [33] the German PUUV strains formed 6 distinct clades comprising strains of human and vole origin corresponding to a different outbreak region. High similarities between human and rodent-derived PUUV strains from the same region and distinct from the others highlight the

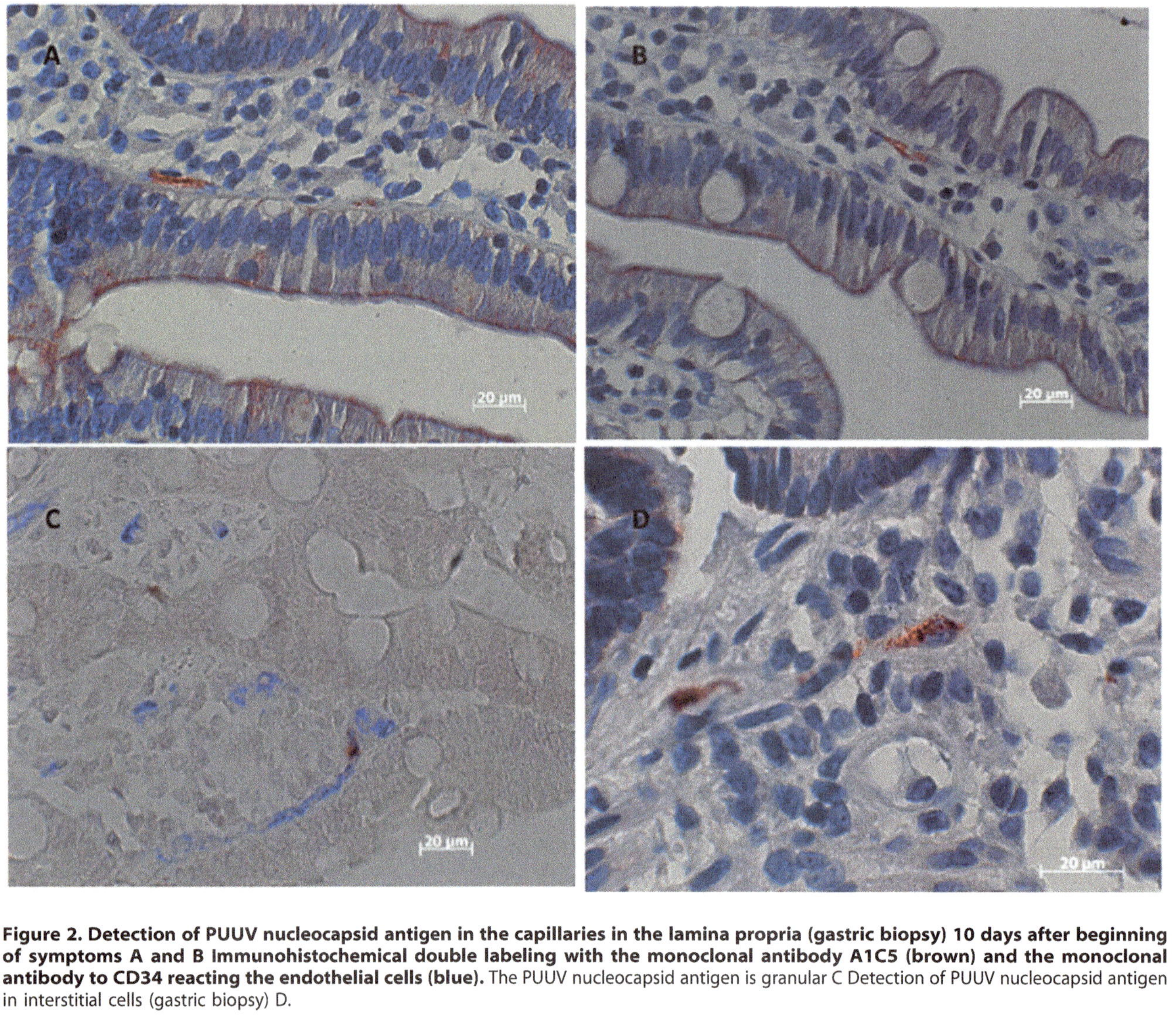

Figure 2. Detection of PUUV nucleocapsid antigen in the capillaries in the lamina propria (gastric biopsy) 10 days after beginning of symptoms A and B Immunohistochemical double labeling with the monoclonal antibody A1C5 (brown) and the monoclonal antibody to CD34 reacting the endothelial cells (blue). The PUUV nucleocapsid antigen is granular C Detection of PUUV nucleocapsid antigen in interstitial cells (gastric biopsy) D.

Table 1. Baseline characteristics of study population during acute phase of NE.

Variable	PUUV nucleocapsid antigen positive (n = 8)	PUUV nucleocapsid antigen negative (n = 5)
n	8	5
Female/male	4/4	1/4
Age at diagnosis (years)	55 (48–65)	51 (38–63)
In-patients/outpatients	8/0	4/1
Duration of hospital stay	9 (7–13)	11 (9–12)
Assumed path of infection		
- Occupational	0	1
- During leisure time	8	4
Symptoms		
Abdominal pain	4/8	3/5
Back pain	3/8	4/5
Pain of the limbs	6/8	3/5
Headache	6/8	4/5
Visual disorders	1/8	0/5
Diarrhea	2/8	2/5
Nausea/Vomiting	5/8	3/5
Clinical signs		
Fever	7/8	5/5
Hemorrhage	0/8	0/5
Urinary analysis at admission	6/8	4/4
- Proteinuria	5/6	3/5
- Hematuria	4/6	1/5
- Leucocyturia	1/6	0/5
Acute Kidney Injury		
Acute Kidney Injury according to RIFLE classification	7/8	3/5
- Risk	5	1
- Injury	0	1
- Failure	2	1

Table 2. Baseline characteristics of study population at follow-up.

Variable	PUUV nucleocapsid antigen positive (n = 8)	PUUV nucleocapsid antigen negative (n = 5)
Number of patients	8	5
Follow-up (months)	10 (7–33)	19 (10–28)
Laboratory findings		
Creatinine (mg/dl [0.5–1.4])	0.9 (0.8–1.0)	0.9 (0.8–0.9)
Platelets (10^9/L [>150])	238 (220–256)	241 (216–258)
Urinary analysis		
- Proteinuria	0/8	0/5
- Hematuria	2/8	0/5
- Leucocyturia	2/8	0/5
- Presence of bacteria	0/8	0/5
Hypertension		
Hypertension at time of presentation	1/8	1/5

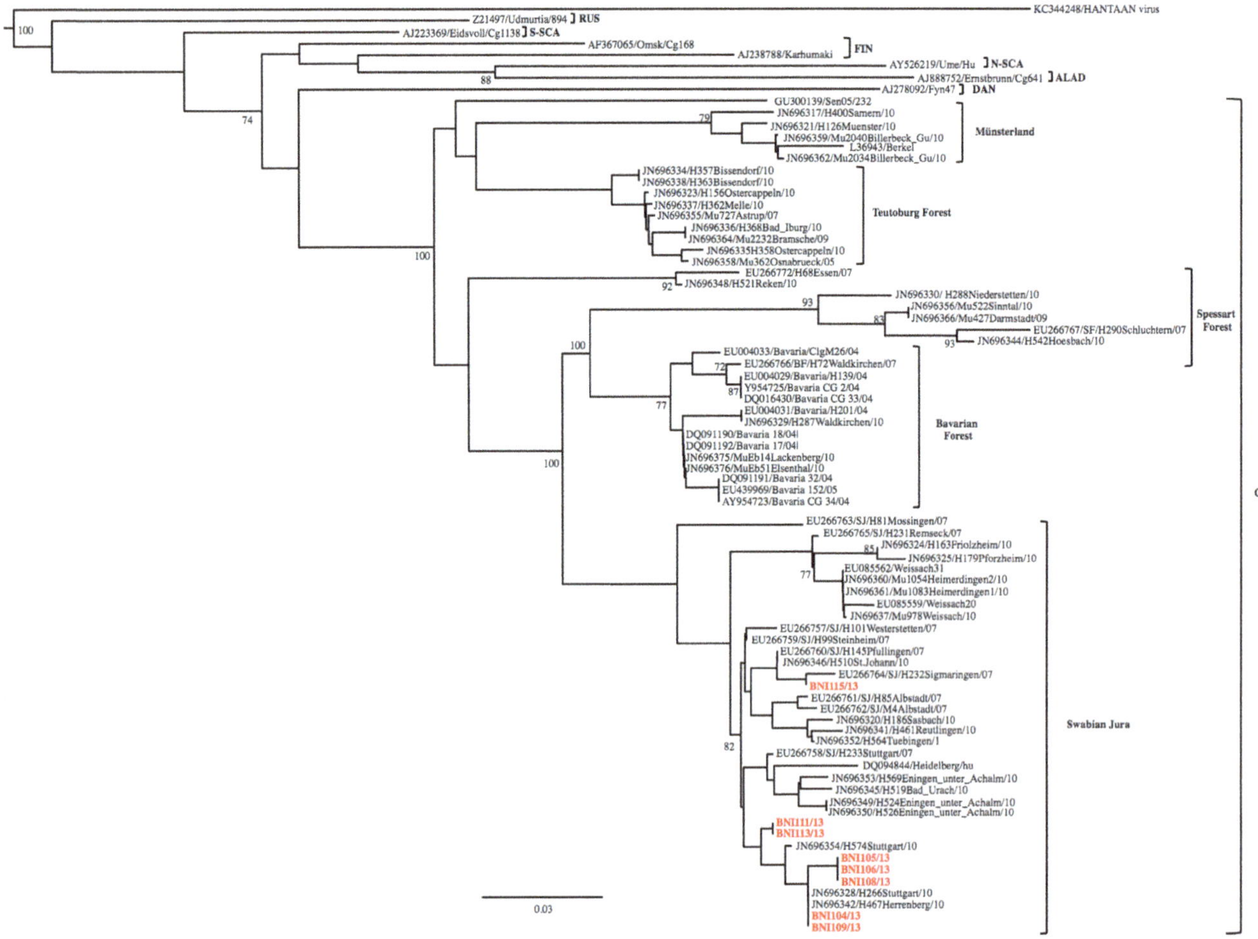

Figure 3. Maximum-likelihood phylogenetic tree of PUUV based on partial (144 bp) sequences of the small segment showing the placement of the PUUV strains from this study into the German subtypes. Bootstrap values >70%, calculated from 10,000 replicates are shown at the tree branches. For clarity, the Central European PUUMV clade include only German strains. Previously characterized PUUMV clades: **ALAD**, Alpe-Adrian; **CE**, Central European; **S-SCA**, South Scandinavian; **FIN**, Finnish; **RUS**, Russian; **N-SCA**, North Scandinavian; **DAN**, Dannish. The tree was rooted using murine-associated hantavirus: Hantaan virus (HNTV). Scale bar indicates mean number of nucleotide substitutions per site. GenBank accession numbers and the name of the strains are shown.

fact that the 2010 epidemic was associated with increased densities and infection rates of the bank voles in several regions of Germany and not determined by countrywide spread of the same PUUV strain [33]. In conclusion, we successfully developed a method to detect PUUV in FFPE tissues by RT-PCR and demonstrated its use as potential diagnostic tool as well as for PUUV molecular epidemiology investigations. Furthermore, it is possible to perform retrospective studies of archived materials from patients where PUUV was not the initial diagnosis.

This is the first study, which investigated biopsies of the human intestine in patients with NE using IHC and molecular approaches. PUUV nucleocapsid antigen and PUUV RNA were frequently detected. This finding might be an expression of a more generalized infection, which is emphasized by high rates of AKI in this study population. The presence of PUUV antigen was not correlated with the extension of abdominal complains. We suggest that a larger patient cohort should be analyzed in future studies to demonstrate possible significant differences and correlations.

Author Contributions

Conceived and designed the experiments: NB JL JSC DC. Performed the experiments: NB JL JSC DK MDA GO KTR PR DC. Analyzed the data: JL NB DK MDA JSC DC. Contributed reagents/materials/analysis tools: KTR PR GO DC. Wrote the paper: JL NB MDA DK JSC DC.

References

1. Schmaljohn CS, Dalrymple JM (1983) Analysis of Hantaan virus RNA: evidence for a new genus of bunyaviridae. Virology 131: 482–491.
2. Kruger DH, Schonrich G, Klempa B (2011) Human pathogenic hantaviruses and prevention of infection. Hum Vaccin 7: 685–693.
3. Lee HW, van der Groen G (1989) Hemorrhagic fever with renal syndrome. Prog Med Virol 36: 62–102.
4. Mertz GJ, Hjelle B, Crowley M, Iwamoto G, Tomicic V, et al. (2006) Diagnosis and treatment of new world hantavirus infections. Curr Opin Infect Dis 19: 437–442.

5. Peters CJ, Simpson GL, Levy H (1999) Spectrum of hantavirus infection: hemorrhagic fever with renal syndrome and hantavirus pulmonary syndrome. Annu Rev Med 50: 531–545.
6. Vapalahti O, Mustonen J, Lundkvist A, Henttonen H, Plyusnin A, et al. (2003) Hantavirus infections in Europe. Lancet Infect Dis 3: 653–661.
7. Kruger DH, Ulrich RG, Hofmann J (2013) Hantaviruses as zoonotic pathogens in Germany. Dtsch Arztebl Int 110: 461–467.
8. Hofmann J, Meisel H, Klempa B, Vesenbeckh SM, Beck R, et al. (2008) Hantavirus outbreak, Germany, 2007. Emerg Infect Dis 14: 850–852.
9. Heyman P, Thoma BR, Marie JL, Cochez C, Essbauer SS (2012) In Search for Factors that Drive Hantavirus Epidemics. Front Physiol 3: 237.
10. Mertens M, Wolfel R, Ullrich K, Yoshimatsu K, Blumhardt J, et al. (2009) Seroepidemiological study in a Puumala virus outbreak area in South-East Germany. Med Microbiol Immunol 198: 83–91.
11. Essbauer SS, Schmidt-Chanasit J, Madeja EL, Wegener W, Friedrich R, et al. (2007) Nephropathia epidemica in metropolitan area, Germany. Emerg Infect Dis 13: 1271–1273.
12. Krautkramer E, Zeier M, Plyusnin A (2013) Hantavirus infection: an emerging infectious disease causing acute renal failure. Kidney Int 83: 23–27.
13. Krautkramer E, Grouls S, Stein N, Reiser J, Zeier M (2011) Pathogenic old world hantaviruses infect renal glomerular and tubular cells and induce disassembling of cell-to-cell contacts. J Virol 85: 9811–9823.
14. Zeier M, Ritz E (1996) [Hantavirus-induced acute renal failure]. Internist (Berl) 37: 1092–1095.
15. Mustonen J, Helin H, Pietila K, Brummer-Korvenkontio M, Hedman K, et al. (1994) Renal biopsy findings and clinicopathologic correlations in nephropathia epidemica. Clin Nephrol 41: 121–126.
16. Groen J, Bruijn JA, Gerding MN, Jordans JG, Moll van Charante AW, et al. (1996) Hantavirus antigen detection in kidney biopsies from patients with nephropathia epidemica. Clin Nephrol 46: 379–383.
17. Muranyi W, Bahr U, Zeier M, van der Woude FJ (2005) Hantavirus infection. J Am Soc Nephrol 16: 3669–3679.
18. Hautala T, Sironen T, Vapalahti O, Paakko E, Sarkioja T, et al. (2002) Hypophyseal hemorrhage and panhypopituitarism during Puumala Virus Infection: Magnetic Resonance Imaging and detection of viral antigen in the hypophysis. Clin Infect Dis 35: 96–101.
19. Hung T, Zhou JY, Tang YM, Zhao TX, Baek LJ, et al. (1992) Identification of Hantaan virus-related structures in kidneys of cadavers with haemorrhagic fever with renal syndrome. Arch Virol 122: 187–199.
20. Kim S, Kang ET, Kim YG, Han JS, Lee JS, et al. (1993) Localization of Hantaan viral envelope glycoproteins by monoclonal antibodies in renal tissues from patients with Korean hemorrhagic fever H. Am J Clin Pathol 100: 398–403.
21. Temonen M, Mustonen J, Helin H, Pasternack A, Vaheri A, et al. (1996) Cytokines, adhesion molecules, and cellular infiltration in nephropathia epidemica kidneys: an immunohistochemical study. Clin Immunol Immunopathol 78: 47–55.
22. Nuutinen H, Vuoristo M, Farkkila M, Kahri A, Seppala K, et al. (1992) Hemorrhagic gastropathy in epidemic nephropathy. Gastrointest Endosc 38: 476–480.
23. Braun N, Haap M, Overkamp D, Kimmel M, Alscher MD, et al. (2010) Characterization and outcome following Puumala virus infection: a retrospective analysis of 75 cases. Nephrol Dial Transplant 25: 2997–3003.
24. Vaheri A, Strandin T, Hepojoki J, Sironen T, Henttonen H, et al. (2013) Uncovering the mysteries of hantavirus infections. Nat Rev Microbiol 11: 539–550.
25. Latus J, Fritzenkotter M, Schmidt-Chanasit J, Tenner-Racz K, Leibold T, et al. (2012) Hantavirus and acute appendicitis—the diagnosis behind the diagnosis? J Clin Virol 53: 156–158.
26. Bellomo R, Ronco C, Kellum JA, Mehta RL, Palevsky P (2004) Acute renal failure - definition, outcome measures, animal models, fluid therapy and information technology needs: the Second International Consensus Conference of the Acute Dialysis Quality Initiative (ADQI) Group. Crit Care 8: R204–212.
27. Pickering TG, Hall JE, Appel LJ, Falkner BE, Graves J, et al. (2005) Recommendations for blood pressure measurement in humans and experimental animals: Part 1: blood pressure measurement in humans: a statement for professionals from the Subcommittee of Professional and Public Education of the American Heart Association Council on High Blood Pressure Research. Hypertension 45: 142–161.
28. Chobanian AV, Bakris GL, Black HR, Cushman WC, Green LA, et al. (2003) The Seventh Report of the Joint National Committee on Prevention, Detection, Evaluation, and Treatment of High Blood Pressure: the JNC 7 report. JAMA 289: 2560–2572.
29. Zoller LG, Yang S, Gott P, Bautz EK, Darai G (1993) A novel mu-capture enzyme-linked immunosorbent assay based on recombinant proteins for sensitive and specific diagnosis of hemorrhagic fever with renal syndrome. J Clin Microbiol 31: 1194–1199.
30. Schwab SJ, Christensen RL, Dougherty K, Klahr S (1987) Quantitation of proteinuria by the use of protein-to-creatinine ratios in single urine samples. Arch Intern Med 147: 943–944.
31. Guindon S, Dufayard JF, Lefort V, Anisimova M, Hordijk W, et al. (2010) New algorithms and methods to estimate maximum-likelihood phylogenies: assessing the performance of PhyML 3.0. Syst Biol 59: 307–321.
32. Darriba D, Taboada GL, Doallo R, Posada D (2012) jModelTest 2: more models, new heuristics and parallel computing. Nat Methods 9: 772.
33. Ettinger J, Hofmann J, Enders M, Tewald F, Oehme RM, et al. (2012) Multiple synchronous outbreaks of Puumala virus, Germany, 2010. Emerg Infect Dis 18: 1461–1464.
34. Clement J, Maes P, van Ypersele de Strihou C, van der Groen G, Barrios JM, et al. (2010) Beechnuts and outbreaks of nephropathia epidemica (NE): of mast, mice and men. Nephrol Dial Transplant 25: 1740–1746.
35. Sironen T, Klingstrom J, Vaheri A, Andersson LC, Lundkvist A, et al. (2008) Pathology of Puumala hantavirus infection in macaques. PLoS One 3: e3035.
36. Maes P, Clement J, Gavrilovskaya I, Van Ranst M (2004) Hantaviruses: immunology, treatment, and prevention. Viral Immunol 17: 481–497.
37. Klempa B, Meisel H, Rath S, Bartel J, Ulrich R, et al. (2003) Occurrence of renal and pulmonary syndrome in a region of northeast Germany where Tula hantavirus circulates. J Clin Microbiol 41: 4894–4897.
38. Klempa B, Schutt M, Auste B, Labuda M, Ulrich R, et al. (2004) First molecular identification of human Dobrava virus infection in central Europe. J Clin Microbiol 42: 1322–1325.
39. Ulrich RG, Imholt C, Kruger DH, Krautkramer E, Scheibe T, et al. (2013) [Hantaviruses in Germany: threat for zoo, pet, companion and farm animals?]. Berl Munch Tierarztl Wochenschr 126: 514–526.

A School-Based Study with Rome III Criteria on the Prevalence of Functional Gastrointestinal Disorders in Chinese College and University Students

Yan-Yan Dong[1,2], Fei-Xue Chen[1], Yan-Bo Yu[1], Chao Du[1], Qing-Qing Qi[1], Han Liu[1], Yan-Qing Li[1]*

1 Department of Gastroenterology, Qilu Hospital, Shandong University, Jinan, Shandong, People's Republic of China, **2** The Key Laboratory of Cardiovascular Remodeling and Function Research, Chinese Ministry of Education and Chinese Ministry of Health, Qilu Hospital, Shandong University, Jinan, Shandong, People's Republic of China

Abstract

Background: Functional gastrointestinal disorders, including functional dyspepsia, irritable bowel syndrome and functional constipation are very common worldwide.

Objective: This research aims to estimate the prevalence and associated factors involved in functional gastrointestinal disorders in Chinese college and university students using the Rome III criteria.

Methods: A total of 5000 students from Shandong University in China were asked in January-May 2012 to complete questionnaires, including the Rome III questionnaire, hospital anxiety and depression scale, and negative life events scale.

Results: Based on the 4638 students who completed the questionnaire, the prevalence of functional dyspepsia, irritable bowel syndrome and functional constipation in college and university students of North China worked out to be 9.25%, 8.34% and 5.45% respectively. They were more frequent in female students. The factors of anxiety (OR 1.07; 95% CI 0.99 to 1.16, $P = 0.002 < 0.05$) and depression (OR 0.55; 95% CI 0.15 to 1.05, $P = 0.045 < 0.05$) indicated a high risk of causing irritable bowel syndrome.

Conclusion: Functional dyspepsia, irritable bowel syndrome and functional constipation were common in college and university students of North China. Psychological disorders such as anxiety and depression provide significant risk factors for irritable bowel syndrome patients.

Editor: Jerson Laks, Federal University of Rio de Janeiro, Brazil

Funding: This study was supported by the Graduate Innovation Foundation of Shandong University (yyx10017). The funders had no role in study design, data collection and analysis, decision to publish, or preparation of the manuscript.

Competing Interests: The authors have declared that no competing interests exist.

* E-mail: liyanqing@sdu.edu.cn

Introduction

Functional gastrointestinal disorders (FGIDs) are very common worldwide [1]. They have a negative impact on health-related quality of life and result in high health care expenditures [2]. The Rome III criteria of FGIDs were updated from the Rome II criteria in 2006 [3]. There are few studies that have estimated the prevalence and associated factors of FGIDs in selected populations using Rome III criteria [4].

Functional dyspepsia (FD), otherwise known as non-ulcer dyspepsia, is clearly the most common cause of dyspeptic symptoms in the upper abdomen [5]. FD is divided into two subgroups according to the Rome III criteria: epigastric pain syndrome (EPS) and postprandial distress syndrome (PDS) [6]. The frequency of FD varied from 8%–23% of the population [7,8]. A similar survey conducted in Korea using Rome III criteria indicated a frequency 8.1% in community population [9]. Most patients with FD complain of several symptoms related to meals. However, the pathophysiology of this disease remains poorly defined.

Irritable bowel syndrome (IBS) is a common, costly and functional gastrointestinal disorder characterized by abdominal pain or discomfort with altered bowel habits, but without any organic damages such as tumor or inflammation [3]. The prevalence of IBS is 15%–24% in the general population of Western countries, while the rate is 5%–10% in Asia [10–12]. It has been shown that some factors, especially psychological factors, such as anxiety and depression, are associated with the onset and course of IBS [13].

Functional constipation (FC) is a common type of FGIDs that manifests itself as persistently difficult, infrequent, or incomplete defecation, which does not meet the IBS criteria [3]. A survey showed the prevalence of FC in the general population of United States was 14.7% [14].

This study aimed to estimate the prevalence and associated factors involved in functional gastrointestinal disorders in Chinese college and university students using the Rome III criteria.

Table 1. Characteristics of students with functional gastrointestinal disorders.

	Total (n = 4638)	Normal (%) (n = 3581)	FD (%) (n = 429)	IBS (%) (n = 387)	FC (%) (n = 253)
Gender					
Male	2215 (47.8)	1767 (49.3)	192 (44.8)	176 (45.5)	84 (33.2)
Female	2423 (52.2)	1814 (50.7)	237 (55.2)	211 (54.5)	169 (66.8)
Branch of learning					
Liberal arts	1637 (35.3)	1236 (34.5)	160 (37.3)	147 (38.0)	101 (39.9)
Science	1546 (33.3)	1199 (33.5)	132 (30.8)	125 (32.3)	93 (36.8)
Medicine	1455 (31.4)	1146 (32.0)	137 (31.9)	115 (29.7)	59 (23.3)
School Level					
Lower	2950 (63.6)	2279 (63.6)	278 (64.8)	238 (61.5)	162 (64.0)
Upper	1688 (36.4)	1302 (36.4)	151 (35.2)	149 (38.5)	91 (36.0)

Data are number (%).
FD: Functional Dyspepsia;
IBS: Irritable Bowel Syndrome;
FC: Functional Constipation.

Materials and Methods

Ethics Statement

All participants gave their written informed consent prior to data collection. The study was approved by the Ethics Committee of Qilu Hospital of Shandong University, China.

Study Setting

This investigation was carried out from January to May 2012 at Shandong University, located in Northern China.

Sample Size

It has been generally reported that the prevalence of FD, IBS and FC is 8.1%, 10%–25%, and 14.7% of the population, respectively. According to the established formula, the sample size of 5000 enrolled in this research is sufficient to achieve a precision of ±2% with a 95% confidence interval (CI) [15].

Participants

A total of 5000 college and university students, randomly recruited from 3 areas of study (liberal arts, science, and medicine), were asked to voluntarily complete questionnaires. Their age span from 18 to 23 years old. Trained staff answered any questions on the spot.

Measures

Chinese version of Rome III questionnaire. The Rome III criteria have been widely used for the diagnosis of functional gastrointestinal disorders. This self-report standard questionnaire is developed by the Rome Foundation Board to identify FGIDs using the Rome III criteria [3]. This questionnaire has been repeatedly tested and very carefully validated [16]. We used the Chinese version of the previously validated Rome III diagnostic questionnaire. During the past years, the Chinese version has been extensively validated in a variety of adolescents and adult populations, including clinical practice and community research, with well-documented good measurement properties [17–19].

Diagnostic criteria of FGIDs. A Rome III diagnostic criterion of FD required one or more of the following symptoms: (1) bothersome postprandial fullness, (2) early satiation, (3) epigastric pain, and (4) epigastric burning. And no evidence of structural diseases (including on upper gastrointestinal endoscopy) that is likely to explain the symptom was necessary. Diagnostic criteria of subtype PDS must include one or both of the following: (1) bothersome postprandial fullness, happening after ordinary-sized meals, at least several times per week and (2) early satiation that prevents finishing a regular meal, at least several times per week. Diagnosis criteria of subtype EPS must include all of the following criteria: (1) pain or burning localized to the epigastrium of at least moderate severity, at least one time per week, (2) the pain to be intermittent, (3) not generalized or localized to other abdominal or chest regions, (4) not relieved by defecation or passage of flatus, and (5) neither criteria for gallbladder nor sphincter of Oddi disorders. All the above criteria fulfilled for the last 3 months with symptom onset at least 6 months prior to FD diagnosis.

To diagnose IBS, patients must have recurrent abdominal pain or discomfort for at least 3 months in the previous 6 months, with 2 or more of the following symptoms: (1) relief with defecation, (2) onset associated with a change in frequency of stool, and (3) onset associated with a change in form (appearance) of stool. The classification of IBS subtypes was based on the predominant stool pattern. IBS with constipation (IBS-C) was defined as having hard or lumpy stool at least 25% of the time and loose (mushy) or watery stools less than 25% of bowel movements. IBS with diarrhea (IBS-D) diagnosis was defined as having loose (mushy) or watery stools at least 25% of the time and hard stools less than 25% of bowel movements. And mixed IBS (IBS-M) was defined as having hard or lumpy stool at least 25% of bowel movements and loose (mushy) or watery stool at least 25% of bowel movements. Unsubtyped IBS means insufficient abnormality of stool consistency to meet criteria other three subtypes.

FC was diagnosed as the presence of defecation discomfort during at least 3 months in past 6 months with 2 or more of these following symptoms: (1) Straining during at least 25% of defecation; (2) Lumpy or hard stools in at least 25% of defecation; (3) Sensation of incomplete evacuation for at least 25% of defecation; (4) Sensation of anorectal obstruction or blockage for at least 25% of defecation; (5) Manual maneuvers to facilitate at least 25% of defecation (e.g. digital evacuation, support of pelvic floor); (6) Fewer than three defecation per week. And (1) loose stools are rarely present without the use of laxatives, (2) insufficient criteria for irritable bowel syndrome are necessary [3].

Hospital anxiety and depression scale (HADS). The hospital anxiety and depression scale (HADS), a specifically reliable scale developed by Zigmond and Snaith [20], can be used in estimating the emotional disorders of anxiety and depression symptomatology in IBS sufferers. It has published for a long time and is a strong clinical measure that is well validated [21,22]. The good reliability and stability of the HADS were demonstrated in Chinese translated versions [23–25]. The HADS is a short, self-reporting questionnaire consisting of 14 questions with two 7-item subscales for anxiety and depression assessment. For each subscale, the scores can be divided into 0–7 (normal cases), 8–10 (borderline cases), and over 11 (severe cases). Moreover, anxiety and depression scores are summed separately.

Red-flag items. Referring to the guidelines for FGIDs recommended by the American Gastroenterological Association, a series of "red flag" or alarm symptom questions used to distinguish structural intestinal disease from FGIDs [3]. They include drastic weight loss, a history of organic bowel disease, a history of digestive surgery, blood in stool, awakening due to abdominal pain during night, anemia, fever or arthralgia.

Table 2. Characteristics of students with functional dyspepsia and irritable bowel syndrome subtypes.

	FD (n = 429)	PDS (%) (n = 265)	EPS (%) (n = 164)	IBS (n = 387)	IBS-C (%) (n = 150)	IBS-D (%) (n = 189)	IBS-M (%) (n = 48)
Gender							
Male	192	122 (63.5)	70 (36.5)	176	66 (37.5)	92 (52.3)	18 (10.2)
Female	237	143 (60.3)	94 (39.7)	211	84 (39.8)	97 (46.0)	30 (14.2)
Branch of learning							
Liberal arts	160	87 (54.4)	73 (45.6)	147	63 (42.9)	65 (44.2)	19 (12.9)
Science	132	80 (60.6)	52 (39.4)	125	50 (40.0)	60 (48.0)	15 (12.0)
Medicine	137	98 (71.5)	39 (28.5)	115	37 (32.2)	64 (55.6)	14 (12.2)
School Level							
Lower	278	173 (62.2)	105 (37.8)	38	96 (40.3)	104 (43.7)	38 (16.0)
Upper	151	92 (60.9)	59 (39.1)	149	54 (36.2)	85 (57.1)	10 (6.7)

Data are number (%).
FD: Functional Dyspepsia;
IBS: Irritable Bowel Syndrome.

Participants who were identified with one or more of these 7 items were excluded from the survey.

Negative life events in childhood. A life events scale was used in this study focusing on IBS. It has been used in two surveys involving large populations [26,27]. Considering the specific situations of college and university students in China, we assessed 5 of the most stressful events in childhood (occurring under the age of 12 years) in the scale. These included the death of a close family member, divorced parents, extreme financial difficulties, experiencing serious illness or major surgery, major natural disaster or other serious setbacks. The presence of each event was totaled (range 0–5). It was divided it into 0 (normal cases), 1–2 (mild cases), 3–4 (moderate cases), and 5 (severe cases).

Baseline information. The remaining questions are about the socio- demographic characteristics, such as age, sex, schooling level, place of birth, health condition, and personal family information.

Statistical Analysis

All eligible questionnaires were coded. Data analysis was performed using the Statistical Package for Social Science Software for Windows (SPSS 15.0 version). All calculated P-values were two-tailed and $P<0.05$ was considered statistically significant. Analysis of variance was used to compare the anxiety, depression and negative life events levels between groups. Possible risk factors were assessed by logistic regression analysis. Odds ratio (OR) with 95% confidence interval (CI) was calculated. Data are presented as mean ± SD.

Table 3. Description of symptoms for students with functional constipation.

Symptoms	Male (%)	Female (%)	Total
Straining	81 (96.4)	156 (92.3)	237 (93.7)
Lumpy or hard stools	74 (88.1)	150 (88.8)	224 (88.5)
Incomplete evacuation	75 (89.3)	165 (97.6)	240 (94.9)
Anorectal obstruction	72 (85.7)	150 (88.8)	222 (87.7)
Manual maneuvers	36 (42.9)	83 (49.1)	119 (47.0)
Fewer defecation	82 (97.6)	167 (98.8)	249 (98.4)

Data are number (%).
FC: Functional Constipation.

Results

Response Rate and Characteristics of Subjects

Of the 5000 enrolled participants, 4860 completed the questionnaires. Valid responses were obtained from 4638 participants, with a response rate of 92.76%. Of the valid 4638 participants, 2215 (47.8%) were males and 2423 (52.2%) were females, with a mean age of 20.64±1.428 years and 20.88±1.572 years, respectively. The average college level of the students was 2.53±0.162. Of the valid 4638 participants, 3461 (74.6%) were natives of Shandong Province. The characteristics of participants are listed in Table 1.

Prevalence of FGIDs

Of the valid 4638 participants, 429 fulfilled criteria for FD, while 387 fulfilled for IBS with a male/female ratio of 1:1.20, and 253 had FC. The prevalence of FD, IBS and FC was 9.25%, 8.34% and 5.45% respectively, with no statistically significant difference among areas of study or schooling level. The detailed FD and IBS subtype characteristics are described in Table 2. Twelve students had both FD and IBS disorders. Participants who fulfilled the criteria of FC were classified according to their symptoms (Table 3).

HADS Scores and Negative Life Events in Childhood of IBS

The hospital anxiety and depression scores were significantly higher for students with IBS (Table 4), especially for those with normal scores (0–7) than for those with abnormal scores (>11). The mean anxiety score were 6.23±4.564 (IBS-C), 6.65±4.934 (IBS-D), and 6.47±4.360 (IBS-M). The mean depression score were 6.76±3.946 (IBS-C), 6.69±4.362 (IBS-D), and 6.96±4.658 (IBS-M). No difference was found in anxiety and depression scores between the 3 subtype groups. No significant difference was found due to negative life events in childhood.

Table 4. Univariate analysis of psychological factors of irritable bowel syndrome and control groups.

Factors		Total (n = 3968)	Normal (%) (n = 3581)	IBS (%) (n = 387)	χ^2	*P* value
Anxiety						
	0–7	3108 (78.3)	2871 (92.4)	237 (7.6)	98.80	0.00
	8–10	552 (13.9)	435 (78.8)	117 (21.2)	3.67	0.06
	≥11	308 (7.8)	275 (89.3)	33 (10.7)	15.08	0.00
Depression						
	0–7	2827 (71.2)	2611 (92.4)	216 (7.6)	208.86	0.00
	8–10	216 (5.4)	134 (62.0)	82 (38.0)	3.66	0.06
	≥11	925 (23.3)	836 (90.4)	89 (9.6)	110.40	0.00
Negative life events in childhood						
	Normal	2025 (51.0)	242 (12.0)	1783 (88.0)	6.58	0.01
	Mild	1306 (32.9)	105 (8.0)	1201 (92.0)		
	Moderate	558 (14.1)	38 (6.8)	520 (93.2)		
	Severe	79 (2.0)	2 (2.5)	77 (97.5)		

Data are number (%). IBS: Irritable Bowel Syndrome.

Risk Factors for IBS

After the univariate analysis, the multivariable logistic regression analysis was adjusted by sex type. The factors of anxiety (OR 1.07; 95% CI 0.99 to 1.16, $P = 0.002 < 0.05$) and depression (OR 0.55; 95% CI 0.15 to 1.05, $P = 0.045 < 0.05$) were independently associated with IBS (Table 5).

Discussion

FGIDs have become prevalent worldwide in recent years [10,11]. Few data has been shown on the systematic epidemiology of FGIDs in student population. Considering as a young adult community, college and university students in China have similar diet, life activity, educational situation and so on. To our knowledge, the present study is the largest population school-based investigation on the epidemiology of FGIDs in college and university students. The results of the present study demonstrate that the prevalence of FD, IBS and FC was found to be 9.25%, 8.34% and 5.45% respectively, with more female students than male students suffering from FGIDs.

The prevalence of FD varied greatly in the general population [7–9]. We found that PDS was the more common subtype compared to EPS and this finding compared well with similar outside research [4,28]. The reason is thought to be that the diagnostic criteria of EPS are too strict and make it difficult to distinguish between heartburn and epigastric burning in the questionnaire procedure [4]. Most of these studies have limited number of population. Our study showed more detailed epidemiological data.

Table 5. Multivariate logistic regression to evaluate psychological factors of IBS.

Variables	Beta	Standard Error.	Wald	OR (95% CI)	P value
Anxiety	0.072	0.023	10.040	1.07 (0.99 to 1.16)	0.002
Depression	−0.605	0.301	4.034	0.55 (0.15 to 1.05)	0.045

Our research showed the epidemiological rate of IBS in college and university students was 8.34%. The prevalence of IBS in community population varied greatly among different investigations. About 10% to 20% of adults have IBS symptoms, and this disorder affects all races throughout the world [29–31]. It suggested that may be due to the different diagnostic criteria such as Rome II and Rome III used. For example, a research in Southeast China assessing the prevalence of IBS among undergraduates reported 4.7% and 10.4% using Rome II and Rome III criteria respectively [18]. Studies suggest that the Rome III criteria are based on a lower frequency and shorter duration of IBS symptoms than the Rome II criteria [32]. Rome II criteria have been used to examine a 12-week period duration in the past 12 months, which is less than a continuous 6-month period, thus expanding the scope of diagnosis and were stricter than the Rome III criteria [33].

In our study, the female/male ratio of IBS was 1.20:1. Gender differences in IBS may be due to several factors including differences in biobehavioral responses to stress, pain stimulating pathways and sex hormone effects on gastrointestinal function [34]. A survey found that rectal discomfort thresholds were significantly lower in female compared to male patients with IBS [35]. The majority of western population studies have reported female-to-male ratios of 2–3:1 [29,36]. Studies in Asia including ours showed less dramatic gender difference [37,38].

We showed IBS of the diarrhea dominant type was more common than the constipation dominant type, similar to a Chinese population study [19]. Dorn and Ersryd also reported IBS-D was the more prevalent subtype, followed by IBS-C [39,40]. One reason may be that cold water intake may lead to lower visceral perception thresholds in Chinese IBS-D patients [41,42]. Irregular intake of cold drinks is common in college and university students.

Similar with previous studies, our study shows psychological disturbance is associated with IBS [43]. A recent research provided first direct evidence to indicate that the brain-gut pathway is bidirectional which means both brain-gut and gut-brain dysfunction may be meanwhile occurring in patients of

FGIDs [44]. Generally, psychological distress is directly related to the severity and degree of impairment in IBS [45]. The stress and negative life events may affect gastrointestinal function, the pain complaint, quality of life, work absenteeism, health care use and social costs [29,46,47].

The prevalence of FC in college students of North China in the present study was 5.45%. Most of the FC patients developed from childhood constipation. Healthy education first trained to children about constipation is inadequate. The children may become scared of the process of defecation and it may lead to the development of chronic constipation into adult [48,49]. The incidence suggests more attention should be paid in childhood management. Our study also found that most students with FC were affected by the straining involved during defecation and others suffered the sensation of incomplete evacuation. The reason is that the college and university students are young and they usually have irregular eating habits, bedtimes and not enough exercise. Considering the Chinese college and university students as a group within specific age and environmental constraints, this result may be considered rational [50,51].

The limitation of this study was based solely on the self-reporting questionnaires, without any further examinations necessary to exclude structural intestinal diseases. Moreover, the survey was restricted to a community of college and university students and was not representative of the similar age group. More risk associations like diet, exercise and other psychological factors could be analyzed in future study.

In conclusion, this is the largest school-based population investigation on the epidemiology of FGIDs using Rome III criteria. Symptoms of FGIDs including FD, IBS and FC are quite prevalent in college and university students of North China, with more female students than male students suffering from FGIDs. Psychological disorders such as anxiety and depression provide significant risk factors for IBS patients.

Author Contributions

Conceived and designed the experiments: YYD YQL. Performed the experiments: YYD FXC YBY. Analyzed the data: CD QQQ. Contributed reagents/materials/analysis tools: HL. Wrote the paper: YYD. Supervised and reviewed the entire study: YQL.

References

1. Halder SL, Locke GR 3rd, Schleck CD, Zinsmeister AR, Melton LJ 3rd, et al. (2007) Natural History of functional gastrointestinal disorders: a 12-year Longitudinal population-based study. Gastroenterology 133: 799–807.
2. Agarwal N, Spiegel BM (2011) The effect of irritable Bowel syndrome on health-related quality of life and health care expenditures. Gastroenterology Clinics of North America 40(1): 11–19.
3. Drossman DA, Corazziari E, Delvaux M, Spiller RC, Talley NJ, et al. (2006) Rome III: The Functional Gastrointestinal Disorders. 3rd Edition. McLean: Degnon Associates.
4. Jae Myung Park, Myung-Gyu Choi, Yu Kyung Cho, In Seok Lee, Jin Il Kim, et al. (2011) Functional Gastrointestinal Disorders Diagnosed by Rome III Questionnaire in Korea. J Neurogastroenterol Motil 17: 279–286.
5. Locke GR 3rd (1998) Prevalence, incidence and natural history of dyspepsia and functional dyspepsia. Baillieres Clin Gastroenterol 12: 435–442.
6. Drossman DA (2006) The functional gastrointestinal disorders and the Rome III process. Gastroenterology 130: 1377–1390.
7. Li Y, Nie Y, Sha W, Su H (2002) The link between psychosocial factors and functional dyspepsia: an epidemiological study. Chin Med J (Engl) 115: 1082–1084.
8. Kawamura A, Adachi K, Takashima T, Murao M, Katsube T, et al. (2001) Prevalence of functional dyspepsia and its relationship with Helicobacter pylori infection in a Japanese population. J Gastroenterol Hepatol 16: 384–388.
9. Noh YW, Jung HK, Kim SE, Jung SA (2010) Overlap of erosive and non-erosive reflux diseases with functional gastrointestinal disorders according to Rome III criteria. J Neurogastroenterol Motil 16: 148–156.
10. Agréus L, Svärdsudd K, Nyrén O, Tibblin G (1995) Irritable bowel syndrome and dyspepsia in the general population: overlap and lack of stability over time. Gastroenterology 109: 671–680.
11. Frank L, Kleinman L, Rentz A, Ciesla G, Kim JJ, et al. (2002) Health-related quality of life associated with irritable bowel syndrome: comparison with other chronic diseases. Clin Ther 24: 675–689.
12. Chang FY, Lu CL (2007) Irritable bowel syndrome in the 21st century: perspectives from Asia or South-east Asia. J Gastroenterol Hepatol 22: 4–12.
13. Faresjö A, Grodzinsky E, Johansson S, Wallander MA, Timpka T, et al. (2007) Psychosocial factors at work and in everyday life are associated with irritable bowel syndrome. Eur J Epidemiol 22: 473–480.
14. Stewart WF, Liberman JN, Sandler RS, Woods MS, Stemhagen A, et al. (1999) Epidemiology of constipation (EPOC) study in the United States: relation of clinical subtypes to sociodemographic features. Am J Gastroenterol 94(12): 3530–40.
15. Wang JL (2001) Clinical epidemiology. 2nd edition ed. Shanghai: Shanghai Science &Technology Press.
16. Talley NJ (2007) Functional gastrointestinal disorders in 2007 and Rome III: something new, something borrowed, something objective. Rev Gastroenterol Disord 7(2): 97–105.
17. Chang FY, Chen PH, Wu TC, Pan WH, Chang HY, et al. (2012) Prevalence of functional gastrointestinal disorders in Taiwan: questionnaire-based survey for adults based on the Rome III criteria. Asia Pac J Clin Nutr 21(4): 594–600.
18. N Dai, Y Cong, H Yuan (2008) Prevalence of irritable bowel syndrome among undergraduates in Southeast China. Digestive and Liver Disease 40: 418–424.
19. Yao X, Yang YS, Cui LH, Zhao KB, Zhang ZH, et al. (2012) Subtypes of irritable bowel syndrome on Rome III criteria: a multicenter study. J Gastroenterol Hepatol 27(4): 760–5.
20. Zigmond AS, Snaith RP (1983) The hospital anxiety and depression scale. Acta Psychiatr Scand 67: 361–370.
21. Vodermaier A, Millman RD (2011) Accuracy of the Hospital Anxiety and Depression Scale as a screening tool in cancer patients: a systematic review and meta-analysis. Support Care Cancer 19(12): 1899–1908.
22. White D, Leach C, Sims R, Atkinson M, Cottrell D (1999) Validation of the Hospital Anxiety and Depression Scale for use with adolescents. Br J Psychiatry 175: 452–4.
23. Chan YF, Leung DY, Fong DY, Leung CM, Lee AM (2010) Psychometric evaluation of the Hospital Anxiety and Depression Scale in a large community sample of adolescents in Hong Kong. Qual Life Res 19: 865–873.
24. Li XJ, He YL, Ma H, Liu ZN, Jia FJ, et al. (2012) Prevalence of depressive and anxiety disorders in Chinese gastroenterological outpatients. World J Gastroenterol 18(20): 2561–8.
25. Martin CR, Thompson DR, Chan DS (2004). An examination of the psychometric properties of the Hospital Anxiety and Depression Scale in Chinese patients with acute coronary syndrome. Psychiatry Research 129(3): 279–288.
26. Matthews KA, Shumaker SA, Bowen DJ, Langer RD, Hunt JR, et al. (1997) Women's health initiative. Why now? What is it? What's new? Am Psychol 52: 101–116.
27. Golden-Kreutz DM, Thornton LM, Wells-Di Gregorio S, Frierson GM, Jim HS, et al. (2005) Traumatic stress, perceived global stress, and life events: prospectively predicting quality of life in breast cancer patients. Health Psychol 24(3): 288–96.
28. Tack J, Bisschops R, Sarnelli G (2004) Pathophysiology and treatment of functional dyspepsia. Gastroenterology 127(4): 1239–55.
29. Drossman DA, Li Z, Andruzzi E, Temple RD, Talley NJ, et al. (1993) U.S. householder survey of functional gastrointestinal disorders. Prevalence, sociodemography, and health impact. Dig Dis Sci 38(9): 1569–80.
30. Saito YA, Schoenfeld P, Locke GR 3rd (2002) The epidemiology of irritable bowel syndrome in North America: a systematic review. Am J Gastroenterol 97(8): 1910–5.
31. Gwee KA (2005) Irritable bowel syndrome in developing countries–a disorder of civilization or colonization? Neurogastroenterol Motil 17(3): 317–24.
32. Sperber AD, Shvartzman P, Friger M, Fich A (2007) A comparative reappraisal of the Rome II and Rome III diagnostic criteria: are we getting closer to the "true" prevalence of irritable bowel syndrome? Eur J Gastroenterol. Hepatol 19: 441–7.
33. Shen L, Kong H, Hou X (2009) Prevalence of irritable bowel syndrome and its relationship with psychological stress status in Chinese university students. J Gastroenterol Hepatol 24: 1885–1890.
34. Taylor SE, Klein LC, Lewis BP, Gruenewald TL, Gurung RA, et al. (2000) Biobehavioral responses to stress in females: tend-and-befriend, not fight-or-flight. Psychol Rev 107(3): 411–29.
35. Chang L, Naliboff B, Schmulson M, Lee OY, Olivas TI, et al. (2001) The role of gender and bowel habit predominance on visceral perception in IBS. Gastroenterology 120: 1236–45.
36. Sandler RS (1990) Epidemiology of irritable bowel syndrome in the United States. Gastroenterology 99(2): 409–15.
37. Xiong LS, Chen MH, Chen HX, Xu AG, Wang WA, et al. (2004) A population-based epidemiologic study of irritable bowel syndrome in South China: stratified randomized study by cluster sampling. Aliment. Pharmacol Ther 19: 1217–24.

38. Gwee KA, Wee S, Wong ML, Png DJ (2004) The prevalence, symptom characteristics, and impact of irritable bowel syndrome in an Asian urban community. Am J Gastroenterol 99: 924–31.
39. Dorn SD, Morris CB, Hu Y, Toner BB, Diamant N, et al. (2009) Irritable bowel syndrome subtypes defined by Rome II and Rome III criteria are similar. J Clin Gastroenterol 43: 214–20.
40. Ersryd A, Posserud I, Abrahamsson H, Simrén M (2007) Subtyping the irritable bowel syndrome by predominant bowel habit: Rome II versus Rome III. Aliment Pharmacol Ther 26: 953–61.
41. Zuo XL, Li YQ, Shi L, Lv GP, Kuang RG, et al. (2006) Visceral hypersensitivity following cold water intake in subjects with irritable bowel syndrome. J Gastroenterol 41(4): 311–7.
42. Zuo XL, Li YQ, Yang XZ, Guo M, Guo YT, et al. (2007) Plasma and gastric mucosal 5-hydroxytryptamine concentrations following cold water intake in patients with diarrhea-predominant irritable bowel syndrome. J Gastroenterol Hepatol 22(12): 2330–7.
43. Drossman DA, McKee DC, Sandler RS, Mitchell CM, Cramer EM, et al. (1988) Psychosocial factors in the irritable bowel syndrome. A multivariate study of patients and nonpatients with irritable bowel syndrome. Gastroenterology 95(3): 701–8.
44. Koloski NA, Jones M, Kalantar J, Weltman M, Zaguirre J, et al. (2012) The brain-gut pathway in functional gastrointestinal disorders is bidirectional: a 12-year prospective population-based study. Gut 61: 1284–1290.
45. Katon W, Lin E, Von Korff M, Russo J, Lipscomb P, et al. (1991) Somatization: a spectrum of severity. Am J Psychiatry 148: 34–40.
46. El-Serag HB, Olden K, Bjorkman D (2002) Health-related quality of life among persons with irritable bowel syndrome: a systematic review. Aliment Pharmacol Ther 16(6): 1171–85.
47. Pinto C, Lele MV, Joglekar AS, Panwar VS, Dhavale HS (2000) Stressful life-events, anxiety, depression and coping in patients of irritable bowel syndrome. J Assoc Physicians India 48(6): 589–93.
48. Nelhans N, Williams R (2010) Education key in tackling childhood constipation. Practitioner. 254(1731): 22–6.
49. Tabbers MM, Boluyt N, Berger MY, Benninga MA (2011) Clinical practice: diagnosis and treatment of functional constipation. Eur J Pediatr 170(8): 955–63.
50. Irvine EJ, Ferrazzi S, Pare P, Thompson WG, Rance L (2002) Health-related quality of life in functional GI disorders: focus on constipation and resource utilization. Am J Gastroenterol 97(8): 1986–1993.
51. Jeong JJ, Choi MG, Cho YS, Lee SG, Oh JH, et al. (2008) Chronic gastrointestinal symptoms and quality of life in the Korean population. World J Gastroenterol 14(41): 6388–94.

3

Validation of the Fibromyalgia Survey Questionnaire within a Cross-Sectional Survey

Winfried Häuser[1,2]*, Eva Jung[1,2], Brigitte Erbslöh-Möller[3], Mechthild Gesmann[4], Hedi Kühn-Becker[5], Franz Petermann[6], Jost Langhorst[7], Thomas Weiss[8], Andreas Winkelmann[9], Frederick Wolfe[10,11]

1 Department Internal Medicine I, Klinikum Saarbrücken, Saarbrücken, Germany, **2** Department of Psychosomatic Medicine and Psychotherapy, Technische Universität München, München, Germany, **3** Rheumatology Medical Practice, Neunkirchen, Germany, **4** Psychosomatic Medicine and Pain Therapy Medical Practice, Herford, Germany, **5** Psychosomatic Medicine and Pain Therapy Medical Practice, Zweibrücken, Germany, **6** Centre of Clinical Psychology and Rehabilitation, Universität Bremen, Bremen, Germany, **7** Department Internal Medicine V (Intergrative Medicine), Kliniken Essen-Mitte, Essen, Germany, **8** Outpatient Clinic Mannheim, Mannheim, Germany, **9** Department of Physical Medicine and Rehabilitation, Klinikum der Universität München, München, Germany, **10** National Data Bank for Rheumatic Diseases, Wichita, Kansas, United States of America, **11** University of Kansas School of Medicine, Wichita, Kansas, United States of America

Abstract

The Fibromyalgia Survey Questionnaire (FSQ) assesses the key symptoms of fibromyalgia syndrome. The FSQ can be administrated in survey research and settings where the use of interviews to evaluate the number of pain sites and extent of somatic symptom intensity and tender point examination would be difficult. We validated the FSQ in a cross-sectional survey with FMS patients. In a cross-sectional survey, participants with physician diagnosis of FMS were recruited by FMS-self help organisations and nine clinical institutions of different levels of care. Participants answered the FSQ (composed by the Widespread Pain Index [WPI] and the Somatic Severity Score [SSS]) assessing the Fibromyalgia Survey Diagnostic Criteria (FSDC) and the Patient Health Questionnaire PHQ 4. American College of Rheumatology 1990 classification criteria were assessed in a subgroup of participants. 1,651 persons diagnosed with FMS were included into analysis. The acceptance of the FSQ-items ranged between 78.9 to 98.1% completed items. The internal consistency of the items of the SSS ranged between 0.75–0.82. 85.5% of the study participants met the FSDC. The concordance rate of the FSDC and ACR 1990 criteria was 72.7% in a subsample of 128 patients. The Pearson correlation of the SSS with the PHQ 4 depression score was 0.52 ($p<0.0001$) and with the PHQ anxiety score was 0.51 ($p<0.0001$) (convergent validity). 64/202 (31.7%) of the participants not meeting the FSDC criteria and 152/1283 (11.8%) of the participants meeting the FSDC criteria reported an improvement (slightly too very much better) in their health status since FMS-diagnosis ($Chi^2 = 55$, $p<0.0001$) (discriminant validity). The study demonstrated the feasibility of the FSQ in a cross-sectional survey with FMS-patients. The reliability, convergent and discriminant validity of the FSQ were good. Further validation studies of the FSQ in clinical and general population settings are necessary.

Editor: Hamid Reza Baradaran, Tehran University of Medical Sciences, Iran (Islamic Republic of)

Funding: The study was financially supported by the German League for People with Arthritis and Rheumatism (www.rheuma-liga.de). The funders had no role in study design, data collection and analysis, decision to publish, or preparation of the manuscript.

Competing Interests: The authors have read the journal's policy and have the following conflicts: Dr. Häuser received honoraria for education lectures from Eli-Lilly, Pfizer and Janssen-Cilag and a congress travel grant by Eli-Lilly. Dr Weiss and Dr. Winkelmann were investigators in a study of pregabalin in FMS, sponsored by Pfizer. The other authors have no conflicts of interest to declare.

* E-mail: whaeuser@klinikum-saarbruecken.de

Introduction

The publication of American College of Rheumatology (ACR) preliminary diagnostic criteria for fibromyalgia syndrome (FDC) [1] eliminated the tender point examination required for the clinical diagnosis of FMS by the ACR 1990 classification criteria [2]. Because most of the ACR 2010 items can be obtained by self-administration, the FDC were slightly modified so that complete self-administration would be possible by the Fibromyalgia Survey Diagnostic Criteria (FSDC). The FSDC were developed in a longitudinal study of patients of the National Data Bank for Rheumatic Diseases by substituting a count of three symptoms for the physician's (0–3) evaluation of the extent of somatic symptom intensity by a questionnaire assessing the number of pain sites and somatic symptom severity. Patients who satisfy FSDC meet the following 3 conditions: 1) Widespread Pain Index (WPI) $\geq 7/19$ pain sites and Symptom Severity Score (SSS) $\geq 5/12$ or WPI between 3–6/19 and SSS $\geq 9/12$; 2) Symptoms have been present at a similar level for at least 3 months; 3) The patient does not have another disorder that would otherwise sufficiently explain the pain [3]. The conditions 1 and 2 can be assessed by the Fibromyalgia survey questionnaire (FSQ) including the WPI and SSS. The sum of the WPI and the SSS constitutes the Fibromyalgianess Scale (FS) or polysymptomatic distress scale as a measure of physical and psychological symptom intensity (distress) which can be applied to every disease. The FS can be used to track disease status. The assessment of the key symptoms of FMS by the FSQ allows administration in survey research and settings where the use of interviews to evaluate the number of pain sites and extent of somatic symptom intensity would be difficult.

In this study we provided the first translation of the FSQ into German language and validated the FSQ for the first time in a cross-sectional survey with FMS-patients in Germany.

Methods

Clinical institutions

Participants of the study were recruited by the two largest German FMS-self help organisations and nine clinical institutions. The specialties of the clinical institutions were pain medicine and psychotherapy (N = 3), rheumatology (N = 2), complementary and alternative medicine (N = 2), physical therapy (N = 1) and pain therapy (N = 1). The settings were outpatient (N = 6), inpatient (N = 2) and day clinic (N = 1). The levels of care were secondary (N = 6) and tertiary care (N = 1) and rehabilitation (N = 1).

From November 1, 2010 to April 30, 2011 all consecutive patients with an established or first diagnosis of FMS of the participating study centres were asked by the physicians of these centres to take part in the study. All participating physicians had more than 10 years exprerience in the management of FMS-patients. The questionnaires were handed out by the physicians of the centres with a standardized letter explaining the focus of the study. The questionnaires were returned by the patients in a closed and anonymous envelope and kept away from the charts. In 4 centres a tender point examination was performed according to a standardised protocol [4].

Self-help organisations

The package of questionnaires was sent by the central office of the German League for people with Arthritis and Rheumatism to their regional offices with the request that the leaders of the local self-help groups distribute the FSQ during the meetings to the group members (FMS-patients). Group members were asked to fill out the questionnaires separately outside the group meetings and not to discuss it with other group members.

The German Fibromyalgia Association included the package in the issue 4/2010 of its member journal "Optimist" dispatched by post to all members.

The questionnaires were returned by the patients by post to the central office. Moreover, the questionnaires were available on the homepages of both self-help organisations. After downloading and completing they could be sent by mail, fax or email to the central offices. Employees of both central offices removed the personal identifying information and sent the questionnaires to the coordinating study centre.

Inclusion- and exclusion criteria

Members of the self-help organisations should report that the diagnosis of FMS had been established by a physician. Participants without (reported) physician diagnosis of FMS were excluded.

The patients of the study centres should have been previously or currently diagnosed with FMS according to the ACR 1990 classification criteria [3] or the Association of the Medical Scientific Societies in Germany (AWMF) criteria [5]. In four study centres the ACR 1990 criteria (2) were reevaluated during study examination. A diagnostic work-up including a complete physical examination and defined laboratory tests according to the German guideline on the management of FMS were performed in every patient of the study centres in the past or during the study [6]. Patients with somatic diseases sufficiently explaining the pain sites of the WPI (e.g. highly active inflammatory rheumatic disease) and patients who were not able to read German were excluded.

Questionnaires

Demographic data (age, sex, family status, educational level, current professional status, member of a FMS-self help organisation) and medical data (Years since chronic widespread pain and FMS-diagnosis] were assessed by a questionnaire used in a previous multicenter FMS – study [5].

Patients were asked how their health status has changed over the years since the diagnosis of FMS according to their opinion (1 = very much worse, 2 = much worse, 3 = slightly worse, 4 = no change, 5 = slightly better, 6 = much better, 7 = very much better).

The FSQ included the Symptom Severity Score (SSS) with 3 major symptoms (fatigue, trouble thinking or remembering, waking up tired [unrefreshed]) which can be coded 0–3 (0 = not present to 3 = extreme) and three additional symptoms (Pain or cramps in lower abdomen, depression, headache), which can be coded to be present (1) or not present (0) (total suscore 0–3). These three items are surrogates for somatic symptom burden item of the ACR 2010 criteria (reference). The SSS ranges from 0–12. The Widespread Pain Index (WPI) includes 19 non-articular pain sites [2] (see table 1). The English version of the SSS had been forward and backtranslated by four German physicians, two of whom had worked for several years in the USA. We used the validated German version of the WPI [7].

The 4-item Patient Health Questionnaire-4 (PHQ-4) is an ultra-brief self-report questionnaire that consists of a 2-item depression scale (PHQ-2) and a 2-item anxiety scale (GAD-2). A score of 3-or-greater on the depression subscale represents a reasonable cut-point for identifying potential cases of major depression or other depressive disorder, a score of 3-or-greater on the anxiety subscale represents a reasonable cut-point for generalized anxiety, panic, social anxiety, and posttraumatic stress disorders. The PHQ 4 total score can serve as measure for psychological distress [8]. We used the validated German version of the PHQ 4 [9].

Validation methods and hypotheses

The methods used to validate the FSQ were as follows: Patient acceptability (acceptance) of the FSQ was assessed by the proportion of missing or invalid items. The proportion of missing or invalid items should be approximately equal to those in surveys of German patients with chronic liver diseases [10] and celiac disease [11].The reliability of the SSS was assessed by internal consistency (Cronbach's α coefficient) which measures the overall correlation between items within a scale. A level of 0.7 and higher is considered desirable [12].Face (content) validity was assessed by the think aloud technique [13] of five phycians (pain medicine, psychosomatic medicine, rheumatology) and five FMS-patients of local self-help groups not participating in the study who verbalized their thoughts processes while filling out the FSQ.Convergent validity of the SSS and FS was determined by the Pearson correlation with the total sum score of the PHQ 4. The convergent validity is fulfilled when the scale scores for related concepts show moderate to high correlation (correlation coefficient 0.4 to 0.8) [12].Convergent validity of the FSDC was determined by comparing the concordance rates of self-reported diagnosis of FMS made by a physician (members of self-help organisations) with the FSDC and of physician - established diagnosis of FMS (participants of clinical centres) with FSDC. Based on previous studies of the concordance rates of different FMS-diagnostic criteria [5,14] we expected concordance rates between 70–80%.Discriminant validity was tested by the following hypothesis: Longitudinal studies demonstrated that persons diagnosed with FMS can switch between criteria positive and criteria negative states [15]. Therefore we assumed, that patients who will not meet

Table 1. Fibromyalgia survey questionnaire.

I. Using the following scale, indicate for each item the level of severity over the past week by checking the appropriate box.		
0: No problem		
1: Slight or mild problems; generally mild or intermittent		
2: Moderate; considerable problems; often present and/or at a moderate level		
3. Severe: continuous, life-disturbing problems		
Fatigue	☐ 0 ☐ 1 ☐ 2 ☐ 3	
Trouble thinking or remembering	☐ 0 ☐ 1 ☐ 2 ☐ 3	
Waking up tired (unrefreshed)	☐ 0 ☐ 1 ☐ 2 ☐ 3	
II. During the past 6 months have you had any of the following symptoms?		
Pain or cramps in lower abdomen	☐ Yes ☐ No	
Depression	☐ Yes ☐ No	
Headache	☐ Yes ☐ No	
III. Joint/body pain		
Please indicate below if you have had pain or tenderness over the past 7 days in each of the areas listed below. Please make an X in the box if you have had pain or tenderness. Be sure to mark both right side and left side separately		
☐ Shoulder, left	☐ Upper leg, left	☐ Lower back
☐ Shoulder, right	☐ Upper leg, right	☐ Upper back
☐ Hip, left	☐ Lower leg, left	☐ Neck
☐ Hip, right	☐ Lower leg, right	
☐ Upper arm, left	☐ Jaw, left	☐ No pain in any of these areas
☐ Upper arm, right	☐ Jaw, right	
☐ Lower arm, left	☐ Chest	
☐ Lower arm, right	☐ Abdomen	
IV. Overall, were the symptoms listed in I–III above generally present for at **least 3 months**?	☐ Yes ☐ No	

the FSDC at the time of evaluation, will report more frequently that their health status has improved since the diagnosis of FMS.

Statistical analysis

The data were entered by four pairs of study assistants into a preconstructed excel-data sheet. The entering of data was checked by two authors at random and on plausibility during descriptive data analysis. Missing items of the SSS, WPI and PHQ 4 were coded as zero. Patients were excluded from analysis if all items of SSS and/or WPI and/or PHQ4 were not answered.

Support

The participants of the study did not receive any reimbursement. Material costs were covered by the participating institutions.

Ethics

The requirements of data protection and medical professional secrecy were respected by all study investigators. All participants gave their informed written consent to the study. The study had been specifically aproved by the ethical committee of the Ludwig Maximilian Universität München and by the review boards of all study centers.

Results

Study participants

There were no data available concerning how many patients contacted by the self-help organisation did not meet the inclusion criteria or refused to take part in the study. The German League for people with Arthritis and Rheumatism estimated that approximately 10 000 of their members were FMS-patients. The German Fibromyalgia Association is reported to have approximately 4000 members with FMS.

123 patients of the clinical samples did not meet the primary inclusion criteria and 40 of contacted patients refused to take part in the study. 1694 persons returned the questionnaires, of which 1143 (69.2%) had been contacted via self-help organisations. 43 of 1694 contacted persons were excluded due to total missing items in the WPI (N = 40) or SSS (N = 3). The questionnaires of at least 10 persons who were excluded due to missing WPI-items did not include the WPI due to an organisational mistake. 1651 persons were included into analysis.

The total study sample was composed of mainly middle-aged women with a long duration of CWP and FMS-diagnosis. In 30 patients, FMS was diagnosed recently for the first time (see table 2). 881/1633 (54.6%) participants scored >=3 on the PHQ 4 depression scale and 889/1633 (54.4%) scored > = 3 on the PHQ 4 anxiety scale.

Validation

Acceptance. The participants included into analysis completed the SSS and PHQ 4 items as follows: Fatigue 1620 (98.1%), trouble thinking 1609 (97.4%), waking up tired 1618 (98.0%), pain in lower abdomen 1449 (87.8%), depression 1589 (96.2%), headache 1303 (78.9%), three months duration of all symptoms 1375 (83.3%), loss of interest 1622 (98.2%), feeling down 1623 (98.3%), nervousness 1632 (98.8%), worries 1612 (97.6%).

Reliability (Internal consistency). Cronbach's alpha of the SSS was 0.65 and of the FS was 0.71.

Face validity. Two patients felt insecure where to indicate pain in the elbows and knees in the WPI because these pain sites were not mentioned. Two physicians felt puzzled by the different time frames of the FSQ. One physician wondered why abdominal pain was assessed both in the SSS and in the WPI.

Convergent validity. The Pearson correlation of the SSS with the PHQ 4 total score was 0.56 ($p<0.0001$) and of the FS with PHQ4 total score was 0.48 ($p<0.001$).

1411 (85.5%) participants of the total sample met the FSDC of FMS. 1351 (95.7%) reported a WPI ≥7 and a SSS ≥5 and 60 (4.4%) reported a WPI 3–6 and a SSS ≥9.

The diagnosis of FMS according to the ACR 1990 criteria was reevaluated at the date of appointment in 128 patients in 4 study centres with previously or actually diagnosed FMS. The mean of TPC was 13.8 (SD 3.5) (range 0–18). 107/128 (83.6%) participants met the ACR 1990 classification criteria of FMS. The concordance rate of the FSDC and ACR 1990 criteria was 72.7% (see table 3).

Discriminant validity. 64/202 (31.7%) of the participants not meeting the FSDC criteria and 152/1283 (11.8%) of the participants meeting the FSDC criteria reported an improvement (slightly too very much better) of their health status since FMS-diagnosis ($Chi^2 = 55$, $p<0.0001$).

Discussion

Summary of main findings

In this study we provided the first translation of the FSQ into another language and validated the FSQ for the first time in a cross-sectional survey with 1651 FMS-patients. The acceptability, reliability and validity of the FSQ met the predefined quality criteria pointed out in the validation hypotheses.

Relation to other studies

The proportion of missing items in the SSS ranged from 1.9 to 21.1%. The item with 21% missing was the headache item. We cannot explain the low completion rate of this item. The range was higher than the one of a disease specific health-related questionnaire in a survey with 522 patients with celiac disease which was 0.2–11.2 [11] and with 202 chronic liver patients was 0.4–2.8% [10].

The overall concordance rate of physician made diagnosis of FMS and FSDC was 85.5%. In a subsample the concordance of

Table 2. Demographic and clinical characteristics of the total study sample.

Variable	N Total	Mean (SD), lowest and highest value	N (%)
Sex female	1647		1562 (94.8)
Age	1644	54.1 (9.8), 19–84	
Living with partner/in family	1641		1562 (77.4)
Educational level	1640		
No school finished			27 (1.7)
Primary school			558 (34.0)
Secondary school			676 (41.2)
High school			131 (8.0)
University			248 (15.1)
Current professional status	1637		
School			10 (0.6)
Working without sick leave			529 (31.1)
Working, sick leave			287 (14.9)
Applying for early retirement due to FMS			151 (8.9)
Without job			21 (1.2)
Homemaker			186 (10.9)
Pensioner			604 (35.6)
Member of a FMS self-help organisation	1640		994 (60.6)
Years since chronic widespread pain	1629	16.4 (11.6), 0.25–61	
Years since FMS-diagnosis	1596	6.5 (5.5), 0–41	
Somatic severity score (0–12)	1653	8.3 (2.6), 0–12	
Widespread pain index (0–19)	1653	11.6 (3.2), 0–19	
Fibromyalgianess Total score (0–31)	1650	19.9 (5.5); 5–31	
Patient Health Questionnaire 4 Total score (0–12)	1652	6.0 (0.1), 0–12	

Table 3. Concordance rate of American College (ACR) 1990 classification criteria and Fibromyalgia Survey Diagnostic criteria (FSDC) (128 patients of four clinical centres).

ACR 1990 and FDSC positive	Only ACR 1990 positive	Only FDSC positive	Neither ACR 1990 and FDSC positive	Concordance rate ACR 1990 and FDSC
88 (68.8%)	15 (11.7%)	20 (15.6%)	5 (3.9%)	72.7%

FSDC with ACR 1990 criteria was 72.7%. These concordance rates were similar with the ones of a study in an US rheumatologic practice in which the concordance rate of the ACR 1990 and clinical criteria of FMS was 72% [14].

The study results highlight the problem of defining cut-off values for continuous symptom disorders such as FMS. 14.5% of the patients who had once been diagnosed with FMS did not meet the FSDC criteria of FMS at the time of the survey. Most notably, 32% of these patients reported an improvement of health status since FMS-diagnosis. In a longitudinal study with 1,555 fibromyalgia patients meeting the FSDC citeria at study entry conversion from and to criteria positive status was common during 7,448 semi-annual observations for up to 11 years. During follow-up 716 patients (44.0%) failed to meet criteria at least once, and at study closure 24.3% failed to meet criteria [1]. In the long-term management of these patients the assessment of the amount of distress ("fibromyalgianess" or polysymptomatic distress) is possible by summing the SSS and the WPI [3].

The study confirms the high levels of distress reported by FMS patients and the concepualisation of FMS a continuum disorder which can be located at the extreme end of the continuum of distress [16,17].

Limitations

The study did not include FMS-patients from primary care settings.

There is no gold standard how to deal with missing values. We decided not to use imputation methods because the percentage of missing values was one criterion of validation.

Testing of the test-retest reliability and responsiveness to change was not possible within a cross-sectional survey. The test-retest reliability of a WPI ≥7 in FMS-patients of different clinical settings was 100% and the intraclass correlation of the WPI was 0.78 over a period of 4–12 weeks [7].

Because there is no gold standard of the clinical diagnosis of FMS [18], the assessment of the criterion validity of the FSDC were not possible. We used the ACR 1990 criteria as a common standard for the assessment of convergent validity. Due to the study design it was not possible to perform a TPC in all patients.

Conclusions

Research. The study demonstrated the feasibility, reliability and validity of the FSQ in a survey with German FMS-patients. Further validation studies of the FSQ in other countries and/or languages are necessary. A standardization of the different time frames of the questions of the FSQ should be considered.

Clinical practice. The FSDC are not be used for self-diagnosis or as substitute for a physician's diagnosis. The FSQ can be used to gather information about the key symptoms of FMS and the extent of somatic symptom reporting, but the interpretation and assessment of questionnaire validity belongs to the physician [19].

Author Contributions

Conceived and designed the experiments: WH FW. Analyzed the data: WH EJ FW. Contributed reagents/materials/analysis tools: WH BEM MG HKB FP JL TW AW. Wrote the paper: WH EJ FW.

References

1. Wolfe F, Clauw DJ, Fitzcharles MA, Goldenberg DL, Katz RS, et al. (1990) The American College of Rheumatology preliminary diagnostic criteria for fibromyalgia and measurement of symptom severity. Arthritis Care Res (Hoboken) 62(5): 600–10.
2. Wolfe F, Smythe HA, Yunus MB, Bennett RM, Bombardier C, et al. (1990) The American College of Rheumatology 1990 Criteria for the Classification of Fibromyalgia. Report of the Multicenter Criteria Committee. Arthritis Rheum 33(2): 160–72.
3. Wolfe F, Clauw DJ, Fitzcharles MA, Goldenberg DL, Häuser W, et al. (2011) Fibromyalgia criteria and severity scales for clinical and epidemiological studies: a modification of the ACR Preliminary Diagnostic Criteria for Fibromyalgia. J Rheumatol 38(6): 1113–22.
4. Okifuji A, Turk DC, Sinclair JD, Starz TW, Marcus DA (1997) A standardized manual tender point survey. I. Development and determination of a threshold point forthe identification of positive tender points in fibromyalgia syndrome. J Rheumatol 24(2): 377–83.
5. Häuser W, Hayo S, Biewer W, Gesmann M, Kühn-Becker H, et al. (2010) Diagnosis of fibromyalgia syndrome-a comparison of Association of the Medical Scientific Societies in Germany, survey, and American College of Rheumatology criteria. Clin J Pain 26(6): 505–11.
6. Häuser W, Eich W, Herrmann M, Nutzinger DO, Schiltenwolf M, et al. (2009) Fibromyalgia syndrome: classification, diagnosis, and treatment. Dtsch Arztebl Int 106(23): 383–91.
7. Häuser W, Schild S, Kosseva M, Hayo S, von Wilmowski H, et al. (2010) [Validation of the German version of the Regional Pain Scale for the diagnosis of fibromyalgia syndrome]. Schmerz 24(3): 226–35. German.
8. Kroenke K, Spitzer RL, Jannett BW, Williams DSW, Löwe B (2009) An Ultra-Brief Screening Scale for Anxiety and Depression: The PHQ–4. Psychosomatics 50: 613–621.
9. Löwe B, Wahl I, Rose M, Spitzer C, Glaesmer H, et al. (2010) A 4-item measure of depression and anxiety: validation and standardization of the Patient Health Questionnaire-4 (PHQ-4) in the general population. J Affect Disord 122(1–2): 86–95.
10. Häuser W, Schnur M, Steder-Neukamm U, Muthny FA, Grandt D (2004) Validation of the German version of the Chronic Liver Disease Questionnaire. Eur J Gastroenterol Hepatol 16(6): 599–606.
11. Häuser W, Gold J, Stallmach A, Caspary WF, Stein J (2007) Development and validation of the Celiac Disease Questionnaire (CDQ), a disease-specific health-related quality of life measure for adult patients with celiac disease. J Clin Gastroenterol 41(2): 157–66.
12. Fletcher A, Gore S, Jones D, Fitzpatrick R, Spiegelhalter D, et al. (1992) Quality of life measures in health care. II: Design, analysis, and interpretation. BMJ 305(6862): 1145–8.
13. Ericsson K, Simon H (1980) Verbal reports as data. Psychol Rev 87(3): 215–251.
14. Katz RS, Wolfe F, Michaud K (2006) Fibromyalgia diagnosis: a comparison of clinical, survey, and American College of Rheumatology criteria. Arthritis Rheum 5: 169–176.
15. Walitt B, Fitzcharles MA, Hassett AL, Katz RS, Häuser W, et al. (2011) The Longitudinal Outcome of Fibromyalgia: A Study of 1555 Patients. J Rheumatol 38(10): 2238–46.
16. Croft P, Burt J, Schollum J, Thomas E, Macfarlane G, et al. (1996) More pain, more tender points: is fibromyalgia just one end of a continuous spectrum? Ann Rheum Dis 55(7): 482–5.

17. Häuser W, Schmutzer G, Brähler E, Glaesmer H (2009) A cluster within the continuum of biopsychosocial distress can be labeled "fibromyalgia syndrome"-evidence from a representative German population survey. J Rheumatol 36(12): 2806–12.
18. Goldenberg DL (2009) Diagnosis and differential diagnosis of fibromyalgia. Am J Med 122(12 Suppl): S14–2.
19. Wolfe F (2011) How to use the new American College of Rheumatology fibromyalgia diagnostic criteria. Arthritis Care Res (Hoboken) 63(7): 1073–4.

4

Effects of Pregabalin on Central Sensitization in Patients with Chronic Pancreatitis in a Randomized, Controlled Trial

Stefan A. W. Bouwense[1], Søren S. Olesen[2], Asbjørn M. Drewes[2,3], Jan-Werner Poley[4], Harry van Goor[1], Oliver H. G. Wilder-Smith[5]*

1 Pain and Nociception Neuroscience Research Group, Department of Surgery, Radboud University Nijmegen Medical Center, Nijmegen, The Netherlands, **2** Mech-Sense, Department of Gastroenterology and Hepatology, Aalborg Hospital, Aarhus University Hospital, Aalborg, Denmark, **3** Center for Sensory-Motor Interaction (SMI), Department of Health Science and Technology, Aalborg University, Aalborg, Denmark, **4** Department of Gastroenterology and Hepatology, Erasmus MC, University Medical Center, Rotterdam, The Netherlands, **5** Pain and Nociception Neuroscience Research Group, Department of Anaesthesiology, Pain and Palliative Care, Radboud University Nijmegen Medical Center, Nijmegen, The Netherlands

Abstract

Background: Intense abdominal pain is the dominant feature of chronic pancreatitis. During the disease changes in central pain processing, e.g. central sensitization manifest as spreading hyperalgesia, can result from ongoing nociceptive input. The aim of the present study is to evaluate the effect of pregabalin on pain processing in chronic pancreatitis as assessed by quantitative sensory testing (QST).

Methods: This randomized, double-blind, placebo-controlled trial evaluated effects of pregabalin on pain processing. QST was used to quantify pain processing by measuring thresholds to painful electrical and pressure stimulation in six body dermatomes. Descending endogenous pain modulation was quantified using the conditioned pain modulation (CPM) paradigm to elicit a DNIC (diffuse noxious inhibitory controls) response. The main effect parameter was the change in the sum of all body pain threshold values after three weeks of study treatment versus baseline values between both treatment groups.

Results: 64 patients were analyzed. No differences in change in sum of pain thresholds were present for pregabalin vs. placebo after three weeks of treatment. For individual dermatomes, change vs. baseline pain thresholds was significantly greater in pregabalin vs. placebo patients for electric pain detection threshold in C5 ($P = 0.005$), electric pain tolerance threshold in C5 ($P = 0.04$) and L1 ($P = 0.05$), and pressure pain tolerance threshold in T4 ($P = 0.004$). No differences were observed between pregabalin and placebo regarding conditioned pain modulation.

Conclusion: Our study provides first evidence that pregabalin has moderate inhibitory effects on central sensitization manifest as spreading hyperalgesia in chronic pancreatitis patients. These findings suggest that QST can be of clinical use for monitoring pain treatments in the context of chronic pain.

Trial Registration: ClinicalTrials.gov NCT00755573

Editor: Sam Eldabe, The James Cook University Hospital, United Kingdom

Funding: Supported by a free grant from Pfizer Research and Development, Hertha Christensen's Foundation, and Christenson-Ceson's Family Foundation. The funders had no role in study design, data collection and analysis, decision to publish, or preparation of the manuscript.

Competing Interests: The study was investigator initiated and Pfizer donated capsules of pregabalin and placebo. The authors have no conflict of interest regarding this manuscript.

* E-mail: o.wildersmith@anes.umcn.nl

Introduction

The treatment of chronic pancreatitis patients can be a major clinical challenge. [1] Achieving control of pain, one of the main symptoms in this disease, can be difficult, and is often unsatisfactory for patients and doctors. [2] An evidence based approach to this pain for these patients does not exist, and to date there are no uniformly accepted guidelines for treatment.

One of the main factors contributing to this problem is the lack of evidence regarding the origin of chronic pancreatitis pain. [3] Complications of pancreatic inflammation such as dilated pancreatic duct, ductal stones and enlarged pancreatic head can be treated endoscopically or surgically, but numerous patients continue to suffer from pain despite technically successful interventions. [4,5] Even bilateral splanchnicectomy, interrupting ascending nociceptive pathways, fails in a substantial number of patients. [6] In the last decade research has suggested that ongoing nociceptive input from the pancreas is not the only explanation for the debilitating abdominal pain in chronic pancreatitis. It is increasingly accepted that changes in central pain processing, e.g.

central sensitization or a shift towards pro-nociceptive pain modulation, may result from chronic nociceptive input, manifest as spreading hyperalgesia.[7–9] Ultimately, this process may become entirely independent of nociceptive input and inhibitory pain modulation, leading to an autonomous pain state. [10].

Medication targeting altered central pain processing, e.g. gabapentinoids such as pregabalin, has been used successfully to treat other chronic pain disorders such as post-herpetic neuralgia and neuropathic pain of central origin.[11–13] In a recent publication, we demonstrated that pregabalin has a significant clinical analgesic effect in chronic pancreatitis patients. [14] Quantitative sensory testing (QST) is a useful tool to quantify pain processing in chronic pain patients, also in relation to the effectiveness of analgesic interventions. [15,16] Apart from one recent study on S-ketamine for chronic pancreatitis pain and one using gabapentin for visceral pain in irritable bowel syndrome [12,17], we are not aware of any studies having used QST to describe the influence of centrally active medication on pain processing in patients suffering from chronic pain disorders.

The aim of the present study is to evaluate the effect of pregabalin as adjuvant pain treatment on pain processing, measured by somatic QST, in patients with chronic pancreatitis. We hypothesized that the hyperalgesia in chronic pancreatitis patients with pain will undergo reduction under pregabalin treatment, but not under placebo treatment.

Methods

Study Overview

The protocol for this trial and supporting CONSORT checklist are available as supporting information; see Checklist S1 and Protocol S1.

This study was part of an investigator initiated double blind, placebo-controlled, parallel-group study of increasing doses of pregabalin conducted in the Netherlands (department of Surgery, Radboud University Nijmegen Medical Center) and Denmark (department of Gastroenterology & Hepatology, Aalborg Hospital, Aarhus University Hospital). [14] The study was approved by the responsible Ethical Committees in both countries (CMO region Arnhem-Nijmegen, Nijmegen, The Netherlands and The local Ethics Committee North Region, Aalborg, Denmark) and all patients provided written informed consent. This article presents a secondary and further analysis of the data obtained in a previous trial [14] focusing primarily on experimental (QST) endpoints.

Patients

For trial inclusion, patients needed to have chronic abdominal pain typical for pancreatitis (i.e. dull epigastric pain more than 3 days per week for at least 3 months) and a diagnosis of chronic pancreatitis based on the Mayo Clinic diagnostic criteria. [18] Another inclusion criterion was the use of a stable regime of concomitant analgesic medication during the trial. Exclusion criteria were: painful conditions other than chronic pancreatitis, an abnormal electrocardiogram at screening visit, severe renal impairment, active (or history of) major depression, hypersensitivity to pregabalin or any of it components and pregnant or lactating patients. All patients that participated in this trial were included in this study and analyzed in an intention to treat analysis.

Clinical endpoints i.e. pain scores and side-effects of the main study are presented in more detail in the original manuscript. [14].

Healthy Controls

A control group was recruited in Denmark for comparison with our chronic pancreatitis group to confirm the presence of spreading hyperalgesia at the baseline pre-medication measurement in the pancreatitis group. The controls were completely healthy and had no history of a medical condition that could interfere with our pain measurements.

Randomization and Treatment

Eligible patients at our outpatient departments were randomly assigned in a one to one ratio to receive either pregabalin or placebo. A pseudo-random code was computer generated for the randomization blocks that had a size of six. Stratification of trial participants was based on the absence or presence of diabetes mellitus to minimize unbalance in distribution of undiagnosed diabetic polyneuropathy. Patients received increasing doses of either pregabalin or matching placebo for the study period of 3 weeks. Initial dose was 75 mg pregabalin twice a day (BID). After three days this was increased to 150 mg pregabalin BID, with a further increase to 300 mg BID after one week and for the rest of the study period. An equivalent regime was followed in the placebo arm. The same oral dosing schedule was prescribed to all patients. Daily dosages were split into two equivalent doses, one administered in the morning between 7 a.m. and 10 a.m. and one in the evening between 7 p.m. and 10 p.m. In the case of unacceptable side effects experienced by patients, a single downward dose titration was allowed. Patients had to stay on that final dosage for the remaining study period. Patients were instructed to taper their study medication after three weeks of treatment, by halving their dose for seven days, and then to stop medication. Patients and those administrating study medication, assessing outcomes, and analyzing data were blinded to group assignment.

Study Visits

Patients considered for participation in this trial were screened for eligibility and physical fitness. A systematic physical examination including a neurological examination was performed to assess for any relevant conditions and neurological disorders. If eligible, they were randomized by their treating physician for placebo or pregabalin on their second visit, one week after their screening visit. During their second visit all patients had a baseline QST measurement, followed by another QST measurement at the end of the study period of three weeks, i.e. before they were instructed to taper their medication. During the whole study period patients were instructed not to change their daily pain medication. They were only allowed to take extra pain medication in the case of a painful exacerbation of their chronic pancreatitis.

Quantitative Sensory Testing

QST took place using a standard temporal test sequence. [7] Testing in females was not standardized with regard to phase of the menstrual cycle because all female pancreatitis patients were amenorrhoeic. Both the examiners (one in Denmark and one in the Netherlands) were trained in and used the same QST protocol. They performed the measurements in the same way and setting. Pressure pain thresholds were based on two measurements and electrical pain thresholds were based on three measurements.

After initial QST training per participating subject, pressure pain thresholds were obtained for muscles overlying bone using a pressure algometer with a 1.0 cm^2 probe (Somedic Sales AB, Horby, Sweden), at each of the following sites on the dominant body side: clavicle (C5 dermatome), sternum (T4 dermatome), pancreatic site (dorsal and ventral T10 dermatome), hip region (L1 dermatome) and knee (L4 dermatome) (Figure 1). The pancreas and more distant dermatomes were chosen to observe segmental and spreading hyperalgesia respectively. Two thresholds were

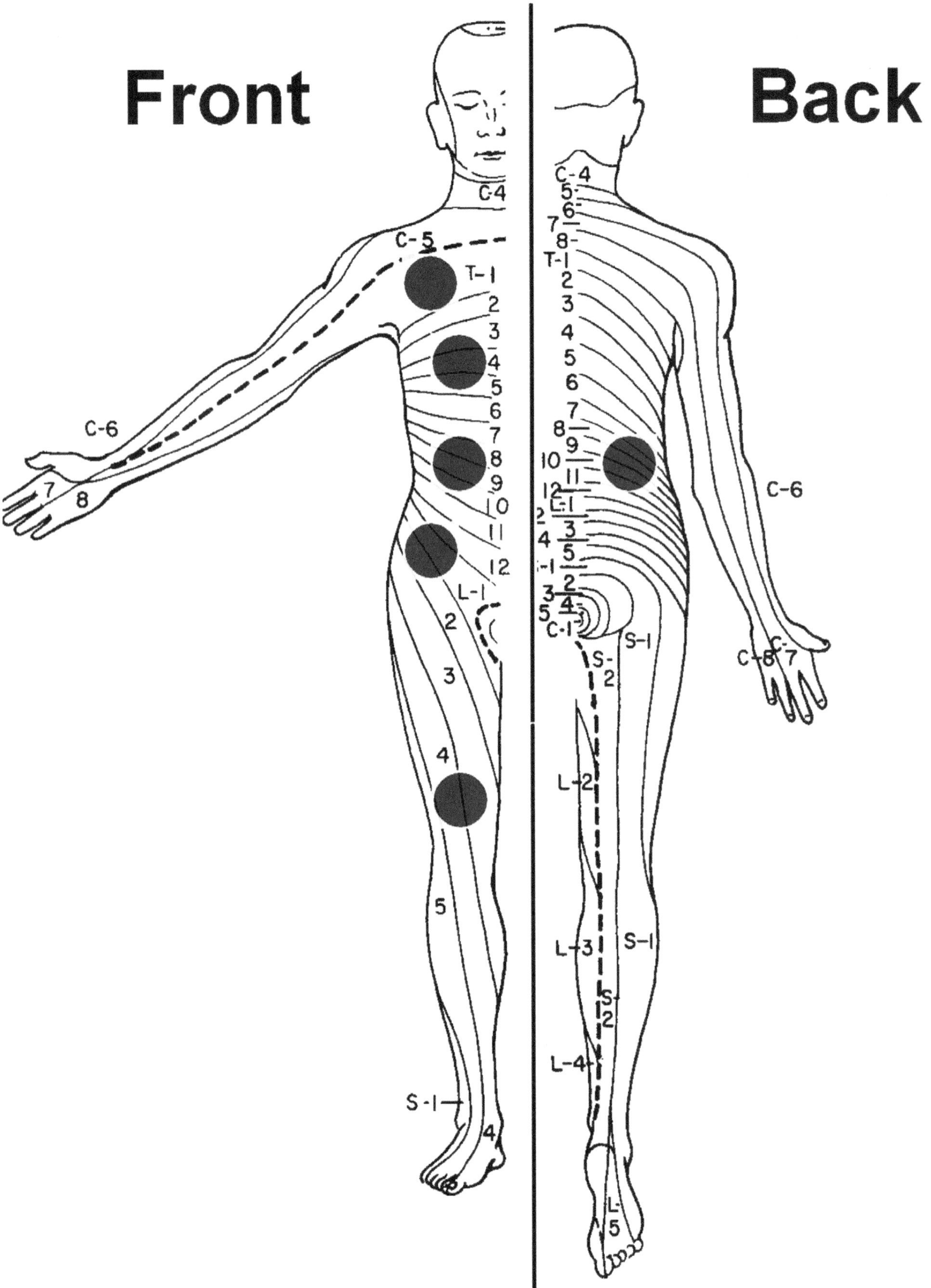
Front
Back
C-4
C-5
T-1
C-6
L-1
S-1
L-2
L-3
L-4
S-2
L-5
C-7
C-8

Figure 1. Dermatomes of measurement for quantitative sensory testing. Quantitative sensory testing was performed on the following sites on the dominant body side (black dots): clavicle (C5 dermatome), sternum (T4 dermatome), pancreatic site (dorsal and ventral T10 dermatome), hip region (L1 dermatome) and knee (L4 dermatome).

measured: pressure pain detection threshold (pPDT) and pressure pain tolerance threshold (pPTT). As the primary endpoint, the sum of all the thresholds across dermatomes was calculated. [17].

Thresholds to electric constant current skin stimulation (Digistim; Biometer A/S, Copenhagen, Denmark; tetanic stimulation at 100 Hz, 0.2-ms square waves, self-adhesive electrodes 3 cm apart) were measured on the dominant side of the body at the same sites as for pressure pain thresholds. Two thresholds were measured: electric pain detection threshold (ePDT) and electric pain tolerance threshold (ePTT). As the primary endpoint, the sum of all the thresholds was again calculated. [17].

The conditioned pain modulation (CPM, previously known as DNIC (diffuse noxious inhibitory control)) paradigm was performed to test the ability of the patient to generate descending inhibitory modulation. [19,20] Thus pressure pain thresholds (pPTT, the test stimulus) were determined before and after the cold pressor task (the conditioning stimulus), and the CPM effect was determined as the relative change (%) in pressure pain thresholds. For the cold pressor task the dominant hand was immersed in ice-chilled water (1.0°C ±0.3°C) continuously stirred by a pump. The patient was told to remove the hand from the water after two minutes of immersion - or sooner if the pain was considered to be intolerable – and the immersion time noted. Immediately after the cold pressor task, the subjects rated the pain experienced during the test by use of a visual analogue scale for quality control purposes. Pressure pain thresholds were obtained in the non-dominant L4 dermatome (knee) immediately before and after ice-water immersion.

Outcome Measures

The primary effect parameter for the study was the between group difference (change) in sum of electric or pressure pain thresholds after three weeks of study medication vs. baseline values. [17] Between group differences in change in individual dermatome thresholds and CPM paradigm results were secondary endpoints.

Statistical Analysis

A *pre hoc* power calculation based on QST as an endpoint was not performed because the study was a part of a randomized clinical trial that investigated pregabalin, powered for a clinical primary endpoint; i.e. change in clinical pain score.

For this mechanistic study we performed an intention to treat analysis. We performed statistical analysis using the Statistica for Windows Software Package (Release 7.0, Statsoft Inc, Tulsa, OK, USA). All baseline characteristics and measurements are given as medians with interquartile ranges. In view of the non-Gaussian data distribution purely non-parametric analysis was performed. Statistical significance was set at $P \leq 0.05$.

The sum of all dermatomes for electric and pressure pain detection and tolerance thresholds and the conditioned pain modulation results were compared between the control and the study group using Mann Whitney U testing to confirm spreading hyperalgesia and pro-nociceptive pain modulation shift in the pancreatitis patients. [14,17].

We calculated differences (change) in sum of thresholds or individual thresholds between values at pre-medication baseline and after three weeks' medication. We then compared these differences between the groups using Mann Whitney U testing. Further analysis consisted of comparison of placebo vs. pregabalin groups at pre-medication baseline and after three weeks' treatment for the sum of thresholds, for individual thresholds, or for conditioned pain modulation values using Mann Whitney U testing.

Results

Enrollment and Baseline Characteristics

From October 2008 to May 2010 a total of 236 patients diagnosed with chronic pancreatitis in the last five years in one of both hospitals were screened and 64 patients were randomized; the study was completed without any incident. The majority of patients not meeting inclusion criteria were free of pain, had passed away or were no longer being treated in either of the hospitals. 64 patients completed the study and were finally analyzed in the intention to treat analysis (Figure 2). The number of patients randomized to pregabalin or placebo treatment was equally distributed between both hospitals. All patients (24 women, 40 men; median age 53 years (IQR (interquartile range) 45–62)) had pain due to chronic pancreatitis and were on a stable analgesic therapy. Their median opioid consumption was 60 mg (IQR 11–150) of morphine equivalents/day. Their median VAS score before start of trial medication was 4 (IQR 2–5) at rest and 5 (IQR 4–7) during activity. Demographic data of the placebo and pregabalin group are provided in Table 1. The healthy control group consisted of 15 volunteers (7 women, 8 men; median age 38 years (IQR 35–49)). Only age was significantly different between the healthy controls and chronic pancreatitis patients ($P = 0.0001$).

Baseline Measurements

Pancreatitis vs. healthy controls. The sum for pressure and electric pain detection and tolerance thresholds of all dermatomes was significantly lower for the pancreatitis group at baseline vs. healthy controls (Table 2). At baseline chronic pancreatitis patients tolerated the cold pressor task for 35 seconds (IQR 24–70) and the healthy controls for 180 seconds (IQR 180–180), ($P = 0.000004$). The healthy control group exhibited a significantly greater CPM response than the pancreatitis patients ($P = 0.008$) (Table 2). These results confirm hyperalgesia and a shift to more pro-nociceptive pain modulation in our pancreatitis patients.

Pregabalin vs. placebo patients. The sum of all dermatomes for pressure and electric pain detection and tolerance thresholds at baseline was similar for the pregabalin vs. placebo groups (Table 3). The same applied to the individual dermatomal thresholds (Table 4).

At baseline, patients in the placebo group tolerated the cold pressor task for 32 seconds (IQR 23–98) and in the pregabalin group for 40 seconds (IQR 23–60), this was not statistically different between groups. Also no significant difference was found in baseline CPM response between the placebo and pregabalin group (Table 4).

Effects of Treatment - Change in Measurements after Three Weeks' Study Medication

Electric pain thresholds. There was no significant difference in differences (change) in *sums* of electric pain detection and tolerance thresholds between the groups (Table 5).

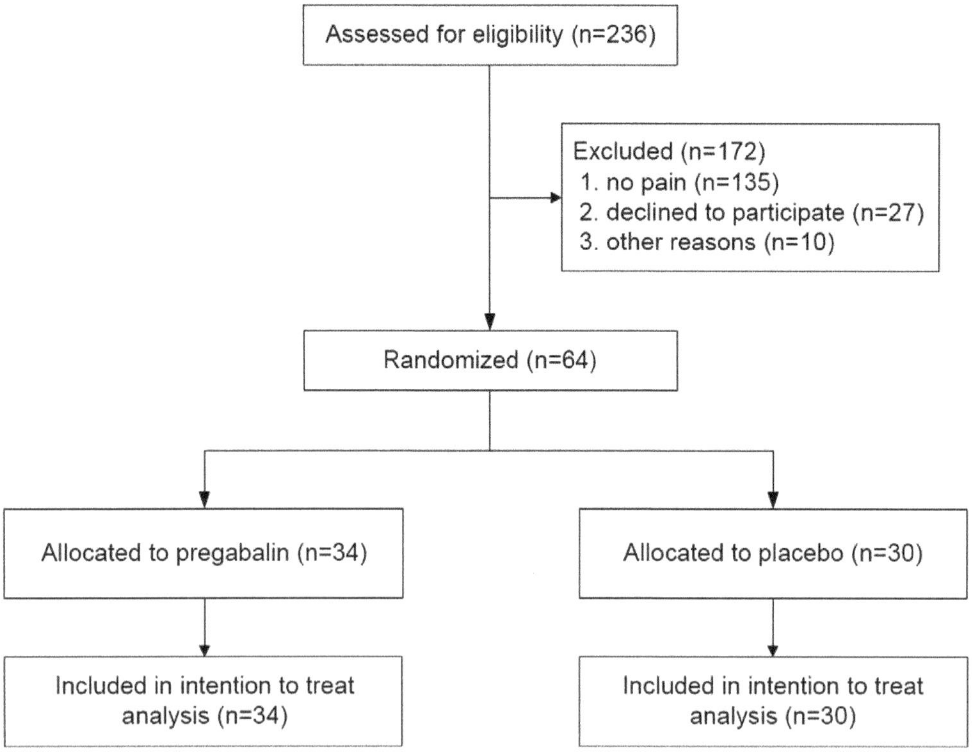

Figure 2. Study enrollment and randomization. The majority of patients not meeting inclusion criteria had passed away, were free of pain or were no longer being treated in either of the hospitals.

For *individual* electric pain detection thresholds, difference (change) in dermatome C5 was significantly higher in the pregabalin group (0.8 vs. −0.1; P = 0.005), with a trend for T10 (P = 0.055) (Table 5).

For *individual* electric pain tolerance thresholds, threshold differences (change) for dermatome C5 (2.0 vs. 0.7; P = 0.04) and L1 (1.9 vs. −0.2; P = 0.05) were significantly higher in the pregabalin group (Table 5).

Pressure pain thresholds. There was no significant difference in differences (change) in *sums* of pressure pain detection and tolerance thresholds between the groups (Table 5).

There was no significant difference in differences (change) in *individual* dermatomal pressure pain detection thresholds between the groups (Table 5).

For *individual* pressure pain tolerance thresholds, threshold differences (change) for dermatome T4 (83 vs. −48; P = 0.004) were significantly higher in the pregabalin group (Table 5).

CPM response. The difference (change) in cold pressor task latency and CPM response was not significantly different between the study groups (Table 5).

Effects of Treatment - Absolute Values after Three Weeks' Study Medication

Electric pain thresholds. After 3 weeks' study medication, *sum* of all dermatomes for electric pain detection thresholds was significantly higher in the pregabalin vs. placebo group (P = 0.01), but not for electric pain tolerance thresholds (Table 3).

For *individual* dermatomes, electric pain detection thresholds were significantly higher in the pregabalin group (T4; P = 0.04, L4; P = 0.05 and T10BACK; P = 0.05) (Table 4). For *individual* dermatomal electric pain tolerance thresholds, C5 (P = 0.05) and L1 (P = 0.03) were significantly higher in the pregabalin group.

Pressure pain thresholds. *Sums* of – or *individual* dermatome – pressure pain detection and tolerance thresholds were similar between groups (Table 3 and 4) after three weeks' study medication.

CPM response. After three weeks of study medication patients in the placebo group tolerated the cold pressor task for 42 seconds (IQR 21–116) and in the pregabalin group for 46 seconds (IQR 27–77); this was not statistically significant. Also no significant difference could be found between groups for CPM response after study medication (Table 4).

Discussion

Our study is the first to demonstrate that a three-week treatment with pregabalin in chronic pancreatitis patients results in a moderate antihyperalgesic effect compatible with a reduction of central sensitization. A shift toward more anti-nociceptive pain modulation appears less likely as mechanism due to the unaltered conditioned pain modulation (CPM) response. Interestingly, this early treatment effect is 1) visible only in dermatomes distant from the referred pancreatic area, and 2) more pronounced for electric skin thresholds than for pressure muscle thresholds. This implies 1) better effects on distant as compared to segmental central sensitization and 2) more effective hyperalgesia reduction in skin compared to deeper tissues. These results suggest that measuring pain sensitivity using quantitative sensory testing (QST) may prove useful in monitoring the effects of pain treatment in chronic pancreatitis and help us to diagnose and manage altered pain processing in chronic pain disorders.

Nociceptive input from the pancreas spreads via ascending pathways to spinal and supraspinal central nervous system structures in chronic pancreatitis. [21,22] Ongoing nociceptive

Table 1. Demographic and clinical characteristics of patients.

	Pregabalin (n = 34)	Placebo (n = 30)
Age (years)	52 (46–58)	55 (42–65)
Males - no. (%)	20 (59)	19 (63)
Etiology - no. (%)		
- Toxic-metabolic	16 (47)	17 (57)
- Idiopathic	11 (32)	11 (37)
- Genetic	2 (6)	0 (0)
- Autoimmune	1 (3)	0 (0)
- Recurrent and severe acute pancreatitis	2 (6)	1 (3)
- Obstructive	2 (6)	1 (3)
Diary pain score (visual analogue scale 0–10)		
- Average pain	4 (2–6)	3 (2–5)
- Maximal pain	6 (4–8)	5 (4–7)
Concomitant analgesics - no. (%)[†]		
- None	3 (9)	2 (7)
- Weak analgesics	7 (21)	11 (37)
- Strong analgesics	24 (71)	17 (57)
MEQ/day	80 (10–158)	49 (13–128)
Duration of chronic pancreatitis (months)	92 (55–132)	83 (60–147)
Diabetes mellitus - no. (%)	10 (29)	10 (33)
Previous interventions for chronic pancreatitis – no. (%)		
- Pancreas resection/drainage procedures	6 (18)	5 (17)
- Thoracoscopic splanchnic denervation	2 (6)	4 (13)
Patients treated with enzymes for pancreatic exocrine insufficiency - no. (%)	18 (53)	13 (43)
Ongoing alcohol abuse - no. (%)[‡]	7 (21)	11 (37)
Current smoker - no. (%)	26 (76)	22 (77)

All values are medians with interquartile ranges unless mentioned otherwise. Percentages may not total 100 due to rounding.
[†]Weak analgesics were defined as NSAIDS, paracetamol, codeine and tramadol. Strong analgesics were defined as opioid based therapies.
[‡]Alcohol abusing patients were defined as female patients drinking >14 units of alcohol per week or male patients drinking >21 units of alcohol per week.
'MEQ' is morphine equivalents, 'pregabalin' is pregabalin study group and 'placebo' is placebo study group.
No statistical differences between groups were observed.

input increases neuronal excitability and synaptic strength, initially at the spinal level, a state characterized by hyperalgesia near the site of injury (segmental hyperalgesia). [3,23] With persisting disease and nociception central sensitization spreads rostrally in the central nervous system. [8] This progression is more marked when descending inhibitory control mechanisms fail or in the presence of descending facilitation, and may in due course result in a widespread hyperalgesic state. [9] Ultimately, these central changes may become independent of peripheral nociceptive input, ending in an autonomous state. [6] Sensitization of the nervous system is not specific for chronic pancreatitis, but is common among other chronic pain disorders.[24–26] Congruently with the described course of events, chronic pancreatitis patients in our study did exhibit widespread hyperalgesia compared to healthy controls.

The treatment of pain in chronic pancreatitis patients is usually based on the WHO pain treatment ladder, which ends with opioid treatment. Opioids can provide effective analgesia in some pancreatitis patients, but may have considerable side effects or even induce hyperalgesia. [27] Recently, pain treatments more directly targeting the central nervous system, e.g. tricyclic antidepressants or gabapentinoids, have been introduced to better control disabling pain and hyperalgesia in chronic pain syndromes. [28] Particularly the use of gabapentinoids has shown clinical results in chronic pain disorders. [12,29,30] The clinical analgesic effect of pregabalin in chronic pancreatitis patients was recently published by our research group. [14] Two studies in an

Table 2. Baseline data for conditioned pain modulation and sum of pain thresholds for pancreatitis patients vs. healthy controls.

	Pancreatitis	Control	P-value
SUM ePDT (mA)	28 (21–41)	47 (21–65)	0.026
SUM ePTT (mA)	44 (34–62)	68 (48–92)	0.017
SUM pPDT (kPa)	1912 (951–2551)	2285 (2018–3018)	0.008
SUM pPTT (kPa)	2694 (2110–3185)	3234 (2785–4018)	0.005
CPM (%)	4.2 (0.0–22.4)	32.6 (10.4–41.8)	0.008

All values are medians with interquartile ranges. 'Control' is healthy control group and 'Pancreatitis' is chronic pancreatitis group. 'ePDT' is electric pain detection threshold, 'ePTT' is electric pain tolerance threshold, 'pPDT' is pressure pain detection threshold, 'pPPT' is pressure pain tolerance threshold and 'CPM' is conditioned pain modulation.

Table 3. Sum of pain thresholds for pregabalin vs. placebo before and after treatment.

	Before		After	
	Pregabalin	**Placebo**	**Pregabalin**	**Placebo**
SUM ePDT (mA)	33.4 (23.6–43.5)	23.4 (18.9–33.8)	37.3 (27.9–51.6) •	26.1 (17.2–39.7)
SUM ePTT (mA)	53.4 (39.2–67.1)	41.7 (32.6–51.6)	52.3 (38.9–73.9)	44.0 (34.9–55.2)
SUM pPDT (kPa)	1936 (1063–2574)	1759 (902–2449)	1817 (1109–3312)	1817 (844–2585)
SUM pPTT (kPa)	2677 (2043–3136)	2720 (2307–3230)	2798 (2355–3945)	2853 (2131–3264)

All values are medians with interquartile ranges. • = Measurements after study treatment were significantly higher in the pregabalin group compared to the placebo group.

Table 4. Conditioned pain modulation and pain thresholds for pregabalin vs. placebo before and after study treatment.

	Before		After	
	Pregabalin	**Placebo**	**Pregabalin**	**Placebo**
ePDT (mA)				
- C5	3.9 (2.5–5.1)	3.5 (2.4–6.0)	4.5 (3.4–5.6)	3.1 (2.1–6.0)
- T4	5.0 (3.0–7.0)	3.5 (2.7–6.3)	6.2 (4.2–8.5) •	3.9 (3.3–7.6)
- T10	5.8 (4.3–8.1)	3.7 (3.0–7.7)	6.5 (4.7–9.2)	4.9 (3.2–7.9)
- L1	4.8 (3.6–6.4)	4.3 (3.1–5.9)	6.6 (4.4–8.9)	4.7 (2.7–8.4)
- L4	5.7 (4.0–8.5)	4.1 (3.2–6.5)	5.8 (4.1–9.1) •	4.4 (3.2–6.6)
- T10 BACK	5.9 (3.8–7.2)	4.8 (3.8–6.9)	5.8 (4.3–10.3) •	4.3 (2.8–7.8)
ePTT (mA)				
- C5	6.9 (5.4–10.7)	5.4 (4.1–9.9)	9.6 (5.4–14.4) •	6.3 (5.0–10.7)
- T4	8.9 (5.6–13.0)	7.6 (5.1–10.7)	10.9 (7.5–16.2)	8.6 (5.6–11.6)
- T10	10.6 (6.1–12.7)	7.3 (3.7–10.7)	8.8 (6.1–15.1)	7.9 (5.6–12.6)
- L1	9.5 (6.5–13.5)	7.2 (5.2–11.1)	9.5 (7.0–14.8) •	7.1 (5.8–12.9)
- L4	9.9 (6.7–13.3)	7.4 (5.1–10.0)	9.1 (6.6–14.9)	7.2 (5.7–10.9)
- T10 BACK	11.7 (6.5–16.3)	9.3 (6.4–12.6)	9.1 (6.6–14.9)	8.9 (6.9–12.5)
pPDT (kPa)				
- C5	263 (142–334)	232 (106–380)	228 (130–321)	245 (115–398)
- T4	281 (195–392)	289 (139–409)	277 (169–421)	268 (147–359)
- T10	166 (97–302)	154 (85–264)	129 (65–328)	157 (61–306)
- L1	376 (207–511)	340 (197–571)	292 (207–566)	424 (168–528)
- L4	406 (235–601)	396 (176–613)	447 (177–689)	332 (204–641)
- T10 BACK	378 (211–474)	276 (162–522)	332 (132–549)	313 (161–480)
pPTT (kPa)				
- C5	421 (313–523)	378 (309–563)	451 (310–614)	459 (358–599)
- T4	481 (307–555)	422 (335–528)	431 (352–691)	371 (284–530)
- T10	246 (165–493)	257 (176–402)	280 (173–570)	236 (156–432)
- L1	578 (454–675)	548 (407–706)	551 (437–716)	581 (479–649)
- L4	608 (530–776)	614 (437–776)	733 (526–933)	700 (508–866)
- T10 BACK	574 (403–699)	561 (476–731)	612 (397–838)	537 (395–635)
CPM response (%)	0.9 (0.0–22.0)	8.9 (0.0–23.8)	0.0 (0.0–22.4)	0.0 (−4.0–19.8)

All values are medians with interquartile ranges. • = Measurements after study treatment were significantly higher in the pregabalin group compared to the placebo group.

experimental pain model in healthy volunteers showed a reduction of hyperalgesia and central sensitization after gabapentin treatment. [31,32] Only two studies, one with S-ketamine in chronic pancreatitis and one with pregabalin in irritable bowel syndrome, showed comparable reductions of hyperalgesia in patients treated with medication active in the central nervous system. [12,17] To

Table 5. Change and percentage change in conditioned pain modulation and pain thresholds for pregabalin vs. placebo after study treatment.

	Pregabalin		Placebo	
	Change	**Percentage change (%)**	**Change**	**Percentage change (%)**
ePDT (mA)				
- C5	0.8 (0.2–1.9) •	24 (5–55)	−0.1 (−0.9–0.5)	2 (−25–16)
- T4	1.5 (−0.7–3.0)	39 (−13–83)	0.7 (−1.1–1.5)	17 (−16–49)
- T10	0.8 (−0.7–3.1)	12 (−11–52)	0.4 (−0.7–1.4)	8 (−9–40)
- L1	1.2 (−0.2–3.8)	25 (−6–71)	0.3 (−0.5–2.3)	11 (−11–51)
- L4	0.9 (−0.8–2.3)	14 (−16–46)	0.7 (−0.9–1.7)	18 (−22–37)
- T10 BACK	0.6 (−1.2–4.3)	16 (−22–75)	−0.6 (−1.4–1.3)	−14 (−29–14)
ePTT (mA)				
- C5	2.0 (−0.1–3.7) •	25 (−1–64)	0.7 (−2.4–1.9)	12 (−27–40)
- T4	2.6 (−0.6–5.1)	41 (−5–60)	1.5 (−0.9–2.9)	15 (−12–46)
- T10	1.0 (−0.8–2.4)	10 (−10–27)	0.8 (−1.2–2.4)	17 (−9–53)
- L1	1.9 (−0.8–4.9) •	29 (−7–59)	−0.2 (−2.3–2.1)	−3 (−28–38)
- L4	1.5 (−2.0–5.2)	22 (−20–53)	−0.3 (−1.2–3.0)	0 (−14–83)
- T10 BACK	1.1 (−1.9–4.8)	10 (−20–57)	−0.5 (−2.8–2.7)	−5 (−21–36)
pPDT (kPa)				
- C5	12 (−79–89)	7 (−39–34)	−13 (−51–50)	−7 (−19–31)
- T4	9 (−91–72)	4 (−34–26)	−3 (−89–45)	−1 (−29–13)
- T10	13 (−31–77)	6 (−31–53)	−1 (−51–26)	0 (−24–15)
- L1	63 (−137–117)	18 (−39–53)	12 (−99–135)	9 (−19–40)
- L4	80 (−129–176)	18 (−30–37)	0 (−50–88)	0 (−13–23)
- T10 BACK	41 (−63–89)	9 (−7–31)	34 (−73–90)	9 (−24–24)
pPTT (kPa)				
- C5	19 (−65–152)	3 (−17–40)	17 (−32–103)	5 (−9–31)
- T4	83 (−24–169) •	18 (−7–43)	−48 (−108–43)	−13 (−21–12)
- T10	10 (−56–111)	5 (−15–53)	20 (−103–56)	7 (−34–23)
- L1	−7 (−82–136)	−1 (−16–32)	69 (−149–144)	16 (−19–28)
- L4	17 (−253–278)	6 (−30–53)	75 (15–225)	12 (3–33)
- T10 BACK	41 (−74–194)	5 (−15–40)	14 (−165–81)	3 (−27–21)
SUM ePDT	6.0 (−1.2–15.0)	19 (−6–62)	2.3 (−1.9–5.8)	9 (−8–19)
SUM ePTT	7.6 (−7.1–13.5)	13 (−14–25)	2.7 (−7.1–10.9)	7 (−15–28)
SUM pPDT	311 (−155–526)	16 (−9–39)	131 (−330–329)	11 (−14–20)
SUM pPTT	226 (−265–593)	10 (−14–20)	193 (−192–380)	8 (−6–17)
CPM response (%)	1 (−4–18)	−18 (−100–134)	−2 (−23–6)	−100 (−136–16)

All values are medians with interquartile ranges. • = Measurements after study treatment were significantly higher in the pregabalin group compared to the placebo group.

date a more prolonged reduction of somatic hyperalgesia and thus central sensitization has not been demonstrated in chronic pain patients in relation to pregabalin treatment.

In this study we failed to show a significant difference between groups regarding our primary outcome measure (change in sum of thresholds). The significant result regarding secondary outcome measure (change in individual dermatomal thresholds) suggests a moderate effect on spreading hyperalgesia. Interestingly, anti-hyperalgesic treatment with pregabalin resulted in a greater increase of electric pain thresholds than of pressure pain thresholds after three weeks treatment. A possible explanation is that pregabalin is initially more effective in reducing skin sensitization, as reflected by electric thresholds, as compared to deep tissue sensitization, as reflected by pressure thresholds. [32,33] If this were true, one might expect greater decreases in deep tissue sensitivity with longer treatment periods in future studies.

In this study no significant improvement in conditioned pain modulation (CPM) could be found, suggesting that the main effect of pregabalin is to directly target central sensitization reflected by hyperalgesia, rather than the pro/anti-nociceptive balance of endogenous modulation. We did, however, demonstrate that before treatment, pancreatitis patients showed less inhibitory pain modulation than healthy controls in accordance with other studies. [9] However, it should be noted that CPM results exhibited considerable variability and are influenced by multiple factors. More research is clearly needed to define the relations between

CPM, disease-related changes in central pain processing, and pain treatment effects. [9,34].

A limitation of this study is the relatively small size of the chronic pancreatitis group. A larger sample of chronic pancreatitis patients would appear necessary to provide more detailed and significant evidence of the relation between pregabalin treatment, changes in pain scores and changes in hyperalgesia. While we did find parallel, separate reductions in pain scores and pain sensitivity in our patient collective, the study was not adequately powered to formally study – or prove – correlations between clinical pain reduction and reduction in hyperalgesia. Definitive proof of such a relationship awaits future larger and longer-lasting trials. It should be noted that most chronic pancreatitis studies are small due to the difficulties in recruiting large groups of uniform chronic pancreatitis patients. Better and larger national and international collaborations are necessary to permit larger and longer population based trials in chronic pancreatitis.

In this study an intention to treat analysis was performed conform the international standard for randomized clinical trials. It can be argued that for the mechanistic endpoints an analysis including only patients fully compliant with the study protocol should be performed (per protocol analysis). We therefore also performed a per protocol analysis, but we did not present these data in this manuscript, because there were no major differences compared to the intention to treat analysis. [14] We checked variability between the study groups and found that standard deviations were comparable between both the groups at the different times. The presence of diabetes mellitus, alcohol consumption and the wide range of morphine dosages might have influenced our results. Certainly some patients might have shown diabetic polyneuropathy or morphine induced hyperalgesia, which could have biased our results. However during the physical examination of trial participants no peripheral sensory or motor disturbances were detected and all baseline characteristics were equally distributed between both treatment groups. There was a significant difference in age between the healthy controls and the chronic pancreatitis patients. The importance of this difference is difficult to assess. Some studies described an increase of pain thresholds during aging [35], others showed no effect [36] and some showed a decrease in thresholds during aging [37].

Another limitation of the study is the absence of a long-term follow-up. We only measured effects after a relatively short treatment period of three weeks. At this time, modest reductions in distant skin hyperalgesia were already noticeable and significant, albeit without return to normal values (i.e. as in healthy volunteers). This reduction in hyperalgesia occurred in a patient population with a long history of chronic pancreatitis, generally regarded as being particularly difficult to manage.

In conclusion our study provides first evidence that pregabalin modestly reduces the spreading hyperalgesia as manifestation of central sensitization associated with chronic pancreatitis pain. This effect was evident after three weeks of pregabalin treatment and was most evident for electric skin pain thresholds. However more research is needed to predict the long-term effects and define effective dosage schemes for pregabalin use in different stages of chronic pancreatitis.

Supporting Information

Checklist S1 CONSORT checklist.

Protocol S1 Trial protocol.

Author Contributions

Conceived and designed the experiments: SAWB SSO AMD HvG OHGW. Performed the experiments: SAWB SSO AMD HvG OHGW. Analyzed the data: SAWB OHG. Contributed reagents/materials/analysis tools: SAWB SSO AMD JWP HvG OHGW. Wrote the paper: SAWB SSO AMD JWP HvG OHGW. Inclusion of patients, acquisition of data: SAWB SSO AMD JWP HvG OHGW.

References

1. Andren-Sandberg A, Hoem D, Gislason H (2002) Pain management in chronic pancreatitis. European journal of gastroenterology & hepatology 14: 957–970.
2. van Esch AA, Wilder-Smith OH, Jansen JB, van Goor H, Drenth JP (2006) Pharmacological management of pain in chronic pancreatitis. Dig Liver Dis 38: 518–526.
3. Drewes AM, Krarup AL, Detlefsen S, Malmstrom ML, Dimcevski G, et al. (2008) Pain in chronic pancreatitis: the role of neuropathic pain mechanisms. Gut 57: 1616–1627.
4. Diener MK, Rahbari NN, Fischer L, Antes G, Buchler MW, et al. (2008) Duodenum-preserving pancreatic head resection versus pancreatoduodenectomy for surgical treatment of chronic pancreatitis: a systematic review and meta-analysis. Ann Surg 247: 950–961.
5. Steer ML, Waxman I, Freedman S (1995) Chronic pancreatitis. The New England journal of medicine 332: 1482–1490.
6. Buscher HC, Schipper EE, Wilder-Smith OH, Jansen JB, van Goor H (2008) Limited effect of thoracoscopic splanchnicectomy in the treatment of severe chronic pancreatitis pain: a prospective long-term analysis of 75 cases. Surgery 143: 715–722.
7. Buscher HC, Wilder-Smith OH, van Goor H (2006) Chronic pancreatitis patients show hyperalgesia of central origin: a pilot study. European journal of pain (London, England) 10: 363–370.
8. Dimcevski G, Sami SA, Funch-Jensen P, Le PD, Valeriani M, et al. (2007) Pain in chronic pancreatitis: the role of reorganization in the central nervous system. Gastroenterology 132: 1546–1556.
9. Olesen SS, Brock C, Krarup AL, Funch-Jensen P, Arendt-Nielsen L, et al. (2010) Descending inhibitory pain modulation is impaired in patients with chronic pancreatitis. Clin Gastroenterol Hepatol 8: 724–730.
10. Buscher HC, Jansen JB, van Dongen R, Bleichrodt RP, van Goor H (2002) Long-term results of bilateral thoracoscopic splanchnicectomy in patients with chronic pancreatitis. The British journal of surgery 89: 158–162.
11. Gilron I, Bailey JM, Tu D, Holden RR, Weaver DF, et al. (2005) Morphine, gabapentin, or their combination for neuropathic pain. N Engl J Med 352: 1324–1334.
12. Houghton LA, Fell C, Whorwell PJ, Jones I, Sudworth DP, et al. (2007) Effect of a second-generation alpha2delta ligand (pregabalin) on visceral sensation in hypersensitive patients with irritable bowel syndrome. Gut 56: 1218–1225.
13. Watson CP, Evans RJ, Reed K, Merskey H, Goldsmith L, et al. (1982) Amitriptyline versus placebo in postherpetic neuralgia. Neurology 32: 671–673.
14. Olesen SS, Bouwense SA, Wilder-Smith OH, van Goor H, Drewes AM (2011) Pregabalin reduces pain in patients with chronic pancreatitis in a randomized, controlled trial. Gastroenterology 141: 536–543.
15. Buscher HC, van Goor H, Wilder-Smith OH (2007) Effect of thoracoscopic splanchnic denervation on pain processing in chronic pancreatitis patients. European journal of pain (London, England) 11: 437–443.
16. Olesen SS, Graversen C, Olesen AE, Frokjaer JB, Wilder-Smith O, et al. (2011) Randomised clinical trial: pregabalin attenuates experimental visceral pain through sub-cortical mechanisms in patients with painful chronic pancreatitis. Aliment Pharmacol Ther 34: 878–887.
17. Bouwense SA, Buscher HC, van Goor H, Wilder-Smith OH (2011) S-ketamine modulates hyperalgesia in patients with chronic pancreatitis pain. Reg Anesth Pain Med 36: 303–307.
18. Layer P, Yamamoto H, Kalthoff L, Clain JE, Bakken LJ, et al. (1994) The different courses of early- and late-onset idiopathic and alcoholic chronic pancreatitis. Gastroenterology 107: 1481–1487.
19. Nir RR, Granovsky Y, Yarnitsky D, Sprecher E, Granot M (2010) A psychophysical study of endogenous analgesia: The role of the conditioning pain in the induction and magnitude of conditioned pain modulation. Eur J Pain.
20. Pud D, Granovsky Y, Yarnitsky D (2009) The methodology of experimentally induced diffuse noxious inhibitory control (DNIC)-like effect in humans. Pain 144: 16–19.
21. Cervero F (2000) Visceral pain-central sensitisation. Gut 47 Suppl 4: iv56–iv57.
22. Liu XG, Sandkuhler J (1998) Activation of spinal N-methyl-D-aspartate or neurokinin receptors induces long-term potentiation of spinal C-fibre-evoked potentials. Neuroscience 86: 1209–1216.
23. Cervero F (1995) Visceral pain: mechanisms of peripheral and central sensitization. Annals of medicine 27: 235–239.

24. Buchgreitz L, Egsgaard LL, Jensen R, Arendt-Nielsen L, Bendtsen L (2008) Abnormal pain processing in chronic tension-type headache: a high-density EEG brain mapping study. Brain 131: 3232–3238.
25. Bolay H, Moskowitz MA (2002) Mechanisms of pain modulation in chronic syndromes. Neurology 59: S2–S7.
26. Fernandez-de-las-Penas C, de la Llave-Rincon AI, Fernandez-Carnero J, Cuadrado ML, Arendt-Nielsen L, et al. (2009) Bilateral widespread mechanical pain sensitivity in carpal tunnel syndrome: evidence of central processing in unilateral neuropathy. Brain 132: 1472–1479.
27. Angst MS, Clark JD (2006) Opioid-induced hyperalgesia: a qualitative systematic review. Anesthesiology 104: 570–587.
28. Finnerup NB, Sindrup SH, Jensen TS (2010) The evidence for pharmacological treatment of neuropathic pain. Pain 150: 573–581.
29. Freynhagen R, Strojek K, Griesing T, Whalen E, Balkenohl M (2005) Efficacy of pregabalin in neuropathic pain evaluated in a 12-week, randomised, double-blind, multicentre, placebo-controlled trial of flexible- and fixed-dose regimens. Pain 115: 254–263.
30. Siddall PJ, Cousins MJ, Otte A, Griesing T, Chambers R, et al. (2006) Pregabalin in central neuropathic pain associated with spinal cord injury: a placebo-controlled trial. Neurology 67: 1792–1800.
31. Arendt-Nielsen L, Frokjaer JB, Staahl C, Graven-Nielsen T, Huggins JP, et al. (2007) Effects of gabapentin on experimental somatic pain and temporal summation. Reg Anesth Pain Med 32: 382–388.
32. Gottrup H, Juhl G, Kristensen AD, Lai R, Chizh BA, et al. (2004) Chronic oral gabapentin reduces elements of central sensitization in human experimental hyperalgesia. Anesthesiology 101: 1400–1408.
33. Dimcevski G, Staahl C, Andersen SD, Thorsgaard N, Funch-Jensen P, et al. (2007) Assessment of experimental pain from skin, muscle, and esophagus in patients with chronic pancreatitis. Pancreas 35: 22–29.
34. Yarnitsky D, Granot M, Nahman-Averbuch H, Khamaisi M, Granovsky Y (2012) Conditioned pain modulation predicts duloxetine efficacy in painful diabetic neuropathy. Pain.
35. Rolke R, Baron R, Maier C, Tolle TR, Treede RD, et al. (2006) Quantitative sensory testing in the German Research Network on Neuropathic Pain (DFNS): standardized protocol and reference values. Pain 123: 231–243.
36. Magerl W, Krumova EK, Baron R, Tolle T, Treede RD, et al. (2010) Reference data for quantitative sensory testing (QST): refined stratification for age and a novel method for statistical comparison of group data. Pain 151: 598–605.
37. Cole LJ, Farrell MJ, Gibson SJ, Egan GF (2010) Age-related differences in pain sensitivity and regional brain activity evoked by noxious pressure. Neurobiol Aging 31: 494–503.

5

Non-Specific Abdominal Pain and Air Pollution: A Novel Association

Gilaad G. Kaplan[1,2,3]⁹, Mieczyslaw Szyszkowicz[4*]⁹, Jakub Fichna[7], Brian H. Rowe[5], Eugeniusz Porada[4], Renaud Vincent[4], Karen Madsen[6], Subrata Ghosh[1,2], Martin Storr[1,2,8]

1 Division of Gastroenterology, University of Calgary, Calgary, Alberta, Canada, **2** Departments of Medicine, University of Calgary, Calgary, Alberta, Canada, **3** Community Health Sciences, University of Calgary, Calgary, Alberta, Canada, **4** Environmental Health Sciences and Research Bureau, Health Canada, Ottawa, Ontario, Canada, **5** Department of Emergency Medicine and School of Public Health, University of Alberta, Edmonton, Alberta, Canada, **6** Department of Medicine, Division of Gastroenterology, University of Alberta, Edmonton, Alberta, Canada, **7** Department of Biomolecular Chemistry, Medical University of Lodz, Lodz, Poland, **8** Department of Medicine, Ludwigs-Maximilians University, Munich, Germany

Abstract

Background: We studied whether short-term exposure to air pollution was associated with non-specific abdominal pain in epidemiologic and animal studies.

Methods: Patients visiting the emergency department with non-specific abdominal pain were identified in Edmonton (1992 to 2002, n = 95,173) and Montreal (1997 to 2002, n = 25,852). We calculated the daily concentrations for ozone (O_3), nitrogen dioxide (NO_2), sulfur dioxide (SO_2), carbon monoxide (CO), and particles <10 (PM_{10}) or <2.5 ($PM_{2.5}$) µm. A case crossover study design was used to estimate the odds ratio (OR) and 95% confidence interval (CI) associated with an increase in the interquartile range of the air pollutants. We investigated differential effects by age and sex. Mice were gavaged with urban particle extracts. In animal models, colonic motility was tested, and visceral abdominal pain was measured using a writhing test, and behavioral response to oil of mustard and neostigmine. Motility and pain was measured acutely (1.5 hours after gavage) and chronically (7-days and 21-days after gavage).

Results: Emergency department visits for non-specific abdominal pain were primarily by women between the ages of 15–24 years. Individuals aged 15 to 24 years were at increased risk of non-specific abdominal pain in Edmonton (same day CO: OR = 1.04, 95% CI = 1.02–1.06; and NO_2: OR = 1.06, 95% CI = 1.03–1.09). The risk of air pollution among 15–24 year olds in Montreal was significantly positive (same day CO: OR = 1.11, 95% CI = 1.05–1.17; NO_2: OR = 1.09, 95% CI = 1.01–1.16; SO_2: OR = 1.17, 95% CI = 1.10–1.25; $PM_{2.5}$: OR = 1.09, 95% CI = 1.04–1.15). Abdominal pain was increased by an acute gavage of pollution extract but not to chronic exposure to pollutants. Colonic transit was delayed following chronic but not acute exposure with the pollutants.

Conclusions: Epidemiological and animal data suggest that short-term exposure to air pollution may trigger non-specific abdominal pain in young individuals.

Editor: Devendra Amre, University of Montreal, Canada

Funding: Funding was provided by Health Canada and The Alberta IBD Consortium. The funders had no role in study design, data collection and analysis, decision to publish, or preparation of the manuscript.

Competing Interests: The authors have declared that no competing interests exist.

* E-mail: mietek.szyszkowicz@hc-sc.gc.ca

⁹ These authors contributed equally to this work.

Introduction

Abdominal pain is the second most common diagnosis (4.2%) claimed by emergency department physicians in the USA. In many cases patients are diagnosed with non-specific abdominal pain, which refers to abdominal pain that is not explained during acute assessment. [1,2] While many patients diagnosed with non-specific abdominal pain are asymptomatic at a later outpatient follow-up [3,4,5], a subset of these patients require recurrent admissions. [6,7,8] Consequently, non-specific abdominal pain is an important clinical presentation associated with impairment in quality of life for patients and significant costs to the health care system. [7,8]

The underlying cause of non-specific abdominal pain is likely multifactorial. non-specific abdominal pain may be due to gastrointestinal diseases such as Crohn's [9] and celiac [10] diseases that are diagnosed after the patient is discharged from the emergency department. Additionally, some patients experience a transient illness such as gastrointestinal infection. Cases of non-specific abdominal pain may also represent a functional disorder such as irritable bowel syndrome. [11] Despite extensive research into the causes of non-specific abdominal pain, risk factors are not known and thus, exploration of triggers of non-specific abdominal pain is warranted.

Air pollution directly effects pulmonary diseases (e.g. asthma) and has been associated with non-pulmonary diseases including cancer and strokes. [12,13,14] Recently, studies have indicated that air pollution may affect gastrointestinal disorders such as the inflammatory bowel diseases and appendicitis. [15,16] Air pollutants can cause systemic effects such as cardiovascular [17] or liver metabolic [18] changes after primary deposition and direct effects in the respiratory compartment. [19] However, most inhaled particles deposited in the nasopharyngeal compartment and airways are removed through mucociliary clearance and swallowed within a day [20] and thus, gastrointestinal effects may be due to direct effects of particles. [19]

Consequently, we investigated whether acute exposure to air pollutants was associated with emergency department visits for non-specific abdominal pain by: 1) evaluating the effect of short-term ambient air pollution exposure in a human population; 2) replicating this epidemiological study in a second population; and 3) exploring the biological plausibility in *in vitro and in vivo* models.

Methods

Phase 1: Epidemiological Studies

Study Population. As described previously [21], the administrative database study was approved by the individual research ethics boards at each participating institution and the data were transferred to the Health Canada following de-identification. No patient contact was made and patients could not be traced. The International Classification for Disease 9th revision was used to identify patients who were discharged from an emergency department with a primary diagnosis of non-specific abdominal pain (789.0×). [2] First, we identified a population-based sample of 95,173 individuals who visited one of 5 emergency department in Edmonton for non-specific abdominal pain from 1992–2002. Second, we identified a replication study population of 25,852 individuals who visited a downtown emergency department in Montreal for non-specific abdominal pain from 1997–2002. Three digit postal codes were used to restrict the study population to residents of the city of Edmonton or Montreal. While the study population from Edmonton was population-based and included all ages, pediatric emergency department visits were underrepresented in Montreal because of the immediate proximity of a Pediatric Hospital. Thus, for the study population from Montreal the analysis was restricted to individuals over the age of 15 years.

Air Pollution and Meteorological Data. The air pollutants measured included sulfur dioxide (SO_2), nitrogen dioxide (NO_2), carbon monoxide CO, ozone (O_3), and particulate matter characterized by an aerodynamic diameter of ≤10 μm (PM_{10}) and of ≤2.5 μm ($PM_{2.5}$). The data on air pollution were supplied by Environment Canada from fixed monitoring stations in Edmonton and Montreal. Environment Canada also supplied hourly data for temperature and relative humidity. For each air pollutant and weather variable, we obtained data on 24 measurements carried out at the monitoring station at hourly intervals. If more than 6 measurements were missing for a specific day, than the data for this monitor was considered as missing. An average was calculated for each monitor to represent daily mean value and average among monitors was used to represent ambient exposure across the city. [22] The distribution of air pollution and weather monitors for both cities can be found in Environment Canada's website. [23] A detailed description of air pollutant and weather measurements, monitor distribution, and correlations among monitors has been previously reported. [24]

Statistical Analysis. We applied a case crossover study design, which is an adaptation of the case–control study whereby cases serve as their own controls. [25] A time-stratified design was used to select referent periods, whereby the referent periods were selected from the same day of the week, month and year as the case's date of hospital visit. Because within-individual comparisons were made, confounding due to time-independent risk factors (e.g. genetics) was reduced. Similarly, the matching of control to case periods by day of week controlled for the influence of "day of week" effects. [25]

We used a conditional logistic regression (subroutine PHREG in SAS) to model the air pollutants and 6 components for natural splines for temperature and relative humidity. Estimates were expressed as the odds ratio (OR) with 95% confidence intervals (CI) associated with an increase in the interquartile range of the air pollutants (SO_2, NO_2, CO, O_3, PM_{10}, and $PM_{2.5}$) after adjusting for temperature and relative humidity. Control for potentially non-linear effects of weather was achieved by including natural spline functions of temperature and relative humidity. The interquartile range was calculated based on the daily mean concentration of each air pollutant during the study period (Table S1). Analyses were performed separately for Edmonton and Montreal. Additionally, the analysis was stratified by: age, categorized as <15 (only Edmonton), 15–24, 25–34, 35–44, 45–64, and >64 years. Different time lags for pollution and weather exposures were used in our analyses including same day, one day before admission (i.e. 1-day lag), and two days before admission (i.e. 2-day lag). Among individuals 15 to 24 years of age we examined for effect modification by sex by incorporating an interaction term (e.g. $PM_{2.5}$ X sex) into the model. All statistical analyses were conducted in SAS (version 8, SAS, Cary, North Carolina, US).

Phase 2: *In Vitro & In Vivo* Studies

Animals. Male Swiss albino mice (CD1, Charles River, Canada), weighing 24–26 g, were used. The animals were housed at a constant temperature (22°C) and maintained under a 12-h light/dark cycle with free access to laboratory chow and tap water. Animal use was approved by the University of Calgary Animal Care Committee.

Particulate Matter Preparation. The urban particles EHC-6802 consisted of a blend of total suspended particulate matter recovered from filters of the single-pass air purification system at the Environmental Health Centre (Tunney's Pasture, Ottawa, ON) in 1996, 1998, 2000, and 2002, as described previously. [26] Particles were mechanically sieved using a 36 μm mesh filter, and combined in equal proportions. EHC-6802 was recovered at the same site and manner as the urban particles EHC-93, and chemical characterization of the EHC-6802 material has confirmed that it was equivalent to the EHC-93 material. [26]

Experimental Design. Animals were randomly assigned to two groups with the same number of animals per treatment group: control (oral tap water, 200 μl/animal, once daily; n = 8) or EHC-6802 (oral 360 μg/200 μl tap water/animal, once daily; n = 8). Gavages were given once daily and experiments were performed in the following protocols: 1) 1.5 h after the gavage; 2) daily for 7 days; and 3) daily for 21 days.

Isolated smooth muscle strips. Full-thickness segments (1 cm) of ileum and distal colon were resected. The preparations were mounted between two platinum electrodes and placed longitudinally in separate organ baths as described previously. [27] One end of each preparation was attached to the bottom of the organ bath, while the other end was connected to a FT03 force displacement transducer (Grass Technologies, West Warwick, RI, USA). Changes in tension were amplified by a P11T amplifier

(Grass Technologies) and recorded on a computer using PolyView software (Polybytes, Cedar Rapids, Iowa).

Electrical field stimulation (EFS; 8 Hz; 60 V; pulse duration 0.5 ms; train duration 10 sec) was applied by a S88X stimulator (Grass Technologies). EFS of isolated smooth muscle strips caused twitch contractions, which were of cholinergic neuronal origin as they were virtually abolished by atropine (10^{-6} M) or TTX (10^{-6} M) (data not shown). In separate experiments the response of ileal and colonic muscle strips to direct muscular activation with stepwise addition of bethanechol (10^{-7} M–3×10^{-5} M) was recorded.

EHC-6802 urban ambient particles were added cumulatively into the organ baths and effects on the EFS-induced contractions were recorded. The mean amplitude of 4 successive twitch contractions was used as an internal control. Changes in contractions were reported as the percentage of the internal control. In control experiments the effects of the vehicle (tap water) were tested to control against possible effects on contractility by adding vehicle..

In separate experiments the response of ileal and colonic muscle strips to (i) neuronal electrical stimulation and (ii) direct muscular activation with stepwise addition of bethanechol (10^{-7} M–3×10^{-5} M) was recorded following 90 min, 7 days and 21 days following oral treatment with EHC-6802 particles.

Colonic expulsion test. Distal colonic expulsion was measured as reported previously. [27] 1.5 hours after receiving tap water (control) or EHC-6802 particle suspension (n = 5–10), a glass bead (2 mm) was inserted 2 cm into the distal colon and the time to bead expulsion was determined.

Behavioural Pain Responses. Behavioural pain responses were tested in 3 models used to study abdominal visceral pain responses (n = 5–10). The writhing test was performed as described by Gach et al. [28] Ninety minutes after oral administration of tap water (control group) or EHC-6802 particle suspension, mice received an intraperitoneal (i.p.) injection (10 ml/kg) of acetic acid solution (0.5%). The total number of writhes was counted 5 minutes after acetic acid injection, during three periods lasting 5 minutes each. The writhing response, considered as a nociceptive behaviour, was characterized by elongation of the body and the development of tension in the abdominal muscles and hind paws.

Behavioural responses to intracolonic (i.c.) oil of mustard (OM) and i.p. neostigmine were determined based on Laird et al. [29] and Eijkelkamp et al. (n = 5–10). [30] For the assessment of the OM-induced pain behaviours, 50 µl of OM (1% in 70% ethanol-30% saline) was administered i.c. under isoflurane anaesthesia. Petroleum jelly was applied to the perianal area to avoid stimulation of somatic areas. After 5 min of recovery, spontaneous behaviours were videotaped for analysis by an observer blinded to the experimental conditions.

In a separate experiment, neostigmine (2.5 µg/kg) or vehicle was administered i.p. and the pain-related behaviours were counted over a 10 minute period after the injection. Postures defined as pain-related behaviours: 1) licking of the abdomen, 2) stretching the abdomen, 3) squashing of lower abdomen against the floor, and 4) abdominal retractions, were each counted as 1.

Statistical Analysis. Statistical and curve-fitting analyses were performed using Prism 4.0 (GraphPad Software Inc., La Jolla, CA, USA). The data are expressed as means ± standard deviation. Student's t-test compared treatment means with control means. Two-sided P-values≤0.05 were statistically significant.

Results

Phase 1: Epidemiological Studies

Nearly 2/3 of emergency department visits for non-specific abdominal pain were by women and the majority of women presented in adolescence and early adulthood (Figure 1A and 1B; Table S1). In Edmonton, where pediatric emergency department visits were available, 61.4% of emergency department visits for non-specific abdominal pain occurred before the age 34 years. In Montreal, patients between the ages of 15 and 34 years accounted for 36.7% of emergency department visits (Table S1).

Table S2 describes the mean daily concentrations and variance of each air pollutant during the study periods. The effect of air pollution exposure was only observed when ages were stratified. In Edmonton, individuals aged 15 to 24 years were at elevated risk for presenting to the emergency department on the same day of higher concentrations of CO (OR = 1.04, 95% CI = 1.02–1.06), NO_2 (OR = 1.06, 95% CI = 1.03–1.09), SO_2 (OR = 1.02, 95% CI = 1.00–1.04), and $PM_{2.5}$ (OR = 1.03, 95% CI = 1.00–1.05). Similar effects were observed in Montreal for CO (OR = 1.11, 95% CI = 1.05–1.17), NO_2 (OR = 1.09, 95% CI = 1.01–1.16), SO_2 (OR = 1.17, 95% CI = 1.10–1.25), and $PM_{2.5}$ (OR = 1.09, 95% CI = 1.04–1.15) (Table 1). Among 15 to 24 year olds, O_3 was negatively associated with emergency department visits for non-

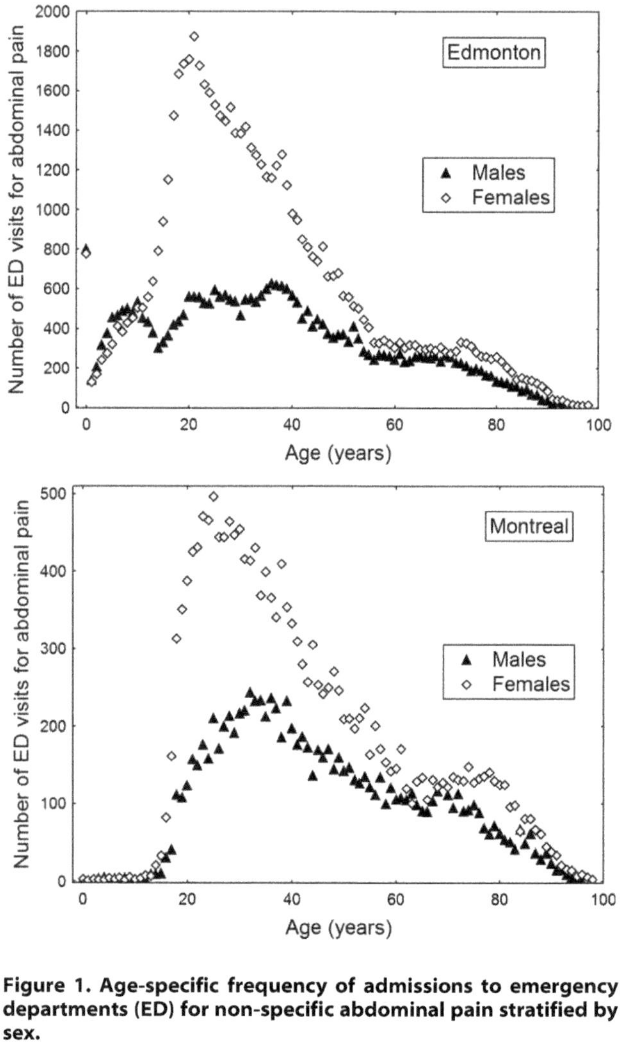

Figure 1. Age-specific frequency of admissions to emergency departments (ED) for non-specific abdominal pain stratified by sex.

specific abdominal pain in Edmonton (OR = 0.95, 95% CI = 0.91–0.99), but not in Montreal (OR = 1.03, 95% CI = 0.95–1.11) (Table 1). The effect of air pollutants on individuals aged 15 to 24 stratified by sex are presented in Table 2. Interaction terms were not significant between sexes (Table 2). The effect of air pollutants with 1-day and 2-day lags stratified by age and sex are presented in Tables S3 and S4, respectively.

Phase 2: *In Vitro* & *In Vivo* Studies

The course of body weight was not significantly different in animals treated with EHC-6802 urban particles by gavage compared to vehicle treated mice (Figure S1).

Gastrointestinal Motility. EHC-6802 (1:100000–1:1) produced a significant, concentration-dependent inhibitory effect on the EFS (8 Hz)-induced twitch contractions in the colon, but not the mouse ileum (Figure 2A). Electrically induced contractions were not changed at any time points (90 min, 7 days, 21 days), compared to bethanechol (10^{-6} M) treatment (Figure S2). Responses to direct muscular activation with bethanechol (10^{-7} M–3×10^{-5} M) were not changed by adding EHC-6802 particles to the organ bath (Figure S1C) at any time point (Figure S2).

In the colonic expulsion test a 7-day treatment with EHC-6802 particles significantly reduced the time to bead expulsion (Figure 2B). Neither acute (1.5 h) nor chronic (21 days) treatment with EHC-6802 significantly affected the colonic bead expulsion time.

Nociception. In our preliminary experiments, we confirmed that the i.p. injection of acetic acid solution, i.e. instillation of OM, and the i.p. injection of neostigmine induced pain behaviors in naïve mice (data not shown). The acute administration of EHC-6802 (1.5 h treatment) significantly increased the number of writhes compared to control group (Figure 3A). 7-day (Figure 3A) and 21-day (data not shown) treatment with EHC-6802 did not modify the response to acetic acid. EHC-6802 administered at 1.5 hour also showed a significantly higher number of spontaneous pain-related behaviours induced by OM (Figure 3B) and neostigmine (Figure 3C), compared to mice after 7- and 21-day treatment (21 days, data not shown).

Discussion

Non-specific abdominal pain is a common clinical presentation to the emergency department, typically involves multiple investigations, and may require admission to hospital. [1] A cause is often not discovered during emergency department visit and in most cases a subsequent organic diagnosis is not made during outpatient follow-up. [3] Although non-specific abdominal pain is a common disorder of the young [31,32], triggers of acute pain are not known. We found that young individuals had the highest prevalence of non-specific abdominal pain and were significantly more likely to visit the emergency department for non-specific abdominal pain when indicators of air pollution were elevated. Furthermore, ingestion of EHC-6802 urban ambient particles by mice led to an acute exacerbation of pain, which did not persist after chronic exposure of the pollutants to the animal. These observations suggest a novel association between air pollution exposure and exacerbation of abdominal pain.

In both Edmonton and Montreal, CO, $PM_{2.5}$, SO2, and NO_2 were associated with non-specific abdominal pain presentations in individuals aged 15 to 24 years. However, PM_{10} was positively associated with non-specific abdominal pain in Edmonton, but null in Montreal. Furthermore, ozone was negatively associated with non-specific abdominal pain in Edmonton, but not in Montreal. Additionally, the risk estimates were generally higher in Montreal than in Edmonton. The heterogeneity of findings between cities may be explained by residents living and/or working in downtown Montreal having greater exposure to air pollutants. In contrast, residents living throughout Edmonton would have been exposed to a wider range of air pollution concentrations. The greater patient-level variability to air pollution exposure experienced in Edmonton may have resulted in non-differential misclassification that would have the effect of biasing the risk estimates towards the null. Furthermore, the fixed monitoring stations are located to represent the background air pollution concentrations in a city; however, misclassifying the air pollution exposure may occur when multiple fixed monitoring sites are averaged into one daily value for the entire city. [22] Thus, future multi-city studies are required to confirm the associations observed in our study and to explore causes of heterogeneity.

Young women are known to have the highest prevalence of non-specific abdominal pain. [31,32] In both Edmonton and Montreal, women aged 15 to 24 years were more likely to visit an emergency department for non-specific abdominal pain. The reason for the disproportionate occurrence of non-specific abdominal pain in women as compared to men is not clear. Abdominal pain may be exacerbated during the menstrual cycle. [33] Furthermore, women have been shown to be more likely to seek medical attention for abdominal pain when compared to men. [34,35] We did not observe effect modification between men and women aged 15 to 24 years, suggesting that the effect of air pollution on non-specific abdominal pain was not sex-specific. However, because the risk estimates observed in our study were modest, we may have not been adequately powered to detect effect modification by sex.

The mechanism by which air pollutants may exacerbate abdominal pain is not known. In one study high concentrations of air pollutants (NO_2, CO, and O_3) impaired gastric basal contractility. [36] However, low-level exposures were not associated with gastric dysmotility. [36] Another study demonstrated that animals fed EHC-6802 had increased IL-8 secretion from the small bowel and experienced changes in the composition of colonic microflora. [37] Our *in vitro* studies demonstrated impaired colonic, but not ileal, contractility after the acute exposure of the ex-vivo tissue with the particulate matter. Neuronally mediated contractility was impaired whereas the direct smooth muscular reactivity was unchanged suggesting that the observed effects involved neuronal rather than muscular mechanisms. *In vivo* reduction of colonic motility was not observed acutely, but a significantly slowed colonic motility was recorded after 7 days, but not after 21 days of daily exposure to the EHC-6802 particles. Overall *in vitro* and *in vivo* effects on intestinal motility by acute and chronic exposure to EHC-6802 particles were negligible.

In contrast, acute exposure to EHC-6802 particles led to significantly increased pain response in mice and this observation was consistent in 3 different behavioral tests of visceral abdominal pain. Chronic exposure to ingested pollutants did not affect the pain response models suggesting that pain adaptation to the pollutants may have occurred over time. The cause for the acute hypersensitivity in mice is not known. The animal studies suggest that the pain response following acute exposure to the pollutants were not driven by intestinal dysmotility. Exposure to air pollution may exacerbate systemic inflammation [38] or lead to oxidative damage of colonic mucosa. [39] Furthermore, air pollution has been shown to mediate dysfunction of endothelial-dependent vasodilation [40] that may contribute to visceral hypersensitivity. Future studies will be needed to explore the exact mechanisms and

Table 1. Odds ratio for presenting to an emergency department with non-specific abdominal pain associated with an interquartile increase in an air pollutant concentration on the same day of ED visit stratified by age.

Pollutant	All Ages OR (95% CI)	<15 years OR (95% CI)	15–24 years OR (95% CI)	25–34 years OR (95% CI)	35–44 years OR (95% CI)	45–64 years OR (95% CI)	>64 years OR (95% CI)
Edmonton							
CO (ppm)	1.01(0.99–1.02)	0.99(0.97–1.02)	1.04(1.02–1.06)	0.99(0.97–1.01)	1.00(0.98–1.02)	1.01(0.99–1.03)	1.01(0.99–1.04)
NO_2 (ppb)	1.02(1.00–1.03)	1.00(0.97–1.04)	1.06(1.03–1.09)	0.99(0.96–1.01)	1.01(0.98–1.04)	1.03(0.99–1.06)	1.00(0.96–1.04)
SO_2 (ppb)	1.01(1.00–1.02)	1.00(0.98–1.03)	1.02(1.00–1.04)	0.99(0.97–1.02)	1.00(0.98–1.02)	1.00(0.97–1.02)	1.04(1.01–1.07)
O_3 (ppb)	0.99(0.97–1.01)	0.98(0.93–1.03)	0.95(0.91–0.99)	1.02(0.98–1.06)	1.02(0.98–1.07)	0.94 (0.90–0.98)	0.99(0.94–1.04)
PM_{10} (mg/m^3)	1.01(1.00–1.02)	1.01(0.98–1.04)	1.04(1.02–1.07)	1.01(0.98–1.03)	0.99(0.97–1.02)	1.00(0.97–1.02)	1.00(0.97–1.03)
$PM_{2.5}$ (mg/m^3)	1.00(0.99–1.01)	1.00(0.97–1.04)	1.03(1.00–1.05)	0.99(0.96–1.02)	0.99(0.96–1.02)	1.00(0.97–1.03)	0.99(0.96–1.03)
Montreal							
CO (ppm)	1.02(0.99–1.04)	NA	1.11(1.05–1.17)	1.04(1.00–1.09)	0.99(0.94–1.04)	1.08(1.04–1.13)	1.01(0.96–1.07)
NO_2 (ppb)	1.02(0.99–1.04)	NA	1.09(1.01–1.16)	1.06(1.00–1.12)	1.00(0.94–1.06)	1.14(1.08–1.20)	1.05(0.99–1.11)
SO_2 (ppb)	1.02(1.00–1.05)	NA	1.17(1.10–1.25)	1.08(1.03–1.14)	1.02(0.96–1.08)	1.13(1.08–1.19)	1.08(1.02–1.14)
O_3 (ppb)	0.99(0.97–1.02)	NA	1.03(0.95–1.11)	1.04(0.98–1.11)	1.09(1.02–1.16)	0.98(0.93–1.04)	1.03(0.96–1.09)
PM_{10} (mg/m^3)	1.01(0.98–1.04)	NA	1.03(0.95–1.11)	1.05(0.98–1.12)	0.97(0.91–1.04)	1.08(1.02–1.15)	0.98(0.91–1.05)
$PM_{2.5}$ (mg/m^3)	1.01(0.99–1.03)	NA	1.10(1.04–1.15)	1.06(1.01–1.10)	1.03(0.99–1.08)	1.08(1.04–1.12)	1.00(0.97–1.05)

NA – not available; CO- carbon monoxide; NO_2 – nitrogen dioxide; SO_2 - sulphur dioxide; O_3 - ozone; PM_{10} - particulate matter <10 microns; $PM_{2.5}$ - particulate matter <2.5 microns; PPM - parts per million; PPB - parts per billion; mg/m^3 - micrograms per meters cubed.

Table 2. Odds ratio for presenting to an emergency department with non-specific abdominal pain associated with an interquartile increase in an air pollutant concentration on the same day of ED visit stratified by gender among individuals aged 15–24 years.

	Edmonton			Montreal		
Pollutant (unit)	Males OR (95% CI)	Females OR (95% CI)	p-Value for Interaction	Males OR (95% CI)	Females OR (95% CI)	p-Value for Interaction
CO (ppm)	0.99(0.95–1.03)	1.05(1.03–1.08)	0.05	1.09(0.96–1.24)	1.10(1.03–1.18)	0.57
NO_2 (ppb)	1.00(0.94–1.06)	1.08(1.04–1.11)	0.07	1.06(0.91–1.22)	1.09(1.01–1.18)	0.10
SO_2 (ppb)	1.02(0.98–1.06)	1.03(1.00–1.05)	0.78	1.16(1.03–1.31)	1.14(1.07–1.23)	0.85
O_3 (ppb)	1.01(0.93–1.09)	0.93(0.89–0.98)	0.18	1.03(0.90–1.20)	1.02(0.93–1.12)	0.10
PM_{10} (mg/m^3)	1.04(1.00–1.09)	1.04(1.02–1.07)	0.66	1.00(0.83–1.21)	1.02(0.93–1.11)	0.26
$PM_{2.5}$ (mg/m^3)	1.06(1.01–1.11)	1.02(0.99–1.05)	0.07	1.09(0.98–1.21)	1.09(1.03–1.15)	0.62

OR – odds ratio; CI – confidence interval; CO- carbon monoxide; NO_2 – nitrogen dioxide; SO_2 - sulphur dioxide; O_3 - ozone; PM_{10} - particulate matter <10 microns; $PM_{2.5}$ - particulate matter <2.5 microns; PPM - parts per million; PPB - parts per billion; mg/m^3 - micrograms per meters cubed.

the associated neuronal circuits involved in triggering abdominal pain.

Several limitations should be considered. First, regional estimates of air pollutants from fixed monitoring stations may not reflect the variability of patient-level exposure to air pollutants. Though, the effects of air pollutants were likely underestimated as measurement errors were presumably non-differential. Second, we attempted to control for confounding through the use of a case crossover study design whereby cases served as their own control; however, residual confounding may have influenced our estimates.

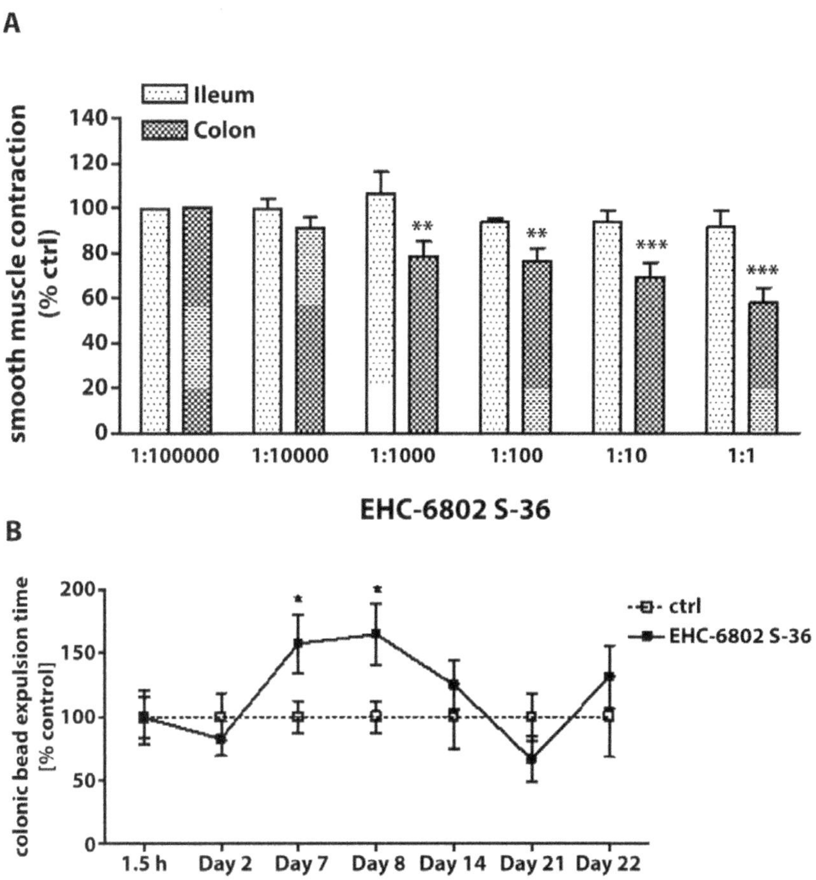

Figure 2. The effect of EHC-6802 on mouse GI motility. A) The effect of EHC-6802 (initial concentration 360 μg/200 μl regarded as 1:1 dilution) on EFS (8 Hz)-stimulated smooth muscle contractions in mouse ileum and colon. Note that EHC-6802 significantly, in a concentration-dependent manner inhibited twitch contractions in mouse colon. Data represent mean ± SEM for n = 8. *P<0.05, as compared with control. B) In vivo effects of EHC-6802 (360 μg/200 μl/animal, QD, p.o.) on colonic bead expulsion time in mice. The results are shown as mean ± SEM of n = 5–10 mice for each experimental group. *P<0.05, as compared with control (animals receiving tap water).

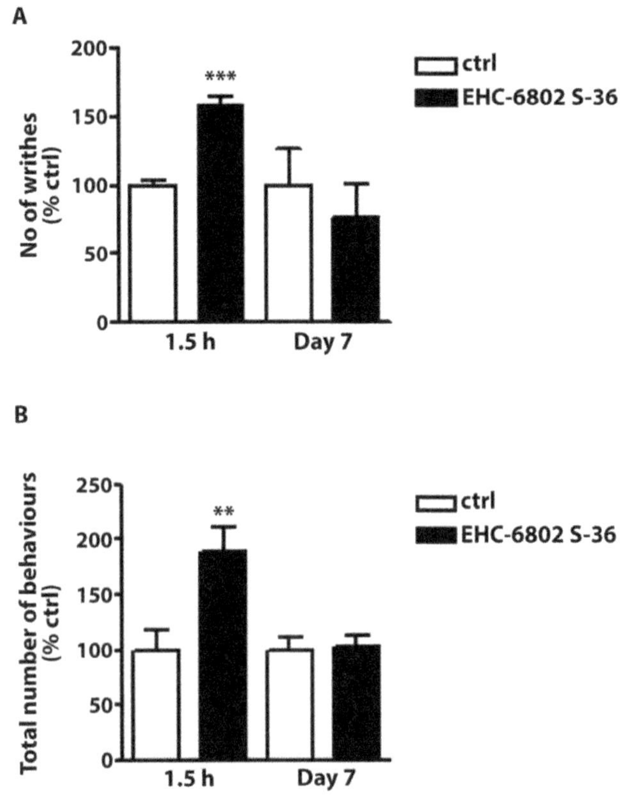

Figure 3. The effect of EHC-6802 (360 μg/200 μl/animal, p.o.) on behavioural pain responses in mice. A) The effect of EHC-6802 in the writhing test in mice. The number of writhes was determined 5 min after acetic acid injection (0.5%, 10 ml/kg, i.p.) over a period of 15 min. Note that a single 1.5 h- treatment with EHC-6802 significantly increased the total number of writhes. Data represent mean ± SEM of 5–10 mice per group. ***$P<0.001$, as compared to control (animals receiving tap water). B) The effect of EHC-6802 on the number of pain-related behaviours (licking of abdomen, stretching, squashing, abdominal contractions) evoked by i.c. administration of oil of mustard (1% in 70% EtOH - 30% saline), determined over a period of 20 min. Note that a single 1.5 h- treatment with EHC-6802 significantly increased the number of pain-related behaviours. Data represent mean ± SEM of 5–10 mice per group. **$P<0.01$, as compared to control (animals receiving tap water). C) The effect of EHC-6802 on the number of pain-related behaviours (licking of abdomen, stretching, squashing, abdominal contractions) evoked by the i.p. administration of neostigmine (2.5 μg/kg), determined over a period of 10 min. Note that a single 1.5 h- treatment with EHC-6802 significantly increased the number of pain-related behaviours. Data represent mean ± SEM of 5–10 mice per group. **$P<0.01$, as compared to control (animals receiving tap water).

For example aeroallergens, which may correlate with air pollution [41], were not evaluated in this study; however, aeroallergens are not known to trigger non-specific abdominal pain. Third, associations were explored in multiple pollutants using several lagged exposures, and stratified to investigate several factors (e.g. age groups). Thus, the probability of observing statistically significant findings by chance is increased. We attempted to minimize multiple comparison errors by including a replication study population and primarily reporting on associations observed in both populations. However, future studies are necessary to confirm our findings. Fourth, some of the non-specific abdominal pain patients may have had an unrecognized organic disease that was diagnosed after discharge from the emergency department. For example, NO_2 exposure (i.e., traffic pollutant) was associated with the development of appendicitis. [15] Furthermore, individuals less than 24 years and living in areas of higher concentration of NO_2 were at a two-fold increased risk of developing Crohn's disease. [16] Because our risk estimates were modest in size, our findings may reflect significant associations among a specific gastrointestinal disorder (e.g., Crohn's disease). Nonetheless, discovering a possible link between air pollution exposure and gastrointestinal disease is an important finding that should motivate further research. Finally, while EHC-6802 particles have been validated to represent daily city exposure of air pollutants [26], our findings should be interpreted cautiously because EHC-6802 particles were gathered in Ottawa and consists of multiple air pollutants.

In conclusion, individuals aged 15 to 24 years were most likely to present to emergency departments with non-specific abdominal pain and this occurred more frequently when the concentration of CO, $PM_{2.5}$, SO2, and NO_2 were elevated in the atmosphere. These findings were observed in a population-based study in Edmonton and replicated in an urban downtown emergency department in Montreal. Additionally, we demonstrated that acute exposure to ingested EHC-6802 particles exacerbated abdominal pain in mice, a response that led to adaptation after chronic exposure. The consistency of the epidemiological and animal studies suggests that air pollution may trigger non-specific abdominal pain in some cases. Thus, future patient-level and basic laboratory studies should be performed to substantiate the findings, further explore possible underlying mechanisms, and identify at risk populations.

Supporting Information

Figure S1 A) In vivo effects of EHC-6802 (360 μg/200 μl/animal, QD, p.o.) or tap water (200 μl/animal, QD, p.o.) during a 21 day treatment course. B) EFS (8 Hz)-stimulated smooth muscle contractions in mouse colon were not changed following 90 min, 7 days or 21 days of treatment with EHC-6802 S-36, as compared to vehicle treated mice. C) Bethanechol (10^{-7} M–3×10^{-5} M) stimulated smooth muscle contractions in mouse ileum (left) and colon (right) were not changed when EHC-6802 (360 μg/200 μl) was added to the organ bath.

Figure S2 Bethanechol (10^{-7} M–3×10^{-5} M) stimulated smooth muscle contractions in mouse ileum and colon were not changed following 90 min, 7 days or 21 days of treatment with EHC-6802 S-36, as compared to vehicle treated mice.

Table S1 Frequency of emergency department visits for non-specific abdominal pain by age group and gender, Edmonton (EDM) and Montreal (MON).

Table S2 Frequency distribution of the daily concentrations of ambient air pollutants and meteorological factors from April 01, 1992 to March 31, 2002 in Edmonton and January 01, 1997 to December 31, 2002 in Montreal.

Table S3 Odds ratio for presenting to an emergency department with non-specific abdominal pain associated with an interquartile increase in an air pollutant concentration stratified by age for 1- and 2-day lags. NA – not available; CO- carbon monoxide; NO_2 – nitrogen dioxide;

SO_2 - sulphur dioxide; O_3 - ozone; PM_{10} - particulate matter <10 microns; $PM_{2.5}$ - particulate matter <2.5 microns; PPM - parts per million; PPB - parts per billion; mg/m^3 - micrograms per meters cubed.

Table S4 Odds ratio for presenting to an emergency department with non-specific abdominal pain associated with an interquartile increase in an air pollutant concentration for 1- and 2-day lag stratified by gender among individuals aged 15–24 years. OR – odds ratio; CI – confidence interval; CO- carbon monoxide; NO_2 – nitrogen dioxide; SO_2 - sulphur dioxide; O_3 - ozone; PM_{10} - particulate matter <10 microns; $PM_{2.5}$ - particulate matter <2.5 microns; PPM - parts per million; PPB - parts per billion; mg/m^3 - micrograms per meters cubed.

Acknowledgments

Dr. Gilaad Kaplan is a Canadian Institutes of Health Research New Investigator and a Population Health Investigator from Alberta-Innovates Health Solutions. Dr. Rowe's research is supported by a Tier I Century Canada Research Chair in Evidence-Based Emergency Medicine from the Canadian Institutes for health Research through the Government of Canada (Ottawa, Ontario).

Author Contributions

Conceived and designed the experiments: M. Szyszkowicz GGK M. Storr BR. Performed the experiments: M. Szyszkowicz GGK JF EP M. Storr. Analyzed the data: M. Szyszkowicz GGK JF EP M. Storr. Contributed reagents/materials/analysis tools: RV. Wrote the paper: M. Szyszkowicz GGK M. Storr KM SG BR RV.

References

1. Sanders DS, Azmy IA, Hurlstone DP (2006) A new insight into non-specific abdominal pain. Ann R Coll Surg Engl 88: 92–94.
2. Nawar EW, Niska RW, Xu J (2007) National Hospital Ambulatory Medical Care Survey: 2005 emergency department summary. Adv Data: 1–32.
3. Jess P, Bjerregaard B, Brynitz S, Holst-Christensen J, Kalaja E, et al. (1982) Prognosis of acute nonspecific abdominal pain. A prospective study. Am J Surg 144: 338–340.
4. O'Byrne JM, Dempsey CB, O'Malley MK, O'Connell FX (1991) Non-specific abdominal pain in pre-menopausal women. Ir J Med Sci 160: 344–346.
5. Lukens TW, Emerman C, Effron D (1993) The natural history and clinical findings in undifferentiated abdominal pain. Ann Emerg Med 22: 690–696.
6. Decadt B, Sussman L, Lewis MP, Secker A, Cohen L, et al. (1999) Randomized clinical trial of early laparoscopy in the management of acute non-specific abdominal pain. Br J Surg 86: 1383–1386.
7. Raheja SK, McDonald PJ, Taylor I (1990) Non-specific abdominal pain–an expensive mystery. J R Soc Med 83: 10–11.
8. Sheridan WG, White AT, Havard T, Crosby DL (1992) Non-specific abdominal pain: the resource implications. Ann R Coll Surg Engl 74: 181–185.
9. Dubinsky MC, Johanson JF, Seidman EG, Ofman JJ (2002) Suspected inflammatory bowel disease–the clinical and economic impact of competing diagnostic strategies. Am J Gastroenterol 97: 2333–2342.
10. Sanders DS, Hopper AD, Azmy IA, Rahman N, Hurlstone DP, et al. (2005) Association of adult celiac disease with surgical abdominal pain: a case-control study in patients referred to secondary care. Ann Surg 242: 201–207.
11. Doshi M, Heaton KW (1994) Irritable bowel syndrome in patients discharged from surgical wards with non-specific abdominal pain. Br J Surg 81: 1216–1218.
12. Brunekreef B, Holgate ST (2002) Air pollution and health. Lancet 360: 1233–1242.
13. Gorham ED, Garland CF, Garland FC (1989) Acid haze air pollution and breast and colon cancer mortality in 20 Canadian cities. Can J Public Health 80: 96–100.
14. Villeneuve PJ, Chen L, Stieb D, Rowe BH (2006) Associations between outdoor air pollution and emergency department visits for stroke in Edmonton, Canada. Eur J Epidemiol 21: 689–700.
15. Kaplan GG, Dixon E, Panaccione R, Fong A, Chen L, et al. (2009) Effect of ambient air pollution on the incidence of appendicitis. Cmaj 181: 591–597.
16. Kaplan GG, Hubbard J, Korzenik J, Sands BE, Panaccione R, et al. (2010) The Inflammatory Bowel Diseases and Ambient Air Pollution: A Novel Association. Am J Gastroenterol.
17. Vincent R, Kumarathasan P, Goegan P, Bjarnason SG, Guenette J, et al. (2001) Inhalation toxicology of urban ambient particulate matter: acute cardiovascular effects in rats. Res Rep Health Eff Inst: 5–54; discussion 55–62.
18. Last JA, Gohil K, Mathrani VC, Kenyon NJ (2005) Systemic responses to inhaled ozone in mice: cachexia and down-regulation of liver xenobiotic metabolizing genes. Toxicol Appl Pharmacol 208: 117–126.
19. Beamish LA, Osornio-Vargas AR, Wine E (2011) Air pollution: An environmental factor contributing to intestinal disease. J Crohns Colitis 5: 279–286.
20. Lippmann M, Yeates DB, Albert RE (1980) Deposition, retention, and clearance of inhaled particles. Br J Ind Med 37: 337–362.
21. Stieb DM, Szyszkowicz M, Rowe BH, Leech JA (2009) Air pollution and emergency department visits for cardiac and respiratory conditions: a multi-city time-series analysis. Environ Health 8: 25.
22. Sajani SZ, Hanninen O, Marchesi S, Lauriola P (2010) Comparison of different exposure settings in a case-crossover study on air pollution and daily mortality: counterintuitive results. J Expo Sci Environ Epidemiol.
23. National Air Pollution Surveillance Program (NAPS) Website. Available: http://www.ec.gc.ca/rnspa-naps/. Accessed 2012 September 30.
24. Zemek R, Szyszkowicz M, Rowe BH (2010) Air pollution and emergency department visits for otitis media: a case-crossover study in Edmonton, Canada. Environ Health Perspect 118: 1631–1636.
25. Maclure M (1991) The case-crossover design: a method for studying transient effects on the risk of acute events. Am J Epidemiol 133: 144–153.
26. Thomson EM, Williams A, Yauk CL, Vincent R (2009) Toxicogenomic analysis of susceptibility to inhaled urban particulate matter in mice with chronic lung inflammation. Part Fibre Toxicol 6: 6.
27. Fichna J, Gach K, Perlikowska R, Cravezic A, Bonnet JJ, et al. (2010) Novel endomorphin analogues with antagonist activity at the mu-opioid receptor in the gastrointestinal tract. Regul Pept 162: 109–114.
28. Gach K, do-Rego JC, Fichna J, Storr M, Delbro D, et al. (2010) Synthesis and biological evaluation of novel peripherally active morphiceptin analogs. Peptides 31: 1617–1624.
29. Laird JM, Martinez-Caro L, Garcia-Nicas E, Cervero F (2001) A new model of visceral pain and referred hyperalgesia in the mouse. Pain 92: 335–342.
30. Eijkelkamp N, Kavelaars A, Elsenbruch S, Schedlowski M, Holtmann G, et al. (2007) Increased visceral sensitivity to capsaicin after DSS-induced colitis in mice: spinal cord c-Fos expression and behavior. Am J Physiol Gastrointest Liver Physiol 293: G749–757.
31. Guthery SL, Hutchings C, Dean JM, Hoff C (2004) National estimates of hospital utilization by children with gastrointestinal disorders: analysis of the 1997 kids' inpatient database. J Pediatr 144: 589–594.
32. Longstreth GF, Thompson WG, Chey WD, Houghton LA, Mearin F, et al. (2006) Functional bowel disorders. Gastroenterology 130: 1480–1491.
33. Heitkemper MM, Jarrett ME (2008) Update on irritable bowel syndrome and gender differences. Nutr Clin Pract 23: 275–283.
34. Ladwig KH, Marten-Mittag B, Formanek B, Dammann G (2000) Gender differences of symptom reporting and medical health care utilization in the German population. Eur J Epidemiol 16: 511–518.
35. Bertakis KD, Azari R, Helms LJ, Callahan EJ, Robbins JA (2000) Gender differences in the utilization of health care services. J Fam Pract 49: 147–152.
36. Roth RP, Tansy MF (1972) Effects of gaseous air pollutants on gastric secretomotor activities in the rat. J Air Pollut Control Assoc 22: 706–709.
37. Kish L, Hotte N, Cheng E, Rioux KP, Kaplan GG, et al. (2011) Orally Ingested Urban Particulate Matter Induces a Pro-Inflammatory Response and Decreases Microflora Diversity. Gastroenterology 140: S-46.
38. Sun Q, Wang A, Jin X, Natanzon A, Duquaine D, et al. (2005) Long-term air pollution exposure and acceleration of atherosclerosis and vascular inflammation in an animal model. Jama 294: 3003–3010.
39. Dybdahl M, Risom L, Moller P, Autrup H, Wallin H, et al. (2003) DNA adduct formation and oxidative stress in colon and liver of Big Blue rats after dietary exposure to diesel particles. Carcinogenesis 24: 1759–1766.
40. Tornqvist H, Mills NL, Gonzalez M, Miller MR, Robinson SD, et al. (2007) Persistent endothelial dysfunction in humans after diesel exhaust inhalation. Am J Respir Crit Care Med 176: 395–400.
41. Bartra J, Mullol J, del Cuvillo A, Davila I, Ferrer M, et al. (2007) Air pollution and allergens. J Investig Allergol Clin Immunol 17 Suppl 2: 3–8.

6

Preference for Different Anchor Descriptors on Visual Analogue Scales among Japanese Patients with Chronic Pain

Junya Yokobe[1]*, Masaki Kitahara[1], Masato Matsushima[2], Shoichi Uezono[1]

1 Department of Anesthesiology, The Jikei University School of Medicine, Minato, Tokyo, Japan, **2** Division of Clinical Epidemiology, The Jikei University School of Medicine, Minato, Tokyo, Japan

Abstract

Context: Although many previous studies have examined the preference of patients for different pain measurement scales, preference for anchor descriptors has not been thoroughly discussed.

Objectives: To examine (1) the preferred end-phrases used in the VAS as anchor labels for Japanese patients with chronic pain, and (2) whether the preference differs according to factors such as age, sex, educational level, duration of pain, and pain intensity.

Methods: We performed an observational study in patients suffering from non-cancer chronic pain for more than 3 months at a pain center in Japan. The patients were asked to rate their pain intensity using four types of VAS that used the following different anchor descriptors: "worst pain" ("Worst"), "worst pain bearable" ("Bearable"), "worst pain imaginable" ("Imaginable"), and "worst pain you have ever experienced" ("Experienced"). They were also asked to rank the four scales according to ease of responding, and asked which descriptor best reflected their perceived pain.

Results: In total, 183 patients participated in the study. They consisted of 119 (65.0%) women and 64 (35.0%) men aged 18–84 years with the mean age of 56.9 years. "Experienced" was most preferred (69.8%), followed by "Bearable" (66.3%), "Worst" (48.8%), and "Imaginable" (16.9%). Factors such as age, sex, educational background, duration of pain, and pain intensity did not significantly affect the results. In 83.1% of patients, the preferred descriptor corresponded to the descriptor that best reflected patients' perceived pain.

Conclusion: The frequently used expression "worst pain imaginable" is considered to be difficult to understand for most patients. Widely preferred descriptors, such as "worst pain you have ever experienced" and "worst pain bearable", should be used when evaluating perceived pain. The preference of anchor descriptors was not significantly affected by the factors such as age, sex, educational level, duration of pain, and pain intensity.

Editor: Masahiko Sumitani, The University of Tokyo Hospital, Japan

Funding: The authors have no support or funding to report.

Competing Interests: The authors have declared that no competing interests exist.

* E-mail: yokobejunya@gmail.com

Introduction

The International Association for the Study of Pain (IASP) states that "Pain is always subjective. Each individual learns the application of the word through experiences related to injury in early life" [1]. Pain is thus an individual experience with multi-dimensional aspects [2–4], and, theoretically speaking, pain intensity is impossible to measure objectively and quantitatively [5]. However, accurate quantitative evaluation of perceived pain intensity is a prerequisite for both clinical practice and research purposes [5–8].

Over the past few decades, several self-reporting unidimensional pain scales have been developed, such as the Visual Analogue Scale (VAS), Numerical Rating Scale (NRS), Verbal Rating Scale (VRS), and the Faces Pain Scale. Of these scales, the VAS and NRS have been used most frequently worldwide because of their outstanding simplicity, and their reliability and validity have been proved [6–10]. These scales are designed to measure pain intensity using extremely painful conditions or situations as a point of reference. However, many descriptors have been used as anchor labels with the VAS and NRS in Japanese as well as other languages, and these descriptors have not yet been standardized [11]. Pain intensity cannot be precisely compared without using standardized anchor descriptors, even if the same pain measurement scale is used.

Several studies have investigated the preferred pain assessment tool among the VAS, NRS, VRS, and so on [8,12–16]. However, very few researchers have paid attention to the descriptors used as anchor labels. Many studies have recommended the use of the NRS [6,12,17–25] and VAS [14,26–28] to evaluate pain intensity; nevertheless, patients are sometimes unable to use these scales to correctly rate their perceived pain intensity in clinical and research settings. Some studies have shown that categorical scales such as the VRS are preferred over the VAS or NRS by elderly patients [2,8,14,29], less educated patients [13], cognitively impaired patients [30], and children [31]. These results might be due not only to difficulties with abstract thinking [2,30–32] but also to the ambiguity of anchor descriptors used in the VAS or NRS. Because appropriate quantitative evaluation of patients' pain intensity requires the patients to be able to obtain a clear image of the situations described in the anchor label, investigation of preferred anchor descriptors is expected to contribute to the improvement of pain intensity evaluations.

The two major purposes of this study are to examine (1) the preferred end-phrases used in the VAS as anchor labels for Japanese patients with chronic pain, and (2) whether the preference differs according to factors such as age, sex, educational level, duration of pain, and pain intensity.

Methods

Participants

The subjects for this study were recruited from chronic pain patients who attended the multi-disciplinary outpatient pain clinic of the Jikei University Hospital between June 2012 and May 2013. Most of the patients who attend the clinic were suffering from multiple types of chronic pain. The clinic consists of doctors, nurses, physiotherapists, clinical psychologists, and acupuncturists. The patients were basically treated with medication, therapeutic exercise, psychophysiological approach, and acupuncture. Inclusion criteria were a diagnosis of chronic non-cancer pain with a duration of more than 3 months and age 18 years or older. Patients who had visual disturbance, were unable to speak Japanese, or were suspected to have impaired cognition (Mini-Mental State Examination (MMSE) score < 23 points) were excluded.

Anchor descriptors

The following four commonly used descriptors of the anchor labels used in the VAS in Japan were selected.

"worst pain" (hereafter "Worst")
"worst pain bearable" (hereafter "Bearable")
"worst pain imaginable" (hereafter "Imaginable")
"worst pain you have ever experienced" (hereafter "Experienced")

An American psychologist who was proficient in Japanese validated the translations of anchor descriptors used in Japanese to make sure that they were consistent with the expressions used in English [11].

Questionnaire

A traditional VAS with a straight, horizontal 10-cm line was used, with the anchor label "no pain" at the left side and one of the translated Japanese descriptors at the right side. The four different VASs were placed on a sheet of paper in fixed order. The participants were asked to mark a vertical line on each VAS corresponding to their perceived average pain during the previous 24 hours. The participants were also asked to rank the scales in order of preference, from first to fourth place, on the basis of ease of responding, and they were also asked which descriptor best expressed their own pain.

Ethics Statement

The protocol of this study was approved by the ethics committees of the Jikei University Hospital, and the study was carried out in accordance with the Declaration of Helsinki. Written informed consent was obtained before study entry from all patients who participated in the study.

Data collection

The questionnaire written in Japanese was distributed to the participants when they gave consent after attending the pain clinic, and was collected on the same day. Age, sex, educational background, duration of pain, VAS, VRS, Hospital Anxiety and Depression Scale (HADS) [33–34], and Pain Catastrophizing Scale (PCS) score [35] data, which were administered on the same day, were obtained from medical records. Because the participants of this study are from the multi-disciplinary pain clinic, it is expected that their psychological factors have severely influenced on their pain condition. Therefore, we used HADS and PCS to verify that we could regard the participants to be the representatives of chronic pain patients in Japan. HADS includes two subscales which are anxiety and depression. The total score of each subscale is 21. The cut-off point of the each subscale of HADS is usually set as 8 and 11. The point between 8 and 10 indicates that the patient probably has anxiety or depression; the point of 11 and over definitely has anxiety or depression. The cut-off point of PCS is usually set as 30. The point of 30 and over indicates that the patient is in pain catastrophizing state.

Statistical analysis

All data were analyzed statistically using the SPSS program (version 21.0, SPSS Inc., Chicago, IL, USA). Data treated as a continuous scale are presented as median and range, and categorical and ordinal data are presented as counts and percentages. Wilcoxon signed-rank test and chi-square test was used to compare the values and proportions between elderly and young group (Table 1). Chi-square test was applied to compare the proportions of preference between two groups (Table 2).

Friedman test was used for analyzing the differences in preference among the different descriptors (Figure 1). Bonferroni correction was employed for *post-hoc* comparison of each pair. Wilcoxon signed-rank test was used for analyzing the relationship between the most-preferred descriptor and best-expressing descriptor (Figure 2). Spearman's rank correlation coefficient was calculated to examine whether the reported VAS pain levels using the different anchor descriptors correlate with each other (Table 3). Wilcoxon signed-rank test of the VAS values between the most-preferred descriptor and the least-preferred descriptor, was also performed to examine if the reported pain level significantly differed depending on the anchor descriptor. P-values less than 0.05 were considered statistically significant.

Results

One hundred and eighty-three patients gave consent to participate in the study. Table 1 shows the demographic characteristics of study participants. Almost all of the participants were able to answer the VASs with four different descriptors; only four participants failed to mark at least one of the four VASs. The HADS score suggested that 27.9% of the respondents were in a depressive state, and 26.8% had anxiety. The PCS score indicated that 60.1% of the respondents were catastrophized.

Table 4 shows the characteristics of the participants' pain (some patients have multiple nature of pain). The majority of the participants are suffering from some of musculoskeletal pain.

Table 1. General characteristics of study participants (n = 183).

	Total (n = 183)	Elderly (n = 87)	Young (n = 96)	p-value
Age, years	59 (18–84)	69 (61–84)	46 (18–60)	< 0.0001**
10–19	1 (0.6)			
20–29	9 (4.9)			
30–39	17 (9.3)			
40–49	33 (18.0)			
50–59	32 (17.5)			
60–69	49 (26.8)			
70–79	34 (18.6)			
80-	8 (4.4)			
Sex				0.42
Female	119 (65.0)	54 (62.1)	65 (67.7)	
Male	64 (35.0)	33 (37.9)	31 (32.3)	
Educational level				0.03*
Junior high school	12 (6.8)	7 (8.5)	5 (5.3)	
High school	79 (44.6)	44 (53.7)	35 (36.8)	
College/University	86 (48.6)	31 (37.8)	55 (57.9)	
Duration of pain, months	36 (3–480)	40 (3–240)	33 (3–480)	0.82
HADS (Anxiety)	7 (0–16)	7 (0–15)	7 (0–16)	0.31
HADS (Depression)	7 (0–20)	7 (0–17)	8 (0–20)	0.35
PCS	32.5 (7–51)	32 (9–51)	33 (7–50)	0.58
VRS				0.27
None	3 (1.7)	2 (2.3)	1 (1.1)	
Mild	62 (34.3)	25 (29.1)	37 (38.9)	
Moderate	96 (53.0)	45 (52.3)	51 (53.7)	
Severe	20 (11.0)	14 (16.3)	6 (6.3)	
VAS ("Worst")	59 (0–100)	65 (0–100)	55 (2–100)	0.27
VAS ("Bearable")	61 (0–100)	59 (0–100)	61.5 (2–100)	0.70
VAS ("Imaginable")	58 (0–100)	68 (0–100)	51 (0–100)	0.03**
VAS ("Experienced")	66 (0–100)	73 (0–100)	55.5 (0–100)	< 0.01**

Values are expressed as the median (range) or as number (percentage).
HADS = Hospital Anxiety and Depression Scale; PCS = Pain Catastrophizing Scale;
VRS = Verbal Rating Scale; VAS = Visual Analogue Scale
*chi-square test statistically significant ($p<0.05$).
**Wilcoxon rank sum test statistically significant ($p<0.05$).

Figure 1 shows the rankings given to the four different descriptors used with the VASs in this study. "Experienced" was most preferred by the largest number of participants (38.5%), followed by "Worst" (33.9%), "Bearable" (24.1%), and "Imaginable" (3.4%). The descriptor ranked as least preferred by most participants was "Imaginable" (38.2%), followed by "Worst" (31.2%), "Experienced" (17.6%), and "Bearable" (12.9%). Friedman test demonstrated the differences among the four different descriptors to be statistically significant ($p<0.001$); Bonferroni *post-hoc* tests demonstrated significant differences between "Imaginable" and "Worst", "Bearable", and "Experienced" ($p<0.05$).

Figure 2 compares percentages between the most-preferred and the best-expressing descriptor. Overall, 83.1% of the descriptors were consistent with each other.

Table 2 shows the percentage of participants that ranked each of the descriptors first or second in terms of preference. "Experienced" and "Bearable" were regarded as preferable by 69.8% and 66.3% of the participants, respectively. Almost half of the participants regarded "Worst" as preferable; "Imaginable" was regarded as preferable by only 16.9% of the participants. As Table 2 shows, approximately the same percentage of preference was observed even when the participants were stratified by age, sex, educational level, duration of pain, and pain intensity, with p-values, analyzed by chi-square test, of 0.41, 0.34, 0.74, 0.87, and 0.87, respectively. Table 3 shows pairwise Spearman's rank correlation coefficient between the pain intensity measured by VASs using the four anchor descriptors. The Spearman's rank correlation coefficient indicated that there were strong correlations between each pair of the anchor descriptors. There was a significant difference between the VAS values with the most-preferred descriptor and the least-preferred descriptor, analyzed by Wilcoxon signed-rank test, with the p-value of 0.038.

Table 2. Percentage of participants who considered each descriptor as preferable (sum of 1st and 2nd place).

	A ("Worst")	B ("Bearable")	C ("Imaginable")	D ("Experienced")	p-value
All (n = 183)	48.8%	66.3%	16.9%	69.8%	
Young (n = 96)	46.2%	66.3%	13.2%	75.0%	0.41
Elderly (n = 87)	51.9%	66.3%	21.0%	63.8%	
Low education (n = 91)	47.8%	60.4%	20.9%	72.8%	0.34
High education (n = 86)	50.0%	72.8%	12.3%	66.3%	
Female (n = 119)	52.2%	62.8%	17.5%	69.3%	0.74
Male (n = 64)	42.4%	72.9%	15.5%	70.7%	
Short duration (n = 94)	48.9%	66.7%	14.6%	71.9%	0.87
Long duration(n = 89)	48.8%	65.9%	19.3%	67.5%	
Low pain intensity (n = 65)	55.0%	63.9%	18.3%	67.2%	0.87
High pain intensity (n = 116)	45.3%	67.6%	17.0%	70.5%	

Elderly, older than 60 years; Young, 60 years or younger;
Low education, junior high school or high school only; high education, college/university or graduate school;
Short duration, thirty six months or less; Long duration, more than thirty six months;
Low pain intensity, sum of "none" and "mild"; High pain intensity, sum of "moderate" and "severe" of Verbal Rating Scale (VRS)

Discussion

The key findings of this study are that (1) Japanese patients with chronic pain show a certain preference concerning the anchor descriptors of extremes; (2) most participants found that one descriptor was both easy to answer and best described their own pain; and (3) preference is not significantly influenced by factors such as age, sex, educational background, duration of pain, and pain intensity of the patient.

Comparison of preference among different anchor descriptors

We found in this study that Japanese patients with chronic pain show a certain preference concerning the descriptors of extremes (Figure 1). The participants preferred "Experienced" and "Bearable" over the other two descriptors, while "Imaginable" was preferred significantly less often than the other descriptors. "Experienced" represents the "real" pain that an individual has actually experienced; almost all individuals, except for some who

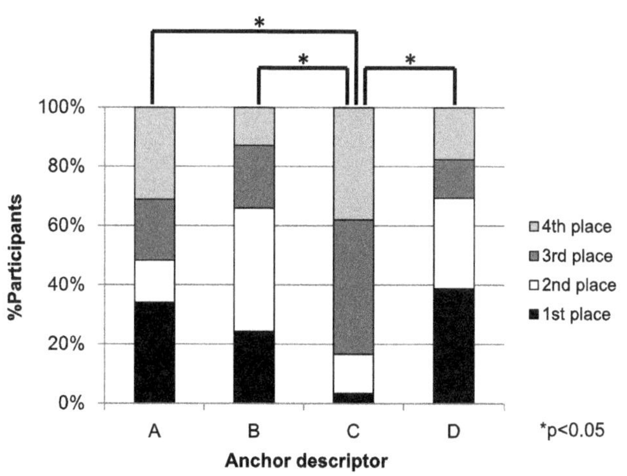

Figure 1. Preference of VAS with the four different descriptors. Friedman test demonstrated a significant difference between the four different descriptors ($p<0.001$); Bonferroni's post-hoc tests demonstrated significant differences between "Imaginable" and "Worst", "Bearable", and "Experienced" ($p<0.05$). A: worst pain ("Worst"). B: worst pain bearable ("Bearable"). C: worst pain imaginable ("Imaginable"). D: worst pain you have ever experienced ("Experienced").

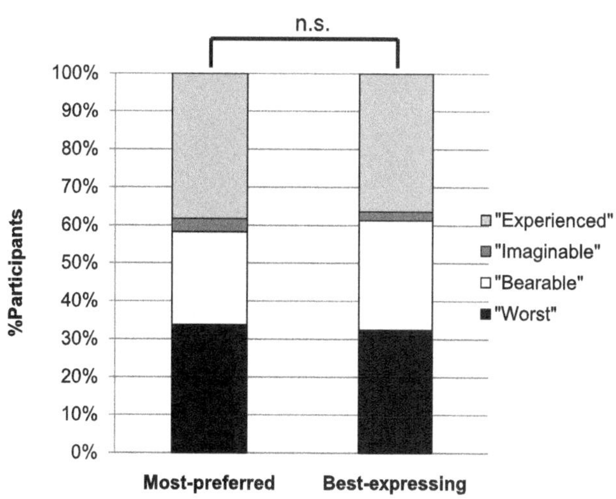

Figure 2. Comparison of percentages between the most-preferred and best-expressing descriptor. n.s., not significant; Wilcoxon's signed rank test, "Worst": worst pain, "Bearable": worst pain bearable, "Imaginable": worst pain imaginable, "Experienced": worst pain you have ever experienced.

Table 3. Pairwise Spearman's rank correlation coefficient between the pain intensity measured by VASs using four anchor descriptors.

	A	B	C	D
A ("Worst")	-			
B ("Bearable")	0.79*	-		
C ("Imaginable")	0.82*	0.78*	-	
D ("Experienced")	0.81*	0.77*	0.87*	-

* Spearman's rank correlation coefficient statistically significant ($p<0.05$).

may have forgotten episodes of severe pain, should be able to remember and imagine such pain. One plausible explanation for the high preference of the descriptors "Experienced" and "Bearable" is that they are relatively easy to relate to.

On the other hand, "Imaginable" required the participants to imagine unexperienced pain, making it difficult to create a concrete image. Some participants mentioned that rather than imagining unexperienced pain, they remembered pain episodes that they had actually experienced.

Interestingly, approximately half of the participants regarded "Worst" as preferable and half as not preferable. Some participants interpreted "the worst pain imaginable" to mean pain they had experienced, while others interpreted this to mean unexperienced pain. The IASP defines pain as "an unpleasant sensory and emotional experience associated with actual or potential tissue damage, or described in terms of such damage" [1]. "Worst" seems to involve affective and emotional aspects more than the other three descriptors, which may have influenced participants' preference.

Table 4. Characteristics of pain (n = 183).

	n
Diagnosis	
Myofascial pain	132
Peripheral neuropathy	19
Spinal degenerative disease	19
Sacroiliac joint dysfunction	18
Failed back syndrome	12
Post-operative pain	9
Postherpetic neuralgia	8
Arthritis	7
Other spinal diseases	6
Complex regional pain syndrome	4
Fibromyalgia	3
Non-specific low back pain	3
Trigeminal neuralgia	3
Headache	2
Type of pain	
Nociceptive	185
Neuropathic	50
Mixed	31
Site of pain	
Face, head, and neck	44
Shoulder and upper extremities	40
Chest and abdomen	16
Back	25
Lumber and buttock	65
Inguinal region and lower extremities	60
Others	5

We also found in this study that participants tended to regard one descriptor as both easy to answer and best to describe their own pain. We defined "preference" as easiest to answer in this study. Peters et al. found that there was little difference between the scales that patients regarded as best describing, "most easy", and "preferred" [8]. Similarly, our results suggest that the anchor label that best described participants' own pain tended to be the one they answered most easily.

As Table 3 showed, the anchor descriptor did not have a great influence on VAS values of the whole group. However, the result of the Wilcoxon signed-rank test indicated that preference of the anchor descriptor could affect the intra-personal pain intensity. Therefore, the easiest descriptor for each patient to understand should be used to evaluate that patient's pain accurately. Moreover, we had probably better not to use the less preferred anchor descriptor, such as "worst pain imaginable" to obtain precise data.

Comparison of preference by subgroups

Although Table 2 shows that participants who were female, younger, and had a low level of education tended to prefer "Experienced" to "Bearable" and, conversely, that male, older, and highly educated participants tended to prefer "Bearable" to "Experienced", the effect of these factors did not reach statistical significance. Previous studies have found that sex influenced the preference of pain scales to a certain extent [8,14–15]. In any case, the percentage of participants that considered "Experienced" to be preferable was similar to the percentage that preferred "Bearable". On the other hand, few participants preferred "Imaginable", and the rank of preference of "Worst" and "Imaginable" did not differ according to subcategories. One plausible explanation is that some patients may have difficulty with the abstract concepts of inexperienced pain such as "Worst" and "Imaginable".

Although "Imaginable" is a frequently used descriptor in Japan, its use as an anchor label in pain measurement may not provide an appropriate evaluation, because "preference" was defined as ease in understanding or answering in this study. Therefore, we consider it more suitable to use descriptors such as "Experienced" or "Bearable" for the evaluation of pain intensity in Japanese patients with chronic pain.

Many previous studies have investigated the preferences of patients for pain assessment tools. However, to the best of our knowledge, very few studies have dealt with the preference for anchor labels. Hjermstad et al.'s review article concerning pain intensity assessment tools written in English reports the use of 24 different descriptors in 239 papers with the VAS and NRS [11]. Thus, a range of non-standardized descriptors are used to evaluate pain intensity both domestically and internationally. Our study indicates that the preference of patients for descriptors can determine how precisely patients are able to communicate their perceived pain intensity.

These results suggest that anchor descriptors should be standardized as soon as possible for more appropriate evaluation of pain intensity. The findings from this study can contribute to more accurate assessment of the intensity of chronic pain. It should be noted that the participants in this study were from a limited population and that factors such as race, ethnicity, and culture are also known to influence pain perception [36]. To what extent our results extend to patients from other racial and cultural backgrounds is unclear and requires further study.

Study limitations

This study has several limitations. First, patients with other types of pain, such as acute pain and cancer pain, were not included. It remains to be clarified whether the findings from this study can be generalized to all Japanese patients.

Second, participants in this study attended a multi-disciplinary pain clinic, introducing a probable selection bias. However, the range of pain intensity measured by the VAS and VRS, as well as psychometric factors such as the HADS and PCS, were distributed widely, so the participants can be considered to represent common Japanese chronic pain patients.

Third, the meaning of the descriptors in Japanese might not necessarily correspond exactly to their English counterparts. However, as the translated descriptors were checked by an American psychologist who is proficient in Japanese, we do not consider this to be a serious problem.

Conclusions

The result of this study indicate that "worst pain you have ever experienced" and "worst pain bearable" are appropriate descriptors for Japanese chronic pain patients. "Worst pain imaginable", though it is frequently used worldwide, may be inappropriate for evaluating pain intensity, at least among Japanese chronic pain patients. Widely preferred descriptors, i.e., most patients can respond without difficulty, should be used when evaluating perceived pain.

The preference of anchor descriptors was not significantly affected by the factors such as such as age, sex, educational level, duration of pain, and pain intensity.

Acknowledgments

We would like to thank Keiko Kojima, Shumpei Kitamura, Makihiko Hirabayashi, Fumitaka Matsuno, and Jin Shinohara for data collection.

We very much appreciate all the patients who participated in this study.

Author Contributions

Conceived and designed the experiments: JY. Analyzed the data: JY MM. Wrote the paper: JY MK SU.

References

1. Taxonomy ITFo (1994) Part III: Pain Terms: A Current List with Definitions and Notes on Usage. In: Merskey H, Bogduk N, editors. Classification of Chronic Pain. 2nd ed. Seattle: IASP Press. pp. 209–214.
2. Kremer E, Atkinson JH, Ignelzi RJ (1981) Measurement of pain: patient preference does not confound pain measurement. Pain 10: 241–248.
3. Melzack R, Katz J (2006) Pain assessment in adult patients. In: McMahon SB, Klotzenburg M, editors. Wall and Melzack's Textbook of Pain. 5th ed. Philadelphia: Elsevier. pp. 291–304.
4. McQuay HJ, Moore A (2006) Methods of therapeutic trials. In: McMahon SB, Klotzenburg M, editors. Wall and Melzack's Textbook of Pain. 5th ed. Philadelphia: Elsevier. pp. 415–425.
5. Loder E, Burch R (2012) Measuring pain intensity in headache trials: which scale to use? Cephalalgia 32: 179–182.
6. Jensen MP, Karoly P, Braver S (1986) The measurement of clinical pain intensity: a comparison of six methods. Pain 27: 117–126.
7. Flaherty SA (1996) Pain measurement tools for clinical practice and research. AANA J 64: 133–140.
8. Peters ML, Patijn J, Lamé I (2007) Pain assessment in younger and older pain patients: psychometric properties and patient preference of five commonly used measures of pain intensity. Pain Med 8: 601–610.
9. Carlsson AM (1983) Assessment of chronic pain. I. Aspects of the reliability and validity of the visual analogue scale. Pain 16: 87–101.
10. Langley GB, Sheppeard H (1985) The visual analogue scale: its use in pain measurement. Rheumatol Int 5: 145–148.
11. Hjermstad MJ, Fayers PM, Haugen DF, Caraceni A, European Palliative Care Research Collaborative (EPCRC), et al. (2011) Studies comparing Numerical Rating Scales, Verbal Rating Scales, and Visual Analogue Scales for assessment of pain intensity in adults: a systematic literature review. J Pain Symptom Manage 41: 1073–1093.
12. Rodriguez CS, McMillan S, Yarandi H (2004) Pain measurement in older adults with head and neck cancer and communication impairments. Cancer Nurs 27: 425–433.
13. Clark P, Lavielle P, Martínez H (2003) Learning from pain scales: patient perspective. J Rheumatol 30: 1584–1588.
14. Herr KA, Mobily PR (1993) Comparison of selected pain assessment tools for use with the elderly. Appl Nurs Res 6: 39–46.
15. Herr KA, Spratt K, Mobily PR, Richardson G (2004) Pain intensity assessment in older adults: use of experimental pain to compare psychometric properties and usability of selected pain scales with younger adults. Clin J Pain 20: 207–219.
16. de C Williams AC, Davies HT, Chadury Y (2000) Simple pain rating scales hide complex idiosyncratic meanings. Pain 85: 457–463.
17. Paice JA, Cohen FL (1997) Validity of a verbally administered numeric rating scale to measure cancer pain intensity. Cancer Nurs 20: 88–93.
18. Gagliese L, Weizblit N, Ellis W, Chan VW (2005) The measurement of postoperative pain: a comparison of intensity scales in younger and older surgical patients. Pain 117: 412–420.
19. Berthier F, Potel G, Leconte P, Touze MD, Baron D (1998) Comparative study of methods of measuring acute pain intensity in an ED. Am J Emerg Med 16: 132–136.
20. Marquie L, Duarte LR, Marine C, Lauque D, Sorum PC (2008) How patients and physicians rate patients' pain in a French emergency department using a verbally administered numerical rating scale and a visual analog scale. Acute Pain 10: 31–37.
21. Brunelli C, Zecca E, Martini C, Campa T, Fagnoni E, et al. (2010) Comparison of numerical and verbal rating scales to measure pain exacerbations in patients with chronic cancer pain. Health Qual Life Outcomes 8: 42.
22. Downie WW, Leatham PA, Rhind VM, Wright V, Branco JA, et al. (1978) Studies with pain rating scales. Ann Rheum Dis 37: 378–381.
23. Bolton JE, Wilkinson RC (1998) Responsiveness of pain scales: a comparison of three pain intensity measures in chiropractic patients. J Manipulative Physiol Ther 21: 1–7.
24. Grotle M, Brox JI, Vollestad NK (2004) Concurrent comparison of responsiveness in pain and functional status measurements used for patients with low back pain. Spine (Phila Pa 1976) 29: E492–501.
25. Larroy C (2002) Comparing visual-analog and numeric scales for assessing menstrual pain. Behav Med 27: 179–181.
26. Seymour RA (1982) The use of pain scales in assessing the efficacy of analgesics in post-operative dental pain. Eur J Clin Pharmacol 23: 441–444.
27. Price DD, Bush FM, Long S, Harkins SW (1994) A comparison of pain measurement characteristics of mechanical visual analogue and simple numerical rating scales. Pain 56: 217–226.
28. Skovlund E, Bretthauer M, Grotmol T, Larsen IK, Hoff G (2005) Sensitivity of pain rating scales in an endoscopy trial. Clin J Pain 21: 292–296.
29. Closs SJ, Barr B, Briggs M, Cash K, Seers K (2004) A comparison of five pain assessment scales for nursing home residents with varying degrees of cognitive impairment. J Pain Symptom Manage 27: 196–205.
30. Radbruch L, Sabatowski R, Loick G, Jonen-Thielemann I, Kasper M, et al. (2000) Cognitive impairment and its influence on pain and symptom assessment in a palliative care unit: development of a Minimal Documentation System. Palliat Med 14: 266–276.

31. Fanurik D, Koh JL, Harrison RD, Conrad TM, Tomerlin C (1998) Pain assessment in children with cognitive impairment. An exploration of self-report skills. Clin Nurs Res 7: 103-119; discussion 120–124.
32. Gabre P, Sjöquist K (2002) Experience and assessment of pain in individuals with cognitive impairments. Spec Care Dentist 22: 174–180.
33. Zigmond AS, Snaith RP (1983) The hospital anxiety and depression scale. Acta Psychiatr Scand 67: 361–370.
34. Bjelland I, Dahl AA, Haug TT, Neckelmann D (2002) The validity of the Hospital Anxiety and Depression Scale. An updated literature review. J Psychosom Res 52: 69–77.
35. Sullivan MJ, Bishop SR, Pivik J (1995) The Pain Catastrophizing Scale: Development and Validation. Psychological Assessment 7: 524–532.
36. Rahim-Williams B, Riley JL 3rd, Williams AK, Fillingim RB (2012) A quantitative review of ethnic group differences in experimental pain response: do biology, psychology, and culture matter? Pain Med 13: 522–540.

7

Influence of the Serotonin Transporter 5HTTLPR Polymorphism on Symptom Severity in Irritable Bowel Syndrome

Rocchina Colucci[1], Dario Gambaccini[2], Narcisa Ghisu[1], Giuseppe Rossi[3], Francesco Costa[2], Marco Tuccori[1], Nicola De Bortoli[2], Matteo Fornai[1], Luca Antonioli[1], Angelo Ricchiuti[2], Maria Gloria Mumolo[2], Santino Marchi[2], Corrado Blandizzi[1]*, Massimo Bellini[2]

1 Division of Pharmacology and Chemotherapy, Department of Clinical and Experimental Medicine, University of Pisa, Pisa, Italy, **2** Unit of Gastroenterology, Department of Translational Medicine, University of Pisa, Pisa, Italy, **3** Unit of Epidemiology and Biostatistics, Institute of Clinical Physiology, National Research Council, Pisa, Italy

Abstract

5HTTLPR polymorphism of serotonin transporter yields short (S) and long (L) alleles. SS and LS genotypes are associated with reduced expression of serotonin transporter. This cross-sectional study investigated the association of 5HTTLPR with symptom severity of irritable bowel syndrome (IBS). Patients with IBS (Rome III) and healthy controls were included. Genomic DNA was extracted from saliva, and 5HTTLPR alleles were assessed by polymerase chain reaction. IBS symptom severity was evaluated by means of IBS-SSS questionnaire. Two hundreds and four IBS patients (159 females; mean age: 39.6±12.3 years; 106 with constipation: C-IBS; 98 with diarrhea: D-IBS) and 200 healthy controls (154 females; mean age: 40.4±15.8 years) were enrolled. The overall IBS-SSS value was higher in LS/SS than LL patients (319.0±71.5 versus 283.8±62.3; P = 0.0006). LS/SS patients had also higher values of abdominal pain (59.7±21.0 versus 51.0±18.8; P = 0.020) and bowel dissatisfaction (80.1±23.9 versus 70.5±22.8; P = 0.035). The overall IBS-SSS values in C-IBS and D-IBS patients were 317.2±68.3 and 296.1±71.4, respectively (P = 0.192), with significantly higher values for abdominal distension (65.0±24.4 versus 51.4±24.8; P = 0.0006), but not for bowel dissatisfaction (80.5±21.7 versus 72.9±25.7; P = 0.138). Frequencies of 5HTTLPR genotypes did not differ significantly when comparing IBS patients (overall or upon stratification in C-IBS and D-IBS) with healthy controls. In conclusion, the LS and SS genotypes are significantly correlated with IBS symptom severity, although their possible direct causal role remains to be proven. In addition, the present findings do not support an association of 5HTTLPR with IBS or its clinical presentation in terms of bowel habit predominance.

Editor: Yvette Tache, University of California Los Angeles, United States of America

Funding: The present work was supported by a grant from the Italian Ministry of Education, University and Research (PRIN 2007, Project number 2007Z292XF_002). The funders had no role in study design, data collection and analysis, decision to publish, or preparation of the manuscript.

Competing Interests: The authors have declared that no competing interests exist.

* E-mail: c.blandizzi@virgilio.it

Introduction

Irritable bowel syndrome (IBS) is a functional digestive disorder characterized by abdominal pain/discomfort and changes in bowel habit (constipation and/or diarrhoea), which can be associated with alterations of gastrointestinal (GI) transit, visceral hypersensitivity and psychopathological comorbidities. [1,2] Owing to its chronicity and substantial lack of effective cures, IBS results in a significant social burden, with a loss of work productivity, impaired quality of life, and a remarkable use of health care resources. [3].

From a pathogenic standpoint, IBS is a complex, heterogeneous disorder, whose development is widely considered as multifactorial in nature. [4,5] Based on current evidence, a gene-environment paradigm has been proposed for IBS, whereby a combination of genetic determinants and environmental factors gives rise to alterations in GI sensation and motor functions, that ultimately account for the occurrence of symptoms. [6,7] In this context, studies on families or twins have given support to the hypothesis of a genetic background in IBS and, consequently, intensive efforts are being made to evaluate whether specific polymorphisms of a number of candidate genes are pathogenically associated with IBS. [6,8] Furthermore, since genetic factors do not act necessarily as risk factors, but they can also impact on clinical phenotypes, great attention is being paid also to possible relationships linking genetic polymorphisms to intermediate phenotypes (e.g., GI transit and pain threshold to rectal distension) or clinical presentation/severity. [9,10,11].

The involvement of serotonin (5-HT) in the pathophysiology of IBS is also an area of active investigation, owing to its presence in both GI tract and brain. Indeed, 5-HT acts as a main regulator of GI motility, secretion and sensory signalling, and plays also a pivotal role in the control of mood at level of the central nervous system (CNS). [12,13] The magnitude and duration of 5-HT actions depend mostly on 5-HT transporter (SERT), which mediates the extracellular reuptake of 5-HT, thus ensuring its recycling and catabolic breakdown. [14,15] Since abnormalities in 5-HT reuptake have the potential of altering the enteric serotonergic signalling, leading to motor, secretory and sensory gut dysfunctions, it has been suggested that genetic or epigenetic

SERT variations might contribute to the pathogenesis or clinical presentation of IBS. [7,16].

The promoter region of human SERT gene contains a polymorphism, designated as '5-HT transporter length polymorphic region' (5HTTLPR), which consists of a 44-base pair deletion/insertion, resulting in a short (S) and long (L) allele. [17,18] The implications of this polymorphism in IBS are currently under evaluation since, as compared with LL genotype, SS or SL genotypes are associated with lower levels of SERT mRNA transcripts, and thereby lower levels of SERT expression and lower efficiency of 5-HT reuptake. [19,20,21] A meta-analysis of association studies has not supported a pathogenic link of 5HTTLPR with IBS. [22] By contrast, some studies have found a significant association when IBS patients were stratified by their predominant bowel habit, [23] or were investigated for pain sensation at rectal distension or somatic symptom scores. [10,24] However, whether 5HTTLPR exerts any influence on symptom severity in IBS remains undetermined. Accordingly, the present study was carried out with the primary purpose of investigating a possible association of 5HTTLPR polymorphism with overall symptom severity in IBS patients.

Methods

Study Aims

The primary objective was to examine the association of 5HTTLPR with the overall symptom severity in IBS patients. The secondary objectives were: 1) to evaluate the association of 5HTTLPR with the severity of different symptoms; 2) to evaluate the overall symptom severity and the severity of different IBS symptoms in patients with predominance of constipation (C-IBS) or diarrhoea (D-IBS); 3) to evaluate the association of 5HTTLPR with IBS in all IBS patients, as well as in the subgroups of C-IBS or D-IBS, by comparisons with healthy controls.

Study Design and Population

This study was conducted on native Italians of Caucasian origin, gender of either sex, age equal or higher than 18 years, and diagnosis of IBS according to Rome III criteria, [1] referred consecutively to the Unit of Gastroenterology from June 2009 to December 2011. Exclusion criteria included: severe organic diseases; history of major abdominal surgery; severe psychiatric disorders; significant alterations of blood chemistry, haematology, and urine analysis; organic lesions at colonoscopy, barium enema, or abdominal ultrasonography; lactose intolerance; treatment with any drug, employed for IBS or affecting the digestive system or CNS, within the previous month. IBS patients with alternation of diarrhea and constipation were also excluded, since changes in the clinical phenotype are common in this subpopulation. [25] To evaluate the association of 5HTTLPR with IBS, healthy volunteers, consisting of native Italians of Caucasian origin, gender of either sex, and age equal or higher than 18 years, were also enrolled. The exclusion criteria included: body mass index lower than 19 or higher than 25 kg/m^2; unremarkable medical history; any functional or organic disease; history of major abdominal surgery; severe psychiatric disorders; food intolerance; any hematologic abnormality.

Experimental Design

At least two samples of saliva were collected from each IBS patient and healthy volunteer in different days and stored at −20°C. All subsequent analytical procedures were performed at the Division of Pharmacology and Chemotherapy. The severity of IBS symptoms was evaluated by the questionnaire IBS-Symptom Severity Score (IBS-SSS). [26] Then all patients received the standard of care. The study protocol was approved by the Ethical Committee of Pisa and was carried out in accordance with the Helsinki Declaration (Edinburgh revision, 2000). A signed informed consent was obtained from each participant.

5HTTLPR Polymorphism Assay

Genomic DNA was isolated from saliva by the alkaline method using QIAamp DNA blood MINI kit (Qiagen, Milano, Italy), quantified by spectrophotometry, and visualized by agarose gel electrophoresis. At the first run, success rates of 97.5% and 95.5% were obtained for DNA extraction in IBS patients and healthy controls, respectively. Additional samples of saliva were then employed or collected again from subjects with extraction failure, and success rates of 100% were achieved at the second run of genomic DNA extraction. In order to avoid and properly manage genotyping errors, for each batch the following cautions were taken as suggested by Pompanon et al. [27]: 1) the laboratory staff was blinded to sample allocation; 2) blanks and duplicate samples of control DNA were included; 3) each sample was assayed in duplicate; 4) cases of genotyping failure in at least one duplicate were resolved by assaying DNA extracted from additional samples of saliva; 5) care was taken to verify whether the genotype distribution was in Hardy-Weinberg equilibrium. The 5HTTLPR polymorphism was typed by polymerase chain reaction (PCR) using the following oligonucleotide primers: forward (LPR-F), 5′-GGCGTTGCCGCTCTGAATGC-3′, spanning from nucleotide −1416 to −1397; reverse (LPR-R), 5′-GAGGGACTGAGCTG-GACAACCAC-3′, spanning from −910 to −888. PCR was performed with the GC-Rich PCR system (Roche Molecular Biochemicals), in a 50-μl reaction containing 1 μl of genomic DNA (20–50 ng), 25 μl of DNAase free H_2O, 1 μl of 10 mM dNTP, 1 μl of 10 mM LPR-F primer, 1 μl of 10 mM LPR-R primer, 10 μl of BUFFER GC resolution, 10 μl of BUFFER 5× DMSO and 1 μl of AmpliTaq polymerase enzyme (ROCHE Diagnostics, Milano, Italy). DNA was denatured at 94°C for 3 min and subjected to 35 cycles of 1 min of denaturation at 94°C, 1 min of annealing at 55°C, 1 min of extension at 72°C, and 7 min of final extension at 72°C. Amplification products were resolved by electrophoresis on 2% agarose gel, and visualized with ethidium bromide staining. The image was acquired by means of a Kodak Image Station 440. The alleles containing the S or L variant of 5HTTLPR yielded PCR products of 528 and 572 base pairs, respectively. Based on PCR results, the enrolled subjects were classified as having the LL, LS or SS genotype.

Evaluation of Symptom Severity

The IBS-SSS questionnaire takes into account the following items: a) presence and severity of abdominal pain or discomfort; b) frequency of abdominal pain or discomfort; c) presence and severity of abdominal distension; d) degree of satisfaction of defecatory behaviour; e) degree of interference of IBS symptoms with daily lifestyle. Each of the above items generates a maximum score of 100, leading to an overall score of 500. [26].

Endpoints

Primary endpoint: overall IBS-SSS value, to compare LL versus LS/SS genotypes in patients. Secondary endpoints: 1) value of each IBS-SSS item, to compare LL versus LS/SS genotypes in patients; 2) overall IBS-SSS value, to compare C-IBS versus D-IBS patients; 3) value of each IBS-SSS item, to compare C-IBS versus D-IBS patients; 4) frequencies of LL and LS/SS genotypes, to compare IBS patients with healthy volunteers; 5) frequencies of LL and LS/SS genotypes, to compare C-IBS patients, D-IBS patients and healthy volunteers.

Statistical Analysis

Data were expressed as mean ± standard deviation (SD) for continuous variables, and as percentage for qualitative variables. Comparisons between groups were performed by analysis of variance (ANOVA) and the non-parametric Wilcoxon unpaired test for continuous variables, and by the Pearson's chi-square or the Fisher's exact test for categorical variables. Adjustments for multiple comparisons were carried out by the Bonferroni correction. Comparisons between groups for IBS-SSS values were also performed by a two-factor (genotype and IBS subgroups) ANOVA, and the two-factor interaction was evaluated. The patients sample size was determined to evaluate a between-groups (LL versus LS/SS genotype) difference of 30 in the mean overall IBS-SSS value, with a standard deviation of 65, a first type error of 0.05 and a power of 0.80. A 2-sided P value <0.05 was considered to be statistically significant. Statistical analysis was performed by JMP 4.0 (SAS Institute Inc., Cary, NC, U.S.A.) and StatXact-4 (Cytel Software Corporation, Cambridge, MA, U.S.A.).

Results

Influence of 5HTTLPR Genotypes on IBS Symptom Severity

Two hundreds and four consecutive patients (45 males, 159 females; mean age: 39.6±12.3 years), with a diagnosis of C-IBS (6 males, 100 females; mean age: 41.2±12.9 years) or D-IBS (39 males, 59 females; mean age: 38.0±11.5 years), were enrolled to assess the relationship between 5HTTLPR genotypes and IBS symptom severity. The C-IBS and D-IBS subgroups differed significantly for male/female proportion (P<0.0001), but not for age. For the purpose of analyzing the primary and secondary endpoints, the subjects with SS and LS genotypes were pooled (LS/SS), since the S allele has been reported to be dominant and both SS and LS genotypes have been associated with a lower SERT expression and reduced efficiency of 5-HT uptake, as compared with the LL genotype. [17,18] However, in order to perform additional exploratory evaluations, subjects with genotypes LS and SS were also analysed as separate groups.

The overall mean symptom severity, as assessed by IBS-SSS, was significantly higher in patients with LS/SS than LL genotype (Table 1). When comparing the mean values obtained for each IBS-SSS item, 'abdominal pain severity' and 'bowel dissatisfaction' were significantly higher in patients with LS/SS than LL genotype, while no significant differences were found with regard for the 'occurrence of pain over the preceding 10 days', 'abdominal distension severity', and 'interference with quality of life' (Table 1). These findings were confirmed also when the P values were adjusted for multiple comparisons by the Bonferroni correction. Of note, an exploratory analysis showed that, when comparing patients with LS and SS genotypes as separate groups, there were no significant differences with regard for the overall symptom severity (P = 0.496) and single-item IBS-SSS values (abdominal pain severity, P = 0.935; occurrence of pain over the preceding ten days, P = 0.348; abdominal distension severity, P = 0.968; bowel dissatisfaction, P = 0.309; interference with quality of life, P = 0.851).

Symptom severity was assessed also in C-IBS and D-IBS patients. The overall mean IBS-SSS values were found to be significantly higher in the C-IBS than D-IBS subgroup, irrespectively of their 5HTTLPR genotype (Table 2). Likewise, when evaluating symptom severity by single items, the score values for 'abdominal distension severity' and 'bowel dissatisfaction' were significantly higher in C-IBS than D-IBS patients (Table 2). However, upon application of Bonferroni correction, the significance of differences in terms of overall symptom severity and bowel dissatisfaction were lost (P = 0.192 and 0.138, respectively), while the significance of differences concerning abdominal distension severity was confirmed (P = 0.0006).

There was a lack of significant interaction between bowel habits (i.e., C-IBS and D-IBS) and 5HTTLPR genotypes, indicating no effect modification and independent effects of bowel habits and genotypes on symptom severity (interaction P values: 0.297 for overall IBS-SSS value; 0.078 for abdominal pain severity; 0.481 for occurrence of pain over the preceding 10 days; 0.811 for abdominal distension severity; 0.379 for bowel dissatisfaction; 0.406 for interference with quality of life).

Association of 5HTTLPR Polymorphism with IBS

In order to evaluate whether 5HTTLPR polymorphism is associated with IBS in the present group of patients, a comparison was made with a group of healthy controls. For this purpose, 200 healthy volunteers (46 males, 154 females; mean age: 40.4±15.8 years) were enrolled in the study. They did not differ significantly in terms of male/female proportion and mean age from the group of IBS patients.

The frequencies of 5HTTLPR genotypes in IBS patients and healthy volunteers are displayed in Table 3. Care was taken to verify that the genotype distribution in healthy volunteers was in Hardy-Weinberg equilibrium (chi-square = 0.21, P = 0.646). In order to allow comparisons with previous observations, the LS and SS genotypes were analyzed either separately or as a pooled group (LS/SS). In both cases, the frequencies of LL, LS, SS or LS/SS genotypes in IBS patients did not differ significantly from those estimated in healthy volunteers (Table 3). Likewise, genotypes frequencies did not differ significantly when the comparisons were conducted on IBS patients after their stratification into two subgroups, according to the predominance of constipation or diarrhea (Table 4).

Discussion

Great attention is currently revolving around the pathogenic bases and pathophysiological mechanisms accounting for the clinical manifestations of IBS, [4,5] and there is consistent evidence suggesting an influence of genetic factors on this disorder. [6,8] In this context, our study provides the first evidence that 5HTTLPR impacts on the severity of IBS symptoms. In particular, our findings point out a higher degree of symptom severity in patients with at least one S allele, and suggest that the S variant affects mainly the severity of abdominal pain and bowel dissatisfaction. Of note, our exploratory analysis showed that IBS-SSS values did not differ significantly when comparing subgroups with LS and SS genotypes, thus suggesting that the group of patients with pooled LS/SS genotypes was a homogeneous population.

The contention that the LS/SS genotypes can increase the severity of IBS symptoms, with particular regard for abdominal pain, is supported by previous investigations. In particular our findings are in line with data from Camilleri et al. [10] who found that the LS/SS genotypes are associated with increased pain sensation at rectal distension. Taken together, these observations [10] and our results are consistent with the notion that the S allele is expected to impair the efficiency of 5-HT reuptake with a consequent prolonged and enhanced activation of serotonergic pathways mediating abdominal pain sensation. Therefore, it can

Table 1. Mean values (± standard deviation) of overall and single-item IBS-SSS in patients with LL versus LS/SS genotype.

	LL (n = 69)	LS/SS (n = 135)	P	P (*)
Abdominal pain severity	51.0±18.8	59.7±21.0	0.004	0.020
Occurrence of pain over the preceding 10 days	50.4±26.4	55.4±29.8	0.089	0.445
Abdominal distension severity	56.4±24.7	59.5±25.9	0.401	1,000
Bowel dissatisfaction	70.5±22.8	80.1±23.9	0.007	0.035
Interference with quality of life	55.7±25.9	62.1±28.3	0.116	0.580
Overall score	283.8±62.3	319.0±71.5	0.0006	

(*) P values after Bonferroni correction.

be argued that the reduced 5-HT re-uptake could induce an overstimulation of extrinsic nerve afferents resulting in neuronal sensory sensitisation, which might occur at peripheral, spinal, or even higher CNS levels. [23,28] In this regard, an interesting study by Fukudo et al. [29], aimed at evaluating the link between 5HTTLPR and differential activation of brain regions by colorectal distention in humans, displayed that individuals with a weak function of serotonin transporter (i.e. S/S genotype) responded to signals from gut with higher intensity in emotion-regulating brain regions, thus suggesting that this functional gene polymorphism may partly predict the individual effects of selective serotonin reuptake inhibitors on visceral pain. [29].

Whether the influence of 5HTTLPR on abdominal pain results mainly from peripheral or central mechanisms, or both, is presently unknown and remains open to future investigations. However, some evidence suggests that central mechanisms may contribute to the enhanced pain perception in IBS patients with LS/SS genotypes: 1) specific brain regions of IBS patients and healthy controls are subjected to differential activation upon application of rectal stimuli; [30] 2) brain regions highly related to pain recognition and emotion (e.g. anterior cingulated cortex) were found to be more activated by distension of descending colon in IBS patients, [9] and altered interactions between anterior cingulated cortex and amygdala have been reported in subjects with LS/SS genotypes; [31] 3) individuals with the SS genotype were more likely to activate these CNS regions, thus suggesting that the S variant can be relevant in brain activation after colorectal distension in IBS patients. [11] Further support to the contribution of central nervous mechanisms on the association of 5HTTLPR with symptom severity in IBS comes from the observations that: 1) in IBS patients, the LS/SS genotypes were associated with high values of somatic symptom scores, suggesting that 5-HTTLPR is implicated in the responses of IBS patients to stress; [24] 2) individuals with the S allele display higher vulnerability to stressful life events and are more prone to develop depressive symptoms. [32]. In this respect, to assess whether the influence of S allele on abdominal pain severity, could be related to differences in patients' psychopathological traits would be of high interest, and this issue deserves future investigations.

In the present study, when the P values were adjusted for multiple comparisons, the analysis for secondary endpoints revealed that the overall symptom severity did not differ in C- and D-IBS patients, while the analysis of single severity items displayed significant differences only for the severity of abdominal distension. Moreover, our analysis showed a lack of significant interaction between bowel habits and 5HTTLPR genotypes. These findings were not completely unexpected, since C-IBS patients are known to complain of abdominal distension more than D-IBS patients. [33] In addition, and most importantly, these data argue against the possibility that the differential influences of 5HTTLPR genotypes on abdominal pain severity might result from differences in bowel habit.

The influence of 5HTTLPR on IBS symptom severity and, particularly, on abdominal pain severity, might have interesting implications for the effectiveness and/or safety of drugs proposed for the therapeutic management of this syndrome. SERT is a specific target of 'selective serotonin reuptake inhibitors' (SSRIs) and there is evidence linking 5HTTLPR to the efficacy and safety of these drugs in patients with depression. [34,35] It is being also appreciated that SSRIs can exert beneficial effects on IBS, with particular regard for the control of abdominal discomfort or pain, [16,36] but whether SERT polymorphisms may influence such therapeutic responses remains unknown.

Table 2. Mean values (± standard deviation) of overall and single-item IBS-SSS in IBS patients with predominance of constipation (C-IBS) or diarrhea (D-IBS).

	C-IBS (n = 106)	D-IBS (n = 98)	P	P (*)
Abdominal pain severity	57.5±20.8	55.9±20.6	0.563	1,000
Occurrence of pain over the preceding 10 days	56.6±30.5	53.3±27.9	0.424	1,000
Abdominal distension severity	65.0±24.4	51.4±24.8	0.0001	0.0006
Bowel dissatisfaction	80.5±21.7	72.9±25.7	0.023	0.138
Interference with quality of life	57.6±27.6	62.5±27.5	0.210	1.000
Overall score	317.2±68.3	296.1±71.4	0.032	0.192

(*) P values after Bonferroni correction.

Table 3. Frequencies of 5HTTLPR genotypes in IBS patients and healthy volunteers (HV).

	IBS (n = 204)	HV (n = 200)	P
LL	69 (33.8%)	60 (30.0%)	0.657 (a)
LS	101 (49.5%)	102 (51.0%)	
SS	34 (16.7%)	38 (19.0%)	
LS/SS	135 (66.2%)	140 (70.0%)	0.455 (b)

(a) comparison by LL, LS and SS subgroups.
(b) comparison by LL and LS/SS subgroups.

Table 4. Frequencies of 5HTTLPR genotypes in IBS patients with predominance of constipation (C-IBS) or diarrhea (D-IBS) and healthy volunteers (HV).

	C-IBS (n = 106)	D-IBS (n = 98)	HV (n = 200)	P
LL	36 (33.9%)	33 (33.7%)	60 (30.0%)	0.594 (a)
LS	56 (52.8%)	45 (45.9%)	102 (51.0%)	
SS	14 (13.3%)	20 (20.4%)	38 (19.0%)	
LS/SS	70 (66.1%)	65 (66.3%)	140 (70.0%)	0.711 (b)

(a) comparison by LL, LS and SS subgroups.
(a) comparison by LL and LS/SS subgroups.

To date, most of the studies on the impact of 5-HT genetics on IBS have investigated the associations of 5HTTLPR with its pathogenesis or clinical presentation. In this regard, the present study was conducted also with the secondary objective of evaluating whether any of such associations could be highlighted in our IBS patients. For this purpose, the frequencies of their 5HTTLPR genotypes were compared with those of healthy controls, selected with similar demographic characteristics, and no significant association was found either for the overall IBS group or for the subgroups of C-IBS and D-IBS patients. Our results are consistent with the majority of previous studies [6,22] which failed in finding a link between 5HTTLPR and IBS. Moreover, while most authors did not find specific links of 5HTTLPR with C-IBS or D-IBS, [24,37,38,39,40] others have reported significant associations of SS with D-IBS, [23,41] SS with C-IBS, [42] or LL with C-IBS. [10,21,43] Among the variety of factors which might account for the heterogeneity of these observations, the most relevant relies perhaps in the different distribution of 5HTTLPR genotypes among different populations. In particular, the allele frequencies between Caucasian and Asian populations are different, since S allele is found in 42% of Caucasians and in 79% of Asians. [44] Furthermore, significant variations in the frequency of 5HTTLPR genotypes can be found even in populations sharing the same Caucasian origin, but belonging to distinct ethnicities. [44] In this respect, both the IBS patients and healthy volunteers evaluated in our study were highly homogeneous, as we enrolled only white Caucasian subjects of Italian origin.

In conclusion, the present study suggests that the LS and SS genotypes are significantly correlated with IBS symptom severity, although their possible direct causal role remains to be proven. In addition, the present findings do not support an association of 5HTTLPR with IBS or its clinical presentation in terms of bowel habit predominance.

Author Contributions

Conceived and designed the experiments: CB MB RC SM NDB. Performed the experiments: RC NG GR. Analyzed the data: RC DG AR MGM NG MF LA MT. Contributed reagents/materials/analysis tools: NG MGM DG. Wrote the paper: MB CB SM FC GR.

References

1. Longstreth GF, Thompson WG, Chey WD, Houghton LA, Mearin F, et al. (2006) Functional bowel disorders. Gastroenterology 130: 1480–1491.
2. Brandt LJ, Chey WD, Foxx-Orenstein AE, Schiller LR, Schoenfeld PS, et al. (2009) An evidence-based position statement on the management of irritable bowel syndrome. Am J Gastroenterol 104 Suppl 1: S1–35.
3. Spiller R (2007) Clinical update: irritable bowel syndrome. Lancet 369: 1586–1588.
4. Ohman L, Simren M (2007) New insights into the pathogenesis and pathophysiology of irritable bowel syndrome. Dig Liver Dis 39: 201–215.
5. Hasler WL (2011) Traditional thoughts on the pathophysiology of irritable bowel syndrome. Gastroenterol Clin North Am 40: 21–43.
6. Saito YA (2011) The role of genetics in IBS. Gastroenterol Clin North Am 40: 45–67.
7. Camilleri M, Katzka DA (2012) Genetic epidemiology and pharmacogenetics in irritable bowel syndrome. Am J Physiol Gastrointest Liver Physiol 302: G1075–1084.
8. Adam B, Liebregts T, Holtmann G (2007) Mechanisms of disease: genetics of functional gastrointestinal disorders–searching the genes that matter. Nat Clin Pract Gastroenterol Hepatol 4: 102–110.
9. Hamaguchi T, Kano M, Rikimaru H, Kanazawa M, Itoh M, et al. (2004) Brain activity during distention of the descending colon in humans. Neurogastroenterol Motil 16: 299–309.
10. Camilleri M, Busciglio I, Carlson P, McKinzie S, Burton D, et al. (2008) Candidate genes and sensory functions in health and irritable bowel syndrome. Am J Physiol Gastrointest Liver Physiol 295: G219–225.
11. Fukudo S, Kanazawa M, Mizuno T, Hamaguchi T, Kano M, et al. (2009) Impact of serotonin transporter gene polymorphism on brain activation by colorectal distention. Neuroimage 47: 946–951.
12. Kim DY, Camilleri M (2000) Serotonin: a mediator of the brain-gut connection. Am J Gastroenterol 95: 2698–2709.
13. Gershon MD (2005) Nerves, reflexes, and the enteric nervous system: pathogenesis of the irritable bowel syndrome. J Clin Gastroenterol 39: S184–193.
14. Chen JX, Pan H, Rothman TP, Wade PR, Gershon MD (1998) Guinea pig 5-HT transporter: cloning, expression, distribution, and function in intestinal sensory reception. Am J Physiol 275: G433–448.
15. Mawe GM, Coates MD, Moses PL (2006) Review article: intestinal serotonin signalling in irritable bowel syndrome. Aliment Pharmacol Ther 23: 1067–1076.
16. Colucci R, Blandizzi C, Bellini M, Ghisu N, Tonini M, et al. (2008) The genetics of the serotonin transporter and irritable bowel syndrome. Trends Mol Med 14: 295–304.
17. Heils A, Teufel A, Petri S, Stober G, Riederer P, et al. (1996) Allelic variation of human serotonin transporter gene expression. J Neurochem 66: 2621–2624.
18. Lesch KP (2001) Variation of serotonergic gene expression: neurodevelopment and the complexity of response to psychopharmacologic drugs. Eur Neuropsychopharmacol 11: 457–474.
19. Lesch KP, Bengel D, Heils A, Sabol SZ, Greenberg BD, et al. (1996) Association of anxiety-related traits with a polymorphism in the serotonin transporter gene regulatory region. Science 274: 1527–1531.
20. Hranilovic D, Stefulj J, Schwab S, Borrmann-Hassenbach M, Albus M, et al. (2004) Serotonin transporter promoter and intron 2 polymorphisms: relationship between allelic variants and gene expression. Biol Psychiatry 55: 1090–1094.
21. Wang YM, Chang Y, Chang YY, Cheng J, Li J, et al. (2012) Serotonin transporter gene promoter region polymorphisms and serotonin transporter expression in the colonic mucosa of irritable bowel syndrome patients. Neurogastroenterol Motil 24: 560–e255.
22. Van Kerkhoven LA, Laheij RJ, Jansen JB (2007) Meta-analysis: a functional polymorphism in the gene encoding for activity of the serotonin transporter protein is not associated with the irritable bowel syndrome. Aliment Pharmacol Ther 26: 979–986.
23. Yeo A, Boyd P, Lumsden S, Saunders T, Handley A, et al. (2004) Association between a functional polymorphism in the serotonin transporter gene and diarrhoea predominant irritable bowel syndrome in women. Gut 53: 1452–1458.
24. Kim HJ, Camilleri M, Carlson PJ, Cremonini F, Ferber I, et al. (2004) Association of distinct alpha(2) adrenoceptor and serotonin transporter

polymorphisms with constipation and somatic symptoms in functional gastrointestinal disorders. Gut 53: 829–837.
25. Garrigues V, Mearin F, Badia X, Balboa A, Benavent J, et al. (2007) Change over time of bowel habit in irritable bowel syndrome: a prospective, observational, 1-year follow-up study (RITMO study). Aliment Pharmacol Ther 25: 323–332.
26. Francis CY, Morris J, Whorwell PJ (1997) The irritable bowel severity scoring system: a simple method of monitoring irritable bowel syndrome and its progress. Aliment Pharmacol Ther 11: 395–402.
27. Pompanon F, Bonin A, Bellemain E, Taberlet P (2005) Genotyping errors: causes, consequences and solutions. Nature Rev Genet 6: 847–59.
28. Mayer EA, Gebhart GF (1994) Basic and clinical aspects of visceral hyperalgesia. Gastroenterology 107: 271–293.
29. Fukudo S, Kanazawa M, Mizuno T, Hamaguchi T, Kano M, et al. (2009) Impact of serotonin transporter gene polymorphism on brain activation by colorectal distention. Neuroimage 47: 946–951.
30. Mertz H, Morgan V, Tanner G, Pickens D, Price R, et al. (2000) Regional cerebral activation in irritable bowel syndrome and control subjects with painful and nonpainful rectal distention. Gastroenterology 118: 842–848.
31. Pezawas L, Meyer-Lindenberg A, Drabant EM, Verchinski BA, Munoz KE, et al. (2005) 5-HTTLPR polymorphism impacts human cingulate-amygdala interactions: a genetic susceptibility mechanism for depression. Nat Neurosci 8: 828–834.
32. Caspi A, Sugden K, Moffitt TE, Taylor A, Craig IW, et al. (2003) Influence of life stress on depression: moderation by a polymorphism in the 5-HTT gene. Science 301: 386–389.
33. Gerson CD, Gerson MJ, Awad RA, Chowdhury A, Dancey C, et al. (2008) Irritable bowel syndrome: an international study of symptoms in eight countries. Eur J Gastroenterol Hepatol 20: 659–667.
34. Smits KM, Smits LJ, Schouten JS, Stelma FF, Nelemans P, et al. (2004) Influence of SERTPR and STin2 in the serotonin transporter gene on the effect of selective serotonin reuptake inhibitors in depression: a systematic review. Mol Psychiatry 9: 433–441.
35. Serretti A, Calati R, Mandelli L, De Ronchi D (2006) Serotonin transporter gene variants and behavior: a comprehensive review. Curr Drug Targets 7: 1659–1669.
36. Ford AC, Talley NJ, Schoenfeld PS, Quigley EM, Moayyedi P (2009) Efficacy of antidepressants and psychological therapies in irritable bowel syndrome: systematic review and meta-analysis. Gut 58: 367–378.
37. Lee DY, Park H, Kim WH, Lee SI, Seo YJ, et al. (2004) [Serotonin transporter gene polymorphism in healthy adults and patients with irritable bowel syndrome]. Korean J Gastroenterol 43: 18–22.
38. Saito YA, Locke GR, 3rd, Zimmerman JM, Holtmann G, Slusser JP, et al. (2007) A genetic association study of 5-HTT LPR and GNbeta3 C825T polymorphisms with irritable bowel syndrome. Neurogastroenterol Motil 19: 465–470.
39. Kohen R, Jarrett ME, Cain KC, Jun SE, Navaja GP, et al. (2009) The serotonin transporter polymorphism rs25531 is associated with irritable bowel syndrome. Dig Dis Sci 54: 2663–2670.
40. Niesler B, Kapeller J, Fell C, Atkinson W, Moller D, et al. (2010) 5-HTTLPR and STin2 polymorphisms in the serotonin transporter gene and irritable bowel syndrome: effect of bowel habit and sex. Eur J Gastroenterol Hepatol 22: 856–861.
41. Park JM, Choi MG, Park JA, Oh JH, Cho YK, et al. (2006) Serotonin transporter gene polymorphism and irritable bowel syndrome. Neurogastroenterol Motil 18: 995–1000.
42. Sikander A, Rana SV, Sinha SK, Prasad KK, Arora SK, et al. (2009) Serotonin transporter promoter variant: Analysis in Indian IBS patients and control population. J Clin Gastroenterol 43: 957–961.
43. Li Y, Nie Y, Xie J, Tang W, Liang P, et al. (2007) The association of serotonin transporter genetic polymorphisms and irritable bowel syndrome and its influence on tegaserod treatment in Chinese patients. Dig Dis Sci 52: 2942–2949.
44. Noskova T, Pivac N, Nedic G, Kazantseva A, Gaysina D, et al. (2008) Ethnic differences in the serotonin transporter polymorphism (5-HTTLPR) in several European populations. Prog Neuropsychopharmacol Biol Psychiatry 32: 1735–1739.

8

Neurologic Manifestations Associated with an Outbreak of Typhoid Fever, Malawi - Mozambique, 2009: An Epidemiologic Investigation

James Sejvar[1]*, Emily Lutterloh[2,3], Jeremias Naiene[4], Andrew Likaka[5], Robert Manda[5], Benjamin Nygren[6], Stephan Monroe[1], Tadala Khaila[5], Sara A. Lowther[2], Linda Capewell[2], Kashmira Date[2], David Townes[2], Yanique Redwood[2], Joshua Schier[7], Beth Tippett Barr[8], Austin Demby[8], Macpherson Mallewa[9], Sam Kampondeni[9], Ben Blount[7], Michael Humphrys[6], Deborah Talkington[6], Gregory L. Armstrong[10], Eric Mintz[6]

1 Division of High-Consequence Pathogens and Pathology, National Center for Emerging and Zoonotic Infectious Diseases (NCEZID), Centers for Disease Control and Prevention (CDC), Atlanta, Georgia, United States of America, **2** Scientific Education and Professional Development Program Office, Epidemic Intelligence Service, CDC, Atlanta, Georgia, United States of America, **3** Current Position, New York State Department of Health, Albany, New York, United States of America, **4** Ministry of Health, Maputo, Mozambique, **5** Ministry of Health, Lilongwe, Malawi, **6** Division of Foodborne, Waterborne, and Environmental Infectious Diseases, NCEZID, CDC, Atlanta, Georgia, United States of America, **7** Division of Environmental Hazards and Health Effects, National Center for Environmental Health (NCEH), CDC, Atlanta, Georgia, United States of America, **8** Global AIDS Program, CDC, Lilongwe, Malawi, **9** Malawi-Liverpool-Wellcome Trust, College of Medicine, Blantyre, Malawi, **10** Division of Viral Diseases, National Center for Immunization and Respiratory Diseases, CDC, Atlanta, Georgia, United States of America

Abstract

Background: The bacterium *Salmonella enterica* serovar Typhi causes typhoid fever, which is typically associated with fever and abdominal pain. An outbreak of typhoid fever in Malawi-Mozambique in 2009 was notable for a high proportion of neurologic illness.

Objective: Describe neurologic features complicating typhoid fever during an outbreak in Malawi-Mozambique

Methods: Persons meeting a clinical case definition were identified through surveillance, with laboratory confirmation of typhoid by antibody testing or blood/stool culture. We gathered demographic and clinical information, examined patients, and evaluated a subset of patients 11 months after onset. A sample of persons with and without neurologic signs was tested for vitamin B6 and B12 levels and urinary thiocyanate.

Results: Between March – November 2009, 303 cases of typhoid fever were identified. Forty (13%) persons had objective neurologic findings, including 14 confirmed by culture/serology; 27 (68%) were hospitalized, and 5 (13%) died. Seventeen (43%) had a constellation of upper motor neuron findings, including hyperreflexia, spasticity, or sustained ankle clonus. Other neurologic features included ataxia (22, 55%), parkinsonism (8, 20%), and tremors (4, 10%). Brain MRI of 3 (ages 5, 7, and 18 years) demonstrated cerebral atrophy but no other abnormalities. Of 13 patients re-evaluated 11 months later, 11 recovered completely, and 2 had persistent hyperreflexia and ataxia. Vitamin B6 levels were markedly low in typhoid fever patients both with and without neurologic signs.

Conclusions: Neurologic signs may complicate typhoid fever, and the diagnosis should be considered in persons with acute febrile neurologic illness in endemic areas.

Editor: Martyn Kirk, The Australian National University, Australia

Funding: U.S. government funding, Centers for Disease Control and Prevention. The funders had no role in study design, data collection and analysis, decision to publish, or preparation of the manuscript.

Competing Interests: The authors have declared that no competing interests exist.

* E-mail: zea3@cdc.gov

Introduction

Typhoid fever is a bacterial disease caused by infection with *Salmonella enterica* serovar Typhi (*Salmonella* Typhi). It is transmitted through the fecal-oral route, generally by contaminated water or food. Typically, it presents as an acute febrile illness often accompanied by signs and symptoms such as headache, abdominal pain, diarrhea or constipation, and malaise [1]. Other, more severe complications of typhoid fever include intestinal perforation, hepatitis, pneumonia, and tissue abscesses [1,2]. Neurologic illness has also been described, most frequently as acute encephalopathy or meningitis [3]. A variety of objective neurologic signs have been documented, including acute neuropsychiatric illness [4,5,6], spasticity and clonus [4,7], ataxia [8,9,10,11,12,13], aphasia [14,15,16], and cerebritis [3,17]. However, these findings have generally appeared as case reports or small case series.

Beginning in June 2009, an outbreak of unexplained febrile illness occurred in villages along the border region between southern Malawi and western Mozambique. This area was known to have a high rate of general mild malnutrition, with most diets high in consumption of wheat, corn, and leafy vegetables. Cassava is consumed, but infrequently. Initial reports described many persons who presented with acute neurologic illness including mental status changes, headache, "difficulty walking", dysarthria, and hyperreflexia. Other neurologic features including seizures and neck stiffness were also described. Gastrointestinal complaints were not prominent among patients early in the outbreak. The investigators initially suspected common etiologies of such neurologic abnormalities in sub-Saharan Africa such as acute encephalitis or heavy metal toxicity, as well as less common etiologies such as neurolathyrism and konzo. However, subsequent investigation revealed the outbreak to be caused by typhoid fever, and after the etiology was determined, persons with signs and symptoms more typical of typhoid fever were increasingly recognized.

We describe the results of an investigation into the clinical, neurologic and laboratory features of persons with typhoid fever during this outbreak. Our investigation suggests that signs of upper motor neuron dysfunction were predominant, neurologic features were generally a later manifestation of typhoid fever, and outcome was generally favorable.

Methods

Patient Identification

The outbreak was first noted in June 2009 by health personnel in Neno District, Malawi, who observed an increase in patients hospitalized at Neno District Hospital with fever and neurologic illness. Ill patients were from villages in Neno District and neighboring Tsangano District, Mozambique. The outbreak occurred in a remote location; the closest health center, Nsambe Health Centre, is approximately 8.5 km away by dirt road over rough terrain. As cases continued, a larger investigation was initiated by the Malawi Ministry of Health (MOH).

Between July and November, 2009, an epidemiologic investigation was conducted [18] that included structured retrospective interviews of previously ill individuals to determine initial signs and symptoms, risk factors, and possible exposures; retrospective hospital record review; structured interview and clinical examination of acutely ill individuals; and verbal autopsy for deceased patients. Questions included specific assessment of dietary habits, sources of drinking water, and other possible exposures that might lead to an infectious or toxic etiology or result in a nutritional deficiency, Based upon initial clinical findings and laboratory results among outbreak patients, a case definition was established for suspected, probable, and confirmed cases [18] (Figure 1). Active surveillance was implemented in affected villages to identify possible patients presenting early in the course of illness.

We identified patients with neurologic illness by several methods. We reviewed medical records at Neno District Hospital for admissions during March through November 2009 for descriptions of objective neurologic findings. From July 22 through November 13, 2009, we prospectively gathered data on persons presenting with illness, and hospitalized patients meeting the case definition underwent neurologic evaluation by one of the authors, a U.S. board-certified neurologist (JJS). When possible, suspected patients meeting clinical case criteria but not hospitalized were evaluated in their villages. When possible, hospitalized patients were serially re-evaluated in order to document progression of illness; a subset of patients underwent re-evaluation approximately 11 months after acute illness to detect the presence of long-term neurologic sequelae.

Laboratory Testing

Cerebrospinal fluid (CSF) white blood cell count (WBC), glucose, and protein level results were reviewed when available. Clinical specimens obtained from acutely ill patients, including serum, blood, urine, and CSF, initially underwent testing for a number of infectious agents including various viruses, bacteria, parasites, and rickettsiae, as well as various toxins at laboratories at CDC (Table S1). Typhoid-specific testing in the field was performed using a rapid diagnostic assay (TUBEX® TF, IDL Biotech, Bromma, Sweden) that detects IgM antibodies against the O9 lipopolysaccharide antigen of *Salmonella* Typhi. Following the establishment of field capacity to collect and transport specimens for culture, confirmatory testing for typhoid was performed by blood or stool culture.

Because some of the neurologic features observed in the patients were similar to those seen in some micronutrient abnormalities, we tested serum specimens on a subset of patients with and without neurologic illness for vitamin B6 and B12 concentrations. Serum B12 concentrations were assessed by electrochemiluminescence immunoassay (ECLIA; Roche Diagnostics Modular Analytics E170) at CDC. Serum B6 concentrations [pyridoxal 5′-phosphate (PLP) and 4-pyridoxic acid (4PA)] were assessed by high-performance liquid chromatography with fluorometric detection [19]. PLP is indicative of longer-term vitamin B6 status, while 4PA is indicative of short-term vitamin B6 intake. Since the neurologic presentation including spasticity and clonus appeared similar to konzo, an illness due to cyanogen toxicity from consumption of improperly cooked bitter cassava, we also tested urine specimens from a subset of patients with and without neurologic illness for urinary thiocyanate levels, a marker for cyanogenic compound exposure. Urine thiocyanate was quantified using isotope dilution tandem mass spectrometry at CDC [20].

Neurodiagnostic Testing

Three patients with neurologic illness underwent brain and spinal cord magnetic resonance imaging (MRI) at the Malawi MRI Facility in Blantyre. Autopsy was performed on one decedent with neurologic illness; tissue from central nervous system, meninges, lung, spleen, kidney, and liver was assessed by routine histology at University of Malawi Medical School, and immunohistochemical staining for leptospira and flaviviruses at CDC.

Data Analysis

Data were entered into an Access™ database. Mean and median concentrations of vitamins B6 and B12 and urinary thiocyanate were calculated; comparisons between patients with and without neurologic illness were made using Wilcoxon rank-sum analysis. SAS software version 9.2 (SAS Institute Inc, Cary, NC) was used for analyses.

Determination of Possible Subclinical Community Neurologic Findings

To determine the possible presence of subclinical or mildly clinical upper motor neuron findings among village populations, persons in two affected villages, who were approximately representative of age group and sex distribution of typhoid cases were evaluated for the presence of objective neurologic findings

Suspected Case:
 	
• Illness in a resident of Neno District, Malawi or Tsangano District, Mozambique
• Onset of illness on or after March 1, 2009
• Fever (documented > 38° C, or subjective)
• AND at least one of the following signs or symptoms
  ○ Gastrointestinal illness (abdominal pain, vomiting, diarrhea, or constipation)
  ○ joint pain
  ○ muscle pain
  ○ headache
  ○ neck pain or stiffness
  ○ difficulty walking or talking
  ○ arms held in flexion
  ○ mental status changes
• AND with no alternative explanation for the illness

Probable Case: • Fever, AND • a positive rapid typhoid test (TUBEX® TF)
Confirmed Case: • Either a blood culture yielding *Salmonella* Typhi, or fever and a stool culture yielding *Salmonella* Typhi

Figure 1. Case definition for typhoid fever used in outbreak investigation, Malawi/Mozambique.

during two village-wide evaluations. These persons underwent a screening neurological evaluation by one of the authors (JJS).

The Malawi MOH conducted the investigation in the context of an outbreak response and a public health intervention, and it was determined by human subjects review at CDC to be public health response evaluation and not research. Verbal consent was obtained from patients or guardians for collection of biological specimens and physical examination.

Results

Demographics

Between March 1 and November 13, 2009, we identified 303 persons meeting the case definition for typhoid fever, including 212 suspected, 45 probable, and 46 confirmed cases. Of these, 40 (13%) persons had objective, focal neurologic findings documented in the medical chart (n = 6) or elicited on examination (n = 34); an additional 27 persons had encephalopathy or altered mental status but did not demonstrate focal neurologic findings and were not included in subsequent analysis. Twenty-six of the 40 cases with neurologic signs met criteria for a suspected case, 10 for a probable case, and 4 for a confirmed case. The median age was 18 years (range: 3–57 years); 53% were female. Age and sex distribution were not significantly different between patients with and without neurologic illness (data not shown). Twenty-seven persons (68%) with neurologic illness were hospitalized, and there were five (13%) deaths; one decedent underwent autopsy. Twenty-one (53%) persons were treated with a variety of antimicrobials at some point during their illness, generally upon hospital admission. The most commonly administered antimicrobials included chloramphenicol (n = 15), lumefantrine-artemether (n = 9), and penicillin G (n = 7). Specific information on dose and duration of antimicrobial therapy was not available.

Clinical Findings

Neurologic signs among cases are shown in Table 1. Ascertainment of exact dates of onset of illness was difficult in this population; however, the mean interval between the best estimate of onset of illness and first documentation of neurologic signs (generally obtained at time of presentation) was 12.4 days (range, 1–35 days). The most common neurologic manifestations were upper motor neuron signs including deep tendon hyperreflexia, spasticity, and sustained ankle clonus; 17 patients had a constellation of all three of these signs. The lower extremities were most frequently affected, and spasticity frequently resulted in gait disturbance. Babinski's signs were present in five patients with other upper motor neuron features; bowel or bladder dysfunction was generally absent. Significant sensory abnormalities, including decrease of vibratory and position sense, were not observed. Twenty patients demonstrated truncal or appendicular ataxia or both, which also resulted in gait abnormalities. Ataxia was unaccompanied by cerebellar signs such as nystagmus or intention tremor. Eight patients demonstrated moderate to severe features of parkinsonism, including bradykinesia, postural instability, facial masking, and decreased arm swing. Other commonly observed neurologic features included flaccid dysarthria with hypophonetic speech (n = 21) and static/kinetic tremor (n = 4). In addition to neurologic signs, many patients described subjective neurologic symptoms including hearing loss and visual problems.

Eleven patients had CSF examination; WBC, protein, and glucose levels were within normal limits in all. No routine blood laboratory parameters were consistently abnormal among patients.

Table 1. Neurologic signs and symptoms among 40 persons with neurologic illness associated with typhoid fever.

Neurologic Sign/Symptom	N	%
Upper Motor Neuron Signs		
Hyperreflexia	22	55
Sustained ankle clonus	16	40
Spasticity	10	25
Babinski's sign	5	13
Dysarthria	21	53
Ataxia	22	55
Encephalopathy/altered mental status	15	38
Headache	15	38
Hearing loss (subjective)	9	23
Parkinsonism	8	20
Tremor	4	10

Extensive diagnostic testing for other viral, bacterial, parasitic, and rickettsial pathogens, including broad-spectrum polymerase-chain reaction (PCR) testing and random-primer sequencing, was performed on 16 of the 303 patients overall and included four patients with neurologic illness. Viral cultures, serologic assays for infectious agents, and PCR for pathogen-specific nucleic acid sequences were negative, and random-primer PCR assays in serum were unremarkable or nonspecific. Autopsy specimens from one decedent with focal neurologic findings, including ataxia, spasticity, and clonus, showed patchy necrosis in the liver; histopathology of cerebral cortex, cerebellum, pons, and medulla were unremarkable and without perivascular cuffing or other signs of acute inflammation. Immunohistochemical assays for leptospira and flaviviruses in all tissues were negative.

Dietary Findings and Laboratory Results

Although chronic malnutrition was present in this poor and rural area, there had been no acute changes in food availability or food type consumption reported by villagers. Cassava consumption was reported in all affected areas, including both bitter and sweet cultivars, but no recent changes in cassava processing were reported. We were unable to elicit a history of pea or legume consumption, or other plants that would be suggestive of *Lathyrus sativus*. Serum vitamin B12 concentrations were assessed in 13 patients with and 10 patients without neurologic signs. The distribution of the 23 levels (range: 175–1540 pg/mL) was mainly within the central 95 percent reference interval generated from a sample of presumably healthy U.S. residents, and the distributions of the two groups were not significantly different from each other (Table 2). Only one patient (without neurologic signs) had a serum vitamin B12 concentration <200 pg/mL, a cutoff value often used to indicate B12 deficiency [21]. Serum PLP and 4-PA concentrations were assessed in eight persons with and nine without neurologic illness. The distribution of these 17 PLP concentrations (range: 0.7–60.4 nmol/L) was lower than the central 95 percent reference interval generated from a U.S. population [22], while the 4PA concentrations (range: 7.4–456 nmo/L) were mainly within this referent range. Fourteen (82%) of the samples had low PLP values (<20 nmol/L) indicative of B6 deficiency, a higher percentage than that seen in the U.S. population (25% of non-supplement users) [22]. The PLP and 4PA concentrations in the two groups were characterized by a large variance, making it difficult to assess statistical differences. However, the group with neurologic signs did not appear to have lower PLP and 4PA values than the group without neurologic signs. Urinary thiocyanate levels among 16 persons without neurologic illness were significantly higher than in 5 persons with neurologic illness ($p = 0.004$, Table 2); however, concentrations in all but one (without neurologic signs) were within the established reference range [23], and no urinary thiocyanate concentrations were above those previously associated with health effects [24].

Neuroimaging Findings

MRI of the brain and spinal cord was performed on three symptomatic persons (two probable, one suspect) with neurologic signs including spasticity, ataxia, and parkinsonism, during their acute illnesses. No signal abnormalities were present, however all three demonstrated generalized cerebral atrophy disproportionate to age (5, 7, and 18 years) (Figure 2).

Short-Term Outcomes

Seventeen typhoid fever patients hospitalized with neurologic illness were serially evaluated for at least 1 week following onset. All had upper motor neuron signs in combination with other neurologic features; seven had parkinsonism. By 1 month after onset, seven had normal neurologic examinations and were symptomatically well with complete resolution of neurologic signs. By 2 months, an additional 6 had resolution of neurologic signs (Table 3). Four continued to display objective neurologic findings—an 18-year-old male with persistent myoclonus, ataxia, and spasticity; a 14-year-old female with persistent ataxia and parkinsonism; and a 7-year-old male and 16-year-old female both of whom had persistent lower extremity hyperreflexia, clonus, and spastic gait. Thirteen of these patients were re-assessed at approximately 11 months after acute illness; none had experienced a recurrence of neurologic illness, but the two patients with hyperreflexia, clonus, and spasticity at one month continued to demonstrate these signs.

Assessment of Subclinical Neurological Illness Among Unaffected Villages

Sixty-five persons from two affected villages who were without a history of illness compatible with typhoid within the previous 6 months, and did not describe a prior history of possible neurologic illness, underwent screening neurologic examination, 35 from Dackson, Mozambique, and 30 from Nseula, Malawi. Median age of these persons was 16 years (range, 4–78 years), and 54% were female, which was similar to the age and sex distribution of patients with neurologic illness (data not shown). Three (5%) persons (median age, 19 years) had brisk deep tendon reflexes with crossed adductors; 1 of these had sustained (>5 beats) ankle clonus. No history of prior neurologic illness could be elicited from these persons. Other nonspecific findings, including physiologic tremors and lower extremity areflexia, were observed in 9 persons.

Discussion

This outbreak of typhoid fever in an area along the Malawi-Mozambique border was associated with a range of objective neurologic findings. Although neurologic complications of typhoid fever have been previously described, the prominence of neurologic illness early in the outbreak initially led to diagnostic confusion and caused investigators to consider numerous other etiologies thought more likely to result in acute febrile neurologic illness. Our investigation benefitted from detailed clinical infor-

Table 2. Levels of serum vitamin B12, vitamin B6 (PLP and 4PA), and urine thiocyanate In typhoid fever patients with and without neurologic signs.

	Neurologic Signs			*No Neurologic Signs*			
Assay	**N**	**Median**	**Mean (95% CI)**	**N**	**Median**	**Mean (95% CI)**	**Referent Range[¥]**
Serum Vitamin B12 (pg/ml)	13	400	597 (367–828)	10	377	415 (280–550)	211–946[¥]
Serum Vitamin B6 (PLP[#]) [nmol/L]	8	2.1	12.6 (0–30.8)[£]	9	3.2	6.5 (0.6–12.3)	11.0–337[^]
Serum Vitamin B6 (4PA[*]) [nmol/L]	8	20.0	72.6 (0–202.2)[£]	9	12.5	26.1 (1.2–51.0)	8.8–464[^]
Urine Thiocyanate (ng/ml)	5	112.5	209.6 (0–446.2)	16	1,185.0	1,407.0 (806.7–2008.5)	1,000–4,000[€]

[¥]Referent ranges for vitamin B12 obtained from kit manufacturer, based upon presumably healthy US population [1].
[^]Referent ranges for vitamin B6 (PLP and 4PA) obtained from a subset of samples from US National Health and Nutrition Examination Survey (NHANES) data among a presumably healthy US population [2].
[€]Referent ranges for urine thiocyanate levels obtained from a sample of non-smoking US residents [3].
[#]PLP – Pyridoxal 5′ phosphate.
*4PA – 4-pyridoxic acid.
[£]Calculated lower confidence interval limits for PLP and 4PA resulted in negative values; for the purposes of reporting, a lower limit of 0 was used as the lower 95% confidence interval limit.

mation, extensive testing for other possible etiologies of neurologic illness, and laboratory confirmation of a large number of temporally and spatially clustered cases.

Thirteen percent of the 303 persons meeting case definition criteria for typhoid fever in this outbreak demonstrated objective neurologic illness. Neurologic signs have been previously described in association with typhoid fever, and have commonly included spasticity and clonus, ataxia, and dysarthria, and less frequently, neuropsychiatric features [5,25,26], cerebellar dysfunction [17], and ophthalmoplegia or other cranial nerve abnormalities [27,28,29]. However, most descriptions of neurologic complications of typhoid fever have been from case reports or small case series, and laboratory confirmation of acute typhoid fever is often absent. To our knowledge, this is the first description of prominent neurologic findings associated with typhoid fever in an outbreak setting. Because outbreaks often result in persons with similar environmental exposures, and, in some cases, genetic factors, being affected, the relatively large number of persons presenting with neurologic illness in this setting may be of etiologic significance.

The most common manifestations in our patients were related to upper motor neuron dysfunction, including spasticity, clonus, and hyperreflexia; a bradykinetic–rigid syndrome; and ataxia. Other manifestations, including seizures, tremors, and dysarthria, were also observed. The presence of variable neurologic manifestations suggests that typhoid produces dysfunction at numerous

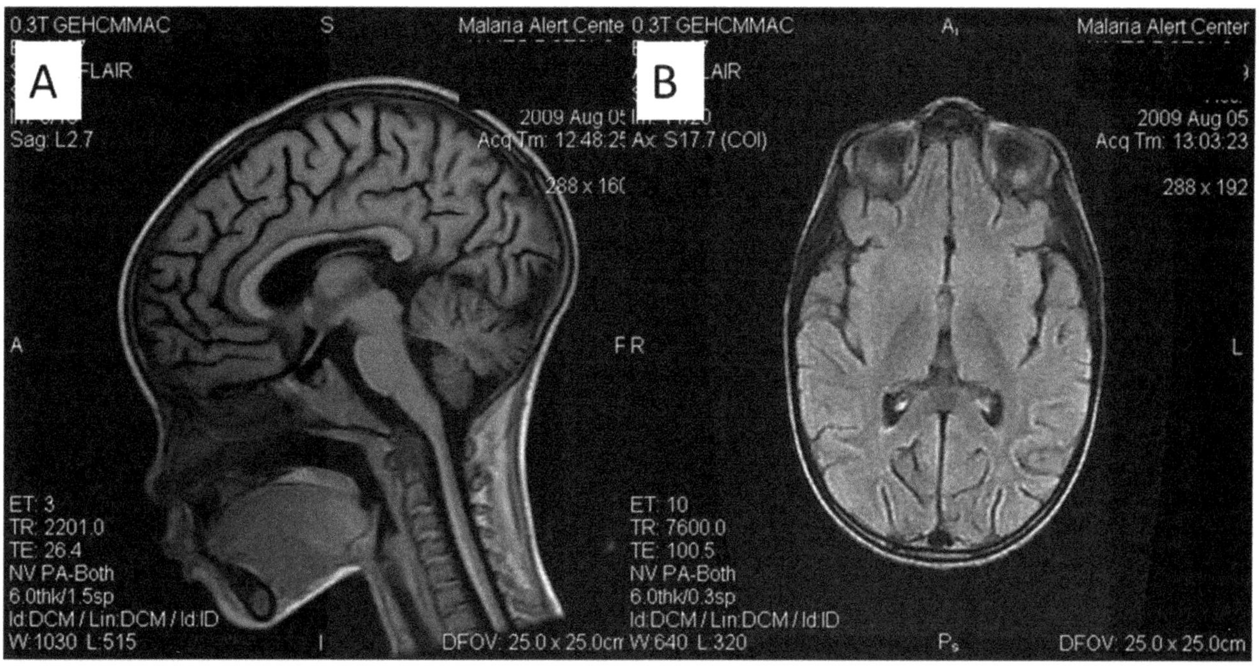

Figure 2. Magnetic resonance imaging (MRI) of a patient with neurologic illness associated with typhoid fever, Malawi. Coronal T1 FLAIR (A) and axial T2 FLAIR (B) MRI Images demonstrating generalized cerebral atrophy, 7 year-old male with neurologic illness associated with acute typhoid fever, Malawi.

Table 3. Demographics, clinical features, and outcomes of 17 persons with typhoid-associated neurologic illness, Malawi-Mozambique, 2009.

Age	Sex	Initial Signs/ Symptoms	Interval, Illness Onset to Neurologic Signs (Approx.)	Neurologic features	Follow-Up	Additional Studies/Comment
5	M	Fever, abdominal pain	5	Hyperreflexia, sustained ankle clonus, diffuse kinetic tremors, severe ataxia	Normal exam at 2 and 11 month evaluations	CSF: WBC 0 cells/mm^3, protein 16 mg/dL, glucose 64 mg/dL MRI: moderate generalized cerebral atrophy
7	M	Fever, headache	12	Hyperreflexia, lower extremity spasticity, sustained ankle clonus, truncal ataxia	Normal exam at 2 and 11 month evaluations	MRI: mild generalized cerebral atrophy
7	M	Fever, abdominal pain, back pain	NK	Lower extremity hyperreflexia, sustained ankle clonus, mild truncal ataxia	Persistent lower extremity hyperreflexia, clonus, spasticity at 1 month; unchanged at 11 months	
10	M		NK	Hyperreflexia, lower extremity spasticity, sustained ankle clonus, parkinsonism	Normal exam at 2 and 11 month evaluations	
13	M	Fever, abdominal pain, backache, leucopenia	28	Lower extremity hyperreflexia, sustained ankle clonus, parkinsonism	Normal exam at 2 and 11 month evaluations	
13	M	Fever, myalgias, back and neck pain, "difficulty walking"	NK	Lower extremity hyperreflexia, sustained ankle clonus, left Babinski's sign	Normal exam at 1 and 11 month evaluations	
14	F	Fever, leg pain	3	Diffuse hyperreflexia, truncal and appendicular ataxia,parkinsonism	Persistent ataxia and parkinsonism at 1 month	
14	M	Fever, myalgias, cough, leg pain	4	Lower extremity hyperreflexia, sustained ankle clonus, truncal ataxia, parkinsonism	Normal exam at 1 and 11 month evaluations	CSF: WBC ND, protein 21 mg/dL, glucose 66 mg/dL
16	F	Fever, abdominal pain, leg pain	13	Lower extremity hyperreflexia, sustained ankle clonus, spasticity, diffuse myoclonus, orthostatic tremor	Persistent lower extremity hyperreflexia, clonus, spasticity at 1 month; unchanged at 11 months	
17	F	Fever, neck and back pain, loose stools	14	Lower extremity hyperreflexia, sustained ankle clonus, altered mental status/ encephalopathy	Normal exam at 2 and 11 month evaluations	
18	F	Fever, headache, abdominal pain, dizziness	21	Lower extremity hyperreflexia, sustained ankle clonus,parkinsonism, myoclonus	Normal exam at 2 and 11 month evaluations	
18	F	Headache	7	Hyperreflexia, sustained ankle clonus, truncal and appendicular ataxia, parkinsonism, confusion/altered mental status, ataxic dysarthria, diffuse kinetic tremors	Normal exam at 2 and 11 month evaluations	CSF: WBC 1 cell/mm^3, protein 20 mg/dL, glucose 52 mg/dL MRI: moderate generalized cerebral and cerebellar atrophy
18	M	Fever, myalgias, back pain, headache, "difficulty walking"	NK	Lower extremity hyperreflexia, lower extremity spasticity, diffuse myoclonus, subjective hearing loss	At 1 month evaluation: clinical status unchanged	
19	M	Fever, backache	35	Hyperreflexia, sustained ankle clonus, truncal ataxia, diffuse kinetic tremors	Normal exam at 2 and 11 month evaluations	
26	F	Fever	30	Hyperreflexia, sustained ankle clonus, truncal and appendicular ataxia,mild parkinsonism	Normal exam at 2 and 11 month evaluations	
52	F	Fever, headache, myalgias, abdominal pain, joint pain	3	Lower extremity hyperreflexia, sustained ankle clonus, lower extremity spasticity, truncal ataxia; subjective hearing loss	Normal exam at 1 month evaluation	
57	F	Fever, chills, general body pain, "difficulty walking"	21	Lower extremity hyperreflexia, sustained ankle clonus; severe hip flexor and extensor weakness	Normal exam at 1 month evaluation	

CSF: Cerebrospinal fluid.
WBC: White blood cell count.
NK: Not known.

sites within the nervous system. Many patients presented with neurologic findings in the absence of encephalopathy or other alteration in mental status, indicating that typhoid may produce focal, as well as generalized, neurologic dysfunction. With few exceptions, the neurologic findings in these subjects resolved over time, sometimes within weeks of acute illness, and long-term or recurrent neurologic sequelae were largely absent among a subset of persons we were able to assess in extended follow-up. Notably, we did not observe some of the other neurologic manifestations that have been frequently mentioned in the setting of typhoid fever, such as acute psychosis [6,25], acute inflammatory polyradiculoneuropathy [15,30], or focal cortical signs [14,15,16].

The reason for the high proportion of cases with neurologic illness during this outbreak is unclear, but there are several possibilities. Surveillance bias is possible; early surveillance and case detection efforts focused on those persons hospitalized with neurologic features. Following recognition of typhoid as the cause of the outbreak, more persons with features typical of typhoid fever, including abdominal pain and other gastrointestinal symptoms, were detected. The involvement of neurologists in the outbreak investigation possibly led to detection of neurologic features that might not be typically assessed or noted by other clinicians. Neurologic manifestations of typhoid have been described as a late manifestation of illness [5,31,32], and the median interval between symptom onset and documentation of neurologic signs in our patients was 12 days. Several factors, including delayed presentation to clinical care and ineffective antimicrobial treatment early in the outbreak because of multi-drug resistance of the causative *Salmonella* Typhi strain [18] may have led to a prolonged course of illness early in the outbreak, resulting in a greater prevalence of neurologic signs. Importantly, following implementation of early diagnostic capabilities and appropriate definitive antimicrobial treatment of typhoid fever with ciprofloxacin, the number of persons presenting with neurologic illness appeared to decrease, suggesting that prompt treatment may avert the onset of neurologic illness.

The mechanism by which typhoid fever may produce neurologic illness is unknown. Rare cases of *Salmonella* Typhi bacterial meningitis, meningo-encephalitis, and intracranial abscesses have been reported both in children and adults [3,33,34]. However, a neuroinvasive bacterial process appears unlikely in our patients; CSF was generally unremarkable and without pleocytosis or protein elevation, features of meningismus were generally absent, and CNS tissue from one confirmed case with neurologic illness, as well as brain and spinal cord MRI on 3 acutely ill patients, did not demonstrate signs of inflammation. This is consistent with prior reports in which neurologic manifestations have largely been unassociated with evidence of CNS inflammation. For these same reasons, a para- or post-infectious immune-mediated inflammatory process in the majority of cases would seem unlikely.

An underlying host factor or environmental exposure that may predispose persons to develop neurologic illness in the setting of severe systemic infection due to typhoid is possible. Many of the predominant signs and symptoms observed in these patients, including spasticity, clonus, hyperreflexia, and ataxia, may be seen with micronutrient abnormalities including vitamin B6 toxicity/deficiency and B12 deficiency [35,36,37,38]. We assessed these micronutrient levels in a subset of persons with and without neurologic signs and did not detect significant differences; however, our sample size was small and variability in the data made it difficult to assess statistical differences. The upper motor neuron findings in this population initially appeared similar to konzo, a neurologic illness seen in tropical areas and associated with thiocyanate toxicity due to consumption of inadequately cooked bitter cassava [39,40,41]. The ataxia demonstrated by some of our patients resembled tropical ataxic neuropathy, also related to the dietary use of large quantities of cassava over long periods of time [42,43]. Although we considered these etiologies because cassava was part of the local diet, the often dramatic and complete resolution of neurologic signs in our patients is inconsistent with konzo or tropical ataxic neuropathy, and measurement of urinary thiocyanate levels did not demonstrate evidence of acute or chronic cyanogen toxicity. Similarly, neurolathyrism seemed unlikely due to improvement in neurologic signs, and we could not obtain a history of consumption of peas or legumes [44,45].

Production of a bacterial toxin may lead to neurologic illness, with toxins produced by *Clostridium botulinum* and *Corynebacterium diphtheriae* being fundamental examples [46]. The diffuse nature of neurologic involvement observed with typhoid-associated disease, and the apparent reversibility of these signs may be suggestive of a bacterial toxic etiology. *Salmonella* Typhi produces a cytolethal toxin, but the role of this toxin in the pathogenesis of typhoid fever is unknown [47,48]. Isolates of *Salmonella* Typhi obtained from cases in this outbreak, including persons with neurologic illness, did not demonstrate significant differences in genetic or bacteriologic properties from other isolates in central Africa [18]; further investigations into the possible presence of a *Salmonella* Typhi-produced neurotoxin are ongoing. Some viral and bacterial infections have been proposed to result in a "cytokinemia" in which hyper-reactive pro- and anti-inflammatory cytokines result in alterations of CNS function with encephalopathy and neurologic illness [49,50,51]. While our investigation did not include assessments of cytokine function, such an indirect effect of *Salmonella* Typhi on the nervous system should be explored in future studies.

Our study has limitations. We did not perform neurologic examinations on all outbreak patients, and the number of cases of neurologic illness may have been underestimated or otherwise biased. Not all patients with suspected illness were positive for or underwent testing for *Salmonella* Typhi infection, and misclassification of some cases is possible. While we initially screened a large number of cases for numerous other infectious and toxic etiologies of neurologic illness, other alternative or concomitant causes of febrile neurologic illness in these persons cannot be entirely excluded. HIV, which could certainly be a contributory factor in neurologic illness occurring in this population, was not routinely tested for. Baseline neurologic status on these patients was unknown, and some may have demonstrated neurologic findings unrelated to their typhoid illness. Specifically, the presence of disproportionate cerebral atrophy on MRI in 3 cases suggests that other host factors, such as nutritional deficiencies, prior cerebral infections, antenatal/perinatal insults, or other factors may result in a background level of mild neurologic illness in this population. It is possible that severe systemic illness caused by typhoid fever, or a *Salmonella* Typhi-specific factor, may exacerbate mild or subclinical neurologic deficits.

Our study demonstrates that persons with typhoid fever may develop acute and severe neurologic illness. The underlying pathophysiological mechanisms producing these features remain unknown. The varying neurologic manifestations observed in this group of patients with typhoid-associated neurologic illness suggest involvement of multiple nervous system localizations. Neurologic illness associated with typhoid fever appears to resolve over time, with few ongoing sequelae, a feature that is important in the prognostic assessment of cases. Acute infection with *Salmonella* Typhi should be included in the differential diagnosis of persons originating or traveling from a typhoid-endemic area with acute febrile neurologic illness, particularly if viral and bacterial etiologies more typically associated with neurologic illness are not apparent. A better understanding of the underlying pathophysiologic mechanisms associated with neurologic illness in typhoid fever is needed.

Supporting Information

Table S1 Initial pathogen testing among ill persons during outbreak of typhoid fever, Malawi – Mozambique, 2009

Video S1 18-year old female with typhoid-associated neurologic illness demonstrating severe truncal and appendicular ataxia and facial masking.

Acknowledgments

The authors would like to thank the following individuals for their valuable contributions to this manuscript: Malawi Ministry of Health: Secretary Chris Kang'ombe, Ben Chilima, Kundai Moyo, and Kapangaza Ntonya; the Neno District Rapid Response Team; Partners in Health: Keith Joseph and Annemarie Ackerman; World Health Organization: F. R. Zawaira, Kelias Msyamboza, and Reggis Kasande; Population Services International; United Nations International Children's Fund; United States Agency for International Development; CDC-Malawi: Dr. Thomas Warne, Rankin Thamanda, Laston Thamangira, Victor Samidu, Ethel Mpagaja, CDC-Mozambique: Amy DuBois, Lisa Nelson; CDC-Nutritional Biomarkers Branch: Christine Pfeiffer, Michael Ryback, Usha Mandava, Huiping Chen, Donna LaVoie, Usha Mandava, Christine Pfeiffer, Daniel Rabinowitz, Michael Rybak, Rosemary Schleicher, Mary Xu, Mindy Zhang; CDC-DASH Laboratory: Nicole Burcher, Michael Dillon; CDC-NCEH Laboratory: Charles Dodson; CDC-Global Disease Detection: Ray Arthur, Rohit Chitale, Kira Christian; CDC-NCEZID: Cheryl Bopp, Michele Parsons, Ermias Belay, Katie Schilling, Sherif Zaki, Wun-Ju Shieh; CDC-NCIRD: Lauren Stockman; and the CDC Emergency Operations Center staff.

The findings and conclusions in this report are those of the authors and do not necessarily represent the views of the U.S. Centers for Disease Control and Prevention/Agency for Toxic Substances and Disease Registry.

Author Contributions

Conceived and designed the experiments: J. Sejvar EL SM J. Schier B. Barr MH GA. Performed the experiments: J. Sevjar EL JN AL RM SM SL LC KD DT YR J. Schier B. Barr SK B. Blount MH. Analyzed the data: J. Sejvar EL BN J. Schier MH GA EM. Contributed reagents/materials/analysis tools: BN SK B. Blount MH DT GA EM. Wrote the paper: J. Sejvar EL JN AL RM BN SM TK SL LC KD DT YR J. Schier B. Barr AD MM SK B. Blount MH DT EM.

References

1. Parry CM, Hien TT, Dougan G, White NJ, Farrar JJ (2002) Typhoid fever. N Engl J Med 347: 1770–1782.
2. Crum NF (2003) Current trends in typhoid Fever. Curr Gastroenterol Rep 5: 279–286.
3. Rajeshwari K, Yadav S, Puri RK, Khanijo CM, Sethi Y (1995) Cerebritis in typhoid fever. Indian Pediatr 32: 1305–1307.
4. Osuntokun BO, Bademosi O, Ogunremi K, Wright SG (1972) Neuropsychiatric manifestations of typhoid fever in 959 patients. Arch Neurol 27: 7–13.
5. Venkatesh S, Grell GA (1989) Neuropsychiatric manifestations of typhoid fever. West Indian Med J 38: 137–141.
6. (1973) Psychiatric symptoms in typhoid fever. Br Med J 2: 436–437.
7. Osuntokun BO, Adeuja AO, Bademosi O (1974) The prognosis of motor neuron disease in Nigerian africans. A prospective study of 92 patients. Brain 97: 385–394.
8. Sachdev HS, Puri MP, Mohan M (1982) Acute cerebellar ataxia in typhoid fever. Indian Pediatr 19: 639–640.
9. Sawhney IM, Prabhakar S, Dhand UK, Chopra JS (1986) Acute cerebellar ataxia in enteric fever. Trans R Soc Trop Med Hyg 80: 85–86.
10. Chand G, Singh K (1988) Acute cerebellar ataxia–a rare complication of enteric fever. J Assoc Physicians India 36: 741.
11. Cheong BM (2008) Typhoid fever presenting as acute cerebellar ataxia and severe thrombocytopenia. Med J Malaysia 63: 77–78.
12. David CB, Tolaymat A (1978) Typhoid fever: unusual presentation. J Pediatr 93: 533.
13. Dewan P, Pooniya V, Kaushik JS, Gomber S, Singhal S (2009) Isolated cerebellar ataxia: an early neurological complication of enteric fever. Ann Trop Paediatr 29: 217–219.
14. Singh S, Gupta A, Marwaha RK (1993) Wenckebach phenomenon and motor aphasia in enteric fever. Indian J Pediatr 60: 147–149.
15. Adehossi E, Parola P, Brouqui P (2003) Febrile Broca's aphasia: a rare presentation of typhoid fever. J Travel Med 10: 192–193.
16. Bansal AS, Venkatesh S, Jones SR, Williams W (1995) Acute aphasia complicating typhoid fever in an adult. J Trop Med Hyg 98: 392–394.
17. Misra GC, Singh SP, Mohapatra MK, Mohapatra RK, Prusty PK, et al. (1985) Typhoid cerebellitis. J Indian Med Assoc 83: 352–353.
18. Lutterloh E, Likaka A, Sejvar J, Manda R, Naiene J, et al. (2012) Multidrug-resistant typhoid fever with neurologic findings on the Malawi-Mozambique border. Clin Infect Dis 54: 1100–1106.
19. Rybak ME, Pfeiffer CM (2004) Clinical analysis of vitamin B(6): determination of pyridoxal 5′-phosphate and 4-pyridoxic acid in human serum by reversed-phase high-performance liquid chromatography with chlorite postcolumn derivatization. Anal Biochem 333: 336–344.
20. Valentin-Blasini L, Blount BC, Delinsky A (2007) Quantification of iodide and sodium-iodide symporter inhibitors in human urine using ion chromatography tandem mass spectrometry. J Chromatogr A 1155: 40–46.
21. Thorpe SJ, Heath A, Blackmore S, Lee A, Hamilton M, et al. (2007) International Standard for serum vitamin B(12) and serum folate: international collaborative study to evaluate a batch of lyophilised serum for B(12) and folate content. Clin Chem Lab Med 45: 380–386.
22. Morris MS, Picciano MF, Jacques PF, Selhub J (2008) Plasma pyridoxal 5′-phosphate in the US population: the National Health and Nutrition Examination Survey, 2003–2004. Am J Clin Nutr 87: 1446–1454.
23. Blount BC, Pirkle JL, Osterloh JD, Valentin-Blasini L, Caldwell KL (2006) Urinary perchlorate and thyroid hormone levels in adolescent and adult men and women living in the United States. Environ Health Perspect 114: 1865–1871.
24. Cliff J, Nicala D, Saute F, Givragy R, Azambuja G, et al. (1999) Ankle clonus and thiocyanate, linamarin, and inorganic sulphate excretion in school children in communities with Konzo, Mozambique. J Trop Pediatr 45: 139–142.
25. Khosla SN, Srivastava SC, Gupta S (1977) Neuro-psychiatric manifestations of typhoid. J Trop Med Hyg 80: 95–98.
26. Ali G, Rashid S, Kamli MA, Shah PA, Allaqaband GQ (1997) Spectrum of neuropsychiatric complications in 791 cases of typhoid fever. Trop Med Int Health 2: 314–318.
27. Ghosh JB (1995) Pharyngeal palsy in enteric fever. Indian J Pediatr 62: 627–628.
28. Kamala CS, Manimegalai S, Kumar S (1991) Palatal paralysis in enteric fever. Indian Pediatr 28: 1213–1214.
29. Nahata MC (1961) Ophthalmoplegia following enteric fever. J Indian Med Assoc 37: 134–135.
30. Ozen H, Cemeroglu P, Ecevit Z, Secmeer G, Kanra G (1993) Unusual neurologic complications of typhoid fever (aphasia, mononeuritis multiplex, and Guillain-Barre syndrome): a report of two cases. Turk J Pediatr 35: 141–144.
31. Chikanza IC, Latif AS, Neill P, Mason P, Olweny CL (1986) Unusual complications of typhoid fever. Cent Afr J Med 32: 31–34.
32. Kanwar K (1962) Symptomatology and treatment of typhoid paratyphoid fevers with special reference to the neurologic manifestations and liver damage. Indian J Child Health 11: 525–539.
33. Suri S, Bhasin A, Srivastava VK (1992) Salmonella typhi meningitis with facial nerve palsy. Indian Pediatr 29: 901–902.
34. Maheshwari VD, Jain MK, Karant VN (2001) Intracerebral haemorrhage as a complication of enteric fever. J Assoc Physicians India 49: 1035.
35. Gdynia HJ, Muller T, Sperfeld AD, Kuhnlein P, Otto M, et al. (2008) Severe sensorimotor neuropathy after intake of highest dosages of vitamin B6. Neuromuscul Disord 18: 156–158.
36. Incecik F, Herguner MO, Altunbasak S, Leblebisatan G (2010) Neurologic findings of nutritional vitamin B12 deficiency in children. Turk J Pediatr 52: 17–21.
37. Mankad K, Kullmann DM, Davagnanam I (2010) Neurological manifestation of vitamin B12 deficiency. Am J Med 123: e1–2.
38. Senol MG, Sonmez G, Ozdag F, Saracoglu M (2008) Reversible myelopathy with vitamin B12 deficiency. Singapore Med J 49: e330–332.
39. Cliff J, Muquingue H, Nhassico D, Nzwalo H, Bradbury JH (2010) Konzo and continuing cyanide intoxication from cassava in Mozambique. Food Chem Toxicol.
40. Cliff J, Nicala D (1997) Long-term follow-up of konzo patients. Trans R Soc Trop Med Hyg 91: 447–449.

41. Tylleskar T, Howlett WP, Rwiza HT, Aquilonius SM, Stalberg E, et al. (1993) Konzo: a distinct disease entity with selective upper motor neuron damage. J Neurol Neurosurg Psychiatry 56: 638–643.
42. Njoh J (1990) Tropical ataxic neuropathy in Liberians. Trop Geogr Med 42: 92–94.
43. Madhusudanan M, Menon MK, Ummer K, Radhakrishnanan K (2008) Clinical and etiological profile of tropical ataxic neuropathy in Kerala, South India. Eur Neurol 60: 21–26.
44. Barceloux DG (2009) Grass pea and neurolathyrism (Lathyrus sativus L.). Dis Mon 55: 365–372.
45. Bradbury JH, Lambein F (2011) Konzo and neurolathyrism: similarities and dissimilarities between these crippling neurodegenerative diseases of the poor. Food Chem Toxicol 49: 537–538.
46. Henkel JS, Baldwin MR, Barbieri JT (2010) Toxins from bacteria. EXS 100: 1–29.
47. von Rhein C, Bauer S, Lopez Sanjurjo EJ, Benz R, Goebel W, et al. (2009) ClyA cytolysin from Salmonella: distribution within the genus, regulation of expression by SlyA, and pore-forming characteristics. Int J Med Microbiol 299: 21–35.
48. von Rhein C, Hunfeld KP, Ludwig A (2006) Serologic evidence for effective production of cytolysin A in Salmonella enterica serovars typhi and paratyphi A during human infection. Infect Immun 74: 6505–6508.
49. Kalita J, Srivastava R, Mishra MK, Basu A, Misra UK (2010) Cytokines and chemokines in viral encephalitis: a clinicoradiological correlation. Neurosci Lett 473: 48–51.
50. Ichiyama T, Morishima T, Isumi H, Matsufuji H, Matsubara T, et al. (2004) Analysis of cytokine levels and NF-kappaB activation in peripheral blood mononuclear cells in influenza virus-associated encephalopathy. Cytokine 27: 31–37.
51. Ichiyama T, Isumi H, Ozawa H, Matsubara T, Morishima T, et al. (2003) Cerebrospinal fluid and serum levels of cytokines and soluble tumor necrosis factor receptor in influenza virus-associated encephalopathy. Scand J Infect Dis 35: 59–61.

9

Identification of a Novel Nonsense Mutation p.Tyr1957Ter of CACNA1A in a Chinese Family with Episodic Ataxia 2

Yafang Hu❡, Haishan Jiang❡, Qun Wang, Zuoshan Xie, Suyue Pan*

Department of Neurology, Nanfang Hospital, Southern Medical University, Guangzhou, People's Republic of China

Abstract

Type 2 episodic ataxia (EA2) is the most common subtype among a group of rare hereditary syndromes characterized by recurrent attacks of ataxia. More than 60 mutations and several gene rearrangements due to large deletions in CACNA1A gene have been reported so far for the cause of EA2. Because CACNA1A gene is a large gene containing 47 exons and there is no hot spot mutation, direct sequencing will be a challenge in clinical genetic testing. In this study, we used next generation sequencing technology to identify a novel nonsense mutation of CACNA1A (p.Tyr1957Ter, NP_001120693.1) resulting in truncated protein without 305 amino acids in the c-terminus. Sanger sequencing confirmed the heterozygous mutation of CACNA1A in a Chinese family with 11 affected individuals. Affected individuals experienced recurrent attacks with or without nystagmus, dysarthria, seizure, myokymia, dystonia, weakness, blurred vision, visual field defects, diplopia, migraine, dizziness, nausea and vomiting, sweating and abdominal pain. This is the first report of EA2 in a Chinese family that carries a novel mutation in CACNA1A gene and had abdominal pain as a novel phenotype associated with EA2.

Editor: Ali Torkamani, The Scripps Research Institute, United States of America

Funding: This work was supported by the chief program funding of Nanfang Hospital, Southern Medical University, China. The funders had no role in study design, data collection and analysis, decision to publish, or preparation of the manuscript.

Competing Interests: The authors have declared that no competing interests exist.

* E-mail: pansuyue82@yahoo.com.cn

❡ These authors contributed equally to this work.

Introduction

Episodic ataxias (EAs) are rare, autosomal dominant disorders characterized by recurrent attacks of imbalance and incoordination [1]. Until now, there have been at least seven distinct subtypes of episodic ataxias based on clinical features and genetics. Mutations of four genes have been linked to different syndromes: KCNA1, CACNA1A, CACNB4, and SLCIA3 for EA1, EA2, EA5 and EA6 respectively [2,3,4,5].

Type 2 episodic ataxia (EA2) is the most common episodic ataxia syndrome. EA2 typically occurs early in life and patients may variably exhibit nystagmus, vertigo, diplopia, tinnitus, dystonia, hemiplegia, dysarthria, nausea, vomiting, migraine and headache [1]. These symptoms last from minutes to days in duration. Patients with EA2 respond well to acetazolamide treatment.

EA2 is caused by heterozygous mutations in CACNA1A, which are also responsible for familial hemiplegic migraine type-1 (FHM1) and spinocerebellar ataxia type-6 (SCA 6) [3,6]. CACNA1A gene (NM_001127221.1) is a large gene spanning approximately 300 kb with 47 exons, which encodes Cav2.1, the main subunit of the P/Q type voltage-gated calcium channel [3]. The full-length CACNA1A protein contains four domains consisting of 6- transmembrane segments, N-terminus, C-terminus, and intracellular loops [7]. Most FHM1 carried missense mutations in CACNA1A gene. More than 60 mutations including missense, nonsense, splice site, small inserts or deletions that span the entire gene have been identified for EA2 [7]. Gene rearrangement due to large genomic deletions is another important cause of EA2 and these deletions are highly variable in size and location [8,9,10,11]. Glutamine-encoding CAG-repeat expansion in the C terminus of CACNA1A causes SCA6 [6].

CACNA1A is heavily expressed throughout the central nervous system and particularly enriched in axon terminals and in Purkinje cells of the cerebellum where it is involved in coupling action potentials with neurotransmitter release [12,13,14,15]. It is generally thought that mutations in CACNA1A result in decreases (mostly in EA2) or increases (FMH1 or SCA6) in CaV2.1 currents [1]. The decrease in Ca2+ entry through CaV2.1 channels results in decreased output from Purkinje cells contributes to EA2 symptoms [16]. On the other hand, increased Ca2+ entry causes aberrant transmitter release and excitotoxicity.

Although EA2 is the best characterized syndrome, no CACNA1A mutation has been found in many patients who present EA2-like symptoms. Because there are no hot mutation sites for large gene like CACNA1A and overlapping clinical features among different types of ataxia, we explored next generation sequencing technology to identify mutations in all exons of four known EAs genes, KCNA1, CACNA1A, CACNB4, and SLCIA3. We have successfully identified a novel mutation of CACNA1A associated with EA2 in a Chinese family with 11 affected individuals.

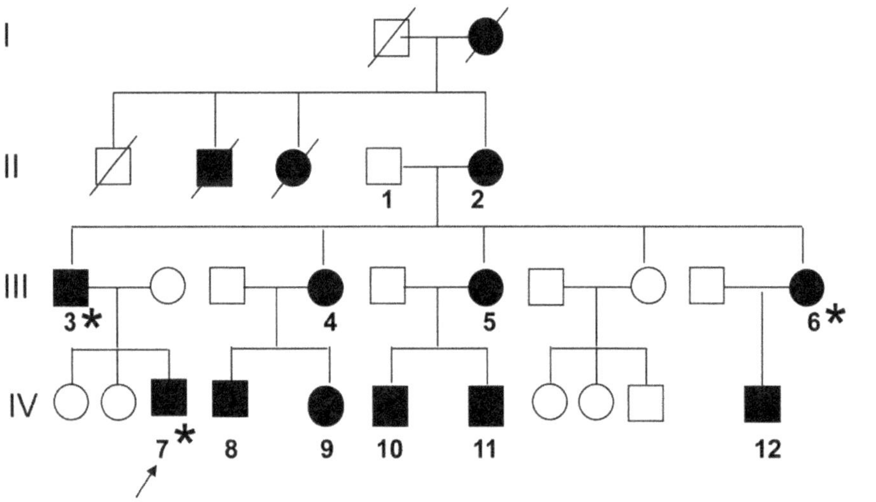

Figure 1. Pedigree of four generation family with EA2. Generations are shown as I to IV. Individuals affected with episodic ataxia are indicated by a black filled circle or square for females or males. Numbers (1–12) were assigned to individuals who agreed to take blood samples. The proband (III-7) is indicated by an array. DNA samples went to next generation sequencing were labeled with Asterisk (*).

Subjects and Methods

Subjects

A 19 year old man from the southern China area (Chinese Han) was hospitalized because of recurrent abdominal pain attacks associated with dysarthria, limb weakness, and imbalance gait with duration of 1 hour. Ten more members in his four-generation family had similar symptoms. Genetic tests were performed for the affected individuals and an unaffected individual as a control.

This study was approved by the ethics committee of Southern Medical University, Guangzhou and all subjects or their guardians provided written consent to get blood samples for genetic testing.

Genetic Test

Because of the clinical features overlapping among the EAs and the novel phenotype presented in this family, four known genes, CACNA1A, KCNA1, CACNB4, SLC1A3, responsible for four EAs, were sequenced by next generation sequencing that was performed by BGI (Shenzhen, China) on subject 3, 6 and 7 (Figure 1a). Experimental procedures included the following three steps. Step 1: library preparation. Genomic DNA was extracted from blood samples and fragmented. Fragments were ligated by adapters and purified. Step2: hybridization. Templates were then amplified by ligation-mediated PCR (LM-PCR) on non-captured samples, purified, and hybridized to a customized 2.1M Human Array from Roche NimbleGen (Madison, USA) for 68–72 hours. After washing, captured LM-PCR was obtained. STEP 3: Sequencing. Captured LM-PCR products were subjected to Agilent 2100 Bioanalyzer and ABI stepOne to estimate the magnitude of enrichment. After quality control, DNA libraries were bound to complementary adapter oligos grafted on the surface of the Illumina sequencing flow cell. The templates were copied from the hybridized primer by 3′ extension using a high fidelity DNA polymerase to create clonal clusters. Each captured library was then loaded on HiSeq2000 platform for sequencing. Data analysis was performed using the Illumina Bioinformatics analysis pipeline. Raw image files were processed by Illumina basecalling Software 1.7 for base-calling with default parameters and the sequences of each individual were generated as 90bp pair-end reads. The suspicious mutation was further confirmed by Sanger sequencing in all affected individuals and one unaffected member. Primers were: forward, CACNA1A-F:5′- CAGAGCC-CACAAGGTCATTC- 3′, reverse, CACNA1A-R:5′-GCTCAGCCACCCTCATATTC-3′. All PCR reactions were performed as following conditions: denaturation at 94°C for 5 min; 30 cycles of 94°C for 30 s, 56°C for 30 s, and 72°C for 35 s; and a final extension at 72°C for 10 min. The predicted size of PCR products was 659 bp.

Results

1. Clinic Features of a Chinese Family with EA-2

The four-generation pedigree was shown as in figure 1. A 19 year old proband (IV-7) visited our hospital in March 2009 when he experienced recurrent abdominal pain around the navel associated with limb weakness, dizziness, difficulty swallowing, dysarthria and diplopia. He had similar attacks for the past 4 years with a frequency once per 2–3 days. The symptoms lasted up to 1 h and disappeared without treatment. No precipitating factors were found. Neurological examination disclosed no obvious sign except for awkwardly rotation and drunken gait. Electroencephalogram recording revealed normal activity during attack. Brain magnetic resonance imaging was normal. During hospitalization, the patient had three attacks with 3–4 days intervals. During attacks, patients suffered abdominal pain, dizziness, dysarthria, and limb weakness. Limb tremor and upward nystagmus were observed once. The patient responded well to acetazolamide.

Family history revealed that 10 other kindred, deceased great-grandmother, deceased grandma's sister and brother also had similar symptoms. Then, affected individuals in the family were evaluated and their symptoms and signs were described in table 1. All visited individuals were numbered (in figure 1) and their DNA samples were obtained. Except for the symptoms and signs reported in the literature, a total of five patients in this family suffered from abdominal pain during attacks (showed in table 1). Most patients recovered from attacks after rest or sleep without any treatment.

Table 1. Clinical features of EA-2 family.

Pt. no	Age	Age of onset	Trigger	Duration	Frequencies	Abdominal pain	Gait ataxia	Additional symptoms	interictal symptoms
2	74	5	–	several; ds	3–4/y	+	+	slurred speech, nystagmus, myokymia, nausea and vomiting	–
3	54	35	emotion, sports	6 hs	1–2/m	–	+	dysarthria, nystagmus, blurred vision, visual field defects, seizure, myokymia, dystonia, weakness, migraine, dizziness, nausea, vomiting, sweating	
4	47	12	–	mins	1/1–4 w	+	+	dysarthria, vertigo, nausea and vomiting	+
5	44	6–7	–	up to 5 mins	1/ys	+	–	nausea and vomiting	+
6	39	7	–	till sleep	½–3 m	–	–	diplopia, headache, vertigo, lower extremity numbness	+
7	21	15	–	1 h	1/2–3 d	+	+	dysarthria,diplopia,dizziness, nausea and vomiting	
8	25	4	emotion, frightened sports	3–4 hs	1/1–2d	–	+	dysarthria,diplopia,defects of visual field, myotonia,myokymia sometime, vertigo, weakness, dizziness, obvious right arm tremor	+
9	21	17	tired	mins	1/1–2 w	–	–	diplopia, migraine, tinnitus sometime	+
10	21	7	frightened, sports	till sleep	irregular		+	dysarthria, diplopia,headaches, vertigo, myokymia, tinnitus palpitation, sweat, unable to hold items	–
11	16	5	–	hs	1/y	+	+	dysarthria, weakness, migraine, nausea and vomiting	
12	16	13	sports	mins	1/m	–	–	dysarthria,diplopia, vertigo, tinnitus (low noise)	–

Pt no = patients number; min = minute; h = hour; d = days; w = week; m = month; y = year.

2. Characterization of CACNA1A Mutation

Even though the patients presented EA2 like symptoms, due to the large size of CACNA1A, lack of no hot mutation spots, and existing abdominal pain not reported in literature, we choose to sequence four known EAs responsible genes CACNA1A, KCNA1, CACNB4, and SLC1A3 with DNA samples from proband (IV-7), his father (III-3) and one aunt (III-6). We found nonsense mutation in CACNA1A (c.6107C>A, exon 40, NM_001127221.1) in all three patients. This mutation introduced a premature stop codon (p.Tyr1957Ter, NP_001120693.1) and caused either loss of 305 aa (amino acids) in the C-tail or nonsense-mediated mRNA decay. Sanger sequencing confirmed the heterozygous genetic defect mutation in all affected patients. The Human Gene Mutation Database Data and literature search revealed a novel mutation in CACNA1A. The sequencing raw data analysis and Sanger sequencing results were shown as in figure 2 and Tables S1.

Discussion

Here we described a Chinese four-generation family with EA2. Recurrent attacks lasted from minutes to days and were associated with or without nystagmus, dysarthria, seizure, myokymia, dystonia, weakness, blurred vision, visual field defects, diplopia, migraine, dizziness, nausea, vomiting, sweating and abdominal pain. All symptoms or signs except for abdominal pain have been reported. Most patients experienced attacks in their childhood and teenage years except for one case, which occurred at age 35. Using next generation sequencing technology, we identified a nonsense mutation of p.Tyr1957Ter in CACNA1A. Sanger sequence confirmed all affected members harbored this heterozygous mutation.

EA2 belongs to the rare hereditary ataxia syndromes. Mutations in CACNA1A currently have been found responsible for a lot of EA2 patients. Due to the large size of the gene, mutations that widely span 47 exons, and existence of genomic rearrangement,

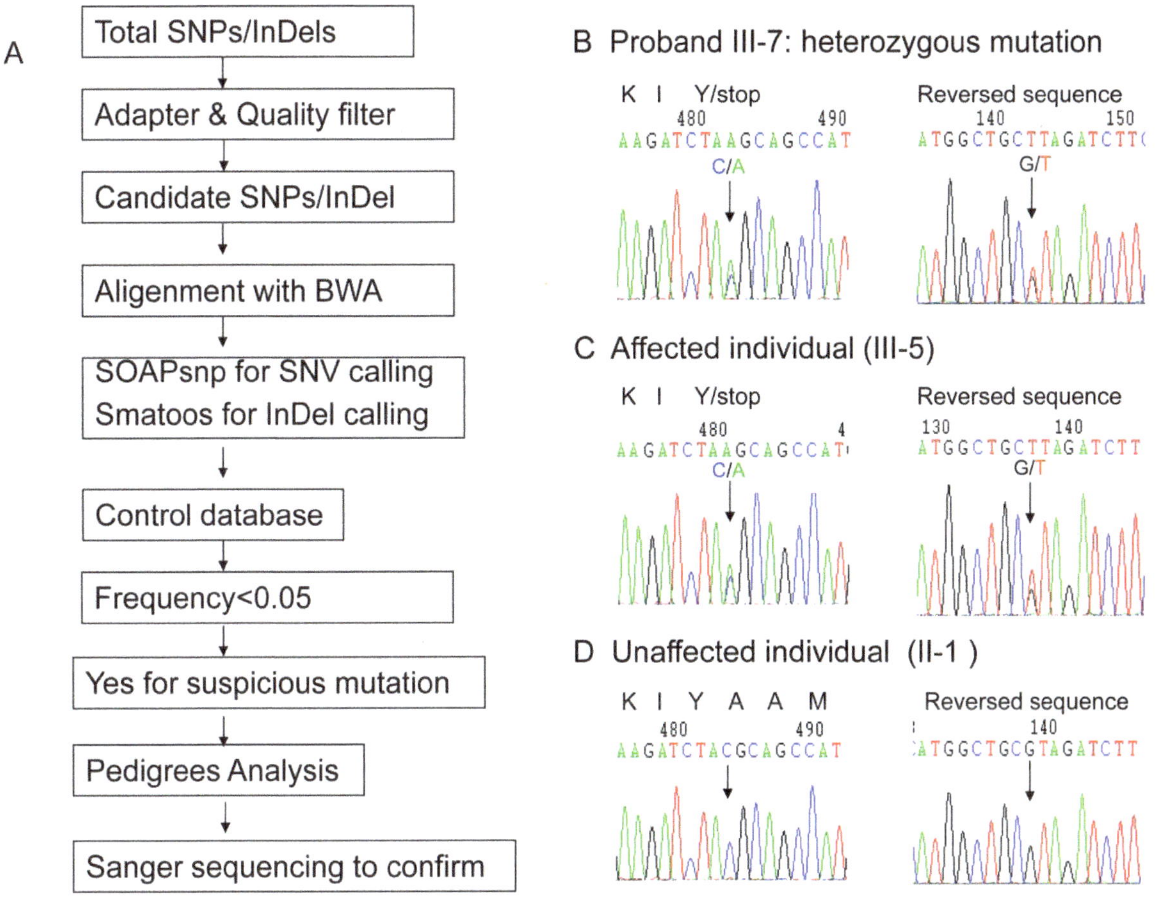

Figure 2. Identification of novel premature mutation (p.Tyr1957Ter) in the c-tail of CACNA1A in a Chinese EA2 family. A. Schematic of the bioinformatics analysis pipeline of data from next generation sequencing to identify nonsense mutation (p.Tyr1957Ter) in CACNA1A. SNP, single nucleotide polymorphism, InDels, insertions or deletions, BWA, Burrows-Wheeler Alignment Tool, SNV, single nucleotide variants. B. Confirmation of a heterozygous mutation in CACNA1A (c.6107C>A, NM_001127221.1, p.Tyr1957Ter, NP_001120693.1) by Sanger sequencing in the proband. C. A heterozygous C/A change at nucleotide 6107 in the affected individual D. C/C sequence at nucleotide 6107 in grandfather (I-1).

genetic detection becomes a challenge. Low numbers of recurrent mutations were found in different studies [3,7,17] and detection rates from direct sequencing range from 13% to 40% [7,18,19]. Detections have only been carried out in advanced countries. The results show there are more than 60 mutations in EA2, the majority characterized in Caucasian families with a few identified in Japanese families [1,7,20]. This is the first genetic analysis study for Chinese family with EA2. However, there are lots of genetic test studies for SCA6, the allelic gene disease of CACNA1A. The detection rate for SCA6 is between 1.86–3.3%, among the largest cohort study in mainland China [21,22].

Although truncating mutations have been reported and are the most common mutations to cause EA2, the truncated mutation of p.Tyr1957Ter in this study becomes interesting because abdominal pain has never been reported elsewhere. Five out of eleven affected members from three generations experienced with abdominal pain around the navel but only one had abnormal electroencephalogram recording. Acetazolamide, but not anti-epilepsy treatment, relieved abdominal pain of the proband. The correlation between the mutation and the phenotype remain unclear. It has recently been suggested that irregular firing of cerebellar Purkinje cells contributes to motor symptoms associated with EA2 [17].The heterozygous mutation in CACNA1A in our cases will probably produce of a mixture of wild type and truncated subunits. There are two hypotheses that suggest the genetic defection cause disease: dominant negative effect or haploinsufficiency. The former suggests that truncated proteins compete with wild type Cav2.1 and play dominant negative effect [23,24,25]. Some investigators support the haploinsufficiency hypothesis because the shortest truncated proteins only have domain 1 intact and large deletions are unlikely to exert a dominant negative effect [7,10]. Since most EA2 mutations disrupt the reading frame, it is unlikely that abdominal pain is caused by "dominant negative effect" of the p.Tyr1957Ter. However, abdominal pain and episodic ataxia can be observed in many metabolic and cerebral ataxia disorders, suggesting a shared mechanism in neuroendocrine dysregulation.

In summary, a novel nonsense mutation of p.Tyr1957Ter in CACNA1A was identified in a four-generation Chinese family. Affected individuals presented typical EA2 like clinical features except for abdominal pain. Targeted sequencing by next generation sequencing technology is an ideal approach for genetic testing for large genes or syndromes with overlapping clinic features.

Acknowledgments

We thank Dr. Jiandong Yang in Children's National Medical Center, Washington, DC, for suggestions in data analysis and manuscript preparation. We thank Dr. Harish Pant, NINDS, NIH for editing our manuscript.

Author Contributions

Conceived and designed the experiments: YH HSJ QW ZSX SYP. Performed the experiments: YH HSJ QW ZSX. Analyzed the data: YH SYP. Contributed reagents/materials/analysis tools: HSJ SYP. Wrote the paper: YH SYP.

References

1. Jen JC, Graves TD, Hess EJ, Hanna MG, Griggs RC, et al. (2007) Primary episodic ataxias: diagnosis, pathogenesis and treatment. Brain 130: 2484–2493.
2. Browne DL, Gancher ST, Nutt JG, Brunt ER, Smith EA, et al. (1994) Episodic ataxia/myokymia syndrome is associated with point mutations in the human potassium channel gene, KCNA1. Nat Genet 8: 136–40.
3. Ophoff RA, Terwindt GM, Vergouwe MN, van Eijk R, Oefner PJ, et al. (1996) Familial hemiplegic migraine and episodic ataxia type-2 are caused by mutations in the Ca2 channel gene CACNL1A4. Cell 87: 543–52.
4. Escayg A, De Waard M, Lee DD, Bichet D, Wolf P, et al. (2000) Coding and noncoding variation of the human calcium-channel beta4-subunit gene CACNB4 in patients with idiopathic generalized epilepsy and episodic ataxia. Am J Hum Genet 66(5): 1531–9.
5. Jen JC, Wan J, Palos TP, Howard BD, Baloh RW (2005) Mutation in the glutamate transporter EAAT1 causes episodic ataxia, hemiplegia, and seizures. Neurology 65: 529–34.
6. Zhuchenko O, Bailey J, Bonnen P, Ashizawa T, Stockton DW, et al. (1997) Autosomal dominant cerebellar ataxia (SCA6) associated with small polyglutamine expansions in the alpha 1A-voltage-dependent calcium channel. Nat Genet 15: 62–9.
7. Mantuano E, Romano S, Veneziano L, Gellera C, Castellotti B, et al. (2010) Identification of novel and recurrent CACNA1A gene mutations in fifteen patients with episodic ataxia type 2. J Neurol Sci 291(1–2): 30–6.
8. Riant F, Mourtada R, Saugier-Veber P, and Tournier-Lasserve E (2008) Large CACNA1A deletion in a family with episodic ataxia type 2. Arch Neurol 65: 817–820.
9. Riant F, Lescoat C, Vahedi K, Kaphan E, Toutain A, et al. (2010) Identification of CACNA1A large deletions in four patients with episodic ataxia. Neurogenetics 11: 101–106.
10. Labrum RW, Rajakulendran S, Graves TD, Eunson LH, Bevan R, et al. (2009) Large scale calcium channel gene rearrangements in episodic ataxia and hemiplegic migraine: implications for diagnostic testing. J Med Genet 46: 786–791.
11. Wan J, Mamsa H, Johnston JL, Spriggs EL, Singer HS, et al. (2011) Large Genomic Deletions in CACNA1A Cause Episodic Ataxia Type 2. Front Neurol 2: 51.
12. Evans RM, Zamponi GW (2006) Presynaptic Ca2+ channels–integration centers for neuronal signaling pathways. Trends Neurosci 29: 617–624.
13. Mori Y, Friedrich T, Kim MS, Mikami A, Nakai J, et al. (1991) Primary structure and functional expression from complementary DNA of a brain calcium channel. Nature 350: 398–402.
14. Stea A, Tomlinson WJ, Soong TW, Bourinet E, Dubel SJ, et al. (1994) Localization and functional properties of a rat brain alpha 1A calcium channel reflect similarities to neuronal Q- and P-type channels. Proc Natl Acad Sci U S A 91: 10576–10580.
15. Usowicz MM, Sugimori M, Cherksey B, Llinas R (1992) P-type calcium channels in the somata and dendrites of adult cerebellar Purkinje cells. Neuron 9: 1185–1199.
16. Walter JT, Alviña K, Womack MD, Chevez C, Khodakhah K (2006) Decreases in the precision of Purkinje cell pacemaking cause cerebellar dysfunction and ataxia. Nat Neurosci 9(3): 389–97.
17. Jen J, Kim GW, Baloh RW (2004) Clinical spectrum of episodic ataxia type 2. Neurology 62: 17–22.
18. Denier C, Ducros A, Vahedi K, Joutel A, Thierry P, et al. (1999) High prevalence of CACNA1A truncations and broader clinical spectrum in episodic ataxia type 2. Neurology 1999 52: 1816–21.
19. Eunson LH, Graves TD, Hanna MG (2005) New calcium channel mutations predict aberrant RNA splicing in episodic ataxia. Neurology 65: 308–10.
20. Matsuyama Z, Murase M, Shimizu H, Aoki Y, Hayashi M, et al. (2003) A novel insertion mutation of acetazolamide-responsive episodic ataxia in a Japanese family. J Neurol Sci 210(1–2): 91–3.
21. Tang B, Liu C, Shen L, Dai H, Pan Q, et al. (2000) Frequency of SCA1, SCA2, SCA3/MJD, SCA6, SCA7, and DRPLA CAG trinucleotide repeat expansion in patients with hereditary spinocerebellar ataxia from Chinese kindreds. Arch Neurol 57(4): 540–4.
22. Wang J, Shen L, Lei L, Xu Q, Zhou J, et al. (2011) Spinocerebellar ataxias in mainland China: an updated genetic analysis among a large cohort of familial and sporadic cases. Zhong Nan Da Xue Xue Bao Yi Xue Ban 36(6): 482–9.
23. Mezghrani A, Monteil A, Watschinger K, Sinnegger-Brauns MJ, Barrere C, et al. (2008) A destructive interaction mechanism accounts for dominant-negative effects of misfolded mutants of voltage-gated calcium channels. J Neurosci 28: 4501–4511.
24. Page KM, Heblich F, Margas W, Pratt WS, Nieto-Rostro M, et al. (2010) N terminus is key to the dominant negative suppression of Ca(V)2calcium channels: implications for episodic ataxia type2. J Biol Chem 285: 835–844.
25. Few AP, Nanou E, Scheuer T, Catterall WA (2011) Molecular determinants of CaV2.1 Channel regulation by calcium- banding protein-1. J Biol Chem 286(49): 41917–23.

10

MicroRNA Profiling in Mucosal Biopsies of Eosinophilic Esophagitis Patients Pre and Post Treatment with Steroids and Relationship with mRNA Targets

Shaolei Lu[1], Vincent A. Mukkada[2], Shamlal Mangray[1], Kelly Cleveland[1], Nick Shillingford[1], Christoph Schorl[3], Alexander S. Brodsky[3], Murray B. Resnick[1]*

1 Department of Pathology and Laboratory Medicine, Rhode Island Hospital, the Alpert School of Medicine, Brown University, Providence, Rhode Island, United States of America, **2** Department of Pediatrics, Hasbro Children's Hospital, Providence, Rhode Island, United States of America, **3** Department of Molecular Biology, Cell Biology and Biochemistry, Brown University, Providence, Rhode Island, United States of America

Abstract

Background: The characterization of miRNAs and their target mRNAs involved in regulation of the immune process is an area of intense research and relatively little is known governing these processes in allergic inflammation. Here we present novel findings defining the miRNA and mRNA transcriptome in eosinophilic esophagitis (EoE), an increasing recognized allergic disorder.

Methods: Esophageal epithelial miRNA and mRNA from five paired biopsies pre- and post-treatment with glucocorticosteroids were profiled using Taqman and Affymetrix arrays. Validation was performed on additional paired biopsies, untreated EoE specimens and normal controls. Differentially regulated miRNAs and mRNAs were generated, within which miRNA-mRNA target pairs with high predicted confidence were identified.

Results: Compared to the post-glucocorticoid treated esophageal mucosa, of all the 377 miRNA sequences examined, 32 miRNAs were significantly upregulated and four downregulated in the pre-treated biopsies. MiR-214 was the most upregulated (150 fold) and miR-146b-5b, 146a, 145, 142-3p and 21 were upregulated by at least 10 fold. Out of 12 miRNAs chosen for validation by qRT-PCR, five (miR-214, 146b-5p, 146a, 142-3p and 21) were confirmed and 11 shared the same trend. When the expression of the 12 miRNAs in the EoE mucosa was compared to unrelated normal mucosa, six (miR-214, 146b-5p, 146a, 21, 203, and 489) showed similar significant changes as in the paired samples and 10 of them shared the same trend. In the same five pairs of samples used to profile miRNA, 311 mRNAs were down-regulated and 35 were up-regulated in pre-treated EoE mucosa. Among them, 164 mRNAs were identified as potential targets of differentially regulated miRNAs. Further analysis revealed that immune-related genes, targeted and non-targeted by miRNAs, were among the most important genes involved in the pathogenesis of EoE.

Conclusions: Our findings add to the accumulating body of data defining a regulatory role for miRNA in immune and allergic processes.

Editor: Sunil K. Ahuja, South Texas Veterans Health Care System and University Health Science Center San Antonio, United States of America

Funding: Molecular Pathology Core of the COBRE Center for Cancer Research Development, funded by the National Institute of General Medical Sciences of the National Institutes of Health under Award Number P20GM103421. The previous segment of this project was supported by the National Center for Research Resources (NCRR) under P20RR017695. The content is solely the responsibility of the authors and does not necessarily represent the official views of the National Institutes of Health. The funders had no role in study design, data collection and analysis, decision to publish, or preparation of the manuscript.

Competing Interests: The authors have declared that no competing interests exist.

* E-mail: mresnick@lifespan.org

Introduction

Eosinophilic esophagitis (EoE) is an increasingly recognized antigen-driven disorder of the esophagus occurring in children and adults [1]. Diagnosis of the disorder is based on clinicopathological correlation between the patient's clinical manifestations and histologic findings on mucosal biopsies. There is increasing evidence to support that EoE can be an aero-and food allergen driven process in which Th2 derived cytokines and chemokines play important roles [2]. Recently published studies have focused on the EoE transcriptome and a number of dysregulated genes influencing key cellular players such as eosinophils, lymphocytes, mast cells, esophageal epithelial cells and subepithelial myofibroblasts have been characterized [3,4].

MicroRNAs (miRNAs) are small, non-coding 19–25 nucleotide long RNAs that constitute the most abundant class of regulators of gene expression [5]. Their primary mechanism of action is post-transcriptional regulation via RNA interference leading to mRNA strand degradation or translational inhibition. MiRNAs participate in the regulation of a wide range of physiological and pathological processes including development, neoplasia, stress response and inflammation. The interplay between miRNA and mRNA is complex as each mammalian genome contains several hundred miRNAs, a single miRNA may regulate several mRNAs and each mRNA may be affected by several different miRNAs [6].

The characterization of miRNAs and their target mRNAs involved in regulation of the immune process is an area of intense research [7]. Although a number of studies have described the miRNA profile in other allergic disorders [8–12], only one recent study addressed the miRNA profile of EoE esophageal mucosa [13].

This goal of this study was to characterize the miRNA profile of well documented EoE mucosal biopsies, before and after successful treatment with glucocorticosteroids, and to correlate this profile with dysregulated mRNA identified using the same cohort. These findings were further verified on an additional cohort of biopsies from patients with EoE as opposed to normal mucosa.

Materials and Methods

Patients and Biopsies

Archival esophageal biopsies from seven pediatric patients before and after treatment for EoE were retrieved from the Department of Pathology at Rhode Island Hospital (Providence, RI). The first five pairs were used for both miRNA and mRNA profiling and all seven were used for validation (Table 1). Eight additional samples from patients newly diagnosed with EoE (from whom no post-treatment sample was available for analysis) and 10 control samples from pediatric patients with normal esophageal mucosa were also obtained (Table 1).

Patient records were reviewed by a pediatric gastroenterologist (V.M.) to ensure that the clinical characteristics of the patients fit the diagnosis of EoE. The slides were reviewed by a pathologist (M.R.) to confirm the presence or absence of EoE. Classic features of EoE consist of numerous intraepithelial eosinophils greater than 15 per high powered field (HPF) (ranging from 35 to over 100 per HPF), superficial eosinophilic microabscesses, basal layer hyperplasia and subepithelial fibrosis. The posttreatment biopsy material consisted of normal appearing squamous mucosa with only rare intraepithelial eosinophils numbering less than 2 per HPF.

A summary of the seven EoE patients' clinical information is presented in Table 1. Of the seven EoE patients evaluated prior to and following corticosteroid therapy five were males and two were females ranging from 16 months of age through 12 years. The presenting symptoms were a combination of abdominal pain, vomiting, dysphagia and chest pain in the older children and vomiting, food refusal and failure to thrive in the younger patients. Five of the seven patients tested positive for other food allergies. All of the patients responded completely to either budesonide or fluticasone.

The study was performed according to a protocol approved by the institutional review board (IRB) of Lifespan/Rhode Island Hospital. The requirement of consent was specifically waived by the IRB committee.

RNA Extraction and Quality Assessment

Eight 10 μm sections were cut from each block and mounted onto plain glass slides. If the biopsy section contained only epithelium, the sections were scraped from the slides and were ready for total RNA extraction. If biopsy sections contained sub-epithelium, the sections were deparaffinized, stained, dehydrated through graded alcohols using the Paradise FFPE reagent System (Applied Biosystems, Foster City, CA) and subjected to LCM within 2 hours of deparaffinization. About 20,000 epithelial cells were captured on LCM Macro CapSure caps (Applied Biosystems) using the Arcturus XT LCM instrument (Applied Biosystems) and the captured cells in the caps were used to extract total RNA. In either case, only the RNA from the epithelial mucosa was extracted. RecoverAll Total Nucleic Acid Extraction Kits for FFPE tissues (Ambion, Austin, TX) were used for extraction. RNA was further purified and concentrated using the RNEasy Minelute Cleanup Kit (Qiagen, Valencia, CA), and then evaluated by the Agilent Bioanalyzer using an RNA 6000 Nano or Pico LabChip (Agilent Technologies Santa Clara, CA) as described previously [14].

MicroRNA Expression Analysis by Taqman Low-density Array

Five nanograms of total RNA was reverse-transcribed using the Taqman MicroRNA Reverse Transcription Kit and the Megaplex RT primer Human Pool A (Applied Biosystems). The reverse-transcribed cDNA was then pre-amplified in 12 cycles of PCR using Taqman PreAmp Master Mix and the Megaplex PreAmp primers, Human Pool A (Applied Biosystems). The cDNAs were then diluted and loaded onto a Taqman Human miRNA Array card A (Applied Biosystems), which contains probes for 377 distinct miRNAs and a housekeeping gene (MammU6). The Array cards were run on an ABI HT7900 quantitative PCR (qPCR) instrument. Ct values were obtained for all miRNAs represented on the cards and fold changes in expression were calculated using the delta delta Ct (ddCt) method. Expression levels of MammU6 on the Array card were used as control for the purpose of ddCt calculation. The expression array data have been deposited in Gene Expression Omnibus (GEO) of National Center for Biotechnology Information (NCBI) and are accessible through GEO series accession number GSE36726.

Confirmation of miRNA Expression Data by qRT-PCR

Expression of miRNAs that demonstrated high differential expression by array card in five matched EoE cases before and after treatment were confirmed again in those same matched cases as well as in two additional matched cases. In addition, the expression of these differentially expressed miRNAs was determined in eight new samples of EoE biopsy material and compared to ten biopsies from unrelated normal esophageal epithelium (Table 1). Five nanograms of total RNA was reverse transcribed using the Taqman MicroRNA Reverse Transcription Kit and a pool of specific RT primers for the 12 miRNAs chosen for confirmation and a housekeeping gene (MammU6) (Applied Biosystems). The RT products were then pre-amplified using the same pool of the PCR primers and the pre-amplified products were used as templates for the individual Taqman miRNA assays which were run on an Agilent MX3005p qPCR instrument. Fold changes were again calculated using the ddCt method.

Amplification of Total RNA for mRNA Expression Analysis by Affymetrix Expression Array and qRT-PCR

Fifty nanograms of total RNA was amplified and reverse-transcribed into cDNA using Ovation FFPE WTA system (Nugen Technologies, San Carlos, CA). Five to ten micrograms of amplified cDNA from the amplification above was fragmented and labeled for Affymetrix array analysis using Encore Biotin Module (Nugen Technologies). Array hybridization and analysis were performed by Genomics Core Facility at the Center for Genomics and Proteomics (Brown University, Providence, RI) according to Affymetrix protocols (Affymetrix Inc, Santa Clara, CA).

Table 1. Clinical features of the eosinophilic esophagitis patients.

Patient Group	No.	Age at Diagnosis	Gender	Presenting Complaint	Food Allergy	Steroid Used
Paired EoE patients	1	11	M	Ab pain	Yes	Bud
	2	5	M	Vomiting, Food refusal	Yes	Bud
	3	2	M	Regurgitation	Yes	Bud
	4	13	F	Dysphagia, Chest pain	Yes	Bud
	5	2	F	Vomiting, FTT	No	Bud
	6	9	M	Vomiting, Food refusal	No	Flu
	7	1.3	M	FTT, Food refusal	Yes	Flu
Untreated EoE	1	5	M	Dysphagia	Yes	
	2	16	M	Dysphagia	Yes	
	3	10	M	Dysphagia, Reflux symptoms	No	
	4	2	M	Food refusal	Yes	
	5	10	M	Reflux symptoms, Ab pain	No	
	6	1.5	M	Dysphagia	Yes	
	7	15	F	Diarrhea	No	
	8	14	F	Ab Pain, Diarrhea	No	
Normal Control	1	13	F	Ab pain, Diarrhea, Wt loss	No	
	2	14	F	Ab pain, Fatigue	No	
	3	15	F	Ab pain	No	
	4	5	M	Ab Pain	No	
	5	6.5	M	Dysphagia,	Yes	
	6	17	F	Nausea	Yes	
	7	17	F	Hematochezia	No	
	8	3	F	Food refusal, Wt loss	No	
	9	16	M	Ab pain	No	
	10	8	F	Ab pain	No	

Abbreviations used: Ab, Abdominal; Wt, weight; FTT, Failure to Thrive; Bud, Budesonide; Flu, Fluticasone.

Bioinformatic Data Analysis

Affymetrix Gene 1.0 ST Array data was analyzed by Genomics Core Facility using Affymetrix Command Console and Expression Control. The expression array data have been deposited in GEO of NCBI and are accessible through GEO series accession number GSE36725.

Functional annotation was performed using Partek Genomics Suite 6.0, Partek Inc, St. Louis, MI). Differentially regulated genes are selected based on the fold-change (FC), false discovery rate (FDR), and statistical significance (P-value of Student's paired t-test). Target genes for miRNA were predicted using Ingenuity Pathway Analysis (IPA, Ingenuity Systems, Inc. Redwood City, CA). The miRNA and mRNA in a pair have to be regulated in opposite directions and their interactions are either "Experimentally observed" or exhibit "High (predicted) Confidence" as defined by IPA. Functional pathway analysis and network analysis were performed using modules within IPA.

Results

Identification of EoE Specific miRNA Transcripts

Total RNA from five pairs of EoE biospies before and after treatment was extracted and miRNA expression levels were quantified by Taqman Low Density Array. Of all the miRNAs tested by the array, 36 of them were differentially regulated based on a paired t-test P-value of less than 0.05. Five transcripts were down-regulated after treatment and 33 were up-regulated. The absolute fold changes range from 1.6 to 151. Some miRNAs share the same target sites so that a total of 31 target sites were identified from all the miRNAs. MiR-373 and miR-520e share the same target sites while miR-373 is up-regulated and miR-520e is down-regulated post treatment and thus are excluded for further analysis. The differentially regulated miRNAs are listed in Table 2, and a heatmap is presented in Figure 1 which includes 36 miRNAs and 30 target sites.

Confirmation of Individual miRNA Expression by Quantitative RT-PCR in Additional EoE Biopsies

To validate the expression of the differentially regulated miRNAs discovered by Taqman Low Density Array in Table 2, the same five paired biopsy specimens from the previous section and two additional paired biopsy specimens for a total of seven samples before and after treatment were evaluated by qRT-PCR. Twelve miRNAs that demonstrated high differential expression by Array card (the top ten upregulated and the bottom two downregulated) were chosen for validation by qRT-PCR. Five miRNAs (miR-214, miR-146b-5p, miR-146a, miR-142-3p and miR-21) were confirmed with statistical significance (P-value <0.05) and 11 of the miRNAs (except miR489) shared the same regulatory trends (Table 3 and Figure 2).

Paired biopsies from the same patient were used to profile the miRNA expression for the purpose of eliminating the inter-

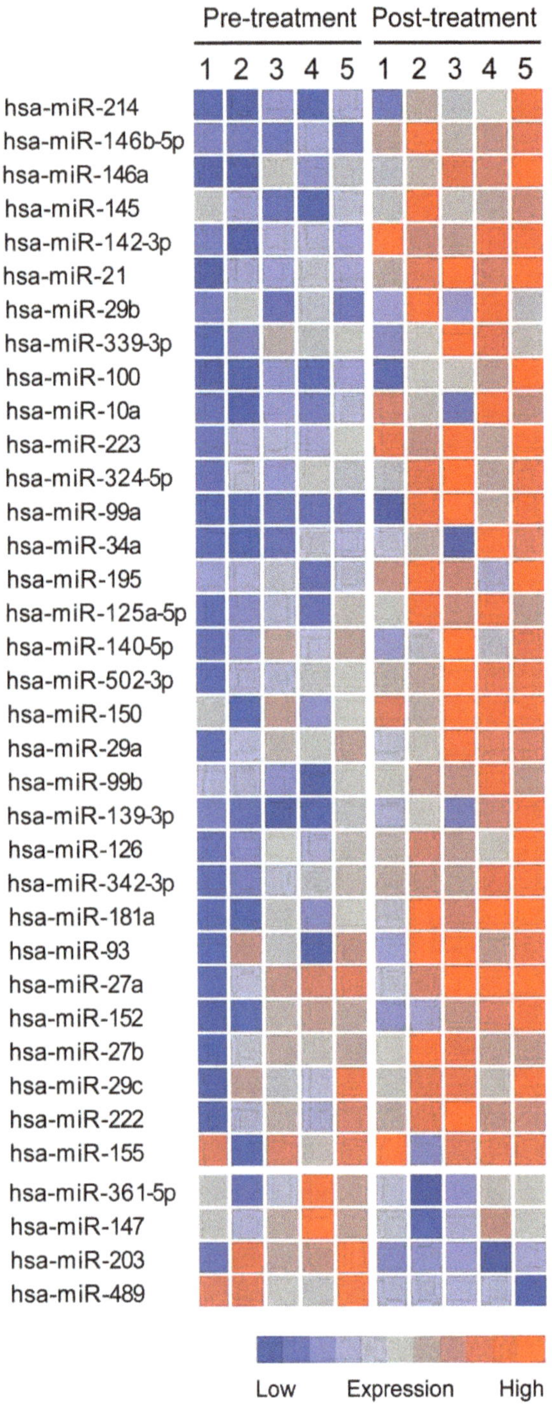

Figure 1. Steroid treatment regulates miRNA expression of EoE mucosa. The heat map illustrates miRNA expression in five paired esophageal epithelium samples of EoE purified before and after treatment. Each column represents one sample. MiRNA expression levels were stratified individually for each miRNA and each square was colorized based on the level of its expression. The overall fold changes pre- and post-treatment are listed in Table 2.

Table 2. Taqman Array data of differentially regulated miRNAs in esophageal epithelium of EoE patients before vs following treatment with glucocorticosteroids.

miRNA ID	Overlapping target sites	P-value*	Fold change**
hsa-miR-214		0.019	151.46
hsa-miR-146b-5p		0.0015	47.15
hsa-miR-146a	Same as miR-146b-5p	0.00045	39.22
hsa-miR-145		0.028	35.95
hsa-miR-142-3p		0.0017	26.55
hsa-miR-21		0.0010	11.51
hsa-miR-29b		0.015	9.43
hsa-miR-339-3p		0.018	7.79
hsa-miR-100		0.025	7.27
hsa-miR-10a		0.048	6.70
hsa-miR-223		0.0028	5.44
hsa-miR-324-5p		0.014	5.34
hsa-miR-99a	Same as miR-100	0.024	5.20
hsa-miR-34a		0.030	4.99
hsa-miR-195		0.0041	4.87
hsa-miR-125a-5p		0.019	4.75
hsa-miR-140-5p		0.017	4.64
hsa-miR-502-3p		0.0020	4.62
hsa-miR-150		0.0043	4.53
hsa-miR-29a	Same as miR-29b	0.0060	4.28
hsa-miR-99b	Same as miR-100	0.033	4.13
hsa-miR-139-3p		0.020	3.86
hsa-miR-126		0.010	3.82
hsa-miR-342-3p		0.0019	3.22
hsa-miR-181a		0.012	3.19
hsa-miR-93		0.019	2.95
hsa-miR-27a		0.0038	2.93
hsa-miR-152		0.0058	2.87
hsa-miR-27b	Same as miR-27a	0.043	2.05
hsa-miR-29c	Same as miR-29b	0.036	1.97
hsa-miR-222		0.026	1.85
hsa-miR-155		0.035	1.58
hsa-miR-361-5p		0.038	−2.22
hsa-miR-147		0.0064	−2.45
hsa-miR-203		0.036	−2.68
hsa-miR-489		0.037	−2.76

*Paired Student's T-test; comparing the expression levels before and after treatment.
**Fold change = expression levels before/after treatment.

individual variation. However, as glucocorticosteroids were the major treatment component in our patient's cohort, miRNA expression following treatment may be related in part to the treatment effect. To test this hypothesis, we compared the miRNA expression of the mucosal biopsies from a new set of eight EoE patients with those from normal mucosa of ten additional pediatric esophageal biopsy samples from patients without any history of EoE. As shown in Table 3 and Figure 3, six out of same 12 miRNAs (miR-214, miR-146b-5p, miR-146a, miR-21, miR-203, and miR489) showed similar significant differential expression as in the paired samples and 10 of them (except for miR-10a and miR-29b) shared the same regulatory trends.

Table 3. qRT-PCR validation of differentially regulated miRNAs in esophageal epithelium of EoE patients pre-vs post-treatment and untreated EoE patients vs normal control.

miRNA	Taqman Array		qRT-PCR Verification			
			Pre- vs post treatment		EoE vs Normal	
	Fold Change	p-value	Fold Change	p-value	Fold Change	p-value
hsa-miR-214	151.45	0.019	26.62	0.02	2.02	0.078
hsa-miR-146b-5p	47.15	0.0015	18.79	0.0031	5.4	0.004
hsa-miR-146a	39.22	0.00045	9.89	0.0022	3.1	0.033
hsa-miR-145	35.95	0.028	3.15	0.079	1.73	0.1
hsa-miR-142-3p	26.55	0.0017	8.61	0.019	1.3	0.12
hsa-miR-21	11.51	0.001	6.67	0.006	4.39	0.003
hsa-miR-29b	9.43	0.015	13.04	0.09	0.97	0.24
hsa-miR-339-3p	7.78	0.018	1.92	0.31	1.21	0.28
hsa-miR-100	7.27	0.025	1.58	0.38	0.93	0.25
hsa-miR-10a	6.7	0.048	1.03	0.49	0.38	0.062
hsa-miR-203	0.37	0.036	0.237	0.072	0.19	0.0006
hsa-miR-489	0.36	0.037	5.27	0.21	0.13	0.042

Bioinformatic Analysis of miRNA Targets

The major role of miRNA is to regulate mRNA expression at the transcriptional and translational level. We wished to determine how much of the mRNA expression in EoE is influenced by miRNAs. To profile the global mRNA changes in EoE, an Affymetrix GeneChip based mRNA gene profiling was conducted on five paired EoE biopsies before and after treatment. Total RNA was extracted from FFPE tissue sections and hybridized to Human Gene ST 1.0 Genechips. The Principle Component Analysis of data demonstrated that gene expression data from biopsies of the same status are highly correlated with each other (Figure 4). To screen for differentially regulated genes, FC >2, FDR<0.05 and P-value <0.05 were used as criteria. Of all the probes on the chip, 415 probes passed the screen resulting in 346 differentially regulated genes, of which 311 genes were down-regulated and 35 genes were up-regulated in EoE. Among them, 164 genes were identified as potential targets of miRNAs listed in Table 2 under stringent conditions using Ingenuity Pathway Analysis. Table 4 lists the mRNAs with the highest fold change for each miRNA. Many of the mRNAs can be targeted by more than one miRNA. A full list of all differentially regulated mRNAs regardless of fold change is available in Table S1. Of these mRNAs, 162 were down-regulated and 2 were up-regulated. The remaining 184 genes out of 346 differentially regulated genes are not targeted by miRNA.

Information regarding the miRNA-mRNA pairs is incorporated into a pathway network analysis on the 346 differentially regulated genes using IPA program. One of the top pathway networks IPA revealed is a gene regulatory network of more than 24 genes involving "inflammatory response", "cell-to-cell

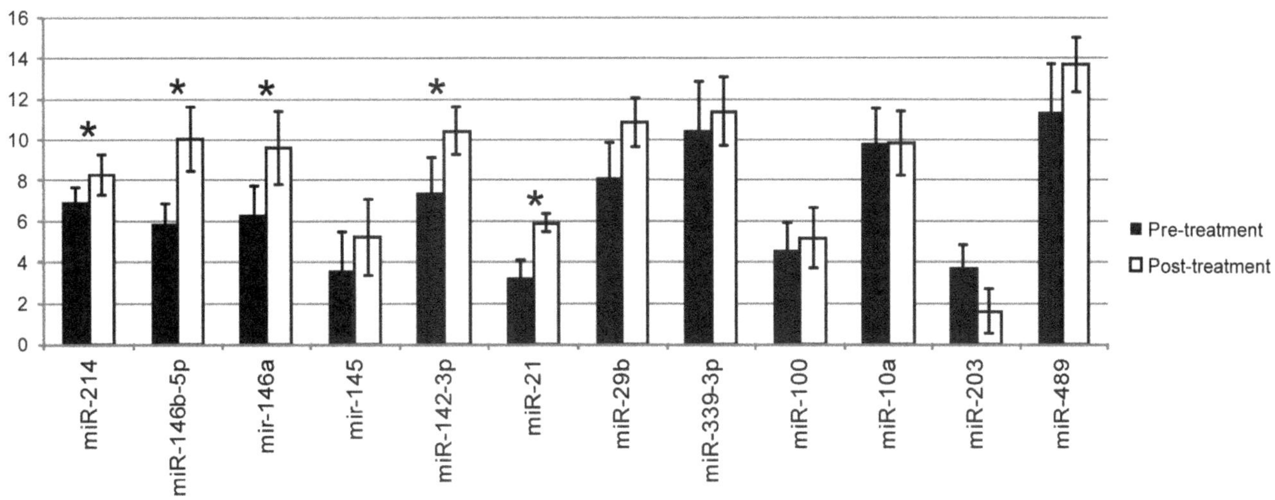

Figure 2. Treatment-induced miRNA expression changes validated by qRT-PCR. Delta Ct values are used to represent selected miRNA expression levels in esophageal epithelium of 7 paired EoE patients pre- vs post-treatment (5 pairs used in miRNA profiling and 2 additional pairs; Table 1). Asterisks indicate statistical significance ($P<0.05$).

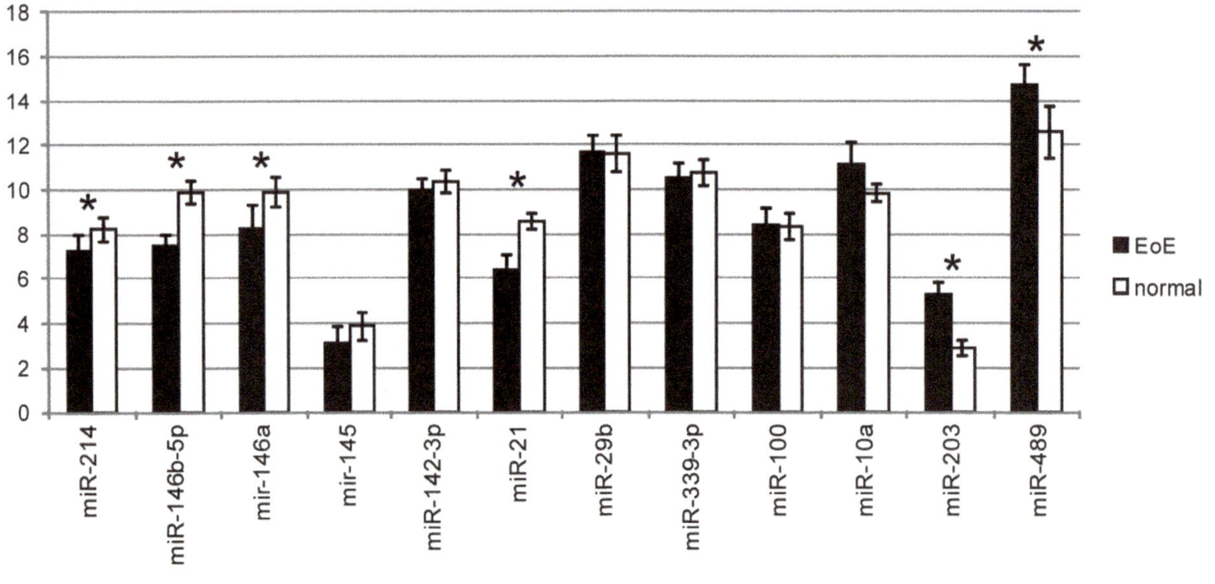

Figure 3. EoE-related miRNA expression changes determined by qRT-PCR. Delta Ct values are used to represent selected miRNAs expression levels in esophageal epithelium of 8 untreated EoE patients versus 10 normal epithelium of control patients (Table 1). Asterisks indicate statistical significance ($P<0.05$).

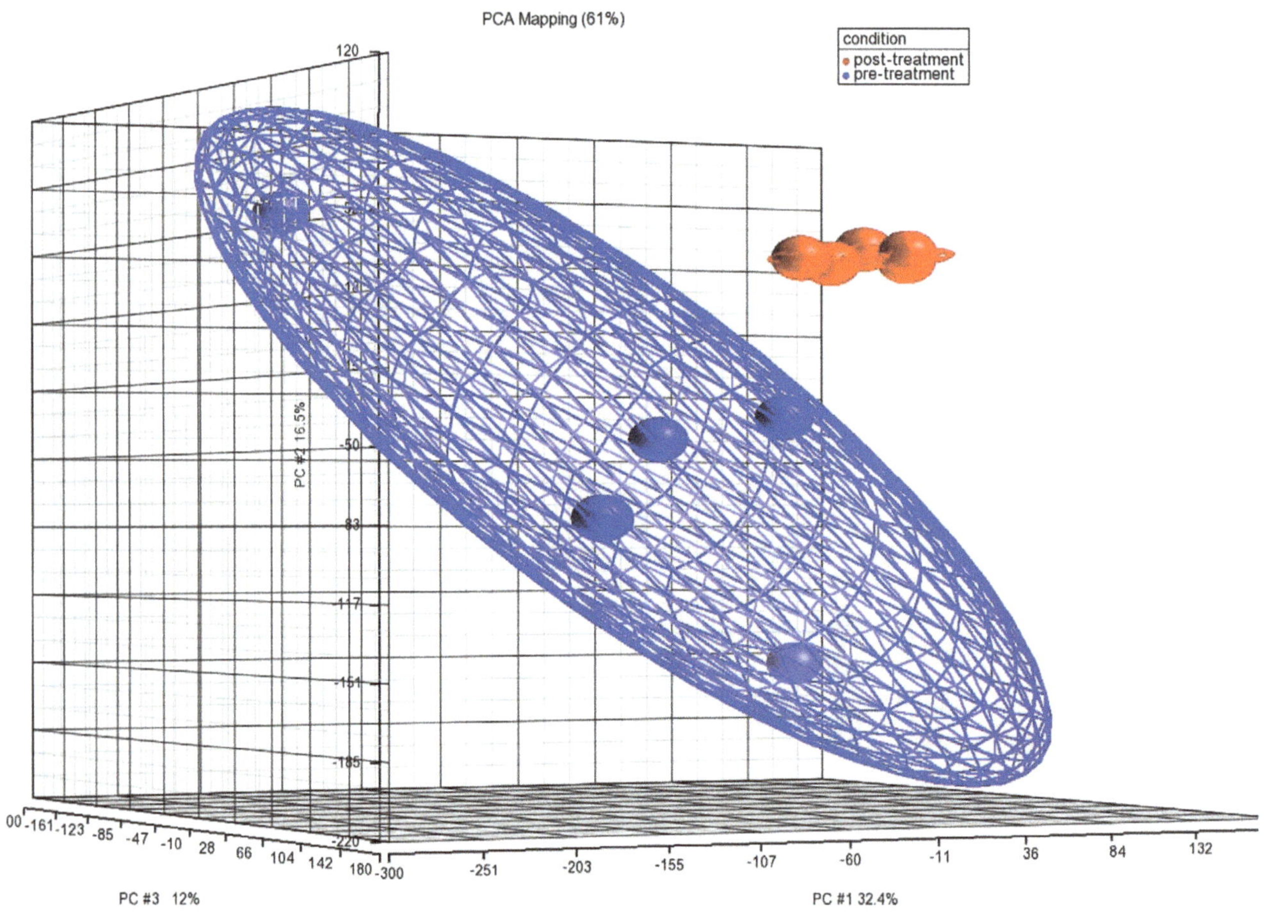

Figure 4. Principle component analysis of mRNA expression before and after treatment of EoE. In this 3-dimentional plot of the first three principle components of all ten samples, samples of the same treatment status were grouped together. Five pre-treatment samples (Blue) and five post-treatment samples (Red) were clearly separated from each other.

Table 4. A total of 164 mRNAs targeted by 31 miRNAs (25 target sites)* differentially regulated in EoE epithelium.

miRNAs and Target mRNAs	Fold Change
hsa-miR-203	**−2.68**
ALOX15	10.30
hsa-miR-147	**−2.45**
CYP2S1,	2.03
hsa-miR-10a	**6.70**
ZFAND5, CNST, RAP2A, ACTG1, TIAM1	−2.78 ~ −2.00
hsa-miR-125a-5p	**4.75**
ETNK2, IL1RN, PRDM1, B4GALT1, GRHL1, TRPS1, FAM129B, RIT1, DOCK3, MEGF9	−4.88 ~ −2.08
hsa-miR-126	**3.83**
TOM1	2.67
hsa-miR-140-5p	**4.64**
PHACTR2, STRADB, SNX16, RALA, RIOK3, C15orf29, PRDM1, MYO6, CAMK2N1, MRPS10	−4.49 ~ −2.24
hsa-miR-142-3p	**26.55**
MGLL, C18orf25, USP6NL, CCDC6, RAB2A, TIPARP, HECTD1, KAT2B, WASL, TWF1, C1orf9	−3.00 ~ −2.00
hsa-miR-145	**35.95**
PADI1, BNIP3, PHACTR2, SNX24, KIF21A, TSPAN6, SAMD5, SRGAP1, TMOD3, AIM1	−6.97 ~ −2.99
hsa-miR-146a and miR-146b-5p	**47.15 ~ 39.22**
S100A12, ZNF117, MYO6, CCDC6, IL1RAP, IL1RL2	−6.70 ~ −2.1
hsa-miR-150	**4.53**
SYNPO2L, PDIA6, EREG, TOM1, CNST, TRPS1, ADIPOR2, CAST, AIFM2, FOPNL	−3.63 ~ −2.20
hsa-miR-152	**2.87**
RMND5A, PHACTR2, EMP1, MXD1, STRADB, B4GALT5, MOSPD1, C18orf25, CLOCK, KIAA0232	−4.82 ~ −2.61
hsa-miR-155	**1.58**
ETNK2, ZNF431, PPL, WNK1, TRPS1, CAB39, PEA15, PTN, ZNF714, TWF1	−4.88 ~ −2.03
hsa-miR-181a	**3.19**
PHACTR2, SASH1, PHLDA1, MOSPD1, SRGAP1, C12orf29, UBL3, PHACTR4, EREG, RALA	−4.49 ~ −2.83
hsa-miR-195	**4.87**
ALOX12, PHACTR2, CGNL1, KIF21A, STRADB, RASGEF1B, TUFT1, PDIA6, SNX16, TRIP10	−8.65 ~ −2.92
hsa-miR-21	**11.51**
IL12A, RMND5A, SASH1, PELI1, TOR1AIP2, SECISBP2L, HIPK3, RFFL, TIAM1	−6.25 ~ −2.00
hsa-miR-214	**151.46**
ABLIM3, DOCK9, ARHGAP10, PIM1, TRPS1, CPEB4, RAB5B, CAPN5, TWF1, KIF1B	−5.08 ~ −2.01
hsa-miR-222	**1.85**
PHACTR4, C18orf25, INPP4B, ZFAND5, KIAA1370, TRPS1, LYPLA1, TIPARP, TP53BP2, MEGF9	−2.89 ~ −2.08
hsa-miR-223	**5.44**
NAMPT, SNX24, MSMO1, PRDM1, CDS1, SECISBP2L, TWF1, ZNF365	−4.01 ~ −2.02
hsa-miR-27a and miR-27b	**2.94 ~ 2.05**
ENDOU, BNIP3, RMND5A, CRISP2, LPIN1, CCNYL1, CAB39L, CPPED1, CNN3, WNK1	−6.94 ~ −2.81
hsa-miR-29a, miR-29b and miR-29c	**9.43 ~ 4.28**
PHACTR2, TUBB2A, EMP1, SNX24, MXD1, AMFR, AIM1, RIOK3, WDR26, DSC2	−4.49 ~ −2,53
hsa-miR-342-3p	**3.22**
RMND5A, SYNPO2L, CAMK2N1, CPEB4, C20orf11, TIAM1	−7.19 ~ −2.00
hsa-miR-34a	**4.99**
ABLIM1,TOM1,CLOCK,NCOA1,AREG, PEA15, MARCH5, DOCK3,RNF169, B4GALR5, AIM1	−2.92 ~ −2.99
hsa-miR-502-3p	**4.62**
B4GALT5,AIM1	−3.36 ~ −2.99
hsa-miR-93	**2.95**
MXD1, SASH1, NPAS2, HIF1A, SLC16A9, MSMO1, SNX9, MGLL, SNX16, TRIP10, EREG	−3.96 ~ −2.99
hsa-miR-99a, miR-9b and miR-100	**5.20**

Table 4. Cont.

miRNAs and Target mRNAs	Fold Change
GRHL1, PPP1CB	−2.58 ~ −2.18

*Only up to 10 mRNAs with the highest fold change are listed under each miRNA.
**miR-339-3p, miR-489, miR-361-5p, miR-324-5p, and miR-139-3p do not have predicted targets in combined gene list.

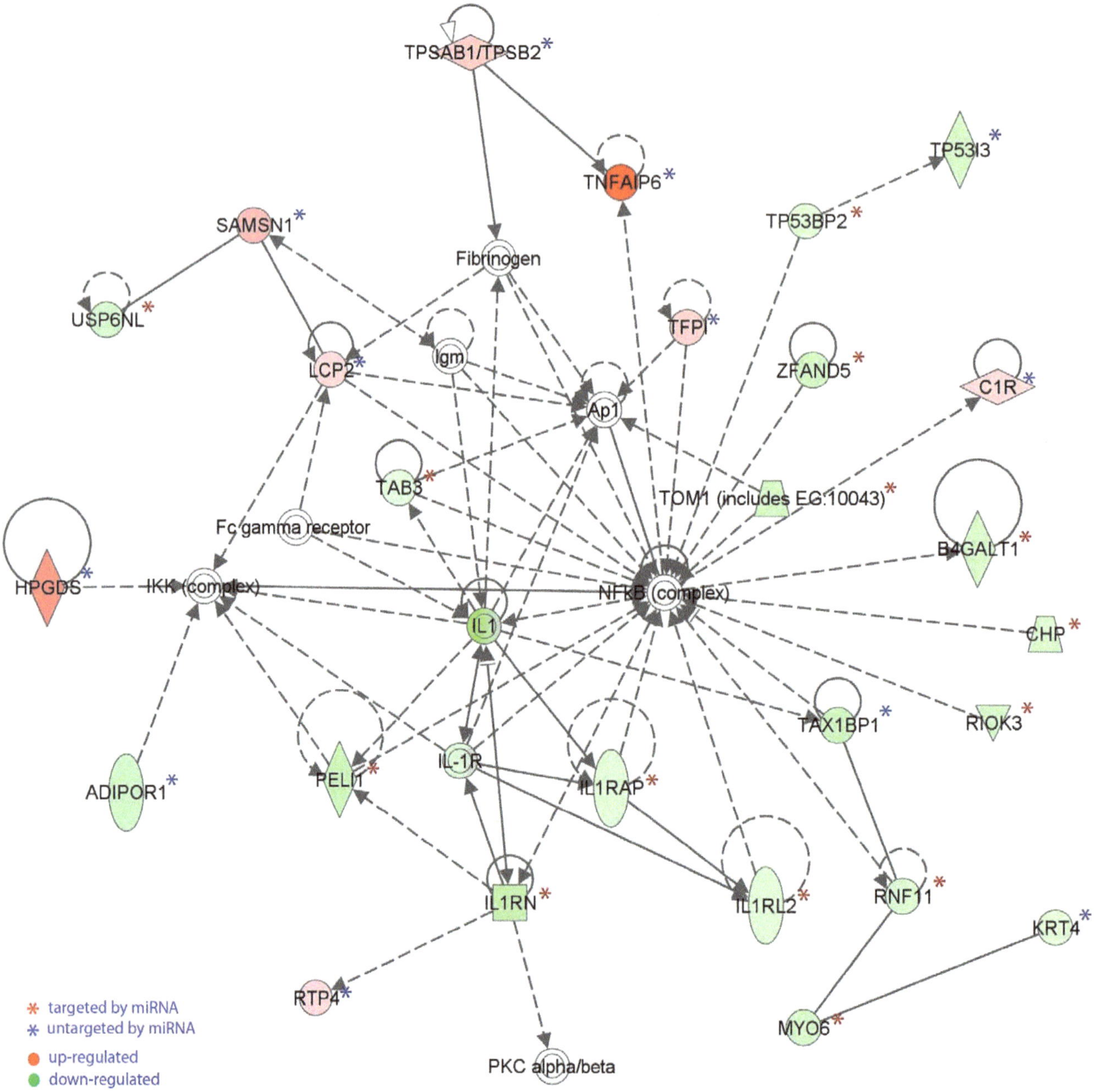

Figure 5. Functional pathway network analysis of 346 differentially regulated mRNAs. One of the primary pathway networks is associated with network functions of "Inflammatory Response, Cell-To-Cell Signaling and Interaction, Hematological System Development and Function".

Table 5. List of 69 Immune related genes targeted by differentially regulated miRNAs in EoE epithelium.

ID	p-value	Fold Change	ID	p-value	Fold Change
ALOX15	0.0012	10.30	B4GALT1	0.00098	−2.59
ALOX12	3.4E-05	−8.65	NCOA1	0.00044	-2.56
S100A12	0.00014	−6.70	DSC2	0.00047	−2.53
IL12A	5.0E-05	−6.25	PIM1	4.3E-05	−2.44
ETNK2	7.7E-05	−4.89	CNST	0.00021	−2.42
LPIN1	6.4E-05	−4.60	KIAA1370	0.00038	−2.41
PHACTR2	4.7E-05	−4.49	TRPS1	0.00013	−2.39
TUBB2A	0.00036	−4.19	CCDC6	1.9E-05	−2.38
NAMPT	0.0011	−4.01	ADIPOR2	0.00042	−2.35
SNX24	0.00017	−4.00	PSD3	0.00049	−2.35
MXD1	0.0012	−3.96	CPEB4	0.00092	−2.33
NPAS2	8.7E-05	−3.58	CYP4F3	1.2E-05	−2.35
CPPED1	0.00096	−3.53	AREG	0.0004	−2.32
HIF1A	0.00020	−3.45	CAST	0.0012	−2.31
SC4MOL	0.00023	−3.33	RAB2A	5.1E-05	−2.30
SAMD5	0.00028	−3.24	ACTG1	0.00027	−2.22
IL1RN	0.00026	−3.16	GNG12	3.8E-05	−2.20
AMFR	2.6E-06	−3.13	PPP1CB	0.00078	−2.18
PELI1	0.00033	−3.13	EPB41L4A	1.7E-06	−2.15
CNN3	0.00064	−3.09	MARCH5	0.00096	−2.14
PDIA6	0.00037	−3.01	DOCK3	0.00024	−2.14
MGLL	6.8E-07	−3.00	WASL	0.00025	−2.12
ABLIM1	4.2E-05	−2.92	GABARAPL2	0.00037	−2.11
UBL3	0.00044	−2.90	IL1RAP	8.0E-05	−2.10
EREG	0.00014	−2.89	RAB5B	0.00077	−2.10
C18orf25	0.00063	−2.86	STK39	0.0011	−2.08
PFKFB3	7.6E-05	−2.84	ZNF714	0.00096	−2.08
INPP4B	0.00014	−2.84	PI4K2A	0.00047	−2.06
RALA	0.00070	−2.83	PLEKHA6	0.00013	−2.06
WNK1	5.16E-06	−2.81	ZNF365	0.00035	−2.02
KRT7	8.21E-06	−2.69	KIF1B	0.00051	−2.01
PLEKHM1	0.00025	−2.69	RNF169	0.00080	−2.00
RIOK3	0.00038	−2.65	IL13RA1	0.0010	−2.00
CLOCK	0.00089	−2.62	TIAM1	8.0E-05	−2.00
PRDM1	0.00063	−2.59			

*Genes related to "hypersensitivity response", "immunological disease", "inflammatory disease", and "inflammatory response" by IPA annotation are selected to represent immune related genes.

Table 6. List of 59 Immune related genes not targeted by differentially regulated miRNAs in the esophageal epithelium of EoE patients.

ID	p-value	Fold Change	ID	p-value	Fold Change
TNFAIP6	0.00033	39.23	WNT5A	0.00099	−3.32
CPA3	7.0E-05	7.70	SCNN1B	5.2E-05	−3.28
HPGDS	3.0E-05	5.87	TMEM57	0.00011	−3.17
SAMSN1	0.00017	3.82	GNG4	0.0011	−2.97
SERPINE2	0.00046	3.15	TAX1BP1	0.00025	−2.94
TPSAB1	0.00069	3.02	MAPK3	1.4E-05	−2.92
TFPI	0.00019	2.82	UACA	0.00011	−2.81
LAPTM5	0.00091	2.6	ZNF92	9.2E-06	−2.63
LCP2	0.00016	2.41	ST3GAL4	1.5E-06	−2.62
CNTN4	0.00020	2.30	ADIPOR1	0.00015	−2.58
HIST1H4K	0.00077	2.24	EFNA5	0.00076	−2.57
C1R	0.00039	2.23	ZDHHC21	0.0012	−2.54
HDC	0.00025	2.21	S100A9	0.00089	−2.36
IGFBP3	0.00097	2.18	NHSL1	0.00016	−2.34
LOX	0.00016	2.15	DOPEY2	0.00031	−2.33
B2M	0.00088	2.08	CD68	0.00046	−2.29
IFITM3	0.00043	2.03	GNA15	0.00041	−2.22
SLURP1	0.000062	−8.13	DYNLL1	0.00024	−2.21
SFTA2	0.00011	−7.87	S100A14	6.6E-05	−2.18
CRYAB	0.00032	−5.74	DSG1	0.00034	−2.15
IL18	0.00015	−5.11	AHCY	0.00036	−2.15
CST6	0.0012	−4.25	RALB	0.00038	−2.14
PSCA	0.00029	−4.14	GPT2	0.0011	−2.12
CXCR2	0.000053	−4.12	PARD3	0.00013	−2.12
ACPP	0.00017	−3.98	LGMN	0.00082	−2.11
C3orf67	1.9E-07	−3.90	PLD1	0.00055	−2.08
CDA	0.001	−3.71	PCSK5	0.00071	−2.08
RHCG	0.00033	−3.7	OSTF1	0.00026	−2.04
MTHFD1L	0.00092	−3.51	CDK7	0.00082	−2.01
TPRG1	0.00081	−3.43			

*Genes related to "hypersensitivity response", "immunological disease", "inflammatory disease", and "inflammatory response" by IPA annotation are selected to represent immune related genes.

signalling and interaction", and "hematological system development and function" (Figure 5). Within this network 14 genes are targeted by miRNAs while 11 are not targeted. Interestingly genes involving the IL1 cytokine pathway are exclusively targeted by miRNAs (Figure 5).

Given the finding that both targeted genes and non-targeted genes are equally represented in the network (Figure 5), we conducted a full search of immune-related genes in the 346 differentially regulated genes. Indeed, immune-related genes were identified in both groups. Out of 164 targeted genes, 69 of them are related to the immune process, of which one gene was up-regulated and the rest were down-regulated (Table 5). Out of 184 untargeted mRNAs, 59 are immune related genes (Table 6).

Discussion

Little is known regarding miRNA regulatory pathways in allergic inflammation in general [8–12] and this is the second report to address differential miRNA expression in EoE [13]. This study is unique in that it correlated miRNA and mRNA expression in the same patient population before and after treatment with glucocorticosteroids, the tissue sampling was restricted to the epithelial layer and it was performed on archival formalin-fixed paraffin embedded tissues.

In our study 36 miRNAs were differentially expressed (32 upregulated and 4 downregulated) in EoE before and following treatment including 25 miRNAs at a level of 3 fold or more.

Differential miRNA expression was correlated with differential mRNA expression in the same patients: 311 genes were found to be downregulated and 35 upregulated when comparing the pretreated to posttreated samples. Several of the mRNAs identified have been shown to play a role in EoE or in other allergic disorders. In general the results of this study are more heavily weighted towards miRNAs with increased expression levels and mRNAs with decreased expression levels in the inflammatory state as opposed to the treated samples. The opposing direction of the miRNA and mRNA expression is in line with miRNA's regulatory role on gene expression [5].

In an attempt to better define how much of the differential regulation of miRNAs in EoE was related to the effect of the glucocorticosteroid treatment on the allergic process as opposed to the allergic process alone we examined the expression levels of the miRNAs originally detected to those in additional material from EoE patients compared to control tissue from histologically normal appearing esophageal mucosa. The fold changes as detected by qPCR were significantly higher in the pre vs posttreatment tissue than in the EoE vs control tissue and not all of the qRT-PCR differential expression reached statistical significance. The differential expression of certain of these miRNAs such as miR-214, miR-142-3p and miR-29b appear to be influenced much more significantly by the treatment as opposed to the allergic process alone.

Another important issue is to determine which cell types are responsible for the differential expression of miRNAs in this study. We purposely dissected areas of epithelium only and avoided submucosal stromal tissue in many cases employing LCM for this purpose. In addition to eosinophils the squamous epithelium in EoE also exhibits increased infiltration by T-cells and mast cells [2]. Based on a recent study by Allantaz et al which determined the expression profile of human immune subsets, the only miRNA that was differentially regulated in our study and found to be differentially regulated by immune cells was miR-223 [15]. In Allantaz's study miR-223 was overexpressed in neutrophils, eosinophils and monocytes [15] whereas in our study there was a five fold increase in biopsies of EoE patients prior to treatment. Thus one may speculate that increased miR-223 in EoE is due to the intraepithelial inflammatory population. Interestingly miR-223 was also shown to be overexpressed in squamous cell carcinomas of the esophagus suggesting that the increased epithelial proliferation characteristic of EoE may also be a contributor to the overexpression of miR-223 [16]. Unfortunately although differential miRNA expression is an area of significant ongoing research in neoplastic processes of the esophagus [16–17] little is known regarding baseline expression of miRNAs by normal squamous epithelium or by actively proliferating esophageal epithelium characteristic of EoE.

A number of miRNAs that were found to be differentially regulated in this study were implicated by others to play a role in allergic and inflammatory disorders [8–13]. There is considerable overlap between the miRNAs that we identified here and those published in the recent report by Lu et al [13], however, a number of differentially miRNAs such as miR-214, miR-145, miR-100 and miR10a were uniquely identified in our study. Furthermore miR-214 was the most significantly elevated miRNA upregulated in EoE patients before treatment. These differences may be attributed to the fact that our study was restricted to harvesting RNA from the epithelial layer alone, at times employing LCM. The submucosal esophageal tissue of EoE patients is rich in inflammatory cells and myofibroblasts thus diluting the influence of epithelial associated mRNA and miRNA. Our study was also based on material that was paraffin embedded and formalin fixed and the initial screen was performed on pretreated vs post-treated biopsy material from the same patient to avoid the variability of comparing pathological material from one source to control tissue from a different source.

Although miR-214 has been implicated in a number of neoplastic disorders, to date a role for miR-214 in inflammatory or allergic disorders has not been described. MiR-214 has been found to be elevated in models of renal injury and may play a role in epithelial mesenchymal transition [18,19]. The epithelial mesenchymal transformation (EMT) pathway likely plays an important role in the subepithelial fibrosis characteristic of airway disease in asthma [20,21]. This pathway might also be involved in the generation of subepithelial fibrosis typically seen in EoE [22–24]. A recent report by Kagawalla et al supports a role for EMT in EoE [25].

Both miR-146a and miR-146b were markedly increased in the epithelium of EoE patients. MiR-146a has been shown to regulate several physiological and pathophysiological pathways in hematopoietic cells as reviewed by Hua et al [26]. MiR-146a has been shown to be induced by the inflammatory mediators TNF-α, IL-8 and IL-1-β in gastric epithelial cells by *Helicobacter pylori* [27] and is regulated by NF-κb [28]. Levels of IL-8 and TNF-β have recently been shown to be increased in pediatric EoE [29]. MiR146b has also been recently found to be upregulated in a murine model of asthma [11].

Increased expression of miR-21 was detected in both the pretreated EoE group as opposed to the post-treated group and in the EoE group as oppose to normal controls. MiR-21 is involved in the regulation of many different pathways and is considered an "oncomir" due to its widespread role in neoplasia. In allergic disorders miR-21 has been shown to be involved in the regulation of allergic lung inflammation by targeting IL12a (IL-12p35) a cytokine that contributes to polarization of Th cells toward Th2 cells [9]. Our finding of a six fold decrease in IL12a mRNA in this study further supports the role of IL12a as a key mediator of the allergic response [30]. MiR-21 has also been shown to play a role via TGF-β1 in pulmonary and renal fibrosis [31,32]. One can speculate that miR-21 plays a similar role in the subepithelial fibrosis seen in EoE. MiR-21 also acts on the S100A12 protein whose gene was down regulated six fold. Seeing that S100A12 has been shown to play a key role in inflammation [33] it would be expected that S100A12 is downregulated in EoE. In addition S100A12 has also been shown to be highly expressed in differentiated esophageal epithelial cells as opposed to basal and proliferating cells [34]. EoE is associated with pronounced basal layer hyperplasia and proliferation so that the levels of S100A12 protein should be lower in EoE as opposed to normal epithelium.

MiR-203 down regulated three fold targets the ALOX15 gene (upregulated 10 fold) which encodes for arachidonate 15 lipoxygenase (15-LO). The 15-LO protein is upregulated in asthma [35] and is expressed both by eosinophils as well as airway epithelial cells [36–38].

As the human genome may encode over 1000 miRNAs, which may target about 60% of mammalian genes, several immune related genes which were dysregulated in our cohort had no complementary regulatory miRNA identified. Of these genes several have been shown to play a role in the pathophysiology of allergic disorders including EoE. TNFAIP6 the most significantly elevated mRNA in the pretreated biopsies as well as CPA a mast cell derived gene were both shown to be significantly upregulated in a previous study of EoE [3]. Functional network analysis in Figure 5 highlighted an NFκB-centered pathway involving both TNFAIP6 and genes in the IL-1 pathway which includes IL-RAP, IL1RN and IL1RL2. All three IL-1 related genes are down-regulated and are targets of differentially regulated miRNAs. As shown in Table 5 and 6, both targeted genes and untargeted genes contain a substantial amount of immune-related genes, indicating miRNAs and mRNAs together build sophisticated interactions contributing to the pathogenesis of EoE.

Our data implicate several miRNAs and miRNA-MRNA gene sets expressed in the epithelial layer in EoE. The identified gene expression changes provide additional diagnostic and therapeutic targets for EoE and other eosinophilic epithelial diseases.

Supporting Information

Table S1 The full list of 346 differentially regulated mRNAs targeted by differentially regulated miRNAs.

Author Contributions

Conceived and designed the experiments: MR VM SL. Performed the experiments: MR KC. Analyzed the data: SL MR KC VM CS AB SM. Contributed reagents/materials/analysis tools: SM NS CS AB. Wrote the paper: MR VM SL KC.

References

1. Liacouras CA, Furuta GT, Hirano I, Atkins D, Attwood SE, et al. (2011) Eosinophilic esophagitis: updated consensus recommendations for children and adults. J Allergy Clin Immunol 128: 3–20.
2. Abonia JP, Rothenberg ME (2012) Eosinophilic esophagitis: rapidly advancing insights. Annu Rev Med 63: 421–434.
3. Blanchard C, Wang N, Stringer KF, Mishra A, Fulkerson PC, et al. (2006) Eotaxin-3 and a uniquely conserved gene-expression profile in eosinophilic esophagitis. J Clin Invest 116: 536–547.
4. Blanchard C, Mingler MK, Vicario M, Abonia JP, Wu YY, et al. (2007) IL-13 involvement in eosinophilic esophagitis: transcriptome analysis and reversibility with glucosteroids. J Allergy Clin Immunol 120: 1292–1300.
5. Bartel DP (2004) MicroRNAs: genomics, biogenesis, mechanism and function. Cell 116: 281–297.
6. Griffiths-Jones S, Saini HK, van Dongen S, Enright AJ (2008) miRBase: tools for micrRNA genomics. Nucleic Acids Res 36: D154–158.
7. O'Connell RM, Rao DS, Baltimore D (2012) MicroRNA regulation of inflammatory responses. Annu Rev Immunol 30: 295–312.
8. Mattes J, Collison A, Plank M, Phipps S, Foster PS (2009) Antagonism of microRNA-126 suppresses the effector function of TH2 cells and the development of allergic airways disease. Proc Natl Acad Sci USA 106: 18704–18709.
9. Lu TX, Munitz A, Rothenberg ME (2009) MicroRNA-21 is up-regulated in allergic airway inflammation and regulates IL-12p35 expression. J Immunol 182: 4994–5002.
10. Collison A, Herbert C, Siegle JS, Mattes J, Foster PS, et al. (2011) Altered expression of microRNA in the airway wall in chronic asthma: miR-126 as a potential therapeutic target. BMC Pulm Med 11: 29.
11. Collison A, Mattes J, Plank M, Foster PS (2011) Inhibition of house dust mite-induced allergic airways disease by antagonism of microRNA-145 is comparable to glucocorticoid treatment. J Allergy Clin Immunol 128: 160–167.
12. Garbacki N, Di Valentin E, Huynh-Thu VA, Geurts P, Irrthum A, et al. (2011) MicroRNAs profiling in murine models of acute and chronic asthma: A relationship with mRNAs targets. PloS ONE 6: e16509.
13. Lu TX, Sherrill JD, Wen T, Plassard AJ, Besse JA, et al. (2012) MicroRNA signature in patients with eosinophilic esophagitis, reversibility with glucocorticoids and assessment as disease markers. J Allergy Clin Immunol 129: 1064–1075.
14. Resnick MB, Sabo E, Meitner PA, Kim SS, Cho Y, et al. (2006) Global analysis of the human gastric epithelial transcriptome altered by Helicobacter pylori eradication in vitro. Gut 55: 1717–1724.
15. Allantaz F, Cheng DT, Bergauer T, Ravindran P, Rossier MF, et al. (2012) Expression profiling of human immune cell subsets identifies miRNA-mRNA regulatory relationships correlated with cell type specific expression. PLoS ONE 7: 29979.
16. Mathé EA, Nguyen GH, Bowman ED, Zhao Y, Budhu A, et al. (2009) MicroRNA expression in squamous cell carcinoma and adenocarcinoma of the esophagus: associations with survival. Clin Cancer Res 15: 6192–6200.
17. Kan T, Meltzer SJ (2009) MicroRNAs in Barrett's esophagus and esophageal adenocarcinoma. Curr Opin Pharmacol 9: 727–732.
18. Godwin JG, Ge X, Stephen K, Jurisch A, Tullius SG, et al. (2010) Identification of a microRNA signature of renal ischemia perfusion injury. Proc Natl Acad Sci USA 107: 14339–14344.
19. Denby L, Ramdas V, McBride MW, Wang J, Robinson H, et al. (2011) miR-21 and miR-214 are consistently modulated during renal injury in rodent models. Am J Pathol 179: 661–672.
20. Hackett TL, Warner SM, Stefanowicz D, Shaheen F, Pechkovsky DV, et al. (2009) Induction of epithelial-mesenchymal transition in primary airway epithelial cells from patients with asthma by transforming growth factor beta. Am J Respir Crit Care Med 180: 122–133.
21. Johnson JR, Roos A, Berg t, Nord M, Fuxe J (2011) Chronic respiratory aeroallergen exposure to mice induces epithelial-mesenchymal transition in the larger airways. PLoS One 6: e16175.
22. Straumann A, Spichtin HP, Grize L (2003) Natural history of primary eosinophilic esophagitis: a follow-up of 30 adult patients for up to 11.5 years. Gastroenterology 125: 1660–1669.
23. Aceves SS, Newbury RO, Dohil R, Bastian JF, Broide DH (2007)Esophageal remodeling in pediatric eosinophilic esophagitis. J Allergy Clin Immunol. 119: 206–212.
24. Chehade M, Sampson HA, Morotti RA, Magid MS (2007) Esophageal subepithelial fibrosis in children with eosinophilic esophagitis. J Pediatr Gastroenterol Nutr 45: 319–328.
25. Kagalwalla AF, Akhtar N, Woodruff SA, Rea B, Masterson JC, et al. (2012) Eosinophilic Esophagitis: Epithelial Mesenchymal Transition Contributes to Esophageal Remodeling and Reverses With Treatment. Journal of Allergy and Clinical Immunology 129: 1387–1396.
26. Hua Z, Chun W, Fang-Yuan C (2011) MicroRNA-146a and hemopoietic disorders. Int J Hematol 94: 224–229.
27. Li N, Xu X, Xiao B, Zhu ED, Li BS, et al. (2011) H. pylori related proinflammatory cytokines contribute to the induction of miR-146a in human gastric epithelial cells. Mol Biol Rep 39: 4655–4661.
28. Taganov KD, Boldin MP, Chang KJ, Baltimore D (2006) NF-kappa-B-dependent induction of microRNA miR-146, an inhibitor targeted to signalling proteins of innate immune responses. Proc Natl Acad Sci USA 103: 12481–12486.
29. Persad R, Huynh HQ, Hao L, Ha JR, Sergi C, et al. (2012) Angiogenic remodeling in pediatric eosinophilic esophagitis is associated with increased levels of VEGFA, angiogenin, IL-8 and activation of the TNF-a-NFkB pathway. J Pediatr Gastroenterol Nutr Feb 10 EPUB.
30. Gavett Sh, O'Hearn DJ, Huang SK, Finkelman FD, Wills-Karp M (1995) Interleukin 12 inhibits antigen induced airway hyperresponsiveness, inflammation, and Th2 cytokine expression in mice. J Exp Med 182: 1527–1536.
31. Liu G, Friggeri A, Yang Y, Milosevic J, Ding Q, et al. (2010) miR-21 mediated fibrogenic activation of pulmonary fibroblasts and lung fibrosis. J Exp Med 207: 1589–1597.
32. Zarjou A, Yang S, Abraham E, Agarwal A, Liu G (2011) Identification of a microRNA signature in renal fibrosis: role of miR-21. Am J Physiol Renal Physiol 301: 793–801.
33. Pieztsch J, Hoppmann S (2009) Human S100A12: a novel key player in inflammation? Amino Acids 36: 381–389.
34. Sato N, Hitomi J (2002) S100P expression in human esophageal epithelial cells: Human esophageal epithelial cells sequentially produce different S100 proteins in the process of differentiation. Anat Rec 267: 60–69.
35. Chu HW, Balzar S, Westcott JY, Trudeau JB, Sun Y, et al. (2002) Expression and activation of 15-lipoxygenase pathway in severe asthma: relationship to eosinophilic phenotype and collagen deposition. Clin Exp Allergy 32: 1558–1565.
36. Sigal E, Grunberger D, Cashman JR, Craik CS, Caughey GH, et al. (1988) Arachidonate 15-lipoxygenase from human eosinophil-enriched leukocytes: partial purification and properties. Biochem Biophys Res Commun 150: 376–383.
37. Nadel JA, Conrad DJ, Ueki IF, Schuster A, Sigal E (1991) Immunocytochemical localization of arachidonate 15-lipoxygenase in erythrocytes, leukocytes, and airway cells. J Clin Invest 87: 1139–1145.
38. Macmillan DK, Hill E, Sala A, Sigal E, Shuman T, et al. (1994) Eosinophil 15-lipoxygenase is a leukotriene A4 synthase. J Biol Chem 269: 26663–26668.

11

Risk Factors for Development of Chronic Kidney Disease following Renal Infarction: Retrospective Evaluation of Emergency Room Patients from a Single Center

Wen-Ling Lin[1], Chen-June Seak[1], Jiunn-Yih Wu[2], Yi-Ming Weng[1], Hang-Cheng Chen[2]*

1 Department of Emergency Medicine, Chang Gung Memorial Hospital, Taoyuan, Taiwan, and Chang Gung University College of Medicine, Taoyuan, Taiwan, **2** Department of Emergency Medicine, Chang Gung Memorial Hospital, Keelung, Taiwan, and Chang Gung University College of Medicine, Taoyuan, Taiwan

Abstract

Background: Previous studies have analyzed factors associated with renal infarction so that patients can be provided with earlier diagnosis and treatment. However, the factors associated with development of chronic kidney disease (CKD) following renal infarction are unknown.

Methods: We retrospectively reviewed the records of patients with a diagnosis of renal infarction based on enhanced computed tomography. All patients were admitted to a single emergency department in Taiwan from 1999 to 2008. Univariate and multivariate analysis were used to assess the effect of different factors on development of CKD based on estimates of the glomerular filtration rate (eGFR) at admission and at 3–12 months after discharge.

Results: Univariate analysis indicated significantly increased risk of CKD in patients older than 50 years, with symptoms for 24 h or less before admission, lower eGFR at admission, APACHE II score greater than 7, SOFA score greater than 1, ASA score greater than 2, and SAPS II score greater than 15. Multivariate analysis indicated that only SOFA score greater than 1 was significantly and independently associated with CKD at follow-up ($p<0.001$).

Conclusions: A total of 32.5% of patients admitted for renal infarction over a ten-year period developed CKD at 3–12 months after discharge. A SOFA score greater than 1 was significantly and independently associated with development of CKD in these patients.

Editor: Giuseppe Remuzzi, Mario Negri Institute for Pharmacological Research and Azienda Ospedaliera Ospedali Riuniti di Bergamo, Italy

Funding: The authors have no support or funding to report.

Competing Interests: The authors have declared that no competing interests exist.

* E-mail: ezn2002@gmail.com

Introduction

Renal infarction is a rare but potentially serious condition that is typically characterized by unilateral flank or abdominal pain, hematuria, and proteinuria. Diagnosis can be difficult because these and other signs and symptoms are non-specific and are often consistent with pyelonephritis, tumor, urolithiasis, and other conditions [1]. Diagnosis is best made by contrast-enhanced computed tomography (CT) and/or renal angiography. CT results typically indicate the presence of a wedge-shaped hypodense area in the peripheral region [2,3]. Thrombosis, embolism, and arterial lesion are the main causes of renal infarction [4].

Prompt initiation of therapy with an anti-coagulant and/or a thrombolytic agent is often the preferred treatment for renal infarction. Catheter-directed intra-arterial thrombolysis may also be effective [5]. However, such treatments are not effective in all patients, possibly due to delays in diagnosis [2]. Patients can recover from renal infarction, but some patients develop irreversible chronic kidney disease (CKD). Many previous case studies and case series have investigated factors associated with renal infarction in order to allow earlier diagnosis [3–8]. However, the factors associated with development of CKD following renal infarction are not yet well-established.

In the present study, we identified factors associated with development of CKD following renal infarction by analysis of patients from a single institution in Taiwan who experienced renal infarction from 1999 to 2008.

Methods

Patient selection

All patients were admitted to the Emergency Department (ED) of Chang Gung Memorial Hospital (Taoyuan, Taiwan) from 1999 to 2008 due to a diagnosis of renal infarction based on enhanced computed tomography (CT). All patients received out-patient follow-up and had serum creatinine measured at admission. Variables were excluded if they were missing in more than 50% of patients, if all subjects had the same value, and if they were not numerically coded. Ultimately, 40 patients were enrolled. The Institutional Review Board of Chang Gung Memorial Hospital approved this retrospective study and the patients provided written informed consent.

Table 1. Baseline characteristics of study subjects admitted to the emergency department for renal infarction (n = 40).

Characteristic	
Age (years), mean ± SD	53.18±15.10
Gender, n (%)	
Female	11 (27.5)
Male	29 (72.5)
Previous renal infarction, n (%)	
No	39 (97.5)
Yes	1 (2.5)
Current Medications	
Aspirin, n (%)	
No	26 (65.0)
Yes	14 (35.0)
Warfarin, n (%)	
No	34 (85.0)
Yes	6 (15.0)
Amiodarone, n (%)	
No	39 (97.5)
Yes	1 (2.5)
Clopidogrel, n (%)	
No	40 (100.0)
Yes	0 (0.0)
Steroid, n (%)	
No	39 (97.5)
Yes	1 (2.5)
Chinese herb, n (%)	
No	39 (97.5)
Yes	1 (2.5)
Hormone replacement therapy, n (%)	
No	38 (95.0)
Yes	2 (5.0)
Clinical symptoms	
Duration (h) of symptoms/signs before admission, median (IQR)	24.0 (12.0–84.0)
Fever, n (%)	
No	34 (85.0)
Yes	6 (15.0)
Chills, n (%)	
No	39 (97.5)
Yes	1 (2.5)
Abdominal pain, n (%)	
No	6 (15.0)
Yes	34 (85.0)
Abdominal fullness, n (%)	
No	36 (90.0)
Yes	4 (10.0)
Dyspnea, n (%)	
No	36 (90.0)
Yes	4 (10.0)
Flank pain, n (%)	
No	23 (57.5)
Yes	17 (42.5)
Back pain, n (%)	
No	37 (92.5)
Yes	3 (7.5)
Nausea, n (%)	
No	26 (65.0)
Yes	14 (35.0)
Vomiting, n (%)	
No	28 (70.0)
Yes	12 (30.0)
Hematuria, n (%)	
No	39 (97.5)
Yes	1 (2.5)
Oligouria, n (%)	
No	40 (100.0)
Yes	0 (0.0)
Anuria, n (%)	
No	40 (100.0)
Yes	0 (0.0)
Etiology, n (%)	
Cardiac or other embolism	18 (45.0)
Thrombosis or coagulation dysfunction	16 (40.0)
Spontaneous renal artery dissection	1 (2.5)
Idiopathic	5 (12.5)
Laboratory test	
eGFR at admission (mL/min per 1.73 m^2), median (IQR)	66.70±31.03
ICU prognostic scores	
APACHE II, median (IQR)	7.0 (4.0–10.0)
SOFA, median (IQR)	1.0 (0.0–2.0)
ASA, median (IQR)	2.0 (1.0–3.0)
SAPS II, median (IQR)	15.0 (13.0–19.0)

Clinical and demographic data

Clinical and demographic data were obtained by retrospective chart review. Serum creatinine was measured by the Jaffe reaction with alkaline picrate. Prognostic scores were calculated upon ED admission (before treatment) based on APACHE II criteria [9], SOFA criteria [10], ASA criteria [11], and SAPS II criteria [12]. These scores were readily available, and although they were not designed to predict the risk of CKD after RI, we investigated their potential use in this new context. CKD was diagnosed based on K/DOQI guidelines [13] and an estimated glomerular filtration rate (eGFR) less than 60 mL/min/1.73 m^2 at ER admission and 3 months after discharge. The eGFR was calculated by the Cockcroft and Gault formula, which was developed in 1976 [14].

Data Analysis

Continuous variables are expressed as means ± SDs if the distribution was normal and as medians with interquartile ranges (IQRs) if the distribution was non-normal. Categorical variables are expressed as frequencies and percentages. The difference in

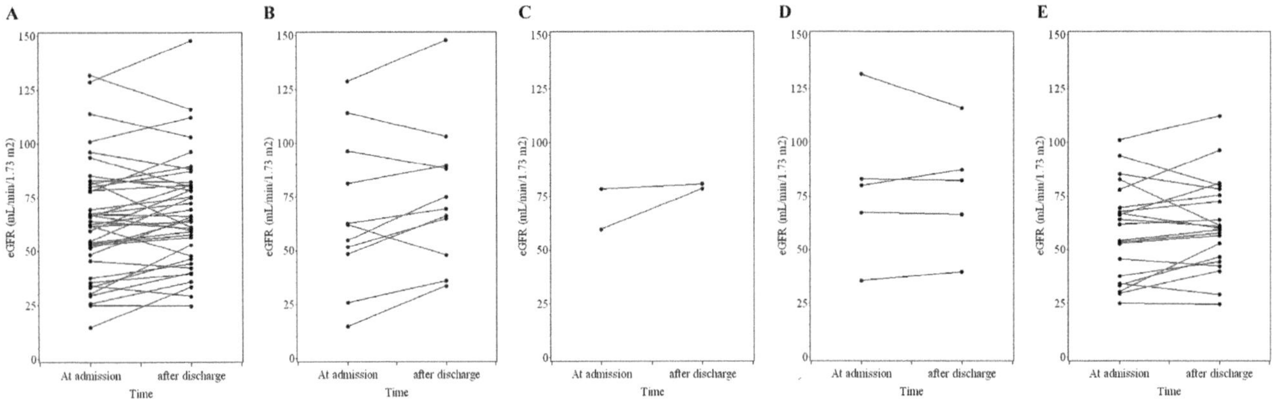

Figure 1. Changes in eGFR for (A) all patients (n = 40), and those evaluated at (B) 3 months after discharge (n = 11), (C) 6 months after discharge (n = 2), (D) 9 months after discharge (n = 6), and (E) 12 months after discharge (n = 21).

eGFR at two time points was assessed by a paired *t*-test. The differences in the presence of CKD in patients with different characteristics were assessed by a Chi-square test or Fisher's exact test, as appropriate. For identification of risk factors associated with CKD, the point estimates and 95% confidence intervals (CIs) of odds ratios (ORs) were calculated by univariate and multivariate logistic regression models. All significant variables in the univariate analysis were used for backward selection in the multivariate logistic regression model; variables that did not improve model fit for a *p*-value less than 0.1 were discarded, but potential confounding variables (age and gender) were forced into the model. All statistical analyses were performed with SAS software version 9.2 (SAS Institute Inc., Cary, NC). A two-tailed *p*-value less than 0.05 was considered statistically significant.

Results

Baseline characteristics of study subjects

A total of 40 patients (29 males [72.5%] and 11 females [27.5%]) who were admitted to our ED for renal infarction, all of whom had eGFR measurements at admission and at 3–12 months after discharge, were included in the analysis (Table 1). The mean patient age was 53.18±15.10 years and the age range was 20 to 78 years. One patient (2.5%) had a previous renal infarction. The most common medications were aspirin (35%) and warfarin (15%). The median (IQR) duration of symptoms/signs before admission was 24.0 h (12.0–84.0). The most common symptoms were abdominal pain (85%) and flank pain (42.5%). Eighteen patients (45%) had an embolism in the heart or other region. The median (IQR) of the APACHE II, SOFA, ASA, and SAPS II scores were 7.0 (4.0–10.0), 1.0 (0.0–2.0), 2.0 (1.0–3.0), and 15.0 (13.0–19.0), respectively. Based on a Kruskal-Wallis test, the distributions of ICU prognostic scores (APACHE II, SOFA, ASA, and SAPS II) did not differ significantly among patients with different etiologies (cardiac or other embolism, n = 18; thrombosis or coagulation dysfunction, n = 16; renal artery dissection, n = 1; idiopathic disease, n = 5).

eGFR at admission and 3 to 12 months after discharge

The eGFRs of all enrolled patients were measured at admission and 3 to 12 months after discharge (Table 2). Eleven patients were evaluated at month-3, 2 at month-6, 6 at month-9, and 21 at month-12 (mean duration: 8.8±3.9 months after discharge) (Figure 1). The results indicate slightly higher mean eGFR after discharge than at admission (66.7±31.0 *vs.* 70.5±28.5 mL/min/1.73 m^2, $p = 0.035$), but no significant change in Cr.

Factors associated with development of chronic kidney disease

A total of 13 patients (32.5%) developed CKD at the last follow-up. Table 3 shows a univariate analysis of risk factors associated with development of CKD. These results indicate significantly increased risk of CKD in patients with the following characteristics: older than 50 years (50.0% *vs.* 11.1%, $p = 0.009$), symptoms for 24 h or less before admission (45.8% *vs.* 12.5%, $p = 0.027$), lower eGFR at admission (per 1 mL/min/1.73 m^2, OR = 0.74, 95% CI: 0.56–0.98, $p = 0.034$), APACHE II score greater than 7 (50.0% *vs.* 18.2%, $p = 0.033$), SOFA score greater than 1 (90.9% *vs.* 10.3%, $p<0.001$), ASA score greater than 2 (71.4% *vs.* 11.5%, $p<0.001$), and SAPS II score greater than 15 (57.9% *vs.* 9.5%, $p = 0.001$).

The final multivariate model was chosen with backward selection for variables that were significant in the univariate analysis. Variables that did not improve model fit ($p<0.1$) were discarded, except for age and gender, which were forced in the

Table 2. Mean (±SD) eGFR and Cr of patients at admission and at 3 to 12 months after discharge (n = 40).

Parameter	At admission	3 to 12 months after discharge	Difference	*p*-value[†]
eGFR (mL/min/1.73 m^2)	66.7±31.0	70.5±28.5	3.8±11.1	0.035
Cr (mg/dL)	1.35±0.64	1.23±0.38	−0.12±0.46	0.115

[†]Paired t-test.

Table 3. Univariate analysis of risk factors associated with chronic kidney disease at follow-up among patients admitted for renal infarction.

Characteristic	CKD/Total (%)	*p*-value	OR (95% CI)	*p*-value
Age (years)				
≦50	2/18 (11.1)	0.009†	1.00 (reference)	
>50	11/22 (50.0)		8.00 (1.48–43.40)	0.016
Gender				
Female	3/11 (27.3)	1.000‡	1.00 (reference)	
Male	10/29 (34.5)		1.40 (0.30–6.49)	0.665
Previous renal infarction				
No	13/39 (33.3)	1.000‡	1.00 (reference)	
Yes	0/1 (0.0)		NA	0.981
Current Medications				
Aspirin				
No	6/26 (23.1)	0.155‡	1.00 (reference)	
Yes	7/14 (50.0)		3.33 (0.83–13.37)	0.089
Warfarin				
No	11/34 (32.4)	1.000‡	1.00 (reference)	
Yes	2/6 (33.3)		1.05 (0.17–6.61)	0.962
Amiodarone				
No	13/39 (33.3)	1.000‡	1.00 (reference)	
Yes	0/1 (0.0)		NA	0.981
Steroid				
No	12/39 (30.8)	0.325‡	1.00 (reference)	
Yes	1/1 (100.0)		NA	0.982
Chinese herb				
No	13/39 (33.3)	1.000‡	1.00 (reference)	
Yes	0/1 (0.0)		NA	0.981
Hormone therapy				
No	12/38 (31.6)	1.000‡	1.00 (reference)	
Yes	1/2 (50.0)		2.17 (0.13–37.64)	0.596
Clinical symptoms				
Duration (h) of symptoms/signs before admission				
≦24[a]	11/24 (45.8)	0.027†	1.00 (reference)	
>24	2/16 (12.5)		0.17 (0.03–0.91)	0.039
Fever				
No	12/34 (35.3)	0.643‡	1.00 (reference)	
Yes	1/6 (16.7)		0.37 (0.04–3.51)	0.384
Chills				
No	13/39 (33.3)	1.000‡	1.00 (reference)	
Yes	0/1 (0.0)		NA	0.981
Abdominal pain				
No	0/6 (0.0)	0.152‡	1.00 (reference)	
Yes	13/34 (38.2)		NA	0.952
Abdominal fullness				
No	12/36 (33.3)	1.000‡	1.00 (reference)	
Yes	1/4 (25.0)		0.67 (0.06–7.11)	0.737
Dyspnea				
No	11/36 (30.6)	0.584‡	1.00 (reference)	
Yes	2/4 (50.0)		2.27 (0.28–18.27)	0.440
Flank pain				
No	5/23 (21.7)	0.091†	1.00 (reference)	

Table 3. Cont.

Characteristic	CKD/Total (%)	*p*-value	OR (95% CI)	*p*-value
Yes	8/17 (47.1)		3.20 (0.81–12.65)	0.097
Back pain				
No	12/37 (32.4)	1.000 ‡	1.00 (reference)	
Yes	1/3 (33.3)		1.04 (0.09–12.66)	0.974
Nausea				
No	9/26 (34.6)	1.000‡	1.00 (reference)	
Yes	4/14 (28.6)		0.76 (0.18–3.11)	0.698
Vomiting				
No	9/28 (32.1)	1.000‡	1.00 (reference)	
Yes	4/12 (33.3)		1.06 (0.25–4.45)	0.941
Hematuria				
No	13/39 (33.3)	1.000‡	1.00 (reference)	
Yes	0/1 (0.0)		NA	0.981
Etiology				
Cardiac or other embolism	8/18 (44.4)	0.379‡	1.20 (0.16–9.01)	0.966
Thrombosis or coagulation dysfunction	3/16 (18.8)		0.35 (0.04–3.08)	0.980
Spontaneous renal artery dissection	0/1 (0.0)		NA	0.971
Idiopathic	2/5 (40.0)		1.00 (reference)	
Laboratory test				
eGFR at admission, per 1 ml/min/1.73 m^2			0.74 (0.56–0.98)	0.034
ICU prognostic scores				
APACHE II				
≦7[a]	4/22 (18.2)	0.033†	1.00 (reference)	
>7	9/18 (50.0)		4.50 (1.08–18.69)	0.038
SOFA				
≦1[a]	3/29 (10.3)	<0.001‡	1.00 (reference)	
>1	10/11 (90.9)		86.67 (8.04–934.35)	<0.001
ASA				
≦2[a]	3/26 (11.5)	<0.001‡	1.00 (reference)	
>2	10/14 (71.4)		19.17 (3.61–101.91)	0.001
SAPS II				
≦15[a]	2/21 (9.5)	0.001†	1.00 (reference)	
>15	11/19 (57.9)		13.06 (2.34–72.82)	0.003
Treatments				
Drug therapy				
None	4/16 (25.0)	0.647‡	1.00 (reference)	
coumadin	0/2 (0.0)		NA	0.958
unfractioned heparin	4/9 (44.4)		2.40 (0.42–13.60)	0.936
LMWH	4/9 (44.4)		2.40 (0.42–13.60)	0.936
coumadin+UFH	0/1 (0.0)		NA	0.969
coumadin+LMWH	1/1 (100.0)		NA	0.932
coumadin+UFH+LMWH	0/1 (0.0)		NA	0.969
UFH+TPA(IV)	0/1 (0.0)		NA	0.969
Surgery				
No	13/36 (36.1)	0.284‡	1.00 (reference)	
Yes	0/4 (0.0)		NA	0.961
Blood pressure control				
No	10/32 (31.3)	1.000‡	1.00 (reference)	
Yes	3/8 (37.5)		1.32 (0.26–6.64)	0.736
Emergent dialysis				

Table 3. Cont.

Characteristic	CKD/Total (%)	*p*-value	OR (95% CI)	*p*-value
No	12/39 (30.8)	0.325‡	1.00 (reference)	
Yes	1/1 (100.0)		NA	0.979
Poor response to opioid				
No	10/29 (34.5)	1.000‡	1.00 (reference)	
Yes	3/11 (27.3)		0.71 (0.15–3.30)	0.665
Pain subsided				
No	6/22 (27.3)	0.435†	1.00 (reference)	
Yes	7/18 (38.9)		1.70 (0.45–6.44)	0.437
Type of renal infarction				
Left renal infarction				
No	9/21 (42.9)	0.142†	1.00 (reference)	
Yes	4/19 (21.1)		0.36 (0.09–1.44)	0.148
Right renal infarction				
No	8/27 (29.6)	0.722‡	1.00 (reference)	
Yes	5/13 (38.5)		1.48 (0.37–5.96)	0.577
Bilateral renal infarction				
No	9/32 (28.1)	0.400‡	1.00 (reference)	
Yes	4/8 (50.0)		2.56 (0.52–12.48)	0.246
Splenic infarction				
No	11/34 (32.4)	1.000‡	1.00 (reference)	
Yes	2/6 (33.3)		1.05 (0.17–6.61)	0.962
Complications				
ESRD				
No	5/21 (23.8)	0.217†	1.00 (reference)	
Yes	8/19 (42.1)		2.33 (0.60–9.03)	0.222
Hospital Stay (day)				
≦10[a]	13/37 (35.1)	0.538‡	1.00 (reference)	
>10	0/3 (0.0)		NA	0.967
ICU Stay (day)				
≦0[a]	13/38 (34.2)	1.000‡	1.00 (reference)	
>0	0/2 (0.0)		NA	0.973
Ventilator use				
No	2/18 (11.1)	0.009†	1.00 (reference)	
Yes	11/22 (50.0)		8.00 (1.48–43.40)	0.016

Abbreviations: OR, odds ratio; CI, confidence interval; NA, non-available; CKD, chronic kidney disease; ESRD, end stage renal disease; LMWH, low molecular weight heparin; TPA, tissue plasminogen activator; UFH, unfractionated heparin.
†Chi-square test; ‡Fisher's exact test.
[a]Median served as the cutoff value.

model for adjustment (Table 4). The results of this analysis indicated that only SOFA score greater than 1 was significantly and independently associated with CKD at follow-up (adjusted OR = 75.60, 95% CI: 5.62–1016.99, $p = 0.001$). In addition, previous hypertension and diabetes mellitus were not significantly associated with CKD (data not shown).

Discussion

We examined the records of 40 patients who were admitted to the ED of Chang Gung Memorial Hospital from 1999 to 2008 with a diagnosis of renal infarction based on enhanced contrast CT. Measurements indicate slightly higher eGFR after discharge than at admission, suggesting a slight improvement in renal function after discharge. A total of 13 patients (32.5%) with renal infarction were diagnosed with CKD after discharge. Univariate analysis indicated that numerous factors were significantly associated with CKD (age >50 years, symptoms for 24 h or less before admission, low eGFR at admission, APACHE II score greater than 7, SOFA score greater than 1, ASA score greater than 2, and SAPS II score greater than 15. However, multivariate analysis indicated that only SOFA score greater than 1 was significantly and independently associated with a diagnosis of CKD. Although the SOFA score was not designed to predict the

Table 4. Multivariate analysis of risk factors associated with chronic kidney disease at follow-up among patients admitted for renal infarction.

Characteristic	Adjusted OR (95% CI)	*p*-value
Age (years)		
≦50	1.00 (reference)	
>50	7.12 (0.54–93.40)	0.135
Gender		
Female	1.00 (reference)	
Male	1.23 (0.11–14.23)	0.868
SOFA		
≦1[a]	1.00 (reference)	
>1	75.60 (5.62–1016.99)	0.001

OR: odds ratio; CI: confidence interval.
[a]Median served as the cutoff value.

risk of CKD after RI, our results suggest a potential new use for this parameter.

It may seem somewhat surprising that our multivariate analysis indicated that SOFA score was independently associated with development of CKD, but that the APACHE II, SAPS II, and ASA scores were not. The SOFA score is an indicator of organ dysfunction and morbidity that was originally developed to assess organ dysfunction in patients with sepsis, but has been validated for assessment of organ dysfunction in general. Although SOFA score is associated with mortality, the APACHE II, SAPS II, and ASA scores place greater emphasis on prediction of mortality. The authors designed the SOFA system with an emphasis on bedside applicability and simplicity based on commonly available variables. These prognostic metrics are widely used to predict outcomes of patients admitted to intensive care units (ICUs) [15]. Although a patient's individual prognostic score is not dispositive, it is often considered in guiding individual treatment decisions and in the distribution of limited medical resources [16]. Moreover, APACHE II, SAPS II, and ASA scores are often more suitable for characterization of patients with diseases that are imminently life-threatening, or the level of anaesthetic risk. Although renal infarction and CKD are serious conditions, appropriate clinical management allows patients to survive.

Our analysis indicated that the post-discharge eGFR was significantly higher than the eGFR at admission. However, it seems doubtful whether this small increase (3.8±11.1 mL/min/1.73 m^2) was clinically significant. Nonetheless, these results indicate an improvement in kidney function, so this result is not surprising [17]. We find it encouraging that the SOFA score is the best predictor of CKD, because this score only requires measurement of 6 parameters (respiratory, cardiovascular, central nervous system, renal, coagulation, and liver). The APACHE II requires measurement of 34 variables and SAPS II requires measurement of 12 variables. We suggest that future studies of the development of CKD in patients admitted with RI consider use of the SOFA score to guide patient follow-up.

Our study had several limitations. First, our sample size was relatively small and all patients were from a single institution. Second, all patients were admitted to the ED and exclusion of out-patients with renal infarction may have provided a biased view of factors associated with development of CKD.

Conclusions

Our retrospective study of patients admitted to a single ED with renal infarction indicated that 32.5% of patients developed CKD within 3 months of discharge. Elevation of serum creatinine at admission and a SOFA score greater than 1? was the factor significantly and independently associated with development of CKD at follow-up.

Author Contributions

Conceived and designed the experiments: CJS. Analyzed the data: WLL HCC. Wrote the paper: WLL. Contributed analysis tools: JYW. Contributed materials: YMW.

References

1. Korzets Z, Plotkin E, Bernhein J, Zissin R (2002) The clinical spectrum of acute renal infarction. IMAJ 4: 781–784.
2. Huang CC, Lo HC, Huang HH, Kao WF, Yen DH, et al. (2007) ED presentations of acute renal infarction. Am J Emerg Med 25: 164–169.
3. Suzer O, Shirkhoda A, Zafar Jafri S, Madrazo BL, Bis KG, et al. (2002) CT features of renal infarction. Eur J Radiol 44: 59–64
4. Tsai SH, Chu SJ, Chen SJ, Fan YM, Chang WC, et al. (2006) Acute renal infarction: a 10-year experience. Int J Clin Pract 61: 62–67.
5. Piffaretti G, Riva F, Tozzi M, Lomazzi C, Rivolta N, et al. (2008) Catheter-directed thrombolysis for acute renal artery thrombosis: report of 4 cases. Vasc Endovascular Surg 42: 375–379.
6. Bolderman R, Oyen R, Verrijcken A, Knockaert D, Vanderschueren S (2006) Idiopathic renal infarction. Am J Med 2006, 119: 356.e9–12.
7. Domanovits H, Paulis M, Nikfardjam M, Meron G, Kürkciyan I, et al. (1999) Acute renal infarction. Clinical characteristics of 17 patients. Medicine (Baltimore) 78: 386–394.
8. Korzets Z, Plotkin E, Bernhein J, Zissin R (2002) The clinical spectrum of acute renal infarction. IMAJ 4: 781–784.
9. Knaus WA, Draper EA, Wagner DP, Zimmerman JE (1985) APACHE II: a severity of disease classification system. Crit Care Med 13: 818–829.
10. Ferreira FL, Bota DP, Bross A, Mélot C, Vincent JL (2001) Serial evaluation of the SOFA score to predict outcome in critically ill patients. JAMA 286: 1754–1758.
11. Keats AS (1978) The ASA classification of physical status—a recapitulation. Anesthesiology 49: 233–236.
12. Le GallJR, Lemeshow S, Saulnier F (1993) A new Simplified Acute Physiology Score (SAPS II) based on a European/North American multicenter study. JAMA 270: 2957–2963.

13. NKF KDOQI Guidelines. Available: http://www.kidney.org/professionals/KDOQI/guidelines_ckd/toc.htm.
14. Cockcroft DW, Gault MH (1976) Prediction of creatinine clearance from serum creatinine. Nephron 16: 31–41.
15. Minne L, Abu-Hanna A, de Jonge E (2008) Evaluation of SOFA-based models for predicting mortality in the ICU: A systematic review. Crit Care 12:R161
16. Lemeshow S, Klar J, Teres D (1995) Outcome prediction for individual intensive care patients: useful, misused, or abused? Intensive Care Med 21: 770–776.
17. Ceriotti F, Boyd JC, Klein G, Henny J, Queraltó J, et al. (2008) Reference intervals for serum creatinine concentrations: assessment of available data for global application. Clin Chem 54: 559–566.

12

Developmental Fluoxetine Exposure Normalizes the Long-Term Effects of Maternal Stress on Post-Operative Pain in Sprague-Dawley Rat Offspring

Liesbeth Knaepen[1], Ine Rayen[2], Thierry D. Charlier[3], Marianne Fillet[4], Virginie Houbart[4], Maarten van Kleef[1], Harry W. Steinbusch[2], Jacob Patijn[1], Dick Tibboel[3], Elbert A. Joosten[1], Jodi L. Pawluski[2,3]*

1 University Pain Center Maastricht, Department of Anesthesiology/Pain Management, Maastricht University Medical Center, Maastricht, The Netherlands, **2** School for Mental Health and Neuroscience, Maastricht University, Maastricht, The Netherlands, **3** University of Liege, GIGA-Neurosciences, Liège, Belgium, **4** Laboratory of Analytical Pharmaceutical Chemistry, Department of Pharmacy, CIRM, University of Liège, Liège, Belgium, **5** Intensive Care and Department of Pediatric Surgery, Erasmus MC-Sophia, Rotterdam, The Netherlands

Abstract

Early life events can significantly alter the development of the nociceptive circuit. In fact, clinical work has shown that maternal adversity, in the form of depression, and concomitant selective serotonin reuptake inhibitor (SSRI) treatment influence nociception in infants. The combined effects of maternal adversity and SSRI exposure on offspring nociception may be due to their effects on the developing hypothalamic-pituitary-adrenal (HPA) system. Therefore, the present study investigated long-term effects of maternal adversity and/or SSRI medication use on nociception of adult Sprague-Dawley rat offspring, taking into account involvement of the HPA system. Dams were subject to stress during gestation and were treated with fluoxetine (2×/5 mg/kg/day) prior to parturition and throughout lactation. Four groups of adult male offspring were used: 1. Control+Vehicle, 2. Control+Fluoxetine, 3. Prenatal Stress+Vehicle, 4. Prenatal Stress+Fluoxetine. Results show that post-operative pain, measured as hypersensitivity to mechanical stimuli after hind paw incision, was decreased in adult offspring subject to prenatal stress alone and increased in offspring developmentally exposed to fluoxetine alone. Moreover, post-operative pain was normalized in prenatally stressed offspring exposed to fluoxetine. This was paralleled by a decrease in corticosteroid binding globulin (CBG) levels in prenatally stressed offspring and a normalization of serum CBG levels in prenatally stressed offspring developmentally exposed to fluoxetine. Thus, developmental fluoxetine exposure normalizes the long-term effects of maternal adversity on post-operative pain in offspring and these effects may be due, in part, to the involvement of the HPA system.

Editor: Judith Homberg, Radboud University, The Netherlands

Funding: This research was funded by a Charge de recherché and Apirant grants from Fonds de la Recherche Scientifique-FNRS, Belgium (to JLP and VH) and by the Pain Knowledge Centers of Maastricht and Rotterdam (to LK). The funders had no role in study design, data collection and analysis, decision to publish, or preparation of the manuscript.

Competing Interests: The authors have declared that no competing interests exist.

* E-mail: j.pawluski@ulg.ac.be

Introduction

Early life events can significantly influence the development of the nociceptive network and pain responses in later life [1]. Recently, maternal adversity in the form of perinatal stress and depression has been shown to affect not only the mother, but also the neonate. Moreover, perinatal maternal stress has been linked to increased nociceptive responses in the newborn [2–4]. For example, exposure to prenatal maternal stress increases a baby's response to a painful heel prick [2]. Perinatal maternal depression, often a stress-related disease, is a major condition which affects 20% of women [5]. However, little is known about the long-term impact of maternal adversity on nociception in offspring.

Preclinical work has shown that perinatal maternal stress results in increased pain sensitivity in adult rat offspring [6,7]. Underlying mechanisms for such long-term effects of maternal adversity on nociception in later life are rather unknown. Clinical and preclinical studies have shown that intra-uterine exposure to high levels of glucocorticoids or maternal stress affect stress responses in offspring [2,8–11]. Furthermore, a dysregulated hypothalamic-pituitary-adrenal (HPA) system has been related to alterations in pain responses [12,13]; decreased cortisol levels have been linked to increased pain symptoms in patients with chronic pain [14]. Glucocorticoid receptors (GRs) are involved in pain processing given their presence on nociceptive neurons in the spinal cord [15,16]. Moreover, these neurons show signs of activation when C-fibers are noxiously stimulated [17] and intrathecal application of a GR antagonist has been shown to attenuate neuropathic pain [18].

Selective serotonin reuptake inhibitor (SSRI) medications, e.g. fluoxetine, are the most common treatment for maternal depression and are prescribed to 5–10% of pregnant mothers [19–21]. SSRIs cross the placenta [22] and are transferred, via breast milk [23], to the infant. Developmental SSRI exposure increases serotonin (5-HT) levels in offspring and may affect the development of the 5-HT-pain inhibitory circuit [1]. Indeed, recent clinical research has shown that infants perinatally exposed to SSRIs have blunted pain responses to a heel prick at two days and two months after birth [24,25], demonstrating an involvement of SSRIs on offspring nociception. Besides having a direct effect on the nociceptive system, 5-HT levels play a prominent role in the development of the HPA-axis [26,27] and perinatal exposure to SSRIs can alter the developing HPA system [28,29]. Therefore SSRIs may impact the developing nociceptive system indirectly via altering the HPA-axis.

The objective of this study was to investigate the effect of maternal stress on nociception in adult offspring. In turn, because SSRIs are commonly used for treatment of maternal stress-related disorders, we investigated the effect of developmental exposure to SSRIs on nociception in adult male offspring taking into account the involvement of the HPA system on these effects. To do this prenatally stressed offspring were exposed to fluoxetine during the perinatal period. Offspring were tested for basal nociception and post-operative nociception after hind paw incision during adulthood. Moreover, circulating corticosterone and corticosteroid binding globulin (CBG) levels were investigated. This work provides important information on the long-term impact of developmental exposure to maternal adversity and SSRI treatment on nociception and sheds light on the underlying physiology related to these changes.

Materials and Methods

Ethical Statement

All animal experiments were performed in accordance with the European Directive for the Protection of Vertebrate Animals Used for Experimental and Other Scientific Purposes (86/609/EEC) and adhered to the Guidelines for the Care and Use of Mammals in Neuroscience and Behavioral Research (National Research Council 2003). The protocol was approved by the Animal Ethics Board of Maastricht University in accordance with Dutch governmental regulations (approval IDs: DEC 2008-184 and DEC 2010-150). All surgery was performed under isoflurane anesthesia, and all efforts were made to minimize suffering.

Animals

In this experiment a total of 20 Sprague-Dawley rats (Charles River Laboratories, France) were used. The animals were housed in a temperature (19–24°C) and humidity (55±15%) conditioned room with a 12:12 light/dark schedule (lights on at 8:00 a.m.) with *ad libitum* access to tap water and rat chow. Breeding of the dams took place by putting one female and one male together in a wire mesh cage. Release of a vaginal plug was considered as gestation day (G) 0.

On G14, dams were randomly assigned to stress (*N* = 9) or control (*N* = 11) groups. Dams in the stress group were individually restrained three times a day (at 8:00 a.m., 11:30 a.m. and 15:30 p.m.) for 45 min in a plastic cylinder under bright light on G14-G20 [11,30,31]. Stress during this period of pregnancy can result in postpartum depressive-like behavior in the dam [32,33]. The day after the last stress exposure (G20) dams were randomly assigned to one of the two treatment groups: fluoxetine (two doses of 5 mg/kg per day) or vehicle, resulting in a total of four groups of dams: 1. Control+Vehicle (CV; *N* = 5), 2. Control+Fluoxetine (CF; *N* = 6), 3. Prenatal Stress+Vehicle (SV; *N* = 4), 4. Prenatal Stress+Fluoxetine (SF; *N* = 5). After weaning at P21, two male offspring per litter were housed together in standard cages and used for behavioral testing, resulting in group sizes of *N* = 8–12. Offspring were weighed at the age of 8 weeks and at 1, 7 and 9 days after surgery. For a timeline of the experiment see Figure 1.

Fluoxetine treatment

During G14–20 dams were trained for oral ingestion of the medication treatment. Dams were fed 1/9th of a vanilla wafer-cookie (Croustifondante, Delacre, Belgium), filled with saline [34]. During feeding dams were not separated from the litter. At G21 treatment was started and dams were fed two times per day (at 9:00 a.m. and 14:00 p.m.) a cookie filled with fluoxetine (Flagron, Belgium) dissolved in vehicle (50% propylenediol in saline; 5 mg/kg) or vehicle solution. Since maternal restraint stress results in postpartum depressive-like behavior, as mentioned before, dams were treated with fluoxetine from G21 until P21. Oral administration via a cookie was preferred instead of oral gavage or injections, which might induce pain and stress in the dam/litter. Since fluoxetine and its active metabolite norfluoxetine are passed to offspring via lactation [35], fluoxetine and norfluoxetine levels were determined at several time-points during lactation (see section 2.3). Exposure of offspring to fluoxetine occurred during a stage of neural development in rodents analogous to that of the third trimester in humans [36], when nociceptive fibers are present but in an immature stage [1].

Fluoxetine and norfluoxetine determination

To determine fluoxetine and norfluoxetine concentrations in rat serum, blood samples were collected by quick decapitation from culled pups on P1, from one female pup on P7 and P14, and from the dam, one female and one male pup at P21. Although, behavioral testing was performed only in male offspring, female offspring were used for drug determinations to provide an indication of the drug levels in the pups at this age. This took place in every litter, where surplus pups were available. Blood samples were centrifuged at 10 000×*g* for 10 minutes and serum was collected. Drug concentrations were determined from serum using liquid chromatography coupled with mass spectrometry (LC-Chip-MS/MS) was used as previously described [37,38]. Briefly, the chromatographic separation was achieved on a 1200 series LC-chip system (Agilent Technologies, Germany) using a Ultra High Capacity chip including a 500 nL trapping column and a 150 mm×75 μm analytical column, both packed with a Zorbax 80SB 5 μm C18 phase (Agilent Technologies). The mobile phase was composed of H2O/FA (100:0.1, v/v) (A) and ACN/H2O/FA (90:10:0.1, v/v/v) (B) and used in gradient elution mode. Mass spectrometric detection was performed using a 6340 Ion Trap equipped with a nanoelectrospray ionization source operating in positive mode (Agilent Technologies, Waldbronn). Finally, an Oasis μElution MCX 96-well plate (Waters, UK) was used to prepare the samples for the analysis. 25 μL serum was needed per experiment and all conditions were performed in duplicate and back-calculated using a calibration curve. Mean drug levels show the presence of fluoxetine and norfluoxetine in offspring serum at the age of P1, P14 and P21 (Table 1) (N = 7–11/group). This shows that fluoxetine is transferred to offspring via lactation.

Nociception behavioral tests

Sensitivity of offspring to mechanical stimuli and thermal stimuli was tested at several time points: basal nociception was tested during development at 4 weeks of age and at the young-adult age of 8 weeks and post-operative hypersensitivity was tested daily in young-adult rats until 9 days after surgery; (Fig. 1). Sensitivity to mechanical stimuli was determined by measuring paw withdrawal thresholds (PWT) using plantar application of 10 von Frey monofilaments (North Coast Medical, Inc., California, USA) with logarithmically incremental stiffness (0.166, 0.407, 0.692, 1.202, 2.041, 3.63, 5.495, 8.511, 15.136 and 28.84 g). Animals were

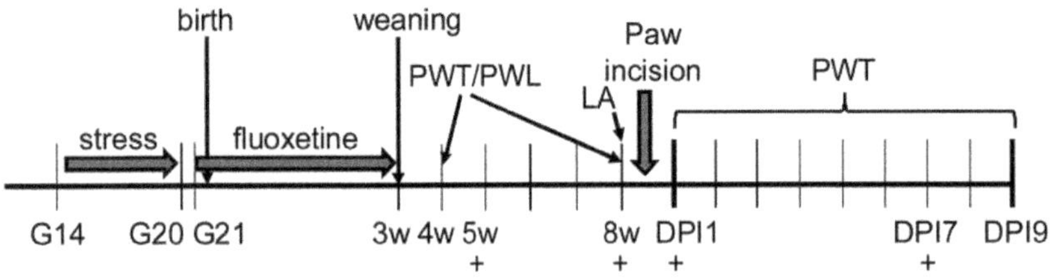

Figure 1. Schematic overview of the study. Pregnant dams were stressed three times per day for 45 minutes from gestational day (G) 14 until G20. The stressor consisted of restraint in a plastic cylinder and exposure to bright light. Fluoxetine was administered orally to the dams from G21 until the day of weaning at three weeks of age (3 w). After weaning, 2 male offspring from control/vehicle, control/fluoxetine, stress/vehicle and stress/fluoxetine dams were subjected to behavioral testing ($N = 8/12$ per group). Their basal paw withdrawal thresholds (PWT) to mechanical stimuli and paw withdrawal latencies (PWL) to heat stimuli were tested at 4 weeks, i.e. a juvenile age during development, and at 8 weeks, when animals were at a young adult age. Also, a locomotor activity (LA) test was performed at the age of 8 weeks. One day after the last behavioral basal test at 8 weeks, all offspring received an incision of the left hind paw, after which PWT were measured daily until 9 days post incision (DPI9). To measure serum levels of corticosterone and corticosterone binding globulin (CBG), tail vein blood was withdrawn at the age of 5 and 8 weeks and at DPI1 and DPI7 (+).

placed in Plexiglass cages on an elevated wire mesh floor and allowed to adapt to the cage for 30 min before testing. Starting with the lowest filament, each filament was applied five times with a duration of one second and inter-application interval of a few seconds to the plantar paw surface. Maximal applied force was defined by maximal withdrawal, i.e. when the animal showed five withdrawal responses. The mechanical force resulting in a 50% withdrawal frequency was considered the PWT and was calculated from a sigmoid curve (withdrawal frequency per filament vs. force log applied) by regression analysis (GraphPad Prism Version 4.00, CA, USA) [39].

Thermal sensitivity was determined using the Hargreaves thermal plantar algesia apparatus at the age of 5 and 8 weeks (Ugo Basile, Collegeville, PA, USA). After an adaptation period of about 30 minutes, an infrared laser beam was placed at the mid-plantar surface of the hind paw. The apparatus measures the paw withdrawal latency (PWL) from the infrared source (intensity of 70) to the nearest 0.1 s. Mean PWL from three measurements per paw (ten minute intervals) was measured with a cut-off time of 20 s. For post-operative testing of hypersensitivity, the Hargreaves apparatus was not used, since mechanical hypersensitivity is reported to be the main outcome for post-incision pain [40]. The researcher performing behavioral testing was blinded to grouping of the animals.

Locomotor activity

Locomotor activity was investigated at 8 weeks of age in offspring to ensure there were no gross differences in locomotion between groups. Animals were placed individually in the center of a 50 cm×100 cm glass arena and their activity was recorded for 10 minutes. All animals were tested between 2:00 and 5:00 p.m. A video-tracking system (Anymaze, Stoelting) was used to measure the distance the animals travelled in the arena. The apparatus was cleaned with 70% ethanol and dried between rats.

Post-operative pain at the age of 8 weeks: plantar hind paw incision

Plantar hind paw incision was performed at the age of 8 weeks, a young-adult age at which alterations in the nociceptive network organization and in hind paw incision pain have been evidenced following neonatal pain exposure [41]. After baseline nociceptive and locomotor activity testing, all male offspring received an injury to the left hind paw, i.e. plantar hind paw incision as a model for post-operative pain [40]. Animals were anesthetised with 3–5% isoflurane (Abbott Laboratories Ltd., Kent, U.K.), mixed with air enriched with 100% oxygen at a constant flow rate of 250 ml/min. Body temperature was maintained at 37.5°C using an automatic heating pad. After making a ±1 cm longitudinal incision through the plantar skin and fascia, the plantaris muscle was elevated and incised at the midline as described previously [40]. Two mattress-sutures with 5–0 nylon on a PS-2 needle (Ethicon, San Lorenzo, P.R.) were used to close the wound. Hypersensitivity to mechanical stimuli after surgery was determined daily by measuring PWT to von Frey filaments until 9 days after surgery.

Corticosterone analysis

To investigate effects of maternal stress and developmental fluoxetine on corticosterone levels in offspring in basal conditions and at one and seven days after hind paw incision, blood samples were collected from the tail vein. Blood samples were centrifuged at 10 000×*g* for 10 minutes and serum was collected. A commercially available corticosterone RIA kit (Corticosterone I^{125} for rats and mice, MP Biomedicals, NY, USA) was used to determine total corticosterone levels in duplicate serum samples. Interassay variability was 7.4%. The lowest detection limit of the kit was 7.7 ng/mL

Table 1. Mean (±SEM) serum levels of fluoxetine (ng/mL) and norfluoxetine (ng/mL) during the postnatal period. (P = postnatal day).

	P1	P7	P14	Male P21	Female P21	Mom P21
Fluoxetine (ng/mL)	19.46 (±22.98)	2.44 (±2.90)	1.76 (±5.38)	2.07 (±3.98)	1.52 (±2.47)	30.65 (±59.14)
Norfluoxetine (ng/mL)	83.01 (±14.45)	16.32 (±17.33)	11.35 (±19.26)	27.41 (±21.03)	33.61 (±21.26)	184.63 (±104.66)

($N = 7–11$).

Table 2. Mean (±SEM) weights (g) of litters and number of male and female pups on postnatal day (PD 1).

	CV	CF	SV	SF
Litter weight at PD1 (g)	96.92 (±5.35)	97.25 (±4.54)	101.60 (±10.55)	92.00 (±7.00)
No. of males	6.80 (±0.49)	5.83 (±0.87)	5.50 (±0.65)	6.40 (±0.87)
No. of females	6.60 (±0.68)	7.83 (±0.75)	8.25 (±1.70)	6.60 (±0.93)

CV: control vehicle, CF: control fluoxetine, SV: stress vehicle, SF: stress fluoxetine, ($N=4$–6/group).

Corticosterone binding capacity

Corticosterone binding capacity was determined by measuring the level of CBG according to an earlier described method [42,43]. Specifically bound CBG counts were calculated by subtracting the non-specific background counts from the average of total bound CBG counts. Interassay variability was 7.3%.

Statistical analysis

All data shown were presented as means±standard error of the mean (SEM). Two-way analysis of variance tests (ANOVA) were used to analyze the effect of group (condition: stress/control, treatment: fluoxetine/vehicle) as independent variables on offspring weight, locomotor activity outcomes, PWT, corticosterone levels, and CBG levels as the dependent variable. Additionally, a mixed design ANOVA was performed with condition (stress/control) and treatment (fluoxetine/vehicle) as the independent variables and time as the repeated measure for CBG and corticosterone serum levels and separately for each paw for PWTs comparisons. Post hoc comparisons were performed for further analysis of single effect comparisons and utilized the Fischer's least significant difference (LSD) test. Correlations were conducted between CBG levels and PWT (log transformed). $P \leq 0.05$ was considered to be statistically significant (Statistica Version 9).

Results

Offspring weight

Total litter weight and the number of male and female pups was not significantly affected by maternal stress and/or fluoxetine exposure ($0.17 \leq P \leq 0.97$) (Table 2). There was a significant main effect of time ($F(3, 108) = 592.36$, $P = 0.001$) for all groups (Table 3) indicating that all animals gained weight during the experiment. However, no effect of stress or treatment was observed ($0.38 \leq P \leq 0.87$).

Locomotor activity

To exclude locomotion problems, which might interfere with nociception behavioral testing, we evaluated overall locomotion and there was no effect of stress or treatment on the distance the animals travelled in the open arena ($0.37 \leq P \leq 0.74$; Table 4).

Basal nociception

There was no significant difference in PWL to thermal stimuli in offspring from mothers exposed to stress and/or fluoxetine at the age of 4 and 8 weeks ($0.21 \leq P \leq 0.91$; Fig. 2). There were also no statistically significant differences associated with condition or treatment in PWT to mechanical von Frey stimuli of male offspring at the age of 4 weeks ($0.16 \leq P \leq 0.85$; Table 5). The PWT at the age of 8 weeks served as the baseline value for post-operative hypersensitivity to mechanical stimuli and the analysis was therefore performed together with the post-operative hypersensitivity data (Fig. 3). At the age of 8 weeks, developmental fluoxetine exposure decreased PWT to von Frey stimuli ($P = 0.0198$; Fig. 3). However, since this decrease was only observed at the left (ipsilateral to the hind paw incision), but not at the right (contralateral) hind paw and was not observed at the age of 4 weeks, it is considered as not consistent.

Post-operative nociception

The effect of hind paw incision on PWT to mechanical stimuli was measured from one day post incision (DPI1) until DPI9. There was a significant interaction effect of time*condition*treatment ($F(9, 324) = 2.41$, $P = 0.012$) on PWT of the incised, i.e. ipsilateral, paw (Fig. 3A). CF offspring had the highest sensitivity to mechanical stimuli, i.e. the lowest PWT after surgery. Post hoc tests showed that CF offspring had lower PWT than SF offspring (^{b} $P = 0.000095$) and CV offspring (^{c} $P = 0.019$) at the baseline (BL), i.e. the day before surgery. Further post hoc tests showed that after incision CF offspring had lower PWT than SV offspring at DPI1, DPI3, DPI4, DPI6, DPI7, DPI8 and DPI9 (DPI1: ^{a} $P = 0.019$, DPI3: ^{a} $P = 0.015$, DPI4: ^{a} $P = 0.0080$, DPI6: ^{a} $P = 0.0076$, DPI7: ^{a} $P = 0.000011$, DPI8: ^{a} $P = 0.0052$, DPI9: ^{a} $P = 0.042$). Also, CF offspring had lower PWT than SF offspring at DPI7 (^{b} $P = 0.00052$) and DPI8 (^{b} $P = 0.000020$) and then CV offspring at DPI7 (^{c} $P = 0.00073$). Moreover SV had higher PWT than all other groups at DPI5 (^{d} $0.002 \leq P \leq 0.009$).

Table 3. Mean (±SEM) weights (g) of male offspring.

Group	8 w weight (g)	DPI1 weight (g)	DPI7 weight (g)	DPI9 weight (g)
CV	323.98 (±6.54)	337.16 (±6.79)	366.71 (±6.85)	376.75 (±6.28)
CF	307.23 (±7.60)	322.39 (±5.77)	355.83 (±4.90)	365.08 (±5.02)
SV	321.11 (±7.52)	331.94 (±8.11)	366.71 (±9.36)	376.75 (±9.81)
SF	303.62 (±10.86)	315.98 (±11.69)	348.13 (±11.59)	365.00 (±11.67)

A statistically significant main effect of time was observed ($F(3, 108) = 592.36$, $P = 0.001$). DPI: days post incision, 8 w: 8 weeks, CV: control vehicle, CF: control fluoxetine, SV: stress vehicle, SF: stress fluoxetine ($N = 8$–12/group).

Table 4. Mean (±SEM) distances that the animals travelled in the open arena at the age of eight weeks.

Group	Distance (m)
CV	12.69 (±0.66)
CF	13.74 (±0.87)
SV	12.68 (±1.26)
SF	12.20 (±0.58)

There were no differences in distances between the groups. CV: control vehicle, CF: control fluoxetine, SV: stress vehicle, SF: stress fluoxetine (N = 8–12/group).

Also, there was a main effect of condition (F(1, 36) = 16.18, P = 0.00028) and treatment (F(1,36) = 10.19, P = 0.0029). There were no significant differences in contralateral PWT at any of the time points measured (0.13≤P≤0.79; Fig. 3B).

We also calculated the area under the curve (AUC) of the post-incision hypersensitivity (Fig. 3C-D). There was a significant main effect of condition on the AUC of the ipsilateral paw, with offspring exposed to maternal stress (SV and SF groups) showing higher AUC compared to offspring from control mothers (CV and CF groups) (F(1, 36) = 18.57, #P = 0.00012; Fig. 3C). Also, there was a significant main effect of treatment with developmental fluoxetine resulting in lower AUC compared to offspring exposed to vehicle treatment (F(1, 36) = 13.83, ##P = 0.00068; Fig. 3C). A trend toward a main effect of condition was observed on the contralateral paw with control animals having a tendency for lower AUC values ($^{\$}P$ = 0.056; Fig. 3D).

Corticosterone levels

There was a significant time*condition interaction effect (F(3, 72) = 2.80, P = 0.046), with control offspring having higher corticosterone levels at the 8 week time point relative to stress offspring, regardless of fluoxetine exposure (*0.00018≤P≤0.019; Fig.4A). There was a significant main effect of time (F(3, 72) = 3.11, P = 0.032) on serum corticosterone levels. Post hoc correction showed that the main effect of time was confined to the increase in serum corticosterone levels at the age of 8 weeks (# 0.0057≤P≤0.028; Fig. 4A). Analysis of the AUC of the corticosterone curves, showed no significant differences (0.16≤P≤0.26; Fig. 4B).

CBG levels

A statistically significant interaction effect of condition*treatment was noted (F(1, 24) = 7.08, P = 0.014; Fig. 4C). Post hoc tests showed that SV offspring had lower serum CBG levels than CV and SF offspring (* 0.031≤P≤0.045; Fig. 4C). There was a main effect of time (F(3, 72) = 9.01, P = 0.000038; Fig. 4C) which was mainly attributable to the decrease in serum CBG levels at DPI1 (# P = 0.0020; Fig. 4C). In the AUC, there was a significant interaction effect between condition and treatment (F(1, 31) = 6.89, P = 0.013) for CBG values, with higher CBG serum levels in SF offspring compared to SV offspring (* P = 0.037; Fig. 4D).

We also found significant positive correlations between CBG levels and basal nociception in the form of paw withdrawal thresholds (PWT) to mechanical stimuli of the ipsilateral (r = 32, P = 047) and contralateral paws on week 8 (r = 33, P = 037) and a tendency for a correlation in the contralateral paw on post incision day 1 (r = 31, P = 051).

Discussion

The present study demonstrates that prenatal maternal stress decreases, and developmental fluoxetine exposure increases, the intensity of post-operative hypersensitivity to mechanical stimuli in adult male offspring. Interestingly, post-operative hypersensitivity was normalized in offspring exposed to maternal stress in combination with fluoxetine exposure during development. Moreover, these effects were, in part, linked to changes in the HPA system.

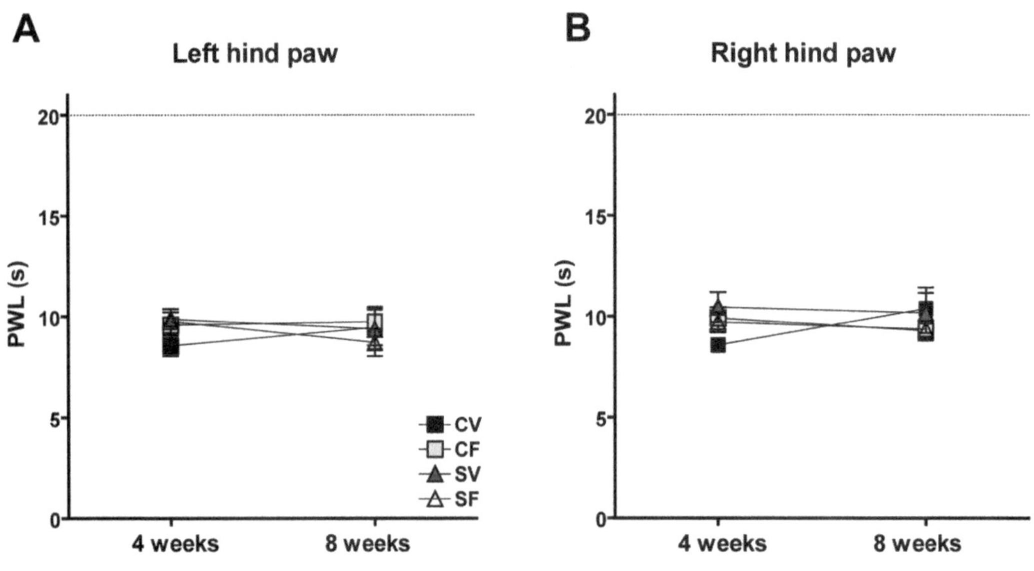

Figure 2. Mean(±SEM) basal nociceptive paw withdrawal latency (PWL) thresholds (s) to heat stimuli. There was no effect of maternal stress or fluoxetine on the PWL to heat stimuli at the left (**A**) or right hind paw (**B**) of male offspring at the age of 4 and 8 weeks. Also, there was no effect of time, since there was no difference in PWL between the age of 4 and 8 weeks. CV: control vehicle, CF: control fluoxetine, SV: stress vehicle, SF: stress fluoxetine (N = 8/12 per group).

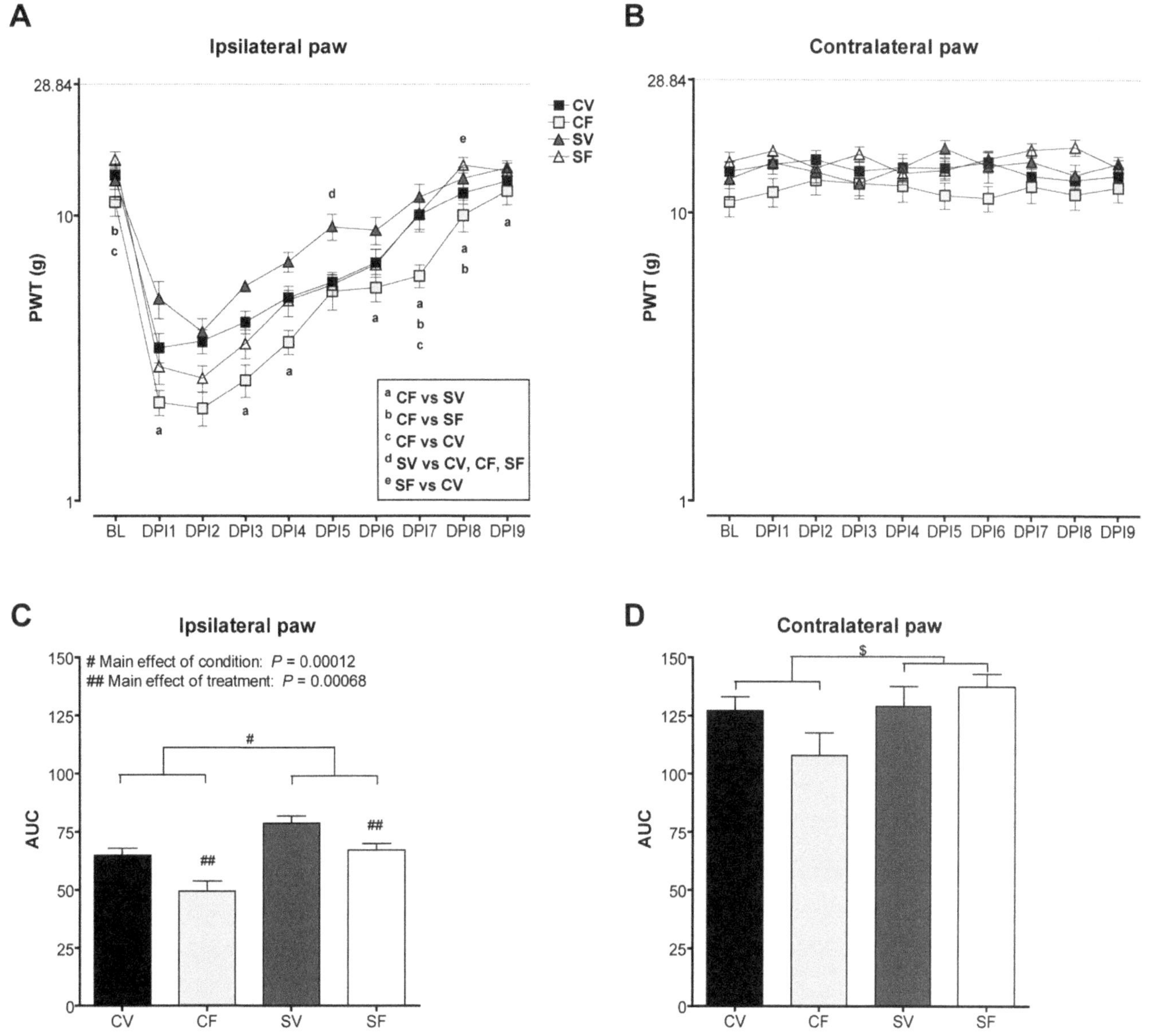

Figure 3. Mean (±SEM) PWTs in male offspring exposed to mechanical stimuli (g) after incision of the left hind paw. There was an overall interaction effect of time*condition*treatment observed for PWT to mechanical stimuli after incision. Also main effects of condition and treatment were observed. Significant differences were shown by post hoc correction and denoted by a, b, c, d and e symbols (A). Contralateral PWT were not affected by paw incision (B), since there were no differences observed between the groups. Area under the curve (AUC) analysis (C) of the ipsilateral PWT graphs in A, showed a main effect of condition (#) and a main effect of treatment (##). Contralateral AUC (D) showed a trend for a main effect of condition with control offspring having a tendency for lower PWT than stress offspring ($). DPI: days post incision, CV: control vehicle, CF: control fluoxetine, SV: stress vehicle, SF: stress fluoxetine ($N = 8/12$ per group).

Prenatal stress and developmental fluoxetine exposure: effects on post-operative pain in adult offspring

Our findings show that maternal prenatal stress decreases post-operative hypersensitivity to mechanical stimuli in offspring at the age of 8 weeks. Although very little work has been done in this area, previous clinical work has shown that maternal stress can increase pain sensitivity in later life with increased somatic pain complaints at 18 months of age and recurrent abdominal pain in 13-year old children [3,4]. Stress exposure in preterm born children affects their HPA-axis response to painful immunization [44] and their HPA system dysfunction has been related to mother behavior [45]. Previous preclinical work has also shown that maternal restraint stress increases inflammatory pain hypersensitivity in newborn and adult offspring [7,46]. Thus, in contrast to our study, maternal stress has been shown to increase pain sensitivity. This difference may depend on the type of pain which is perceived, i.e. incisional pain in our study and inflammatory and abdominal pain in the above mentioned studies. A decrease in post-operative sensitivity to mechanical stimuli, as noted in our study, may be beneficial and indicate a faster recovery from paw incision. However, one study has shown that decreased post-operative pain might be detrimental as it can result in inadequate wound healing [47]. In the previously mentioned study, decreasing post-operative hypersensitivity to mechanical stimuli, after hind paw incision, with an analgesic treatment resulted in animals continually placing weight on the incised paw and consequently

Table 5. Mean (±SEM) PWTs to von Frey stimuli (g), reflecting sensitivity of the hind paws to mechanical stimuli at the age of 4 weeks.

Group	Left hind paw PWT (g)	Right hind paw PWT (g)
CV	12.14 (±1.68)	12.12 (±1.67)
CF	12.05 (±1.45)	12.25 (±1.45)
SV	13.92 (±2.29)	13.92 (±2.29)
SF	15.01 (±1.23)	14.68 (±1.20)

No differences were observed in PWT for the left and right hind paw between the groups. CV: control vehicle, CF: control fluoxetine, SV: stress vehicle, SF: stress fluoxetine ($N = 8–12$/group).

impaired wound apposition occurred [47]. We did not measure the degree of wound healing in the present study, but it is possible that there were differences in the rate of wound healing between offspring exposed to prenatal stress and control offspring.

We found that prenatally stressed offspring exposed to maternal fluoxetine treatment had normalized post-operative hypersensitivity to mechanical stimuli. Surprisingly, we observed that developmental fluoxetine exposure in the absence of prenatal stress increased post-operative hypersensitivity to mechanical stimuli in adult offspring. This highlights the need to investigate the effects of these medications using appropriate models of maternal adversity in order to draw suitable conclusions and clearly parallel the clinical situation. It has been shown that infants from depressed mothers treated with SSRIs have blunted pain responses at two days and two months of age [24,25]. No other studies have investigated the effects of developmental SSRI exposure on post-

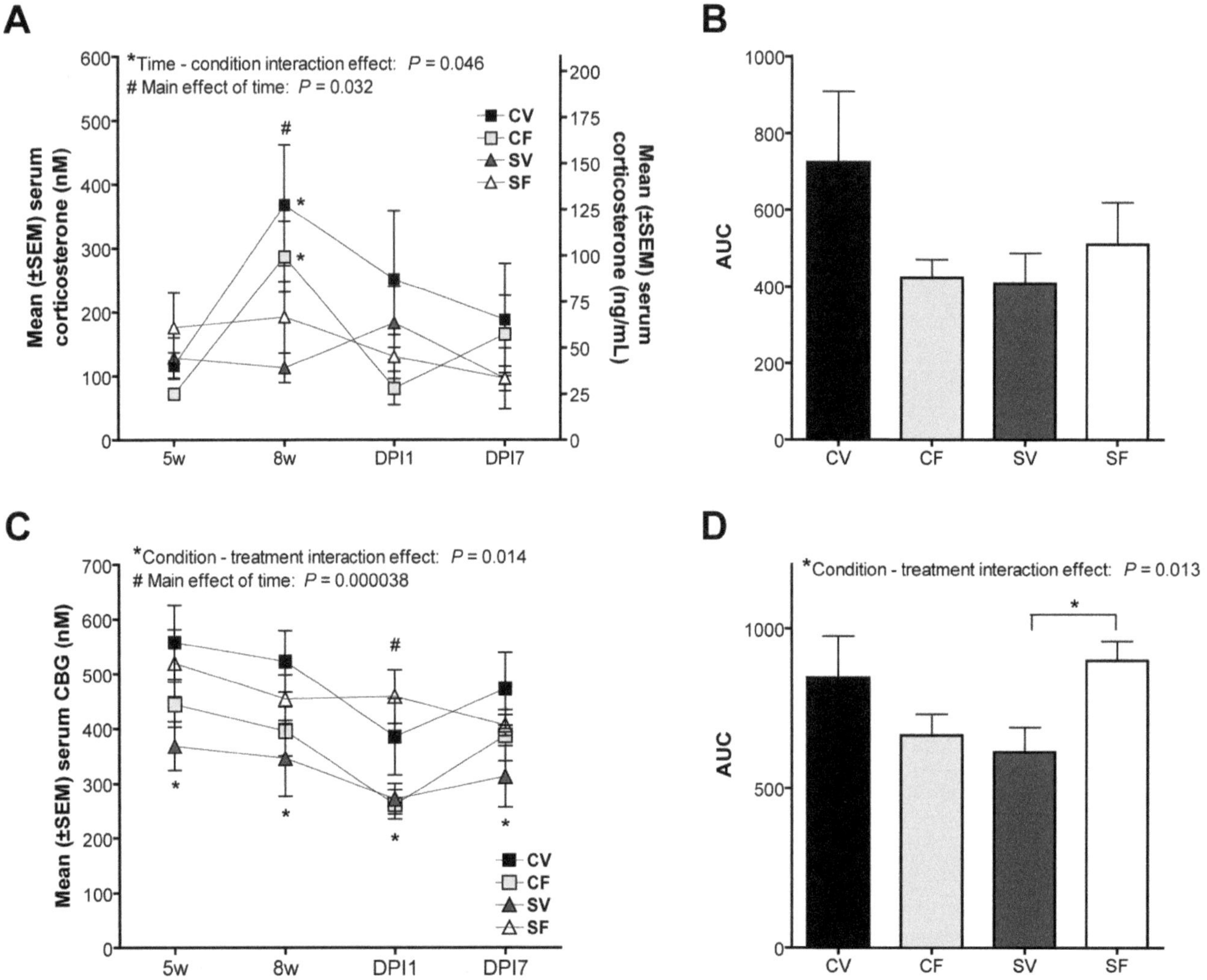

Figure 4. Mean (±SEM) and AUC of serum levels of corticosterone and CBG of male offspring. A time*condition interaction effect was observed in control offspring, but not stress offspring, having a higher corticosterone level at the 8 week time-point (**A**, *). There was a main effect of time on serum corticosterone levels and post hoc corrections showed that the levels at 8 weeks were significantly higher than levels at all other time-points (**A**, #). No effect of condition or treatment was observed on AUC of serum corticosterone levels (**B**). A condition*treatment interaction effect, with lower serum CBG levels in SV offspring, compared to SF and CV offspring (**C**, *). A main effect of time was observed and post hoc correction showed that this was attributable to the decrease in serum CBG at DPI1 (**C**, #). A significant interaction effect of condition*treatment was shown in AUC of CBG serum levels, with lower AUC values for SV offspring, compared to SF offspring (**D**, *). DPI: days post incision, CV: control vehicle, CF: control fluoxetine, SV: stress vehicle, SF: stress fluoxetine ($N = 8/12$ per group).

operative hypersensitivity to pain or the long-term impact of perinatal SSRI exposure on pain sensitivity in any regard. However, developmental exposure to buspirone, a 5-HT1A receptor agonist, was shown to normalize the increased pain hypersensitivity in prenatally stressed adult offspring [7]. More research is needed to investigate how children, prenatally exposed to SSRIs, respond to painful stimuli in later life.

Although beyond the scope of this study, it should be noted that prenatal maternal stress and/or fluoxetine may have affected aspects of maternal care. Although previous work by our group has shown no marked changes in gross maternal care of offspring with prenatal maternal stress or fluoxetine treatment [11], we have also shown that fluoxetine exposure, but not prenatal stress, increases arched-back nursing of pups [38]. However, it is unknown how changes in arched-back nursing, without concomitant changes in licking behavior, may alter pain sensitivity in adult offspring.

Involvement of the HPA system

In the present study we found that hind paw incision resulted in a decrease in serum CBG levels in adult offspring. Interestingly, offspring exposed to maternal prenatal stress alone showed overall lower serum CBG levels compared to prenatally stressed offspring developmentally exposed to fluoxetine and control offspring. This CBG profile is paralleled in their post-operative pain profiles, i.e. lower post-operative pain hypersensitivity in prenatally stressed offspring, and suggests a potential link between the HPA system and post-operative pain. Moreover, prenatally stressed offspring exposed to fluoxetine show serum CBG levels which are comparable with the levels of offspring from control mothers and thus, these levels may parallel effects of normalization of post-operative pain hypersensitivity by developmental fluoxetine exposure in prenatally stressed offspring. Fluoxetine exposure alone appeared to decrease serum CBG levels in adult offspring, as previously described [29], but did not parallel post-operative pain hypersensitivity. Therefore, there may be a relationship between circulating CBG levels and post-operative pain, at least in prenatally stressed male offspring. We did not find a significant correlation between overall CBG levels and pain sensitivity after paw incision. It is likely that a number of factors are mediating this relationship and it also may be that CBG levels at the point of the incision would better clarify the relationship between CBG and post-operative pain sensitivity.

SSRIs increase 5-HT levels in the newborn and 5-HT levels play a prominent role in the development of the HPA-axis [26,27] and therefore SSRIs may impact on the nociceptive system indirectly via the HPA-axis. Interestingly this work suggests that serum CBG levels can be indicative of post-operative pain hypersensitivity, but only when fluoxetine exposure is not present. This is perhaps not surprising as clinical work has shown that the action of antidepressant medications may act to alter CBG levels [48]. Thus developmental exposure to SSRIs may differentially alter the function of CBG with regards to pain sensitivity.

We did not find an effect of hind-paw incision on circulating levels of total corticosterone levels. The absence of an effect of surgery on corticosterone levels in the present study is in line with previous work showing no increase in circulating serum corticosterone levels at 24 hours after open thorax surgery in a rat [49]. However, in humans, increased serum cortisol levels have been shown after major colonic and abdominal surgery [50,51]. Discrepancies between these findings may be related to the severity of the surgical intervention that determines the increase in circulating corticosterone levels or to the timing of blood withdrawal after surgery.

Prenatal stress and developmental fluoxetine exposure: effects on basal nociceptive thresholds in offspring

Besides a small effect of developmental fluoxetine on ipsilateral PWT at 8 weeks, we did not find any significant effect of prenatal stress and/or developmental fluoxetine exposure on basal nociceptive thresholds to mechanical and thermal stimuli in juvenile and adult male offspring. Although these parameters were previously not specifically investigated, research has shown that basal hypersensitivity in response to mechanical stimulation of muscles or viscera can occur in adult offspring following repeated postnatal stress, via maternal separation or exposure to limited bedding material [6,52,53]. The impact of SSRIs during development on basal sensory thresholds has not been widely investigated. Our observation of unaltered thresholds to mechanical and thermal stimuli in fluoxetine-exposed offspring is in line with earlier findings describing unaltered thermal thresholds in adult offspring (at P70) following oral fluoxetine administration to non-stressed pregnant mothers [54]. However, this is in contrast with previous work showing that administering fluoxetine directly to neonatal pups via daily injections increased thermal threshold in adolescent rats (at P35) [55]. Thus, basal nociception outcomes may be dependent on the perinatal stress model, route of SSRI administration or behavioral test used.

Conclusions

The present study is the first to investigate long-term effects of combined prenatal maternal stress and developmental fluoxetine exposure. We show here that both prenatal stress and developmental fluoxetine exposure affect the intensity of post-operative pain differentially in offspring at the age of 8 weeks. Maternal stress decreases and developmental fluoxetine increases post-operative pain hypersensitivity at this age. However, when maternally stressed dams were treated with fluoxetine offspring showed normal post-operative pain profiles, thus SSRI treatment for maternal adversity may normalize nociception in adult offspring. These changes were paralleled, in part, by modulation of the HPA system. Clearly there is a marked long-term effect of maternal adversity and developmental SSRI exposure on post-operative pain in offspring. However, before conclusions can be made about the benefits and risks of perinatal SSRI exposure on offspring development further research is needed.

Acknowledgments

The authors wish to thank Mr. Wiel Honig for his assistance with blood withdrawal procedures.

Author Contributions

Conceived and designed the experiments: LK J. Pawluski EAJ. Performed the experiments: LK J. Pawluski TDC MF VH IR. Analyzed the data: LK J. Pawluski. Contributed reagents/materials/analysis tools: HWS MvK DT J. Patijn. Wrote the paper: LK J. Pawluski EAJ.

References

1. Fitzgerald M (2005) The development of nociceptive circuits. Nat Rev Neurosci 6: 507–520.
2. Davis EP, Glynn LM, Waffarn F, Sandman CA (2011) Prenatal maternal stress programs infant stress regulation. J Child Psychol Psychiatry 52: 119–129.

3. Helgeland H, Sandvik L, Mathiesen KS, Kristensen H (2010) Childhood predictors of recurrent abdominal pain in adolescence: A 13-year population-based prospective study. J Psychosom Res 68: 359–367.
4. Wolff N, Darlington AS, Hunfeld J, Verhulst F, Jaddoe V, et al. (2010) Determinants of somatic complaints in 18-month-old children: the generation R study. J Pediatr Psychol 35: 306–316.
5. Leung BM, Kaplan BJ (2009) Perinatal depression: prevalence, risks, and the nutrition link-a review of the literature. J Am Diet Assoc 109: 1566–1575.
6. Green PG, Chen X, Alvarez P, Ferrari LF, Levine JD (2011) Early-life stress produces muscle hyperalgesia and nociceptor sensitization in the adult rat. Pain 152: 2549–2556.
7. Butkevich I, Mikhailenko V, Vershinina E, Semionov P, Makukhina G, et al. (2011) Maternal buspirone protects against the adverse effects of in utero stress on emotional and pain-related behaviors in offspring. Physiol Behav 102: 137–142.
8. O'Connor TG, Bergman K, Sarkar P, Glover V (2012) Prenatal cortisol exposure predicts infant cortisol response to acute stress. Dev Psychobiol. Epub ahead of print
9. Green MK, Rani CS, Joshi A, Soto-Pina AE, Martinez PA, et al. (2011) Prenatal stress induces long term stress vulnerability, compromising stress response systems in the brain and impairing extinction of conditioned fear after adult stress. Neuroscience 192: 438–451.
10. Abe H, Hidaka N, Kawagoe C, Odagiri K, Watanabe Y, et al. (2007) Prenatal psychological stress causes higher emotionality, depression-like behavior, and elevated activity in the hypothalamo-pituitary-adrenal axis. Neurosci Res 59: 145–151.
11. Rayen I, van den Hove DL, Prickaerts J, Steinbusch HW, Pawluski JL (2011) Fluoxetine during development reverses the effects of prenatal stress on depressive-like behavior and hippocampal neurogenesis in adolescence. PLoS One 6: e24003.
12. Goodin BR, Smith MT, Quinn NB, King CD, McGuire L (2012) Poor sleep quality and exaggerated salivary cortisol reactivity to the cold pressor task predict greater acute pain severity in a non-clinical sample. Biol Psychol. Epub ahead of print
13. Benedetti M, Merino R, Kusuda R, Ravanelli MI, Cadetti F, et al. (2012) Plasma corticosterone levels in mouse models of pain. Eur J Pain 16: 803–815.
14. McLean SA, Williams DA, Harris RE, Kop WJ, Groner KH, et al. (2005) Momentary relationship between cortisol secretion and symptoms in patients with fibromyalgia. Arthritis Rheum 52: 3660–3669.
15. Cintra A, Zoli M, Rosen L, Agnati LF, Okret S, et al. (1994) Mapping and computer assisted morphometry and microdensitometry of glucocorticoid receptor immunoreactive neurons and glial cells in the rat central nervous system. Neuroscience 62: 843–897.
16. Fuxe K, Harfstrand A, Agnati LF, Yu ZY, Cintra A, et al. (1985) Immunocytochemical studies on the localization of glucocorticoid receptor immunoreactive nerve cells in the lower brain stem and spinal cord of the male rat using a monoclonal antibody against rat liver glucocorticoid receptor. Neurosci Lett 60: 1–6.
17. Cintra A, Molander C, Fuxe K (1993) Colocalization of Fos- and glucocorticoid receptor-immunoreactivities is present only in a very restricted population of dorsal horn neurons of the rat spinal cord after nociceptive stimulation. Brain Res 632: 334–338.
18. Wang S, Lim G, Zeng Q, Sung B, Yang L, et al. (2005) Central glucocorticoid receptors modulate the expression and function of spinal NMDA receptors after peripheral nerve injury. J Neurosci 25: 488–495.
19. Oberlander TF, Warburton W, Misri S, Aghajanian J, Hertzman C (2006) Neonatal outcomes after prenatal exposure to selective serotonin reuptake inhibitor antidepressants and maternal depression using population-based linked health data. Arch Gen Psychiatry 63: 898–906.
20. Ververs T, Kaasenbrood H, Visser G, Schobben F, de Jong-van den Berg L, et al. (2006) Prevalence and patterns of antidepressant drug use during pregnancy. Eur J Clin Pharmacol 62: 863–870.
21. Cooper WO, Willy ME, Pont SJ, Ray WA (2007) Increasing use of antidepressants in pregnancy. Am J Obstet Gynecol 196: 544 e541–545.
22. Rampono J, Simmer K, Ilett KF, Hackett LP, Doherty DA, et al. (2009) Placental transfer of SSRI and SNRI antidepressants and effects on the neonate. Pharmacopsychiatry 42: 95–100.
23. Panchaud A, Garcia-Bournissen F, Csajka C, Kristensen JH, Taddio A, et al. (2011) Prediction of infant drug exposure through breastfeeding: population PK modeling and simulation of fluoxetine exposure. Clin Pharmacol Ther 89: 830–836.
24. Oberlander TF, Eckstein Grunau R, Fitzgerald C, Ellwood AL, Misri S, et al. (2002) Prolonged prenatal psychotropic medication exposure alters neonatal acute pain response. Pediatr Res 51: 443–453.
25. Oberlander TF, Grunau RE, Fitzgerald C, Papsdorf M, Rurak D, et al. (2005) Pain reactivity in 2-month-old infants after prenatal and postnatal serotonin reuptake inhibitor medication exposure. Pediatrics 115: 411–425.
26. Andrews MH, Matthews SG (2004) Programming of the hypothalamo-pituitary-adrenal axis: serotonergic involvement. Stress 7: 15–27.
27. Laplante P, Diorio J, Meaney MJ (2002) Serotonin regulates hippocampal glucocorticoid receptor expression via a 5-HT7 receptor. Brain Res Dev Brain Res 139: 199–203.
28. Pawluski JL, Brain UM, Underhill CM, Hammond GL, Oberlander TF (2012) Prenatal SSRI exposure alters neonatal corticosteroid binding globulin, infant cortisol levels, and emerging HPA function. Psychoneuroendocrinology 37: 1019–1028.
29. Pawluski JL, Rayen I, Niessen NA, Kristensen S, van Donkelaar EL, et al. (2012) Developmental fluoxetine exposure differentially alters central and peripheral measures of the HPA system in adolescent male and female offspring. Neuroscience 220: 131–141.
30. Ward IL, Weisz J (1984) Differential effects of maternal stress on circulating levels of corticosterone, progesterone, and testosterone in male and female rat fetuses and their mothers. Endocrinology 114: 1635–1644.
31. Van den Hove DL, Blanco CE, Aendekerk B, Desbonnet L, Bruschettini M, et al. (2005) Prenatal restraint stress and long-term affective consequences. Dev Neurosci 27: 313–320.
32. Smith JW, Seckl JR, Evans AT, Costall B, Smythe JW (2004) Gestational stress induces post-partum depression-like behaviour and alters maternal care in rats. Psychoneuroendocrinology 29: 227–244.
33. O'Mahony SM, Myint AM, van den Hove D, Desbonnet L, Steinbusch H, et al. (2006) Gestational stress leads to depressive-like behavioural and immunological changes in the rat. Neuroimmunomodulation 13: 82–88.
34. Powers BE, Widholm JJ, Lasky RE, Schantz SL (2006) Auditory deficits in rats exposed to an environmental PCB mixture during development. Toxicol Sci 89: 415–422.
35. Pohland RC, Byrd TK, Hamilton M, Koons JR (1989) Placental transfer and fetal distribution of fluoxetine in the rat. Toxicol Appl Pharmacol 98: 198–205.
36. Romijn HJ, Hofman MA, Gramsbergen A (1991) At what age is the developing cerebral cortex of the rat comparable to that of the full-term newborn human baby? Early Hum Dev 26: 61–67.
37. Houbart V, Servais AC, Charlier TD, Pawluski JL, Abts F, et al. (2012) A validated microfluidics-based LC-chip-MS/MS method for the quantitation of fluoxetine and norfluoxetine in rat serum. Electrophoresis 33: 3370–3379.
38. Pawluski JL, Charlier TD, Fillet M, Houbart V, Crispin HT, et al. (2012) Chronic fluoxetine treatment and maternal adversity differentially alter neurobehavioral outcomes in the rat dam. Behav Brain Res 228: 159–168.
39. Ren K, Anseloni V, Zou SP, Wade EB, Novikova SI, et al. (2004) Characterization of basal and re-inflammation-associated long-term alteration in pain responsivity following short-lasting neonatal local inflammatory insult. Pain 110: 588–596.
40. Brennan TJ, Vandermeulen EP, Gebhart GF (1996) Characterization of a rat model of incisional pain. Pain 64: 493–501.
41. Knaepen L, Patijn J, van Kleef M, Mulder M, Tibboel D, et al. (2013) Neonatal repetitive needle pricking: Plasticity of the spinal nociceptive circuit and extended postoperative pain in later life. Dev Neurobiol 73: 85–97.
42. Hammond GL, Lahteenmaki PL (1983) A versatile method for the determination of serum cortisol binding globulin and sex hormone binding globulin binding capacities. Clin Chim Acta 132: 101–110.
43. Pawluski JL, Charlier TD, Lieblich SE, Hammond GL, Galea LA (2009) Reproductive experience alters corticosterone and CBG levels in the rat dam. Physiol Behav 96: 108–114.
44. Grunau RE, Tu MT, Whitfield MF, Oberlander TF, Weinberg J, et al. (2010) Cortisol, behavior, and heart rate reactivity to immunization pain at 4 months corrected age in infants born very preterm. Clin J Pain 26: 698–704.
45. Brummelte S, Grunau RE, Zaidman-Zait A, Weinberg J, Nordstokke D, et al. (2011) Cortisol levels in relation to maternal interaction and child internalizing behavior in preterm and full-term children at 18 months corrected age. Dev Psychobiol 53: 184–195.
46. Butkevich IP, Barr GA, Vershinina EA (2007) Sex differences in formalin-induced pain in prenatally stressed infant rats. Eur J Pain 11: 888–894.
47. Hamalainen MM, Subieta A, Arpey C, Brennan TJ (2009) Differential effect of capsaicin treatment on pain-related behaviors after plantar incision. J Pain 10: 637–645.
48. Barden N, Reul JM, Holsboer F (1995) Do antidepressants stabilize mood through actions on the hypothalamic-pituitary-adrenocortical system? Trends Neurosci 18: 6–11.
49. Berguer R, Dalton M, Ferrick D (1998) Adrenocortical response and regional T-lymphocyte activation patterns following minimally invasive surgery in a rat model. Surg Endosc 12: 236–240.
50. Motamed S, Klubien K, Edwardes M, Mazza L, Carli F (1998) Metabolic changes during recovery in normothermic versus hypothermic patients undergoing surgery and receiving general anesthesia and epidural local anesthetic agents. Anesthesiology 88: 1211–1218.
51. Kotani N, Hashimoto H, Sato Y, Sessler DI, Yoshioka H, et al. (2001) Preoperative intradermal acupuncture reduces postoperative pain, nausea and vomiting, analgesic requirement, and sympathoadrenal responses. Anesthesiology 95: 349–356.
52. Moloney RD, O'Leary OF, Felice D, Bettler B, Dinan TG, et al. (2012) Early-life stress induces visceral hypersensitivity in mice. Neurosci Lett 512: 99–102.
53. Tsang SW, Zhao M, Wu J, Sung JJ, Bian ZX (2011) Nerve growth factor-mediated neuronal plasticity in spinal cord contributes to neonatal maternal separation-induced visceral hypersensitivity in rats. Eur J Pain. Epub ahead of print
54. Lisboa SF, Oliveira PE, Costa LC, Venancio EJ, Moreira EG (2007) Behavioral evaluation of male and female mice pups exposed to fluoxetine during pregnancy and lactation. Pharmacology 80: 49–56.
55. Lee IJ (2009) Neonatal fluoxetine exposure affects the neuronal structure in the somatosensory cortex and somatosensory-related behaviors in adolescent rats. Neurotox Res 15: 212–223.

13

Concordance of Sleep and Pain Outcomes of Diverse Interventions

Anthony G. Doufas[1,2], Orestis A. Panagiotou[3], John P. A. Ioannidis[4,5,6]*

1 Department of Anesthesia, Stanford University School of Medicine, Stanford, California, United States of America, 2 Outcomes Research Consortium, Cleveland, Ohio, United States of America, 3 Department of Hygiene and Epidemiology, University of Ioannina School of Medicine, Ioannina, Greece, 4 Stanford Prevention Research Center, Department of Medicine, Stanford University School of Medicine, Stanford, California, United States of America, 5 Department of Health Research and Policy, Stanford University School of Medicine, Stanford, California, United States of America, 6 Department of Statistics, Stanford University School of Humanities and Sciences, Stanford, California, United States of America

Abstract

Background/Objective: Pain influences sleep and vice versa. We performed an umbrella review of meta-analyses on treatments for diverse conditions in order to examine whether diverse medical treatments for different conditions have similar or divergent effects on pain and sleep.

Methods: We searched published systematic reviews with meta-analyses in the Cochrane Database of Systematic Reviews until October 20, 2011. We identified randomized trials (or meta-analyses thereof, when >1 trial was available) where both pain and sleep outcomes were examined. Pain outcomes were categorized as headache, musculoskeletal, abdominal, pelvic, generic or other pain. Sleep outcomes included insomnia, sleep disruption, and sleep disturbance. We estimated odds ratios for all outcomes and evaluated the concordance in the direction of effects between sleep and various types of pain and the correlation of treatment effects between sleep and pain outcomes.

Results: 151 comparisons with 385 different trials met our eligibility criteria. 96 comparisons had concordant direction of effects between each pain outcome and sleep, while in 55 the effect estimates were in opposite directions ($P<0.0001$). In the 20 comparisons with largest amount of evidence, the experimental drug always had worse sleep outcomes and tended to have worse pain outcomes in 17/20 cases. For headache and musculoskeletal pain, 69 comparisons showed concordant direction of effects with sleep outcomes and 36 showed discordant direction ($P<0.0001$). For the other 4 pain types there were overall 27 vs. 19 pairs with concordant vs. discordant direction of effects ($P=0.095$). There was a weak correlation of the treatment effect sizes for sleep vs. headache/musculoskeletal pain ($r=0.17$, $P=0.092$).

Conclusions: Medical interventions tend to have effects in the same direction for pain and sleep outcomes, but exceptions occur. Concordance is primarily seen for sleep and headache or musculoskeletal pain where many drugs may both disturb sleep and cause pain.

Editor: Giorgio F. Gilestro, Imperial College London, United Kingdom

Funding: No specific and/or direct funding was received for this study. No funding bodies played any role in the design, writing or decision to publish this manuscript. The authors were personally salaried by their institutions during the period of writing though no specific salary was set aside or given for the writing of this paper. There are no current external funding sources for this study.

Competing Interests: The authors have declared that no competing interests exist.

* E-mail: jioannid@stanford.edu

Introduction

Sleep is a critical process of life that is often under threat by acute or chronic pain. Dysfunctional sleep and chronic pain are two major, yet unmet, public health challenges with an enormous societal cost [1–4]. Over a third of the US population is affected by a chronic pain condition, while a fifth suffer from sleep disorders, which degrade daily function and may lead to metabolic and cardiovascular morbidity [2,4]. Twenty percent of adults report that pain disturbs their sleep a few nights a week or more [5], while back pain, headaches, and muscle aches are the most common types of pain experienced at night [6]. Approximately 10% of patients seen in primary care report major insomnia [7] and sleep disturbances exist in 50–89% [8–10] or more [11,12] patients with chronic pain. Reciprocally, patients with primary sleep disorders [13–15] are far more likely to suffer from chronic pain diseases like fibromyalgia, rheumatoid arthritis, temporomandibular joint disorder, or headaches [16]. Both experimental [15–19] and preliminary clinical [20–22] evidence support a complicated, circular model of influence between the functions of sleep and pain [17,23]. Patients with impaired sleep may possess genetic or physiological traits that facilitate the development or exacerbate certain types of chronic pain behavior with or without the occurrence of an opportune acute injury [20–22,24–26]. Ultimately, unremitting pain may further disrupt sleep perpetuating a vicious cycle.

Many treatments given for diverse conditions may cause sleep or pain problems or may aim at improving pain and/or sleep as primary or secondary outcomes. It is unknown whether the effects of different treatments in diverse settings on sleep and pain are concordant, and whether situations exist where responses in these two outcomes are different or even in the opposite direction. It would be useful to dissect the concordance between these outcomes for different types of pain. To explore these issues, we performed an umbrella review that encompassed a large number of systematic reviews with meta-analysis of clinical trials on topics where data on both pain- and sleep-related outcomes were available.

Methods

Eligibility Criteria

We considered Cochrane systematic reviews including separate data on binary pain- and sleep-related outcomes during follow-up for the comparison of the same experimental treatment against the same comparator (placebo, no treatment, or other treatment). We included comparisons regardless of the number of trials with data for each outcome. We also accepted comparisons for any disease or condition. We excluded protocols; reviews where the assessed outcomes did not include at least one pain-related and at least one sleep-related outcome; and comparisons where it was unclear which one was the experimental intervention among those compared (comparisons of different doses/formulations of the same intervention, different agents in the same class, or different interventions where it was unclear which one is the standard of care).

Whenever assessments for either pain or sleep were performed at several different time points we retained the data for the time points with the largest number of studies. We accepted reviews regardless of whether the pain- or sleep-related assessments pertained to the evaluation of outcome status or change (improvement or deterioration).

Search strategy. We searched the Cochrane Library database (last search performed October 20, 2011) using the terms "sleep" and "insomnia" for sleep, and "pain", "headache", "migraine", "myalgia", "arthralgia", "backache", and "ache" for pain. Whenever reviews contained >1 eligible comparison, these were considered separately.

Sleep and Pain Outcomes

Eligible sleep-related assessments were considered together and included outcomes classified as insomnia, sleep disruption and sleep disturbance. We excluded outcomes named somnolence, drowsiness, sedation, abnormal dreams, and hypersomnia. Pain-related outcomes were categorized into 6 groups: headache, musculoskeletal, abdominal, pelvic, generic, and other pain. A detailed description of the specific assessments contained under these categories appears in Table S1 and Table S2. When a pain outcome was listed as generic, we examined carefully the context to see whether it belonged in any of the 5 specific categories.

Extracted Data

Two authors independently documented eligible comparisons and discrepancies were settled with discussion. In each eligible comparison we recorded the trials with data on the eligible pain and sleep outcomes, noting any overlap and capturing the year of publication, first author, and outcome definitions. Finally, we extracted the 2×2 tables for outcome status or change from baseline. When both were available, we preferred change from baseline.

Standardization of Outcome Metrics

We estimated the odds ratio (OR) for all outcomes. We consistently coined the comparisons to reflect the contrast of the experimental treatment versus control and consistently to reflect pain or sleep problems or worsening in pain or sleep problems. This means that when the data reflected the number of patients who had no pain (e.g., 10/36), we took the complementary counts (i.e., 26/36); and whenever the data reflected the number of patients with improvement in pain, we took again the complementary counts. The same rule was applied to sleep outcomes. Therefore, whenever the experimental treatment is better, the OR is <1.00.

Analyses

Multiple trials on the same comparison were synthesized per fixed-effect models [27]. Sensitivity analyses used random-effects [27] and the results are highly similar (not shown in detail), because in most topics there was either only one trial or a few trials and no demonstrable between-trial heterogeneity. We evaluated whether the point estimates for pain and sleep outcomes were in the same or opposite direction and whether they were nominally statistically significant in the same or opposite direction. Direction of effect pertains to the point estimates of the treatment effects and these have large uncertainty when there are limited data. Therefore, we also examined how often the 95% confidence intervals (CIs) excluded a null-effect for both outcomes, and, if so, whether these effects were in the same or opposite direction; how many of the 95% CIs of pain and sleep outcomes did not overlap; and how many of the 95% CIs of pain and sleep outcomes differed beyond chance ($p<0.05$).

To assess whether the magnitude of the treatment effect size correlated for pain and sleep outcomes, we estimated the Pearson correlation coefficients weighted by the inverse of the sum of the variances (squares of the standard errors) of the effects for pain and sleep. This means that observations with limited amount of evidence on either sleep or pain carried less weight in the calculations. We also estimated correlation coefficients without weighting.

There is clinical [14,16,17,21,28–32] and experimental [15,18,33,34] evidence that sleep tends to co-exist more with headache and musculoskeletal pain in particular. Therefore, we hypothesized that headache and musculoskeletal pain may have stronger concordance with sleep outcomes than other types of pain. These two types of pain were considered together and the other types of pain were considered as a separate group. We also hypothesized that the concordance between sleep and pain outcomes may be stronger when these are primary outcomes. Thus, we evaluated separately comparisons where the pain or sleep outcome(s) were considered primary outcomes of the systematic review; and those where neither was among the primary outcomes. We also performed sensitivity analyses limited to trials with data on both sleep and pain outcomes; double-blinded trials; and comparisons of active treatments against no treatment or placebo.

All analyses were performed in STATA 11.2. p-values are two tailed.

Results

Eligible Data

Sixty-eight Cochrane reviews met the eligibility criteria (Figure S1). These reviews corresponded to 385 different trials pertaining to 151 sleep-pain comparisons (headache, n = 80; musculoskeletal pain, n = 25; abdominal pain, n = 24; pelvic pain, n = 2; generic pain, n = 13; other type of pain, n = 7). The included trials were published between 1961 and 2010 (median 1999; interquartile range, IQR, 1996–2004). The median (IQR) sample size across the 151 comparisons was 432 (127–1999) for pain and 310 (108–968) for sleep outcomes. Table 1 shows the 20 pairs with the largest amount of evidence. They all pertained to drug treatments. Full data on all 151 pairs appear in Table S3.

Concordance of Direction of Effects

Ninety-six comparisons had concordant direction of effects between each pain outcome and sleep disturbance, and 55 had point estimates of effects in opposite direction (binomial test for concordant vs. discordant direction $p<0.0001$) when all pain outcomes were considered (94 vs. 57 by random-effects calculations).

Among the 20 pairs with the largest amount of evidence, 17 (85%) had effect estimates in the same direction for the two outcomes (Table 1). In all 20 pairs the experimental drug tended to worsen sleep versus the control (statistically significantly so in all but 4 cases). The experimental drug also tended to worsen pain versus the control in 17/20 pairs, and the difference in pain between experimental and control treatment was nominally significant in 3 cases. Effect estimates for sleep and pain outcomes were in the same direction in 14/15 cases where headache or musculoskeletal pain was involved.

Statistically Significant Effects in the Same and Opposite Direction

We found 6 situations where the pain and sleep disturbance outcomes had nominally statistically significant effects in the same direction. In 5 cases, the experimental interventions worsened both outcomes (sleep and abdominal pain, n = 3 [cholinesterase inhibitor for Alzheimer's disease [35], naltrexone for alcohol dependence [36], sertraline for depression [37]]; sleep and headache, n = 1 [cholinesterase inhibitor for Alzheimer's disease [35]]; and sleep and pelvic pain, n = 1 [goserelin versus oral contraceptives for pain associated with endometriosis [38]]), whereas in 1 situation it improved both sleep and musculoskeletal pain (ozzlo pillow for preventing and treating pelvic and back pain in pregnancy [39]). Conversely, there were 3 situations where the pain and sleep disturbance outcomes had nominally statistically significant results in opposite directions. Sertraline versus tricyclics for depression [37] worsened sleep but improved generic pain; GnRH analogs vs placebo worsened sleep, but improved endometriosis-related pelvic pain [40]; and atovaquone-proguanil improved sleep but had worse abdominal pain than amodiaquine when given for uncomplicated malaria [41]. The picture was similar with random effects calculations, except for GnRH analogs versus placebo.

The 95% CIs of the pain and sleep outcomes did not overlap in 12 cases (8%), and the effect estimates differed beyond chance in 23 cases (15%).

Table 1. Treatment effects for sleep and pain outcomes for the 20 comparisons with largest amount of evidence[a].

Review	Comparison	OR (95% CI) for sleep	OR (95% CI) for pain	Type of pain
CD000440	Risperidone vs. typical neuroleptic medication for schizophrenia	1.05 (0.83–1.34)	1.06 (0.84–1.36)	Headache
CD001190	Donepezil vs. placebo for dementia due to Alzheimer's disease	2.16 (1.53–3.04)	1.25 (0.97–1.60)	Headache
CD001396	SSRIs vs. placebo for premenstrual syndrome	1.80 (1.32–2.47)	1.18 (0.92–1.51)	Headache
CD001765	SSRIs vs. placebo for obsessive compulsive disorder	1.96 (1.57–2.45)	1.06 (0.85–1.33)	Headache
CD001867	Naltrexone vs. placebo for alcohol dependence	1.36 (1.04–1.77)	1.01 (0.85–1.19)	Headache
			1.08 (0.76–1.52)	Musculoskeletal pain
			2.30 (1.61–3.27)	Abdominal pain
			1.25 (0.89–1.76)	Generic pain
CD005445	Ribavirin/Interferon vs. interferon for chronic hepatitis C	1.61 (1.37–1.90)	0.84 (0.69–1.04)	Headache
			0.79 (0.59–1.06)	Abdominal pain
			0.95 (0.85–1.06)	Musculoskeletal pain
CD005593	Cholinesterase inhibitor (optimum dose) vs. placebo for Alzheimer's disease	1.47 (1.10–1.97)	1.47 (1.19–1.82)	Headache
			1.90 (1.40–2.58)	Abdominal pain
CD006103	Varenicline (1.0 mg 2/d) vs. placebo for smoking cessation	1.73 (1.44–2.08)	1.20 (0.99–1.45)	Headache
CD006117	Sertraline vs. TCAs for depression	1.67 (1.21–2.31)	1.31 (0.99–1.74)	Headache
CD006369	Paliperidone - any dose or flexible doses vs. quetiapine (flexible dose all short term) for schizophrenia	1.22 (0.60–2.47)	1.26 (0.65–2.41)	Headache
CD006564	Dopamine agonists vs. placebo/L-dopa in early Parkinson's disease	1.28 (1.00–1.62)	1.27 (0.95–1.68)	Headache
CD006622	Aripiprazole vs. placebo for schizophrenia	1.12 (0.84–1.50)	1.16 (0.88–1.54)	Headache
CD007621	Natalizumab + interferon vs. interferon for relapsing remitting multiple sclerosis	1.07 (0.79–1.45)	1.09 (0.86–1.37)	Headache
			1.17 (0.94–1.46)	Musculoskeletal pain

[a]Amount of evidence is defined by the weight (sum of the inverse variances of the pain and sleep outcome effect sizes), OR>1.00 signifies worse outcome with the experimental versus control treatment.
SSRIs, selective serotonin reuptake inhibitors; OR, odds ratio; CI, confidence interval:, TCA, tricyclic antidepressants.

Concordance of Direction of Effects and Correlation of Effect Sizes According to type of Pain

For headache and musculoskeletal pain, 69 interventions showed concordant direction of effect estimates between pain and sleep disturbance outcomes and 36 showed discordant direction ($p<0.0001$). As shown in Figure 1 and in Table 2, there was some modest correlation in the effect sizes for headache versus sleep disturbance in both weighted and unweighted analyses, and in weighted analyses for musculoskeletal pain versus sleep disturbance, but this was not nominally statistically significant. When both headache and musculoskeletal pain were considered together against sleep, weighted correlation was 0.17 ($p = 0.092$).

For the other 4 pain types there were 27 interventions with concordant direction of effect estimates and 19 with discordant direction ($p = 0.095$). As shown in Figure 2 and Table 2, there was no evidence for correlation between effect sizes.

Primary and Non-primary Outcomes

There were very limited data where both pain and sleep were primary outcomes (n = 5 comparisons), and sparse data where at least one of the two was a primary outcome (n = 17 comparisons) to allow any conclusive inferences (Table 3). However, even when both pain and sleep disturbance were non-primary outcomes, it was more likely for the direction of the effect estimates to be in concordant vs. discordant direction for sleep and headache (49 vs. 30, $p = 0.003$) and musculoskeletal pain (16 vs. 4, $p = 0.047$), but not for the other types of pain. Treatment effect sizes did not seem to correlate for pain and sleep.

Other Sensitivity and Subgroup Analyses

Among trials with data on both pain and sleep, there were 90 comparisons with concordant direction of effects and 48 with opposite direction of effects ($p<0.0001$). The preponderance of concordant results was observed for headache (48 vs. 27, $p = 0.0006$) and musculoskeletal pain (15 vs. 6, $p = 0.006$), but also for others types of pain (27 vs. 15, $p = 0.01$). Among double-blinded trials, there were 79 comparisons with concordant direction of effects and 46 with discordant direction of effects ($p<0.0001$). The preponderance of concordant results was driven by headache (43 vs. 26, $p = 0.004$) and musculoskeletal pain (13 vs. 3, $p = 0.0004$), and not by others types of pain (23 vs. 17, $p = 0.18$). Finally, among trials that had compared an active intervention against an inactive control (placebo/no treatment) there were 58 comparisons with concordant direction of effects and 29 with discordant direction of effect ($p<0.0001$).

Discussion

Across 151 treatment comparisons with pain and sleep outcomes, it was almost twice more common to see concordance in the direction of the treatment effects between sleep and pain rather than point estimates in opposite directions. Sleep outcomes were mostly concordant with headache and musculoskeletal pain. In the evaluated topics where most evidence was available, drug treatments that worsened sleep almost always also tended to worsen headache or musculoskeletal pain. Correlations in the magnitude of the effect size for sleep and pain were weak, but the strongest hints were again seen for headache and musculoskeletal pain. The concordant pattern was seen even though in most trials sleep and pain were not primary outcomes. The same picture emerged when we limited analyses to trials that provided data on both sleep and pain, double-blinded trials and trials with inactive controls.

Current evidence suggests a bidirectional relationship between sleep and pain where pain results in sleep disturbance and disturbed sleep enhances pain [17,20–22,26] with 50–89% of

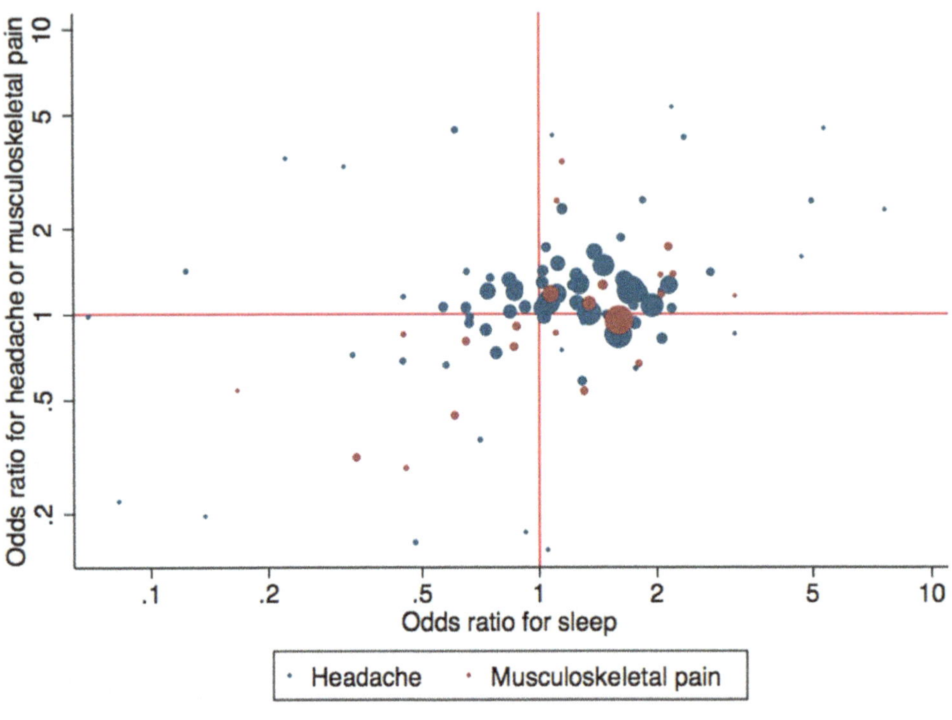

Figure 1. Correlation between treatment effect size (odds ratio) for sleep vs. headache or musculoskeletal pain. Not shown are 6 (3 on each type of pain) comparisons that have effects outside the range.

Table 2. Correlations of the effect sizes for sleep versus pain outcomes.

	Unweighted analyses		Weighted analyses	
Type of pain	**Correlation coefficient**	***p*-value**	**Correlation coefficient**	***p*-value**
Headache	0.28	0.013	0.11	0.35
Musculoskeletal pain	−0.03	0.89	0.32	0.12
Abdominal pain	−0.13	0.55	−0.08	0.72
Pelvic pain	NP	NP	NP	NP
Generic pain	−0.09	0.77	0.10	0.74
Other type of pain	0.19	0.69	−0.06	0.9
Headache & musculoskeletal pain	0.14	0.15	0.17	0.092
All other 4 types of pain	0.06	0.69	−0.08	0.62

NP, not pertinent, because only two comparisons were available.

chronic pain patients also experiencing concomitant sleep problems [42]. Several chronic disease states including headache [43], and musculoskeletal syndromes (back pain [8,10], fibromyalgia [11,24,25,44], and temporomandibular joint disorder [15]) manifest both pain and sleep disturbance as major symptoms [16,45]. Furthermore, poor sleep in fibromyalgia patients could predict pain at 1 year follow up [24], while longitudinal evidence from 12,350 healthy women has shown that sleep problems increased the risk of fibromyalgia in a dose–dependent manner [25]. The presence of restorative sleep in patients suffering from fibromyalgia predicted the resolution of pain at 15 months [44].

We found substantial evidence to support that sleep and pain outcomes are concordant predominantly when headache or musculoskeletal pain were involved. In the typical situation we encountered, drugs with poor sleep outcomes also had more headache or musculoskeletal pain. These findings confirm our hypothesis and prior evidence from both the general population [6] and chronic pain patients in specific [9,16,46]. Insomnia is a common symptom in patients with headache [43] and information on sleep disturbances is crucial in the clinical investigation of these patients [28]. Similarly, musculoskeletal pain is the most frequent complain for sleep disturbance in the general population [6], and, these two are major manifestations of common pain disorders like chronic back pain, fibromyalgia, and osteoarthritis [16].

The evidence for concordance of sleep with other types of pain outcomes was weak. For some cases where both sleep and abdominal pain worsened significantly, this could be attributed to specific side effects of the corresponding drugs. Sleep disturbance, gastrointestinal upset, stomach pain/cramps, and headaches are known side-effects of cholinesterase inhibitors, naltrexone [47], and sertraline, whereas goserelin can also cause sleep disturbance [48]. The choice of comparator may affect sometimes the concordance of sleep and pain outcomes. For example, goserelin

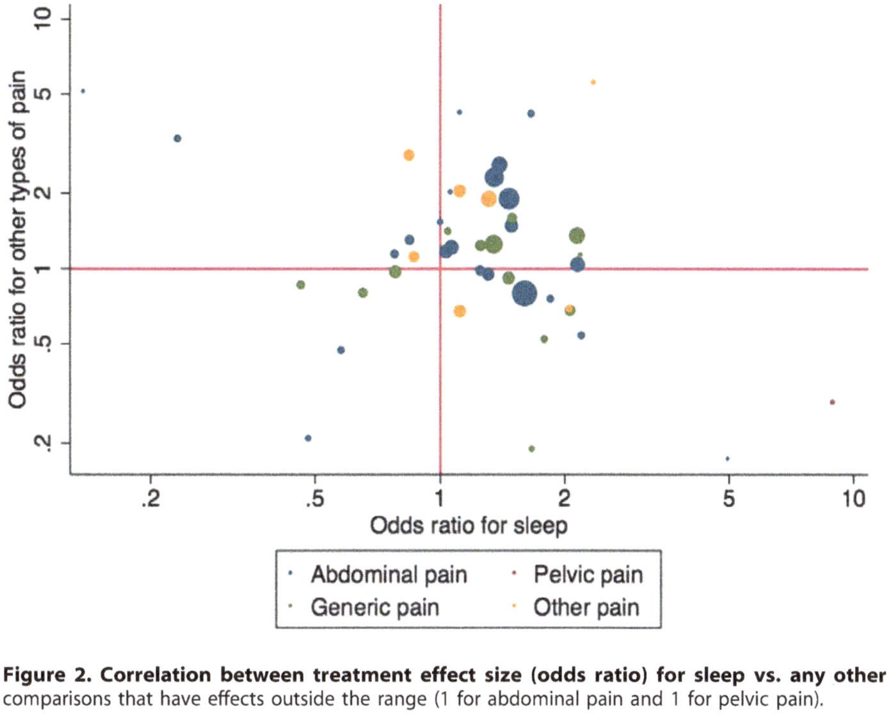

Figure 2. Correlation between treatment effect size (odds ratio) for sleep vs. any other type of pain outcome. Not shown are 2 comparisons that have effects outside the range (1 for abdominal pain and 1 for pelvic pain).

Table 3. Analyses for primary vs. non-primary outcome.

Sleep and pain outcomes	Type of pain	Concordant direction of effects	Discordant direction of effects	*p*-value for binomial test	Weighted correlation coefficient	*p*-value for correlation
Both non-primary outcomes	Headache	49	30	0.003	0.09	0.43
	Musculoskeletal pain	16	4	0.047	0.25	0.28
	Abdominal pain	14	10	0.25	−0.08	0.72
	Generic pain	9	4	0.05	0.10	0.74
	Other type of pain	3	4	0.59	−0.06	0.90
One or both of them primary outcomes	Headache	4	3	0.59	0.07	0.88
	Musculoskeletal pain	5	2	0.11	0.03	0.95
	Abdominal	0	1	NA	NA	NA
	Pelvic	1	1	NA	NA	NA

NA, not applicable.

was worse than oral contraceptives in both sleep outcome and pain control for endometriosis [38] but it was worse for sleep and better for pain when compared with placebo [40]. While we found many examples, where medical treatments worsened both pain and sleep, we found sparse conclusive data on medical treatments that can improve both of these outcomes. The observed beneficial effect of ozzlo pillow on both sleep and back pain is probably not surprising given the strong bidirectional relationship of the two outcomes [49].

Additionally, we identified nominally significant effects in the opposite direction for sleep disturbance and generic pain and abdominal pain with sertraline and atovaquone-proguanil respectively. For the case of sertraline, disturbed sleep has been identified as a common side effect of all SSRIs, whereas pain may be a common symptom for the conditions that it is indicated for. On the contrary, atovaquone-proguanil is known to cause abdominal pain, while amodiaquine, the active comparator, demonstrates insomnia as one of its main toxicities [48].

We should acknowledge some limitations in our work. First, although we accumulated data from 385 trials, most of them were small, and thus many of the effect estimates carried large uncertainty. This introduces noise in the effect size and may also affect the direction of the estimate. Noise would weaken, if anything, the observed concordance of outcomes and correlation of effect sizes. Second, both pain and sleep are influenced by a multitude of other factors and many of these are intervention-specific or disease-specific. However, overarching patterns emerge when many conditions and treatments are examined. Third, we limited our analyses to binary outcomes for consistency, but a perusal of the Cochrane database suggested that very few topics would have been added, if we had included also continuous outcomes. Fourth, we cannot exclude the possibility of selective reporting for some outcomes in several trials. For example, perhaps some outcomes were more likely to be reported, if they had statistically significant results. Although many trials did not report both sleep and pain outcomes, a sensitivity analysis limited to trials reporting both yielded similar inferences. Fifth, each of the pain categories included different types of pain that may be quite different and may not have the same exact relationship with how they might affect sleep outcomes. Moreover, some types of pain syndromes were not represented in our data, e.g. fibromyalgia.

Acknowledging these caveats, this empirical assessment identifies a common thread with concordance between headache and musculoskeletal types of pain and sleep outcomes. The concordance is not absolute, there are exceptions to this pattern, and it is not possible to predict reliably the exact magnitude of the effect of an intervention on pain based on the magnitude of its effect on sleep and vice versa for most medical interventions. However, it seems that several drugs may cause both sleep and pain problems. Many trials and systematic reviews currently address only one of these two outcomes. More routine assessment of both of these types of outcomes may need to be integrated in evaluating the response of patients to diverse treatments, since these adverse effects may coexist. Conversely, more prospective clinical trials are needed to identify the extent to which treatments that provide effective pain relief can also enhance sleep and whether patients with chronic pain disorders could potentially benefit from interventions at the level of sleep.

Supporting Information

Figure S1 Flow chart for the selection of eligible reviews.

Table S1 Eligible sleep-related outcomes which were all considered together under the inclusive term sleep disturbance.

Table S2 Eligible pain-related outcomes.

Table S3 The eligible comparisons on sleep and pain. Trials have been synthesized under fixed-effects.

Author Contributions

Identified the eligible reviews and performed the data extraction: AGD OAP JPAI. Conceived and designed the experiments: AGD JPAI. Performed the experiments: AGD OAP JPAI. Analyzed the data: OAP JPAI. Wrote the paper: AGD OAP JPAI.

References

1. Daley M, Morin CM, LeBlanc M, Gregoire JP, Savard J (2009) The economic burden of insomnia: direct and indirect costs for individuals with insomnia syndrome, insomnia symptoms, and good sleepers. Sleep 32: 55–64.
2. Institute of Medicine (US) Forum on Advancing Pain Research, Care, and Education (2011) Relieving Pain in America: A Blueprint for Transforming Prevention, Care, Education, and Research; Policy BoHS, editor: Washington (DC): National Academies Press (US).
3. Latham J, Davis BD (1994) The socioeconomic impact of chronic pain. Disabil Rehabil 16: 39–44.
4. Institute of Medicine (US) Forum on Sleep Medicine and Research (2006) Sleep Disorders and Sleep Deprivation: An Unmet Public Health Problem; Policy BoHS, editor: Washington (DC): National Academies Press (US).
5. National Sleep Foundation (2000) Omnibus Sleep in America Poll. In: National Sleep Foundation, editor. Washington, DC.
6. National Sleep Foundation (2000) 1997 Survey on Sleeplessness, Pain and the Workplace. In: National Sleep Foundation, editor. Washington, DC.
7. Simon GE, VonKorff M (1997) Prevalence, burden, and treatment of insomnia in primary care. Am J Psychiatry 154: 1417–1423.
8. Marty M, Rozenberg S, Duplan B, Thomas P, Duquesnoy B, et al. (2008) Quality of sleep in patients with chronic low back pain: a case-control study. Eur Spine J 17: 839–844.
9. McCracken LM, Iverson GL (2002) Disrupted sleep patterns and daily functioning in patients with chronic pain. Pain Res Manag 7: 75–79.
10. Tang NK, Wright KJ, Salkovskis PM (2007) Prevalence and correlates of clinical insomnia co-occurring with chronic back pain. J Sleep Res 16: 85–95.
11. Rohrbeck J, Jordan K, Croft P (2007) The frequency and characteristics of chronic widespread pain in general practice: a case-control study. Br J Gen Pract 57: 109–115.
12. Theadom A, Cropley M, Humphrey KL (2007) Exploring the role of sleep and coping in quality of life in fibromyalgia. J Psychosom Res 62: 145–151.
13. Alattar M, Harrington JJ, Mitchell CM, Sloane P (2007) Sleep problems in primary care: a North Carolina Family Practice Research Network (NC-FP-RN) study. J Am Board Fam Med 20: 365–374.
14. Okura K, Lavigne GJ, Huynh N, Manzini C, Fillipini D, et al. (2008) Comparison of sleep variables between chronic widespread musculoskeletal pain, insomnia, periodic leg movements syndrome and control subjects in a clinical sleep medicine practice. Sleep Med 9: 352–361.
15. Smith MT, Wickwire EM, Grace EG, Edwards RR, Buenaver LF, et al. (2009) Sleep disorders and their association with laboratory pain sensitivity in temporomandibular joint disorder. Sleep 32: 779–790.
16. Menefee LA, Cohen MJ, Anderson WR, Doghramji K, Frank ED, et al. (2000) Sleep disturbance and nonmalignant chronic pain: a comprehensive review of the literature. Pain Med 1: 156–172.
17. Okifuji A, Hare BD (2011) Do sleep disorders contribute to pain sensitivity? Curr Rheumatol Rep 13: 528–534.
18. Edwards RR, Grace E, Peterson S, Klick B, Haythornthwaite JA, et al. (2009) Sleep continuity and architecture: Associations with pain-inhibitory processes in patients with temporomandibular joint disorder. Eur J Pain 13: 1043–1047.
19. Smith MT, Edwards RR, McCann UD, Haythornthwaite JA (2007) The effects of sleep deprivation on pain inhibition and spontaneous pain in women. Sleep 30: 494–505.
20. Edwards RR, Almeida DM, Klick B, Haythornthwaite JA, Smith MT (2008) Duration of sleep contributes to next-day pain report in the general population. Pain 137: 202–207.
21. Smith MT, Haythornthwaite JA (2004) How do sleep disturbance and chronic pain inter-relate? Insights from the longitudinal and cognitive-behavioral clinical trials literature. Sleep Med Rev 8: 119–132.
22. Smith MT, Klick B, Kozachik S, Edwards RE, Holavanahalli R, et al. (2008) Sleep onset insomnia symptoms during hospitalization for major burn injury predict chronic pain. Pain 138: 497–506.
23. Lavigne GJ, Nashed A, Manzini C, Carra MC (2011) Does sleep differ among patients with common musculoskeletal pain disorders? Curr Rheumatol Rep 13: 535–542.
24. Bigatti SM, Hernandez AM, Cronan TA, Rand KL (2008) Sleep disturbances in fibromyalgia syndrome: relationship to pain and depression. Arthritis Rheum 59: 961–967.
25. Mork PJ, Nilsen TI (2012) Sleep problems and risk of fibromyalgia: longitudinal data on an adult female population in Norway. Arthritis Rheum 64: 281–284.
26. O'Brien EM, Waxenberg LB, Atchison JW, Gremillion HA, Staud RM, et al. (2011) Intraindividual variability in daily sleep and pain ratings among chronic pain patients: bidirectional association and the role of negative mood. Clin J Pain 27: 425–433.
27. Lau J, Ioannidis JP, Schmid CH (1997) Quantitative synthesis in systematic reviews. Ann Intern Med 127: 820–826.
28. Rains JC, Poceta JS (2010) Sleep and headache. Curr Treat Options Neurol 12: 1–15.
29. Rasmussen BK (1993) Migraine and tension-type headache in a general population: precipitating factors, female hormones, sleep pattern and relation to lifestyle. Pain 53: 65–72.
30. Wilson KG, Watson ST, Currie SR (1998) Daily diary and ambulatory activity monitoring of sleep in patients with insomnia associated with chronic musculoskeletal pain. Pain 75: 75–84.
31. Wittig RM, Zorick FJ, Blumer D, Heilbronn M, Roth T (1982) Disturbed sleep in patients complaining of chronic pain. J Nerv Ment Dis 170: 429–431.
32. Kelman L, Rains JC (2005) Headache and sleep: examination of sleep patterns and complaints in a large clinical sample of migraineurs. Headache 45: 904–910.
33. Haack M, Lee E, Cohen DA, Mullington JM (2009) Activation of the prostaglandin system in response to sleep loss in healthy humans: potential mediator of increased spontaneous pain. Pain 145: 136–141.
34. Smith MT, Quartana PJ, Okonkwo RM, Nasir A (2009) Mechanisms by which sleep disturbance contributes to osteoarthritis pain: a conceptual model. Curr Pain Headache Rep 13: 447–454.
35. Birks J (2006) Cholinesterase inhibitors for Alzheimer's disease. Cochrane Database Syst Rev: CD005593.
36. Rosner S, Hackl-Herrwerth A, Leucht S, Vecchi S, Srisurapanont M, et al. (2010) Opioid antagonists for alcohol dependence. Cochrane Database Syst Rev: CD001867.
37. Cipriani A, La Ferla T, Furukawa TA, Signoretti A, Nakagawa A, et al. (2010) Sertraline versus other antidepressive agents for depression. Cochrane Database Syst Rev: CD006117.
38. Davis L, Kennedy SS, Moore J, Prentice A (2007) Modern combined oral contraceptives for pain associated with endometriosis. Cochrane Database Syst Rev: CD001019.
39. Pennick VE, Young G (2007) Interventions for preventing and treating pelvic and back pain in pregnancy. Cochrane Database Syst Rev: CD001139.
40. Brown J, Pan A, Hart RJ (2010) Gonadotrophin-releasing hormone analogues for pain associated with endometriosis. Cochrane Database Syst Rev: CD008475.
41. Osei-Akoto A, Orton L, Owusu-Ofori SP (2005) Atovaquone-proguanil for treating uncomplicated malaria. Cochrane Database Syst Rev: CD004529.
42. Fine PG (2011) Long-term consequences of chronic pain: mounting evidence for pain as a neurological disease and parallels with other chronic disease states. Pain Med 12: 996–1004.
43. Lateef T, Swanson S, Cui L, Nelson K, Nakamura E, et al. (2011) Headaches and sleep problems among adults in the United States: findings from the National Comorbidity Survey-Replication study. Cephalalgia 31: 648–653.
44. Davies KA, Macfarlane GJ, Nicholl BI, Dickens C, Morriss R, et al. (2008) Restorative sleep predicts the resolution of chronic widespread pain: results from the EPIFUND study. Rheumatology (Oxford) 47: 1809–1813.
45. Sivertsen B, Krokstad S, Overland S, Mykletun A (2009) The epidemiology of insomnia: associations with physical and mental health. The HUNT-2 study. J Psychosom Res 67: 109–116.
46. Pilowsky I, Crettenden I, Townley M (1985) Sleep disturbance in pain clinic patients. Pain 23: 27–33.
47. Ciraulo DA, Piechniczek-Buczek J, Iscan EN (2003) Outcome predictors in substance use disorders. Psychiatr Clin North Am 26: 381–409.
48. National Library of Medicine (2008) DailyMed: Current medication information. May 19, 2008 ed: U.S. National Library of Medicine, National Institutes of Health.
49. Marin R, Cyhan T, Miklos W (2006) Sleep disturbance in patients with chronic low back pain. Am J Phys Med Rehabil 85: 430–435.

Enhanced Auditory Brainstem Response and Parental Bonding Style in Children with Gastrointestinal Symptoms

Shizuka Seino[1], Satoshi Watanabe[1], Namiko Ito[1], Konosuke Sasaki[2], Kaori Shoji[2], Shoko Miura[4], Kanoko Kozawa[4], Kunihiko Nakai[3], Hiroshi Sato[3], Motoyori Kanazawa[1], Shin Fukudo[1]*

1 Department of Behavioral Medicine, Tohoku University Graduate School of Medicine, Sendai, Japan, **2** Health Science, Tohoku University Graduate School of Medicine, Sendai, Japan, **3** Department of Environmental Health Science, Tohoku University Graduate School of Medicine, Sendai, Japan, **4** Department of Clinical Physiology, Tohoku University Hospital, Sendai, Japan

Abstract

Background: The electrophysiological properties of the brain and influence of parental bonding in childhood irritable bowel syndrome (IBS) are unclear. We hypothesized that children with chronic gastrointestinal (GI) symptoms like IBS may show exaggerated brainstem auditory evoked potential (BAEP) responses and receive more inadequate parental bonding.

Methodology/Principal Findings: Children aged seven and their mothers (141 pairs) participated. BAEP was measured by summation of 1,000 waves of the electroencephalogram triggered by 75 dB click sounds. The mothers completed their Children's Somatization Inventory (CSI) and Parental Bonding Instrument (PBI). CSI results revealed 66 (42%) children without GI symptoms (controls) and 75 (58%) children with one or more GI symptoms (GI group). The III wave in the GI group (median 4.10 interquartile range [3.95–4.24] ms right, 4.04 [3.90–4.18] ms left) had a significantly shorter peak latency than controls (4.18 [4.06–4.34] ms right, $p = 0.032$, 4.13 [4.02–4.24] ms left, $p = 0.018$). The female GI group showed a significantly shorter peak latency of the III wave (4.00 [3.90–4.18] ms) than controls (4.18 [3.97–4.31] ms, $p = 0.034$) in the right side. BAEP in the male GI group did not significantly differ from that in controls. GI scores showed a significant correlation with the peak latency of the III wave in the left side (rho = −0.192, p = 0.025). The maternal care PBI scores in the GI group (29 [26–33]) were significantly lower than controls (31 [28.5–33], $p = 0.010$), while the maternal over-protection PBI scores were significantly higher in the GI group (16 [12–17]) than controls (13 [10.5–16], $p = 0.024$). Multiple regression analysis in females also supported these findings.

Conclusions: It is suggested that children with chronic GI symptoms have exaggerated brainstem responses to environmental stimuli and inadequate parental behaviors aggravate these symptoms.

Editor: Antje Timmer, Bremen Institute of Preventive Research and Social Medicine, Germany

Funding: This research was supported by a Grant-in-Aid for Scientific Research from Ministry of Ministry of Education, Culture, Sports, Science and Technology Ministry of Health, Labour and Welfare, Japan. The funders had no role in study design, data collection and analysis, decision to publish, or preparation of the manuscript.

Competing Interests: The authors have declared that no competing interests exist.

* E-mail: sfukudo@med.tohoku.ac.jp

Introduction

Irritable bowel syndrome (IBS) is the most common functional gastrointestinal (GI) disorder (FGID) [1]. IBS is characterized by altered bowel habits and is associated with chronic abdominal pain and discomfort [2]. On the other hand, recurrent abdominal pain (RAP) during childhood is one of the most common pediatric disorders [3], [4], with epidemiological studies suggesting that 7–25% of school-age children suffer from RAP [5], [6]. RAP in childhood has been known to have visceral hypersensitivity sharing the pathophysiological features of childhood IBS [7] and to develop into adult IBS [8]. The prevalence of RAP increases with age into adolescence [8]. Age and gender have been shown to influence the prevalence of RAP, with an equal gender ratio in early childhood, with symptoms reported by girls predominately by late childhood [6], [9]. However, the pathogenesis and pathophysiology of IBS/RAP in childhood is complex and incompletely understood. It is not clear whether there is sex difference of pathophysiology of childhood IBS/RAP and the process of development into IBS.

In IBS patients, visceral hypersensitivity is one of the representative pathophysiology phenomena [10], [11]. Several studies using rectal barostats have confirmed the presence of visceral hypersensitivity by showing lower pain thresholds in children with IBS [4], [7], [12]. This enhanced sensitivity may underlie the multiple IBS mechanisms including increased attention, arousal, and emotion [13], [14]. Several brain imaging studies also observed greater activation of the dorsal pons and midbrain region in IBS patients to rectal distention [15]. In the dorsal brainstem, down-regulation is inhibited in IBS patients during cued expectation [16]. During anticipated conditions, down-regulation is maximal within the dorsal pons after habituation [16]. From this evidence, it appears that IBS patients show different brainstem activities.

IBS patients also show altered central nervous system (CNS) responses to stimuli unrelated to the GI tract [17], [18]. Berman et al. [18] reported a pre-attentive disorder of non-visceral sensory gating as measured by event related potential (ERP). IBS patients show hypersensitivity to various stimuli (such as an exaggerated startle response) and deficits in the ability to habituate to adverse information [17], [18]. Hypersensitivity and deficits to control experimental stimuli may be the key feature of IBS and play an important role in central pain amplification [11]. Therefore, IBS patients have not only visceral hypersensitivity but also hypersensitivity to stimuli unrelated to the GI tract.

The sensitivity of children's brainstems can be examined using the brainstem auditory evoked potential (BAEP) [19], [20]. The amplitude and latency of several electroencephalogram (EEG) waveforms recorded from scalp electrodes in response to specific sensory events are physiological measures of CNS [19], [20]. In particular, the latency of the BAEP wave is an indicator of sensory processing and estimates CNS responsiveness [19], [20]. Although several previous studies evaluated central sensitivity using ERP [18], none have investigated BAEP in children with GI symptoms. Moreover, childhood is an important period for neurodevelopment and is characterized by increased vulnerability to stressors [21], [22]. IBS/RAP children experience more stressful life events in the year before the onset of their symptoms [22], [23], and stressful life events may be associated with abdominal pain in IBS/RAP children [5], [24].

Levy et al. [25] indicated that environmental factors have an equal or greater influence on the development of IBS than genetic factors. Parental overprotection [26] or an unusually high degree of parental anxiety has been shown to have an effect on children's health [27], [28]. Previous studies revealed that patients with psychiatric disorders are apt to receive low parental care or excessive over-protection [28–30]. Therefore, it is suspected that alterations of neural pathways along the brain-gut axis could lay the physiological foundations for the integration of life experiences such as sustained parental bonding. However, it is not clear how GI symptoms in children and parental bonding interact with each other. Moreover, how BAEP response in children is influenced by parental bonding style has not been investigated.

In the present study, we investigated the pathogenesis and pathophysiology with neurophysiological features of children at seven. We regarded the age 7 as important period to construct the neurological foundation and the valid period because this age is known to be the pediatric onset of IBS [6]. Moreover, age 7 was used as a reliable age to complete the neurobehavioral testing in the previous study [20]. The aim of this study was to explore the pathogenesis and pathophysiology of FGID in childhood. We tested the primary hypothesis that children with GI symptoms like FGID show exaggerated BAEP responses. We also tested the secondary hypothesis that children with GI symptoms receive more inadequate parental bonding from their parents and the tertiary hypothesis that BAEP response in children is influenced by parental bonding style.

Materials and Methods

Subjects

A total of 141 mother-child pairs (73 male children and 68 female children) participated in this study. The healthy participants were recruited without desease, serious mental retardation and mental illness. All children were just 84 months old at the experimental time point and had no audiometric or neurological complaints. Subjects were screened using a medical checklist to exclude current epilepsy or psychoactive medication treatment. No children had inflammatory or other structural diseases as assessed by medical interview. Verbal and written informed consent was obtained from the caretakers of all subjects. This study is part of the Tohoku study of child development but tested hypotheses were completely different from the published study [31]. The present study was approved by Tohoku University Ethics Committee and is performed in accordance with the ethical standards laid down in the Declaration of Helsinki.

Brainstem auditory evoked potential (BAEP) recordings

The entire experimental session lasted about 2 h. After familiarization with the testing equipment and subsequent equipment fitting, the subjects sat on a chair in a resting state with eyes open in a sound-attenuated air-conditioned and dimly lit room during electroencephalogram (EEG) recording, which has been reported previously [32]. In brief, according to the international 10–20 system, original EEG signals were recorded from scalp Ag/AgCl electrodes and separate ear electrodes A1 and A2. Impedance of electrodes/skin was kept below 5 kΩ.

Segments containing eye movements, blinks, and muscle activity were excluded from analysis. The subjects were instructed to minimize eye blinks and refrain from making movements during the experimental session. On demand, some parents sat beside their children in the testing room during the experimental session. Necessary announcements were given via intercom. The subjects were monitored outside the testing room by a camera system.

The experimental session consisted of two blocks. The first block started with a 75 dB click noise in the right ear and 45 dB white noise masking the opposite ear via headphones; these noises were exchanged from side to side. Stimuli of 75 dB were presented at 0.1 ms duration with a frequency of 20 Hz and an interval of 50 ms. The second block started with a 90 dB click noise in the left ear using the same procedure. Two blocks of 1,000 repetitions were recorded for about 100 s. Data were analyzed using a computer program (Signal Processor 7T-18; NEC Sanei Instruments, Ltd, Tokyo, Japan) and software (EPLYZER, BIMUSTAS; Kissei Comtec, Nagano, Japan) with a 100 ms recording window starting 10 ms after the stimulus onset. Responses were averaged from 2,000 stimuli. All BAEP data were assessed through computerized procedures. Two independent researchers identified BAEP waveforms and measured the latency. Peak latencies were measured in relation to the stimulus [33].

GI Symptoms and Parental Bonding

The subjects' mothers were administered the Children's Somatization Inventory (CSI) and the Parental Bonding Instrument (PBI) before commencement of the BAEP.

Children's Somatization Inventory

The Children's Somatization Inventory (CSI) [34], [35] is a self-report questionnaire comprising 35 items and requiring individuals to report the extent to which they experienced each symptom in the previous two weeks: 0 = not at all, 1 = a little, 2 = somewhat, 3 = a lot, 4 = a whole lot. The total CSI score (maximum 140) is the sum of all items reflecting both the range and intensity of experienced symptoms. The CSI has previously been shown to have adequate good internal reliability with coefficient alphas in excess of 0.90. There are four factors in this inventory: pseudoneurological symptoms, cardiovascular symptoms, gastrointestinal symptoms, and pain weakness symptoms.

There are seven items related to GI symptoms like FGID in the CSI questionnaire including abdominal pain, constipation, diarrhea, and abdominal bloating. Using the questionnaire, the children were divided into two groups. Those with a GI score of one or more were classified as the "GI group" and the other children with no GI score were classified as "controls".

Parental Bonding Instrument

The Parental Bonding Instrument (PBI) is a well-validated inventory [36], [37] that has also been widely used in medical studies [26], [30]. It is a self-report questionnaire with 25 items that measures parental styles recalled by the responders from the first 16 years of their childhood. The PBI is scored separately for fathers and mothers to subjectively evaluate the relationship between children and each of their parents. Responders were asked to score their attitudes or behaviors using four-point Likert scales (very much like, moderately like, moderately unlike, very unlike). The PBI consists of two factors: the over-protection factor (13 items, a maximum score of 39 and cut-off score 13.5 for mother and 12.5 for father) and the care factor (12 items, a maximum of 36 and cut-off score 27 for mother and 24 for father). Mothers of all subjects completed the PBI both for themselves and the children's fathers.

Statistical Analyses

All mothers (n = 141) filled out the CSI, but two did not complete the PBI values. Some BAEP values from the right (n = 9) or left side (n = 6) were incomplete because children dropped out during the experimental session because of anxiety or the inability to sit still for a long time.

The Statistical Package for Social Sciences (SPSS), version 12.0 for Windows, was used in all analysis. Results are expressed as the median [interquartile ranges]. Comparisons of differences between two groups were performed by Mann-Whitney U-test. Correlation coefficients were calculated with Spearman's Rho. Multiple regression analysis was performed to determine the relationship between GI scores and BAEP parameters, parental care, parental overprotection, and CSI scores, with the exception of GI scores. Statistical significance was judged by a p-value less than 0.05.

Results

Children with GI symptoms screened by CSI

There were 66 (42%) children (37 males and 29 females) without GI symptoms (controls). Seventy-five (58%) children (36 males and 39 females) had one or more GI symptoms and were classified as the GI group. GI scores of the GI group ranged from 1 to 21 with a mean of 2.3 and a SD of 2.7.

Comparison of BAEP peak latency between controls and GI group

We obtained remarkable and positive I, III, and V waves in ipsilateral recordings of the stimulated sides and vague wave forms in contralateral recordings of the opposite sides (**Figure 1**). In the ipsilateral recordings, the original III wave form of the GI group showed a shorter latency than that of controls.

In the right side, the latency of the III wave in the GI group (4.10 [3.95–4.24] ms) had a significantly shorter peak latency than that in controls (4.18 [4.06–4.34] ms, $p = 0.032$) (**Figure 2A**). In the left side, the latency of the III wave in the GI group (4.04 [3.90–4.18] ms) had a significantly shorter peak latency than that in controls (4.13 [4.02–4.24] ms, $p = 0.018$) (**Figure 2B**). By contrast, there was no significant difference in I and V waves between the two groups (**Table 1**).

BAEP peak latency in female and male GI groups

The female GI group had a significantly shorter peak latency of the III wave in the right side (4.00 [3.90–4.18] ms) than controls (4.18 [3.97–4.31] ms, $p = 0.034$) (**Figure 3A**). There was a tendentially but not significantly shorter peak latency of the III wave in the left side of the female GI group (3.94 [3.84–4.06] ms) than that of controls (4.08 [3.93–4.19] ms, $p = 0.059$) (**Figure 3B**). By contrast, the male GI group showed the same peak latency of the III wave in the right side (4.21 [4.02–4.34] ms) and left side (4.10 [4.02–4.20] ms) compared with the controls in the right side (4.21 [4.08–4.37] ms, $p = 0.668$) and left side (4.16 [4.02–4.25] ms, $p = 0.279$) (**Figure 3C, 3D**). There was no significant difference in the other components between the two female groups or two male groups (**Table 1**).

Correlation between GI symptoms and BAEP latency of III wave

The number of GI symptoms slightly but significantly correlated with the peak latency of the III wave on the left side (rho = −0.19, $p = 0.028$). GI scores also showed a significant correlation with the peak latency of the III wave on the left side (rho = −0.19, $p = 0.025$).

BAEP peak latency and somatization

We divided children into two groups according to the median (5) total CSI score. There was no significant difference in the peak

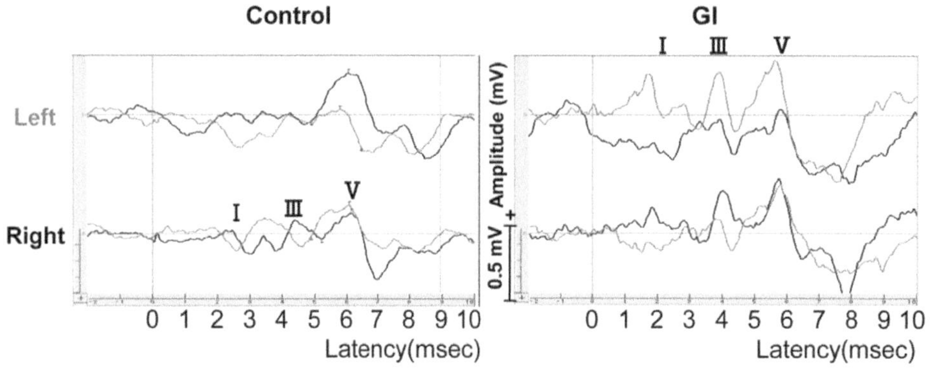

Figure 1. Actual wave forms of the brainstem auditory evoked potential (BAEP) in controls and FGID children. Upper lines are BAEPs with left ear stimulation, lower lines are BAEPs with right ear stimulation. Gray lines indicate recordings of left side, black lines show those of right side. Note remarkable and positive I, III, and V waves in ipsilateral recordings of stimulated sides, and vague wave forms in contralateral recordings of opposite sides. Note shorter latency of III wave in GI child compared with control.

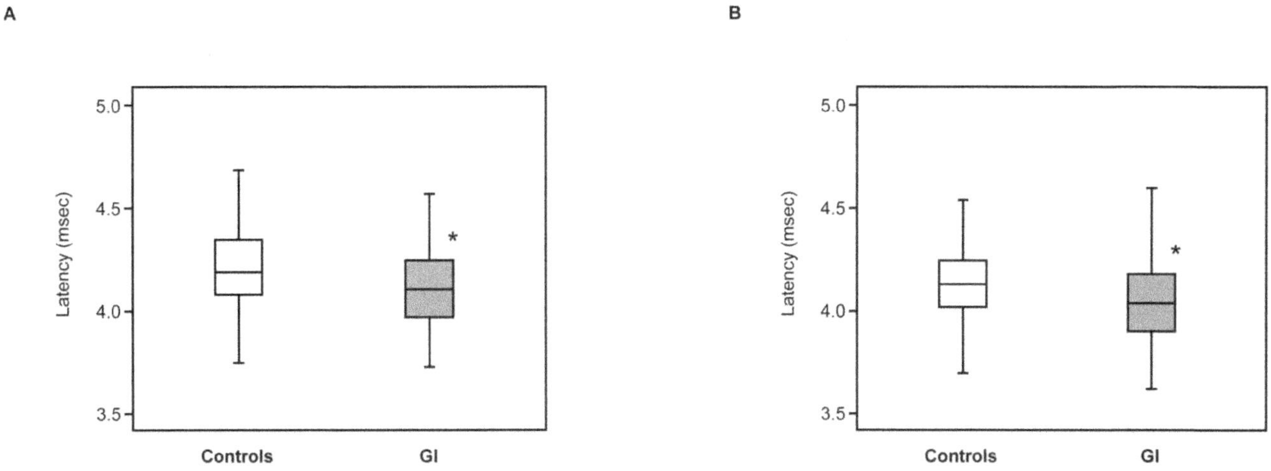

Figure 2. Peak latency of BAEP III wave in all children. **A**: right ear, □open box: controls (n = 63), ■shaded box: GI group (n = 69). **B**: left ear, □open box: controls (n = 62), ■shaded box: GI group (n = 73). Values (msec) are given as median [interquartile range] (minimum-maximum). Asterisk (*) indicates significant difference versus controls at $p = 0.032$ in the right and $p = 0.018$ in the left.

latency in any component between children with high somatization and those with low somatization (data not shown).

PBI and GI symptoms

The maternal care PBI scores in the GI group (29 [26–33]) were significantly lower than those of controls (31 [28.5–33], $p = 0.010$) (**Figure 4A**). In addition, the PBI maternal care score showed a significantly negative correlation with GI scores (rho = −0.22, $p = 0.010$). The maternal over-protection PBI scores in the GI group (16 [12–17]) were significantly higher than those of controls (13 [10.5–16], $p = 0.024$) (**Figure 4B**) and showed a significantly positive correlation with GI scores (rho = 0.19, $p = 0.023$). There was no significant difference in paternal care between GI group and controls.

Table 1. Latency of I and V Waves of the Brainstem Auditory Evoked Potential.

Latency (msec)	controls	GI	p-value
All subjects (number)	63 (right)/62 (left)	69 (right)/73 (left)	
I wave (right)	1.96 (1.83–2.10)	1.94 (1.84–2.04)	0.629
I wave (left)	1.85 (1.72–2.04)	1.82 (1.74–2.00)	0.563
V wave (right)	5.88 (5.79–6.06)	5.88 (5.74–6.02)	0.460
V wave (left)	5.84 (5.74–6.00)	5.82 (5.66–5.96)	0.405
Female (number)	27 (right)/27 (left)	35 (right)/37 (left)	
I wave (right)	1.96 (1.84–2.07)	1.90 (1.81–2.02)	0.303
I wave (left)	1.86 (1.79–2.12)	1.78 (1.72–1.90)	0.133
V wave (right)	5.82 (5.76–5.87)	5.84 (5.75–5.92)	0.594
V wave (left)	5.76 (5.67–5.88)	5.76 (5.54–5.92)	0.629
Male (number)	36 (right)/35 (left)	34 (right)/36 (left)	
I wave (right)	1.96 (1.83–2.22)	1.98 (1.88–2.14)	0.659
I wave (left)	1.84 (1.71–2.02)	1.84 (1.76–2.02)	0.519
V wave (right)	6.00 (5.87–6.11)	5.95 (5.74–6.12)	0.394
V wave (left)	5.90 (5.80–6.03)	5.87 (5.72–6.02)	0.743

Data are expressed with median [interquartile range].

Correlation between PBI and BAEP latency of III wave

There was no significant correlation between PBI scores and BAEP latency of III wave (data not shown).

Multivariate analysis between GI symptoms and CSI/PBI/BAEP

Multiple regression analysis revealed that GI scores were significantly predicted by CSI (except GI) score ($\beta = 0.833$, $p = 0.0001$), maternal care ($\beta = -0.160$, $p = 0.014$) and paternal care ($\beta = 0.174$, $p = 0.007$) and tendentially but not significantly predicted by latency of III wave in the left side ($\beta = -0.163$, $p = 0.058$) ($R^2 = 0.699$, $p = 0.0001$)(**Table 2**). Moreover, multiple regression analysis in female revealed that GI scores were significantly predicted by CSI (except GI) score ($\beta = 0.550$, $p = 0.0001$), maternal care ($\beta = -0.384$, $p = 0.001$), paternal care ($\beta = 0.345$, $p = 0.003$) and latency of III wave in the right side ($\beta = -0.257$, $p = 0.015$) ($R^2 = 0.495$, $p = 0.0001$). By contrast, multiple regression analysis in male revealed that GI scores were only predicted by CSI (except GI) score ($\beta = 0.873$, $p = 0.0001$) ($R^2 = 0.775$, $p = 0.0001$).

Discussion

This is the first study to demonstrate an exaggerated response in the brainstem to auditory stimuli in children with GI symptoms. The shorter latency of the BAEP III wave in children with GI symptoms at supports our main hypothesis. By contrast, regarding somatization, there is no significant difference in peak latency of all components compared with controls. Therefore, differences in the peak latency of the III wave may be related to IBS-like symptoms. Peaks of the I, III, and V waves are thought to reflect volume-conducted electrical activity from the acoustic nerve, pons (superior olivary nucleus), and midbrain (inferior colliculi) [33]. The latency of the peak III component of BAEP reflects the brainstem response [33] and is known to increase with age [38]. In previous studies [20], the latency of the BAEP III wave in seven-year-old Japanese children positively correlated with their hair mercury concentration, reflecting neurodevelopmental toxicity caused by methylmercury exposure. The latency of the III wave was previously shown to be negatively correlated with the number of cigarettes smoked during the three months prior to pregnancy

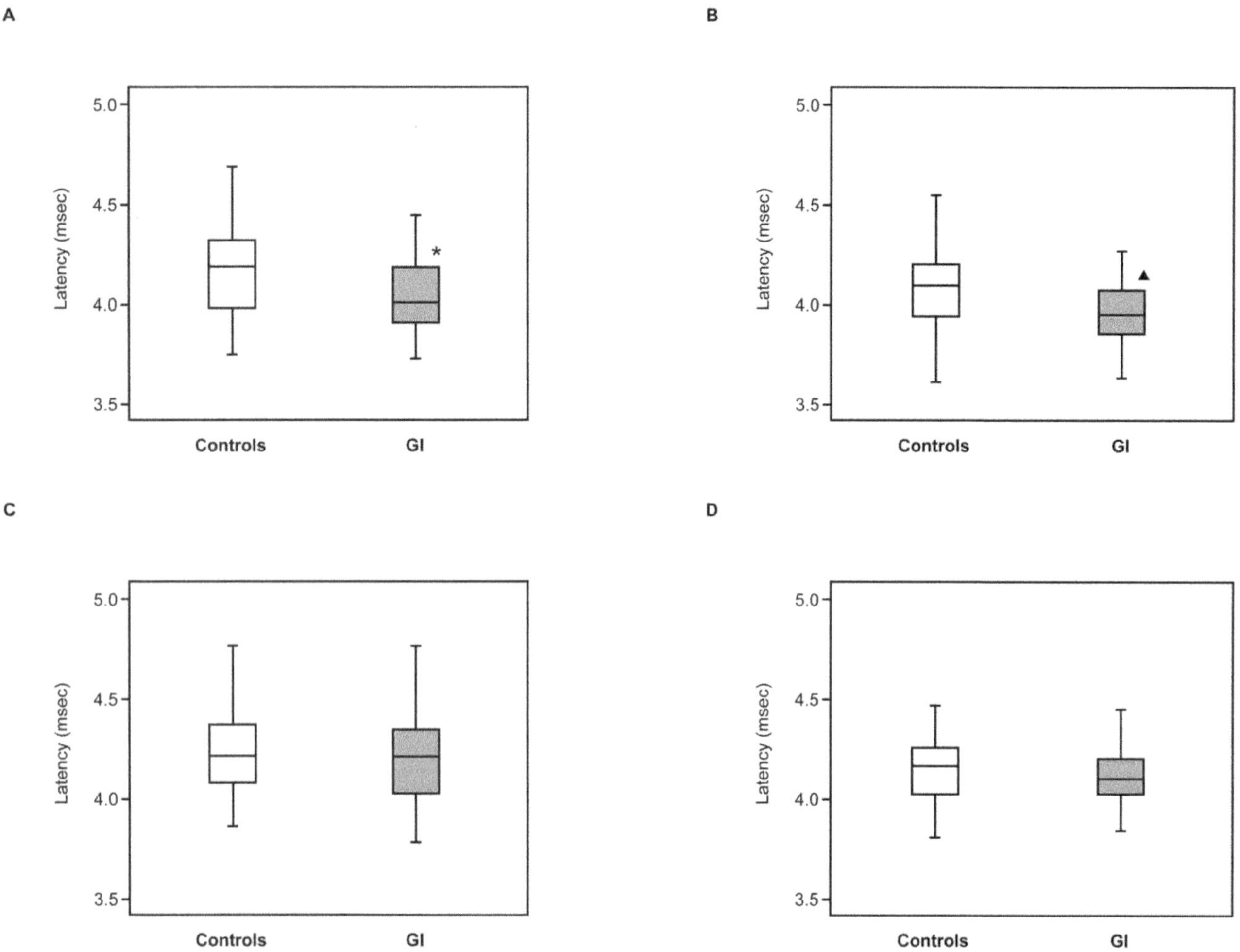

Figure 3. Peak latency of BAEP III wave in females and males. A: female, right ear, □open box: controls (n = 27), ■shaded box: GI group (n = 35), **B**: female, left ear, □open box: controls (n = 27), ■shaded box: GI group (n = 37), **C**: male, right ear, □open box: controls (n = 36), ■shaded box: GI group (n = 34), **D**: male, left ear, □open box: controls (n = 35), ■shaded box: GI group (n = 36). Values (ms) are given as median [interquartile range] (minimum-maximum). Asterisk (*) indicates significant difference versus controls at $p = 0.034$. Solid triangle (▲) indicates tendentially but not significantly different from controls at $p = 0.059$.

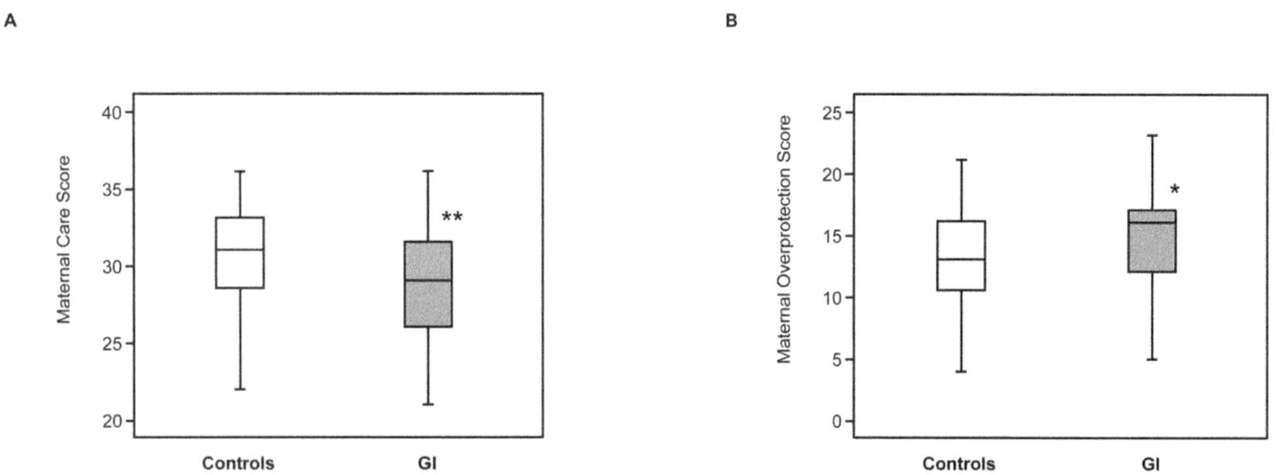

Figure 4. The care score and over-protection score of Parental Bonding Instrument in controls and FGID children. A: maternal care, **B**: maternal overprotection, □open box: controls (n = 64), ■shaded box: GI group (n = 75). Values (ms) are given as median [interquartile range] (minimum-maximum). Double asterisk (**) indicates significant difference versus controls at $p = 0.010$ (A). Asterisk (*) indicates significant difference versus controls at $p = 0.024$ (B).

Table 2. Multiple regression analysis for total sample.

independent variable	standardized β	*p*-value
CSI (except GI) score	0.833	0.0001
paternal care	0.174	0.007
maternal care	−0.160	0.014
latency of III wave (left)	−0.163	0.058
latency of V wave (left)	0.083	0.411
maternal overptotection	−0.054	0.429
latency of I wave (right)	−0.032	0.702
latency of V wave (right)	0.033	0.741
paternal overprotection	0.021	0.754
latency of III wave (right)	−0.022	0.826
latency of I wave (left)	−0.010	0.896

GI symptoms as dependent variable and CSI (except GI) score, parental care, over-protection, and latencies of BAEP as independent variables. $R^2 = 0.699$, $p = 0.0001$.

[39]. Wang et al. [40] also revealed a positive relationship between BAEP and the clinical state of cognition in Alzheimer's disease. Given this background, our findings may reflect a developmental deficit of the brainstem as well as an exaggerated response to auditory stimuli but not minor brain damage.

The BAEP findings in the present study are in the same direction with the earlier studies. Berman et al. [18] revealed that IBS patients show an enhanced large P_1 of ERP due in part to the activity of the pontine region associated with the cholinergic ascending arousal system. The brainstem locus coeruleus is the primary source of ascending noradrenergic projections that mediate arousal and form a positive feedback loop with corticotropin-releasing hormone-containing neurons in the amygdala [41], [42]. There is no clear explanation of female predominant shorter latency of BAEP III wave. However, the locus coeruleus is known to be larger in females than in males [43]. Moreover, brain imaging studies showed that female IBS patients were unable to downwardly regulate the homeostatic afferent processing that occurs during normal anticipation of visceral pain [16], and demonstrate increased activation in the dorsal brainstem and anterior cingulate cortex [16]. The biological substrate functioning as top-down or bottom-up modulation to external stimuli in IBS/RAP children may contribute to enhanced brainstem responsiveness, while the shorter latency of the BAEP III wave clearly seen in female children with GI symptoms may be due to altered perceptual responses to afferent signals. Thus, our main hypothesis was partially supported by results from female children with GI symptoms. Further study is needed to reject the shorter latency of BAEP III wave in male children with GI symptoms.

Our CSI and PBI results support the secondary hypothesis that this study set out to test, namely that children with GI symptoms receive more inadequate parental bonding, such as imbalance of parental bonding, reduced maternal care, excessive paternal care, or overprotection from their parents. The tertiary hypothesis that PBI scores relate to BAEP was not supported. Therefore, inadequate parental bonding and BAEP are independent factors that affect GI symptoms. Adverse childhood experiences are proven risk factors for the development of many diseases [26], [29], [30] and an association between adverse parenting and abnormal cortisol levels has been reported in previous studies [44], [45]. Alterations in the hypothalamic-pituitary-adrenal (HPA) axis and sympathetic nervous system (SNS) have been reported in several stress-related disorders [46], [47]. Many studies revealed that maladaptive HPA responses and SNS function relate to FGID such as IBS [48–50]. Exposure to adverse environments such as inadequate parenting during childhood may lead to serious life-long effects due to impaired brain development and dysregulation of the brain-gut axis [1], [51]. Moreover, chronic sustained stress, particularly as a primary life event, has been demonstrated to be an important factor in both FGID onset and modulation [49], [52]. The mother's parental style during childhood may be associated with dysregulation of emotional inhibition [53], [54] and the onset of GI symptoms [55], [56].

In this study, maternal overprotection beyond normal range and reduced maternal care even within normal range among inadequate parental behaviors are likely to play some roles in childhood GI symptoms. Clinical and epidemiological studies suggest that adverse parenting characterized by low care is a significant risk factor in the development of depressive disorder [30]. Some studies reported that adverse experiences in childhood are mediated by other long-standing vulnerability factors [30], [45]. For example, Walker et al. [23] reported that child patients with abdominal pain have higher levels of anxiety and depression than those without pain, while Levy et al. [25] clarified the mechanism of frequent GI complaints in children based on solicitous responses to illness from their mothers. Childhood and adolescence are important periods for neurodevelopment and maturation of brain regions [57]. While our study researches a similar area to these previous investigations, it builds on the earlier studies by depicting specific parenting styles that increase the risk of developing FGID.

Linear regression analysis revealed that paternal care and maternal care are the predictable factors associated with GI symptoms. In this study, it is not clear why the score of maternal care was negatively related to GI symptoms, but paternal care was positively related to GI score. It is possible that the responders' recall bias may affect these opposite result. Janssens et al [26]. reported that parental bonding may play a role in the development of functional somatic symptoms, and several studies indicated that IBS patients have a hypervigilance for symptom-relevant sensations [58], [59]. The number of GI symptoms is likely to be associated with hypersensitivity. IBS patients show a decreased ability to refocus attention away from bothersome stimuli under chronic heightened autonomic arousal [16]. Hypersensitivity may therefore be associated with attentional and affective modulation of perception in IBS [51]. Neuroplastic and structural alterations have been observed in the CNS in response to sustained severe life stress [46], [47], including presynaptic and postsynaptic changes in ascending monoaminergic arousal systems and the HPA axis [46], [47], which are likely to be related to functional GI symptoms. The relationship between bonding and GI symptoms may go in both directions: either the way of parental bonding changes because the child has GI symptoms (and as a reaction the mother is more over-protective etc.) or the child develops GI problems because of bad parenting. Further research to testify the influence of generation, culture, and gender of caregiver on parental bonding and GI symptoms of children will be available.

This study has some limitations. First, PBI was retrospectively used for measuring the behavior of parents and as such we could not avoid recall bias. However, PBI reliability has been confirmed in previous studies [26], [29], [30], so this limitation is in line with the earlier works. Second, we cannot rule out the possibility that the fact itself that their children had GI symptoms might influence the mothers' replies to PBI. In addition, the mothers' replies to PBI about their husband might be influenced by their relationship. Third, it is difficult to use a questionnaire to measure emotion in seven-year-old children, and therefore this state could not be assessed. Last, we assessed children with IBS-like symptoms using reports from their mothers rather than the results of colonoscopy, radiological examination, or histological biopsy. However, colonic cancer and inflammatory bowel disease among this population is negligible [60]. This study design was done from an ethical point of view to prevent risk to the children.

In conclusion, our study suggests that children with GI symptoms show exaggerated BAEP responses and that they receive more inadequate parental bonding from their parents. Further studies are warranted to explore the pathogenesis and pathophysiology of FGID in childhood together with neurodevelopment.

Acknowledgments

This study is based in part on the research from Tohoku Study of Child Development provided by Environmental Health Science, Tohoku University Graduate School of Medicine. The authors express sincere gratitude to Ms Nozomi Tatsuta of Environmental Health Science, Tohoku University Graduate School of Medicine and Mr Taiki Hattori of Health Science, Tohoku University Graduate School of Medicine for data collection and data management. Think SCIENCE KK assisted writing the manuscript.

Author Contributions

Conceived and designed the experiments: SF KN HS SW SS. Performed the experiments: SS SW NI K. Sasaki K. Shoji SM KK . Analyzed the data: SS MK SW NI K. Sasaki K. Shoji SM KK SF. Contributed reagents/materials/analysis tools: SS SW MK. Wrote the paper: SF SS MK.

References

1. Chang L, Toner BB, Fukudo S, Guthrie E, Locke GR, et al. (2006) Gender, age, society, culture, and the patient's perspective in the functional gastrointestinal disorders. Gastroenterology 130: 1435–1446.
2. Longstreth GF, Thompson WG, Chey WD, Houghton LA, Mearin F, et al. (2006) Functional bowel disorders. Gastroenterology 130: 1480–1491.
3. Plunkett A, Beattie RM (2005) Recurrent abdominal pain in childhood. J Royal Soc Med 98: 101–106.
4. Vlieger AM, Van den Berg MM, Menko-Frankenhuis C, Bongers ME, Tromp E, et al. (2010) No change in rectal sensitivity after gut-directed hypnotherapy in children with functional abdominal pain or Irritable bowel syndrome. Am J Gastroenterol 105: 213–218.
5. Campo JV, Bridge J, Ehmann M, Altman S, Lucas A, et al. (2004) Recurrent abdominal pain, anxiety, and depression in primary care. Pediatrics 113: 817–824.
6. Howell S, Poulton R, Talley NJ (2005) The natural history of childhood abdominal pain and its association with adult irritable bowel syndrome: birth-cohort study. Am J Gastroenterol 100: 2071–2078.
7. Di Lorenzo C, Youssef NN, Singudsson L, Scharff L, Griffiths J, et al. (2001) Visceral hyperalgesia in children with functional abdominal pain. J Pediatr 139: 838–843.
8. Walker LS, Guite JW, Duke M, Barnard JA, Greene JW (1998) Recurrent abdominal pain: a potential precursor of irritable bowel syndrome in adolescents and young adults. J Pediatr 132: 1010–1015.
9. Zuckerman B, Stevenson J, Bailey V (1987) Stomachaches and headaches in a community sample of preschool children. Pediatrics 79: 677–682.
10. Whitehead WE, Holtkotter B, Enck P, Hoelzl R, Holmes KD, et al. (1990) Tolerance for rectosigmoid distention in irritable bowel syndrome. Gastroenterology 98: 1187–1192.
11. Munakata J, Naliboff B, Harraf F, Kodner A, Lembo T, et al. (1997) Repetitive sigmoid stimulation induces rectal hyperalgesia in patients with irritable bowel syndrome. Gstroenterology 112: 55–63.
12. Fature C, Wieckowska A (2007) Somatic referral of visceral sensations and rectal sensory threshold for pain in children with functional gastrointestinal disorders. J Pediatr 150: 66–71.
13. Mayer EA, Naliboff BD, Craig DB (2006) Neuroimaging of the brain-gut axis: from basic understanding to treatment of functional GI disorders. Gastroenterology 131: 1925–1942.
14. Fukudo S, Nomura T, Muranaka M, Taguchi F (1993) Brain-gut response to stress and cholinergic stimulation in irritable bowel syndrome. A preliminary study. J Clin Gastroenterol 17: 133–141.
15. Naliboff BD, Berman S, Suyenobu B, Labus JS, Chang L, et al. (2006) Longitudinal change in perceptual and brain activation response to visceral stimuli in irritable bowel syndrome patients. Gastroenterology 131: 352–365.
16. Berman SM, Naloboff BD, Suyenobu JL, Labus JS, Stains J, et al. (2008) Reduced brainstem inhibition during anticipated pelvic visceral pain correlates with enhanced brain response to visceral stimulus in women with irritable bowel syndrome. J Neurosci 28: 349–359.
17. Dickhaus B, Mayer EA, Firooz N, Stains J, Conde F, et al. (2003) Irritable bowel syndrome patients show enhanced modulation of visceral perception by auditory stress. Gastroenterology 98: 135–143.
18. Berman SM, Naliboff BD, Chang L, Fitzgerald L, Antolin T, et al. (2002) Camplone A, Mayer EA. Enhanced preattentive central nervous system reactivity in Irritable bowel Syndrome. Am J Gastroenterol 97: 2791–2797.
19. Ambrosini A, De Pasqua V, Afra J, Sandor PS, Schoenen J (2001) Reduced gating of middle-latency auditory evoked potentials (P50) in migraine patients: Another indication of abnormal sensory processing? Neurosci Lett 306: 132–134.
20. Murata K, Sakamoto M, Nakai K, Weihe P, Dakeishi M, et al. (2004) Effects of methylmercury on neurodevelopment in Japanese children in relation to the Madeiran study. Int Arch Occup Environ Health 77: 571–579.
21. Ovtscharoffjr W, Helmeke C, Braun K (2006) Lack of parental care affects synaptic development in the anterior cinglate cortex. Brain Res 1116: 58–63.
22. Robinson JO, Alverez JH, Dodge JA (1990) Life events and family history in children with recurrent abdominal pain. J Psychosom Res 34: 171–181.
23. Walker LS, Garber J, Van Slyke DA, Greene JW (1995) Long-term health outcomes in patients with recurrent abdominal pain. J Pediatric Psychol 20: 233–245.
24. Hodges K, Kline J, Barberoand G, Woodruff C (1985) Anxiety in children with recurrent abdominal pain and their parents. Psychosomatics 26: 859–866.
25. Levy RL, Jones KR, Whitehead WE, Feld SI, Talley NJ, et al. (2001) Irritable bowel syndrome in twins: Heredity and social learning both contribute to etiology. Gastroenterology 2001; 121: 799–804.
26. Janssens KM, Oldehinkel AM, Rosmalen GM (2009) Parental overprotection predicts the development of functional somatic symptoms in young adolescents. J Pediatr 154: 918–923.
27. Weydert JA, Ball TM, Davis MF (2003) Systematic review of treatment for recurrent abdominal pain. Pediatrics 111: 1–11.
28. Feldman R, Gordon I, Schneiderman I, Weisman O, Zagoory-Sharon O (2010) Natural variations in maternal and paternal care are associated with systematic changes in oxytocin following parent-infant contact. Psychoneuroendocrinology 35: 1133–1141.
29. Enns MW, Cox BJ, Clara I (2002) Parental bonding and adult psychopathology: results from the U.S. National comorbidity survey. Psychol Med 32: 997–1008.
30. Sato T, Uehara T, Narita T, Sakado K, Fujii Y (2000) Parental bonding and personality in relation to lifetime history of depression. Psychiat Clin Neurosci 54: 121–130.
31. Suzuki K, Nakai K, Sugawara T, Nakamura T, Ohba T, et al. (2010) Neurobehavioral effects of prenatal exposure to methylmercury and PCBs, and seafood intake: Neonatal behavioral assessment scale results of Tohoku study of child development. Environ Res 110: 699–704.
32. Watanabe S, Hattori T, Kanazawa M, Kano M, Fukudo S (2007) Role of histaminergic neurons in hypnotic modulation of brain processing of visceral perception. Neurogastroenterol Motil 19: 831–838.
33. Stockard JJ, Stockard JE, Sharbrough FW (1986) Brainstem auditory evoked potentials in neurology: methodology, interpretation, and clinical application. In: Aminoff MJ, ed. Electrodiagnosis in Clinical Neurology, 2nd edition. Churchill Livingstone, New York. pp 467–503.
34. Meesters C, Muris P, Ghys A, Reumerman T, Rooijmans M (2003) The Children Somatization Inventory: further evidence for its reliability and validity in a pediatric and community sample of Dutch children and adolescents. J Pediatr Psychol 28: 413–422.
35. Vila M, Kramer T, Hickey N, Dattani M, Jefferis H, et al. (2009) Assessment of somatic symptoms in British secondary school children using the children's somatization inventory. J Pediatr Psychol 34: 989–998.
36. Parker G, Tupling H, Brown LB (1979) A parental bonding instrument. Br J Med Psychol 52: 1–10.
37. Kitamura T, Suzuki T (1993) A validation study of the parental bonding instrument in Japanese population. Jpn J Psychiatry Neurol 47: 29–36.
38. Rosenthall U, Bjorkman G, PeSersen K, Kall A (1985) Brainstem auditory evoked potentials in different age groups. Electroencephalogr Clin Neurophysiol 62: 426–430.
39. Kable JA, Coles CD, Lynch ME, Carroll J (2009) The impact of maternal smoking on fast auditory brainstem responses. Neurotoxicol Teratol 31: 216–224.
40. Wang NY, Su JF, Dong HQ, Jia JP, Han DM (2005) Hearing impairment in patients with mild cognitive impairment and Alzheimers disease. Zhonghua Er Bi Yan Hou Tou Jing Wai Ke Za Zhi 40: 279–282.
41. Valentino RJ, Pavcovich LA, Hirata H (1995) Evidence for corticotropin-releasing hormone projections from Barrington's nucleus to the periaqueductal

gray region and dorsal motor nucleus of vagus in the rat. J Comp Neurol 363: 402–422.
42. Valentino RJ, Chen S, Zhu Y, Aston-Jones G (1996) Evidence for divergent projections to the brain noradrenergic system and the spinal parasympathetic system from Barrington's nucleus. Brain Res 732: 1–15.
43. Gorski RA (2000) Sex differentiation of the nervous system. In; Kandel ER, Schwartz JH, Jessell TM, eds. Principles of Neural Science, fourth edition, McGraw-Hill, New York. pp 1131–1148.
44. Nicolson NA (2004) Childhood parental loss and cortisol levels in adult men. Psychoneuroendocrinology 29: 1012–1018.
45. Luecken LJ, Appelhans BM (2006) Early parental loss and salivary cortisol in young adulthood: the moderating role of family environment. Dev Psychopathol 18: 295–308.
46. Tafet GE, Smolovich J (2004) Psychoneuroendocrinological studies on chronic stress and depression. Ann N Y Acad Sci 1032: 276–278.
47. Belmaker RH, Agam G (2008) Major depressive disorder. N Engl J Med 358: 55–68.
48. Fukudo S, Nomura T, Hongo M (1998) Impact of corticotropin-releasing hormone on gastrointestinal motility in normal subjects and patients with irritable bowel syndrome. Gut 42: 845–849.
49. Videlock EJ, Adeyemo M, Licudine A, Hirano M, Ohning G, et al. (2009) Childhood trauma is associated with hypothalamic-pituitary-adrenal axis responsiveness in irritable bowel syndrome. Gastroenterology 137: 1954–1962.
50. Hattori T, Watanabe S, Kano M, Kanazawa M, Fukudo S (2010) Differential responding of autonomic function to histamine H1 antagonism in irritable bowel syndrome. Neurogastroenterol Motil 22: 1284–1291.
51. Creed F, Levy RL, Bradley LA, Francisconi C, Drossman DA, et al. (2006) Psychosocial aspects of functional gastrointestinal disorders. In: Drossman DA, Corazziari E, Delvaux M, Spiller RC, Talley NJ, Thompson WG, Whitehead WE, eds. Rome III: the Functional Gastrointestinal Disorders, Third Edition, Degnon Associates, McLean, Virginia. pp 295–368.
52. Drossman DA, Leserman J, Nachman G, Li ZM, Gluck H, et al. (1990) Sexual and physical abuse in women with functional or organic gastrointestinal disorders. Ann Intern Med 113: 828–833.
53. Blandon AY, Calkins SD, Keane SP, Brien MO (2008) Individual differences in trajectories of emotion regulation processes. Dev Psychol 44: 1110–1123.
54. Shipman KL, Zeman J (2001) Socialization of children's emotion regulation in mother-child dyads: a developmental psychopathology perspective. Dev Psychopathol 13: 317–336.
55. Mayer EA, Craske M, Naliboff BD (2001) Depression, anxiety, and the gastrointestinal system. J Clin Psychiatry 62: 28–36.
56. Dufton LM (2009) Anxiety and somatic complaints in children with recurrent abdominal pain and anxiety disorders. J Pediatr Psychol 34: 176–186.
57. Cruz DA, Lovallo E, Stockton S, Rasband M, Lewis DA (2009) Postnatal development of synaptic structure proteins in pyramidal neuron axon initial segments in monkey prefrontal cortex. J Comp Neurol 514: 353–367.
58. Castilloux J, Noble A, Fayre C (2008) Is visceral hypersensitivity correlated with symptom severity in children with functional gastrointestinal disorders? Pediat Gastroenterol Nut 46: 272–278.
59. Van der Veek PP, Van Rood YR, Masclee AA (2008) Symptom severity but not psychopathology predicts visceral hypersensitivity in irritable bowel syndrome. Clin Gastroenterol Hepatol 6: 321–328.
60. Durno CA, Gallinger S (2006) Genetic predisposition to colorectal cancer: new pieces in the pediatric puzzle. J Pediatr Gastroenterol Nutr 43: 5–15.

15

Catechol-O-Methyltransferase val158met Polymorphism Predicts Placebo Effect in Irritable Bowel Syndrome

Kathryn T. Hall[1,2]*, Anthony J. Lembo[2,3], Irving Kirsch[2,4], Dimitrios C. Ziogas[5], Jeffrey Douaiher[6], Karin B. Jensen[2,7], Lisa A. Conboy[2], John M. Kelley[2,7,8], Efi Kokkotou[2,3], Ted J. Kaptchuk[1,2]

1 Division of General Medicine and Primary Care, Beth Israel Deaconess Medical Center and Harvard Medical School, Boston, Massachusetts, United States of America, **2** Program in Placebo Studies, Beth Israel Deaconess Medical Center and Harvard Medical School, Boston, Massachusetts, United States of America, **3** Department of Gastroenterology, Beth Israel Deaconess Medical Center and Harvard Medical School, Boston, Massachusetts, United States of America, **4** School of Psychology, University of Plymouth, Devon, United Kingdom, **5** Department of Internal Medicine, University of Athens, Athens, Greece, **6** Department of Surgery, Johns Hopkins, Baltimore, Maryland, United States of America, **7** Department of Psychiatry, Massachusetts General Hospital, Harvard Medical School, Boston, Massachusetts, United States of America, **8** Endicott College, Beverly, Massachusetts, United States of America

Abstract

Identifying patients who are potential placebo responders has major implications for clinical practice and trial design. Catechol-O-methyltransferase (COMT), an important enzyme in dopamine catabolism plays a key role in processes associated with the placebo effect such as reward, pain, memory and learning. We hypothesized that the COMT functional val158met polymorphism, was a predictor of placebo effects and tested our hypothesis in a subset of 104 patients from a previously reported randomized controlled trial in irritable bowel syndrome (IBS). The three treatment arms from this study were: no-treatment ("waitlist"), placebo treatment alone ("limited") and, placebo treatment "augmented" with a supportive patient-health care provider interaction. The primary outcome measure was change from baseline in IBS-Symptom Severity Scale (IBS-SSS) after three weeks of treatment. In a regression model, the number of methionine alleles in COMT val158met was linearly related to placebo response as measured by changes in IBS-SSS ($p = .035$). The strongest placebo response occurred in met/met homozygotes treated in the augmented placebo arm. A smaller met/met associated effect was observed with limited placebo treatment and there was no effect in the waitlist control. These data support our hypothesis that the COMT val158met polymorphism is a potential biomarker of placebo response.

Editor: Anthony W.I. Lo, The Chinese University of Hong Kong, Hong Kong

Funding: The funding received for this study came from NCCAM-NIH grants # R01 AT004662, K24 AT004095, 3R01AT004662-02S1, T32 AT000051 and R21 AT002860. The funders had no role in study design, data collection and analysis, decision to publish, or preparation of the manuscript.

Competing Interests: The authors have declared that no competing interests exist.

* E-mail: kthall@bidmc.harvard.edu

Introduction

Placebo treatments have been shown to lead to clinical improvement in a broad spectrum of disorders [1]. Although advances have been made in understanding the neurobiology of placebo [2], our understanding of the genetic modulators of the placebo response remains a critical knowledge gap. Identifying the characteristics of placebo responders and non-responders is key to managing underlying placebogenic factors for patient benefit and to optimizing the design and interpretation of clinical trials.

Studies investigating brain activity associated with placebo response in pain, Parkinson's disease and depression, point to dopamine as a possible integrator of the placebo response [2,3,4,5]. Dopamine is a catecholamine synthesized from tyrosine by tyrosine hydroxylase and dopamine decarboxylase. Once synthesized, dopamine is packaged into presynaptic vesicles and released into the synaptic cleft upon depolarization. Dopamine is cleared from the synapse either by the dopamine reuptake transporter (DAT), or degradation by monoamine oxidases A and B, or catechol-O-methyltransferase (COMT). Whereas reuptake is the primary mechanism of dopamine clearance in the striatum, in the prefrontal cortex, DAT is less abundant, rendering COMT activity critical in regulating prefrontal dopamine signaling [6,7].

Among the genetic polymorphisms in the dopamine pathway, the COMT val158met polymorphism has been studied most extensively in clinical trials for its potential association with treatment responses. COMT val158met, is a G to A transition leading to amino-acid substitution at codon 158 in the transmembrane form of the enzyme [8]. The methionine isoform has reduced thermostability, resulting in a three to four-fold decrease in activity relative to the ancestral valine isoform [9]. This functional polymorphism has been correlated with variations in memory function [10,11], cognition [12], attentional processing [13], affect [14], confirmation bias [15], pain processing and sensitivity [16,17,18,19]. Met/met individuals have higher levels of performance in cognitive tests, which measure executive function as well as increased sensitivity to experimental and chronic pain relative to val/met and val/val individuals [16,19,20,21,22].

Given that COMT has an effect on dopamine levels in the prefrontal cortex, a brain region activated during placebo response, we hypothesized that the functional COMT val158met polymorphism is a placebo response variant. To our knowledge, no previous study has reported an association between COMT and response to placebo treatment in irritable bowel syndrome (IBS). IBS, a common gastrointestinal disorder affecting 10 to 15% of North Americans [23,24] is characterized by abdominal pain or discomfort associated with altered bowel function, bloating, and a sensation of incomplete evacuation after bowel movements [25,26]. IBS is a condition known to have a high placebo response rate and meta-analyses report an average placebo induced global improvement of approximately 40% [27,28,29].

Previously, our team investigated IBS placebo responses in a clinical trial which had three arms: 1) a no-treatment arm that controlled for regression to the mean and normal fluctuations in illness ("waitlist"), 2) a placebo treatment arm which used a validated placebo acupuncture device administered in a business-like no frills clinical context ("limited placebo"), and 3) a limited placebo arm augmented with a supportive warm provider who expressed confidence in the effectiveness of the treatment ("augmented placebo"). Overall, we found a robust clinical response to the placebo treatments; validated IBS outcome measures showed augmented placebo was significantly more effective than limited placebo, which in turn was more effective than the no-treatment waitlist control [30].

Our parent IBS clinical trial was ideal for the study of genetic associations with placebo effects because it included a waitlist (observation alone) control and two different "doses" of placebo (limited and augmented). The waitlist control allowed for separation of regression to the mean and the natural waxing and waning of illness from the effects of placebo treatment. The two types of placebo interventions, limited and augmented, created a comparison of incremental components of the placebo effect in a manner that could be considered analogous to dose dependent.

Here we present the first study to support the hypothesis that the COMT val158met polymorphism is a potential genetic marker of placebo response.

Materials and Methods

Study populations

A randomized clinical trial investigating placebo effects in IBS patients (Trial registration – NCT00065403) was conducted. Details of the design and outcomes of the trial are provided elsewhere [30,31]. The 3-week trial enrolled 262 patients (75% women) $\geq$18 years and diagnosed by IBS Rome II criteria score of $>$150 on the Irritable Bowel Syndrome Symptom Severity Scale (IBS-SSS) [32].

Randomization and Interventions

Patients were randomized to one of three treatment arms: (1) no-treatment control ("waitlist"); (2) placebo acupuncture ("limited"); (3) placebo acupuncture plus a supportive patient-provider ("augmented"). A validated sham acupuncture device was used to deliver placebo acupuncture in 20 minute sessions, twice weekly for three weeks.

Ethics Statement

A subgroup of patients (n = 112) gave consent for genetic analysis from blood samples included in this study. The Institutional Review Board at Beth Israel Deaconess Medical Center (Boston, MA) approved the main study and the genetic follow-up study presented here. All studies were conducted in accordance with the Declaration of Helsinki. Participants provided written consent for this genetic study. The ethics committee approved this procedure.

Outcomes

Three validated IBS research measures from the previous trial, which assessed clinical outcomes, were used in this study. The primary outcome measure was the IBS-SSS, which consists of five 100-point scales (abdominal pain severity, abdominal pain frequency, abdominal distention severity, dissatisfaction with bowel habits, and quality of life disruption) that contribute equally to the final score, yielding a theoretical range of 0–500 [32]. Higher scores reflected a more severe condition. IBS-SSS was measured at baseline and after 3 weeks of treatment. Change in IBS-SSS was determined by subtracting 3-week IBS-SSS score from baseline IBS-SSS. We selected IBS-SSS as our primary outcome because the two secondary measures, Adequate Relief (AR) and the Global Improvement Scale (GIS) did not have baseline measures. Adequate Relief was assessed by a single dichotomous question at 3-weeks, which asked: "Over the past week have you had adequate relief of your IBS symptoms?" [33]. The GIS asked: "Compared to the way you felt before you entered the study, have your IBS symptoms over the past 7 days been: (1) = substantially worse, (2) = moderately worse, (3) = slightly worse, (4) = no change, (5) = slightly improved, (6) = moderately improved, or (7) = substantially improved" [34,35]. These latter two measures were considered secondary because they do not have baseline assessments, thus opening the door to regression artifacts [36]. To mitigate this problem, we controlled for IBS-SSS baseline scores in analyses of AR and GIS.

Genotyping

Of the 262 original study participants, 112 gave consent for genetic screening. Eight patients missing IBS-SSS data at 3-weeks were excluded from the analyses. Two additional patients were missing data for AR and GIS and were excluded from analysis of AR and GIS. Genomic DNA was extracted from whole blood using Qiagen Blood kit (Valencia, CA) following the manufacturer's protocol. Based on the association of COMT SNP rs4633 with COMT expression and activity [37], this SNP was genotyped in addition to rs4680 (val158met). TaqMan SNP Genotyping assays for rs4680 (val158met) and rs4633 were purchased from Applied Biosystems, (Foster City, CA). Quantitative PCR was performed at the Biopolymers Facility at Harvard Medical School, (Boston, MA) following the manufacturer's protocol on an Applied Biosystems 7900HT instrument, using SDS version 2.4 software.

Statistical Analysis

Hardy–Weinberg Equilibrium (HWE) and Linkage Disequilibrium were calculated using the Online Encyclopedia for Genetic Epidemiology studies [38,39]. Statistical analyses were performed using IBM SPSS Statistics version 20 (Chicago, IL).

We used an additive genetic model to investigate the linear effect of increases in the presence of the COMT met allele. We created a variable, "COMT genotype", that coded each patient's val158met genotype as follows: 1 = met/met; 0 = val/met; −1 = val/val. Using standard coding for polynomial trends, we used multiple regression to examine linear and quadratic effects of COMT genotype (number of met alleles) on placebo responses as measured by changes from baseline IBS-SSS, and on AR and GIS. We controlled for initial disease severity by including baseline IBS-SSS as a covariate in the regression models. In addition, we created variables to test for linear and quadratic effects of treatment, conceiving these as ascending "doses" of non-specific effects (waitlist, limited placebo, augmented placebo) to test for interactions between COMT genotype effects and treatment received.

Results

The clinical and demographic characteristics of the subset of genotyped patients (n = 104) relative to the original clinical trial (n = 262) [30] are shown in Table 1. Age, gender, race and marital status of the genotyped patients did not differ significantly from the distribution in the original study; duration, IBS type and baseline IBS-SSS were also similar. Eighty percent of the genotyped patients were women and 94% were white. Furthermore there were no significant differences in demographics and disease characteristics of genotyped patients across the COMT val158met genotypes. The number of patients genotyped and analyzed from each treatment arm (waitlist, 29%; limited, 32%; and augmented, 39%) was similar to the overall distribution in the original trial (waitlist, 33%; limited, 34%; and augmented, 33%).

Based on its association with rs4680, COMT expression and enzymatic activity we also genotyped rs4633 [37]. Rs4633 was found to be in strong linkage disequilibrium with rs4680 (D' = .94 and r2 = .9), such that the two SNPs were almost perfectly correlated: met/met, val/met and val/val of rs4680 corresponded to the T/T, T/C and C/C of rs4633. Therefore we focused on COMT val158met in further analyses. The minor allele frequency of COMT val158met was 0.46 and the SNP was in Hardy–Weinberg Equilibrium (p = .502).

In this study, IBS Symptom Severity Scale (IBS-SSS) was our *a priori* primary clinical outcome. IBS-SSS is a multidimensional measure that captures the full spectrum of IBS disease including abdominal pain severity, abdominal pain frequency, abdominal distention severity, dissatisfaction with bowel habits, and disruption in quality of life and has a theoretical range of 0–500 [32].

Both linear and quadratic effects of COMT alleles and treatment arm (waitlist, limited, augmented) were tested. As there were no significant main effects or interactions involving quadratic tests, results reported here are for a trimmed model with only linear effects and interactions included.

IBS-Symptom Severity Scale (IBS-SSS)

Change in IBS-SSS was associated with a main effect of COMT genotype (number of met alleles) (Figure 1). Number of COMT val158met met alleles showed a significant linear effect on IBS-SSS (beta = 0.17; p = .032). Patients with the met/met genotype had the greatest level of improvement whereas val/val patients had the least, and val/met patients were intermediate (Figure 1). As in the original study [30], there was a main effect of treatment arm on improvement, with patients in the augmented treatment improving most and those on waitlist improving least (beta = 0.19, p = .019).

These linear effects on IBS-SSS were qualified by significant interactions between COMT genotype and treatment arm (beta = 0.17; p = .035). COMT predicted responses in only the augmented placebo arm. In response to a high dose placebo treatment, patients homozygous for met alleles (met/met), showed the greatest improvement; val homozygotes (val/val) showed the least improvement and heterozygote (val/met) patients had an intermediate response (Figure 2).

Adequate Relief

The secondary validated measure of Adequate Relief uses a single dichotomous question at 3-weeks which asked: "Over the past week have you had adequate relief of your IBS symptoms?" [33]. The responses were coded as 0 = No, I did not have Adequate Relief and 1 = Yes, I had Adequate Relief. As expected from the previous study, there was a significant linear effect for treatment arm (beta = 0.32, p = .001), in which patients in the augmented placebo arm showed most improvement and those in the waitlist arm showed the least [30]. Although there was no main effect for COMT genotype, there was a significant interaction between COMT genotype and treatment arm (beta = 0.25, p = .009). In the augmented placebo arm, the met/met patients reported an average Adequate Relief score of 0.88 compared to 0.63 for val/met patients and 0.56 for val/val patients (Figure 3). Conversely, in the waitlist group, val/val patients had an average score of 0.50, whereas the met/met patients had an average score of 0.00, that is no met/met patients on the waitlist arm reported Adequate Relief.

Table 1. Baseline characteristics of genotyped IBS patients compared to participants in the parent randomized clinical trial.

Characteristics	All IBS patients* (n = 262)	Genotyped patients (n = 112)	p value	met/met (n = 20)	val/met (n = 55)	val/val (n = 29)	p value
Demographics							
Age in years (SD)	38 (14)	37 (13)	0.53	40 (12)	36 (13)	38 (14)	0.44
Women (%)	218 (83)	83 (80)	0.51	16 (80)	45 (81)	22 (76)	0.82
White (%)	252 (96)	98 (94)	0.17	20(100)	52 (95)	26 (89)	0.20
Married/living together (%)	101 (39)	32 (31)	0.42	8 (42)	16 (41)	8 (33)	0.79
IBS symptoms and baseline characteristics							
Type of IBS			0.56				0.80
Constipation (%)	74 (28)	35 (34)		5 (25)	21 (39)	9 (31)	
Diarrhea (%)	65 (25)	18 (17)		4 (20)	8 (15)	6 (21)	
Mixed (%)	139 (53)	40 (38)		11 (55)	25 (46)	14 (48)	
Disease for >5 years (%)	103 (39)	63 (61)	0.18	12 (60)	34 (62)	17 (59)	0.96
Baseline IBS-SSS (SD)	273 (73)	270 (66)	0.72	291 (78)	261 (64)	272 (61)	0.23

*Participants in parent clinical trial previously reported [30].

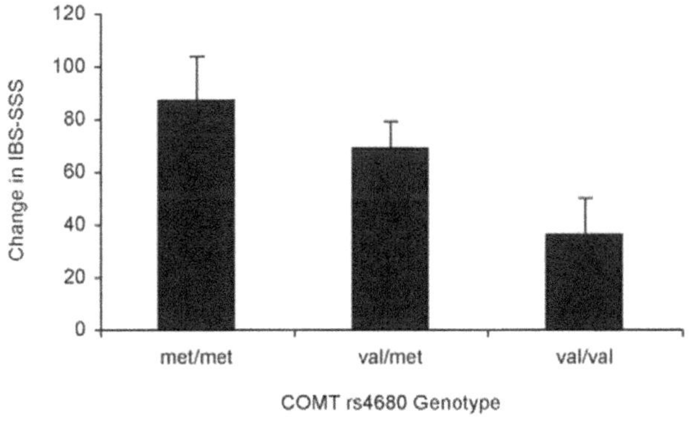

Figure 1. Effect of COMT genotype on change in IBS-SSS. Number of val158met met alleles showed a significant linear effect on IBS-SSS (beta = 0.17; p = .032). IBS-SSS includes abdominal pain severity, abdominal pain frequency, abdominal distention severity, dissatisfaction with bowel habits, and disruption of quality of life. Change in IBS-SSS = (IBS-SSS at baseline – IBS-SSS at 3-weeks). Regression model included COMT genotype (number of met alleles) and baseline IBS-SSS. Error bars indicate the standard error of the mean. N = 104.

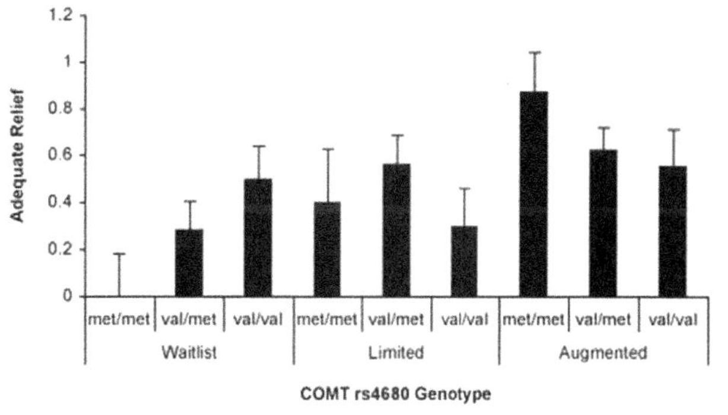

Figure 3. Interaction effect of COMT genotype and treatment arm on Adequate Relief. The interaction (COMT genotype x treatment arm) was statistically significant (beta = 0.25; p = .009), but not COMT genotype (beta = 0.01; p = .954). Adequate Relief was assessed by a single dichotomous categorization at three weeks, which asked patients: "Over the past week have you had adequate relief of your IBS symptoms?" Regression model parameters included: COMT genotype (number of met alleles), treatment arm and their interaction (COMT genotype x treatment arm). Error bars are standard error of the mean. N = 102.

Global Improvement Scale

The other secondary validated measure was Global Improvement Scale (GIS) which asked: "Compared to the way you felt before you entered the study, have your IBS symptoms over the past 7 days been: (1) = substantially worse, (2) = moderately worse, (3) = slightly worse, (4) = no change, (5) = slightly improved, (6) = moderately improved, or (7) = substantially improved" [34]. As in the case of IBS-SSS and Adequate Relief, there was an expected significant linear effect for treatment arm (beta = 0.31, p = .002), in which patients in the augmented placebo arm showed most improvement and those in the waitlist arm showed the least [30]. There was a trend in improvement associated with COMT genotype (beta = 0.18, p = .063) but no interaction of COMT genotype with treatment arm (beta = 0.07, p = .477).

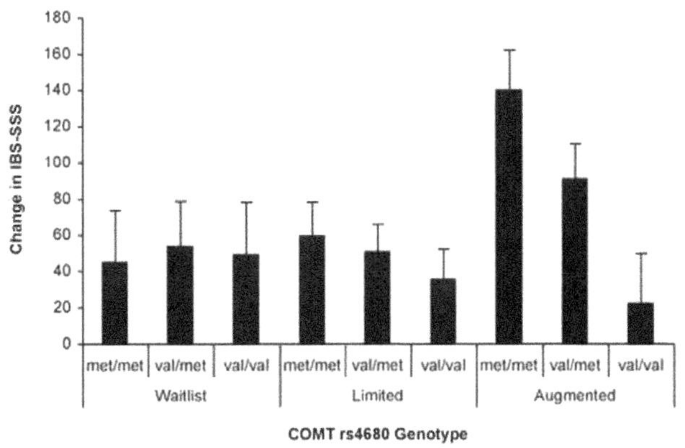

Figure 2. Interaction effect of COMT genotype and treatment arm on change in IBS-SSS. The interaction between COMT genotype (number of met alleles) and treatment arm was statistically significant (beta = 0.17; p = .035). Regression model included the following parameters: COMT genotype (number of met alleles), treatment arm, baseline IBS-SSS and their interaction (COMT genotype x treatment arm). Error bars indicate the standard error of the mean. N = 104.

Discussion

In this study, we demonstrated that IBS patients homozygous for the COMT val158met methionine allele (met/met) were the most responsive to placebo treatment. Heterozygous (val/met) patients showed an intermediate response, and homozygous valine (val/val) patients showed essentially no placebo mediated symptom improvement. To our knowledge, this is the first study to demonstrate genetic modulation of true placebo effects disassociated from changes related to disease natural history and regression to the mean. It is also the first study to demonstrate a relationship between different levels of placebo treatment and COMT genotype.

Our regression analysis showed that as the number of COMT val158met met alleles increased progressively from 0 to 1 to 2, and COMT activity decreased, theoretically making more dopamine available in the prefrontal cortex, placebo responses increased in a linear fashion. Further, there was a significant interaction between number of methionine alleles and placebo treatment arm. Examination of the interactions illustrated in Figures 2 and 3, showed that the relationship between number of COMT met alleles and placebo response occurred primarily in the augmented placebo arm, with a smaller effect in the limited placebo arm, and no effect (IBS-SSS) or a reverse effect (Adequate Relief) in the waitlist control arm. Taken together, these results strongly suggest that COMT val158met, specifically the met/met genotype, is a potential marker for placebo responders in IBS. Furthermore the finding that this genotype is associated with a positive outcome only in groups given a placebo (and not in the waitlist control group) is of particular importance, as it indicates that it is a predictor of the placebo effect, not just improvement in general.

To date, the search for placebo biomarkers has been elusive. The three previous studies we are aware of which looked for a genetic link to the placebo response lacked the critical no-treatment control [21,40,41]. Neither of the two studies that examined the relationship between COMT and placebo response found a statistically significant relationship [21,41]. The third study on severe anxiety disorder (SAD) found that polymorphisms in two serotonin-related genes, the serotonin transporter-linked polymorphic region (5-HTTLPR) and the G703T polymorphism of tryptophan hydroxylase-2, had a significant effect on placebo [40]. However the involvement of the amygdala and these two serotonin-related enzymes suggests that these associations may be unique to SAD and not necessarily generalizable to the placebo response mechanism. Furthermore in the absence of a no-treatment control that would have allowed a clear separation between placebo effects and such phenomenon as regression to the mean, spontaneous remission or the natural waxing and waning of illness, these studies could not rule out whether their findings were a result of a genuine psychobiological process or merely improvement that would have happened without placebo treatment.

Four other placebo-controlled studies designed to examine the effects of tolcapone, a COMT inhibitor, looked at the association between COMT val158met genotype, cognition and information processing [42,43,44,45]. Mentioned *en passant* in their reports was the observation that the met/met subjects had a statistically significant placebo effect, whereas the val/val subjects were unresponsive to placebo treatment. Although this research paradigm is distinctly different from IBS, these findings support our hypothesis and suggest that the COMT mediated placebo response pathway might be generalizable across multiple conditions. Nonetheless, other replications of our study that prospectively hypothesize a COMT involvement with placebo effects and include a no treatment control will be critical to confirm our findings.

Positioned at the intersection of catecholamine metabolism, memory [46], reward processing [47], confirmation bias [15] and pain regulation [16], COMT presents an interesting candidate for a placebo response marker. The inverted U-shaped dopamine response curve, reported in many COMT functional studies suggests a narrow range for optimum dopamine cortical function [48,49]. One might therefore hypothesize that drugs that interfere with the dopaminergic pathway might affect the observed response to treatment by shifting the component of the treatment response resultant from placebo. Indeed several studies that examine the effect of amphetamine [41] or tolcapone [42,43,44,45] relative to a placebo treatment have observed that met/met subjects tend be unresponsive or worsen relative to placebo response when treated with these drugs, suggesting there is an optimum level of dopamine associated with placebo effect. Identifying biological characteristics of placebo responders and non-responders could be key to managing underlying placebogenic factors to benefit patients by delivering personalized medicine, for example by adjusting the dose of medication in accordance to the subject's placebo susceptibility or selecting a different class of drugs for the individualized patient.

Our study illuminates the persistent failure to identify reliable characteristics of placebo responders [50,51,52]. Beyond using a no-treatment control another unique feature of our study was the inclusion of an augmented therapeutic relationship. The therapeutic relationship is considered an active component of non-specific placebo treatment [30]; its presence may be needed to identify reliable predictors of the placebo effect [53]. Prior studies did not include an arm in which the placebo was administered within the context of an augmented therapeutic relationship. Indeed, many of these studies were done with volunteer subjects in experimental rather than clinical contexts in which there was no therapeutic relationship at all. Although this unique design of our study is an asset, it also poses a limitation on using other studies to retrospectively validate our findings, as most clinical trials do not include a no-treatment control. Another limitation of this study is its small sample size and the absence of a power calculation. Given that our study was a secondary data analysis of an existing dataset, the sample size was already fixed. Although a small sample size increases the risk of a type II error (failing to find a significant difference that exists in the population), it does not challenge the validity of results showing significant effects. Hence, our results deriving from a clear hypothesis are still reliable.

It is unlikely that a single locus like COMT, fully accounts for a complex behavioral phenotype like placebo response. However, given that COMT val158met is a functional polymorphism, which results in a three to four-fold reduction in prefrontal dopamine, it has a greater potential to contribute to behavioral variability than other non-functional or noncoding polymorphisms. That COMT has been implicated in multiple disorders i.e. major depressive disorder, Parkinson's and pain, might be deemed as a weakness in its candidacy for a placebo response marker. However we argue that this wide association with disease and drug treatments might be why it is such a powerful potential target for modulating placebo effects.

IBS is a functional condition characterized by a diversity of symptoms measured by subjective instruments, which also poses another limitation to our study. It should be noted though, that placebo treatment is especially thought to influence the experience and perception of subjective symptoms such as depressed mood and pain, rather than directly modifying disease pathophysiology [54,55].

Finally, the power of the patient-doctor interaction to enhance healing is one of the hallmarks of clinical medicine, and increasingly resources are devoted to teaching clinicians how to communicate warmth and caring to their patients [56,57]. Our findings reinforce this healing benefit for met/met patients and raise an interesting question. Despite their best efforts, many a warm and caring physician has had patients that seemed to derive minimum benefit from their empathic attentions. Our findings that val/val patients are less influenced by the placebo treatment, regardless of whether it is delivered in an augmented or limited context, potentially shed some light on this clinical challenge.

Acknowledgments

We thank Benjamin Raby and Michele Hacker from Harvard Catalyst, Roger Davis from Beth Israel Deaconess Medical Center, and Valerie Stone from Massachusetts General Hospital for helpful discussions.

Author Contributions

Hypothesis generation: KJ KH TK. Managed genotyping: KH DZ JD. Experimental design: AL KH KJ TK EK KJ. Data analysis: KH AL TK IK JK LC. Manuscript preparation: KH JD TK EK JK IK.

References

1. Finniss DG, Kaptchuk TJ, Miller F, Benedetti F (2010) Biological, clinical, and ethical advances of placebo effects. Lancet 375: 686–695.
2. Zubieta JK, Stohler CS (2009) Neurobiological mechanisms of placebo responses. Annals of the New York Academy of Sciences 1156: 198–210.
3. Scott DJ, Stohler CS, Egnatuk CM, Wang H, Koeppe RA, et al. (2007) Individual differences in reward responding explain placebo-induced expectations and effects. Neuron 55: 325–336.
4. Scott DJ, Stohler CS, Egnatuk CM, Wang H, Koeppe RA, et al. (2008) Placebo and nocebo effects are defined by opposite opioid and dopaminergic responses. Archives of general psychiatry 65: 220–231.
5. Zubieta JK, Bueller JA, Jackson LR, Scott DJ, Xu Y, et al. (2005) Placebo effects mediated by endogenous opioid activity on mu-opioid receptors. The Journal of neuroscience: the official journal of the Society for Neuroscience 25: 7754–7762.
6. Meyer-Lindenberg A, Kohn PD, Kolachana B, Kippenhan S, McInerney-Leo A, et al. (2005) Midbrain dopamine and prefrontal function in humans:

interaction and modulation by COMT genotype. Nature neuroscience 8: 594–596.
7. Yavich L, Forsberg MM, Karayiorgou M, Gogos JA, Mannisto PT (2007) Site-specific role of catechol-O-methyltransferase in dopamine overflow within prefrontal cortex and dorsal striatum. The Journal of neuroscience: the official journal of the Society for Neuroscience 27: 10196–10209.
8. Lachman HM, Papolos DF, Saito T, Yu YM, Szumlanski CL, et al. (1996) Human catechol-O-methyltransferase pharmacogenetics: description of a functional polymorphism and its potential application to neuropsychiatric disorders. Pharmacogenetics 6: 243–250.
9. Lotta T, Vidgren J, Tilgmann C, Ulmanen I, Melen K, et al. (1995) Kinetics of human soluble and membrane-bound catechol O-methyltransferase: a revised mechanism and description of the thermolabile variant of the enzyme. Biochemistry 34: 4202–4210.
10. Diamond A (2007) Consequences of variations in genes that affect dopamine in prefrontal cortex. Cerebral cortex 17 Suppl 1: i161–170.
11. Solis-Ortiz S, Perez-Luque E, Morado-Crespo L, Gutierrez-Munoz M (2010) Executive functions and selective attention are favored in middle-aged healthy women carriers of the Val/Val genotype of the catechol-o-methyltransferase gene: a behavioral genetic study. Behavioral and brain functions: BBF 6: 67.
12. Winterer G, Goldman D (2003) Genetics of human prefrontal function. Brain research Brain research reviews 43: 134–163.
13. Truong T, Kilpatrick L, Naliboff B, Dandekar S, Papp J, et al. (2009) COMT Genetic Polymorphism Is Associated with Alterations in Attentional Processing in Patients with IBS and Other Functional Pain Syndromes. Gastroenterology 136: A-74, 2009) 136: A–74.
14. Massat I, Kocabas NA, Crisafulli C, Chiesa A, Calati R, et al. (2011) COMT and age at onset in mood disorders: a replication and extension study. Neuroscience letters 498: 218–221.
15. Doll BB, Hutchison KE, Frank MJ (2011) Dopaminergic genes predict individual differences in susceptibility to confirmation bias. The Journal of neuroscience: the official journal of the Society for Neuroscience 31: 6188–6198.
16. Diatchenko L, Slade GD, Nackley AG, Bhalang K, Sigurdsson A, et al. (2005) Genetic basis for individual variations in pain perception and the development of a chronic pain condition. Human molecular genetics 14: 135–143.
17. Dai F, Belfer I, Schwartz CE, Banco R, Martha JF, et al. (2010) Association of catechol-O-methyltransferase genetic variants with outcome in patients undergoing surgical treatment for lumbar degenerative disc disease. The spine journal: official journal of the North American Spine Society 10: 949–957.
18. Tchivileva IE, Lim PF, Smith SB, Slade GD, Diatchenko L, et al. (2010) Effect of catechol-O-methyltransferase polymorphism on response to propranolol therapy in chronic musculoskeletal pain: a randomized, double-blind, placebo-controlled, crossover pilot study. Pharmacogenetics and genomics 20: 239–248.
19. Zubieta JK, Heitzeg MM, Smith YR, Bueller JA, Xu K, et al. (2003) COMT val158met genotype affects mu-opioid neurotransmitter responses to a pain stressor. Science 299: 1240–1243.
20. Loggia ML, Jensen K, Gollub R, Wasan AD, Edwards R, et al. (2011) The catechol-O-methyltransferase(COMT) val158met polymorphism affects brain responses to repeated painful stimuli. PloS one 6: e27764.
21. Jensen KB, Lonsdorf TB, Schalling M, Kosek E, Ingvar M (2009) Increased sensitivity to thermal pain following a single opiate dose is influenced by the COMT val(158)met polymorphism. PloS one 4: e6016.
22. Rakvag TT, Klepstad P, Baar C, Kvam TM, Dale O, et al. (2005) The Val158Met polymorphism of the human catechol-O-methyltransferase (COMT) gene may influence morphine requirements in cancer pain patients. Pain 116: 73–78.
23. Drossman DA, Camilleri M, Mayer EA, Whitehead WE (2002) AGA technical review on irritable bowel syndrome. Gastroenterology 123: 2108–2131.
24. Saito YA, Schoenfeld P, Locke GR 3rd (2002) The epidemiology of irritable bowel syndrome in North America: a systematic review. The American journal of gastroenterology 97: 1910–1915.
25. Chang L, Drossman DA (2010) Rome Foundation Endpoints and Outcomes Conference 2009: Optimizing Clinical Trials in FGID. The American journal of gastroenterology 105: 722–730.
26. Mayer EA, Bushnell MC, International Association for the Study of Pain (2009) Functional pain syndromes: presentation and pathophysiology. Seattle: IASP Press. xviii, 580 p.
27. Dorn SD, Kaptchuk TJ, Park JB, Nguyen LT, Canenguez K, et al. (2007) A meta-analysis of the placebo response in complementary and alternative medicine trials of irritable bowel syndrome. Neurogastroenterology and motility: the official journal of the European Gastrointestinal Motility Society 19: 630–637.
28. Ford AC, Moayyedi P (2010) Meta-analysis: factors affecting placebo response rate in the irritable bowel syndrome. Alimentary pharmacology & therapeutics 32: 144–158.
29. Patel SM, Stason WB, Legedza A, Ock SM, Kaptchuk TJ, et al. (2005) The placebo effect in irritable bowel syndrome trials: a meta-analysis. Neurogastroenterology and motility: the official journal of the European Gastrointestinal Motility Society 17: 332–340.
30. Kaptchuk TJ, Kelley JM, Conboy LA, Davis RB, Kerr CE, et al. (2008) Components of placebo effect: randomised controlled trial in patients with irritable bowel syndrome. BMJ 336: 999–1003.
31. Conboy LA, Macklin E, Kelley J, Kokkotou E, Lembo A, et al. (2010) Which patients improve: characteristics increasing sensitivity to a supportive patient-practitioner relationship. Social science & medicine 70: 479–484.
32. Francis CY, Morris J, Whorwell PJ (1997) The irritable bowel severity scoring system: a simple method of monitoring irritable bowel syndrome and its progress. Alimentary pharmacology & therapeutics 11: 395–402.
33. Mangel AW, Hahn BA, Heath AT, Northcutt AR, Kong S, et al. (1998) Adequate relief as an endpoint in clinical trials in irritable bowel syndrome. The Journal of international medical research 26: 76–81.
34. Gordon S, Ameen V, Bagby B, Shahan B, Jhingran P, et al. (2003) Validation of irritable bowel syndrome Global Improvement Scale: an integrated symptom end point for assessing treatment efficacy. Digestive diseases and sciences 48: 1317–1323.
35. Lembo T, Wright RA, Bagby B, Decker C, Gordon S, et al. (2001) Alosetron controls bowel urgency and provides global symptom improvement in women with diarrhea-predominant irritable bowel syndrome. The American journal of gastroenterology 96: 2662–2670.
36. Campbell DT, Kenny DA (1999) A primer on regression artifacts. New York: Guilford Press. xxi, 202 p.
37. Nackley AG, Shabalina SA, Tchivileva IE, Satterfield K, Korchynskyi O, et al. (2006) Human catechol-O-methyltransferase haplotypes modulate protein expression by altering mRNA secondary structure. Science 314: 1930–1933.
38. Gaunt TR, Rodriguez S, Zapata C, Day IN (2006) MIDAS: software for analysis and visualisation of interallelic disequilibrium between multiallelic markers. BMC bioinformatics 7: 227.
39. Gaunt TR, Rodriguez S, Day IN (2007) Cubic exact solutions for the estimation of pairwise haplotype frequencies: implications for linkage disequilibrium analyses and a web tool 'CubeX'. BMC bioinformatics 8: 428.
40. Furmark T, Appel L, Henningsson S, Ahs F, Faria V, et al. (2008) A link between serotonin-related gene polymorphisms, amygdala activity, and placebo-induced relief from social anxiety. The Journal of neuroscience: the official journal of the Society for Neuroscience 28: 13066–13074.
41. Leuchter AF, McCracken JT, Hunter AM, Cook IA, Alpert JE (2009) Monoamine oxidase a and catechol-o-methyltransferase functional polymorphisms and the placebo response in major depressive disorder. Journal of clinical psychopharmacology 29: 372–377.
42. Apud JA, Mattay V, Chen J, Kolachana BS, Callicott JH, et al. (2007) Tolcapone improves cognition and cortical information processing in normal human subjects. Neuropsychopharmacology: official publication of the American College of Neuropsychopharmacology 32: 1011–1020.
43. Farrell SM, Tunbridge EM, Braeutigam S, Harrison PJ (2012) COMT Val(158)Met genotype determines the direction of cognitive effects produced by catechol-O-methyltransferase inhibition. Biological psychiatry 71: 538–544.
44. Giakoumaki SG, Roussos P, Bitsios P (2008) Improvement of prepulse inhibition and executive function by the COMT inhibitor tolcapone depends on COMT Val158Met polymorphism. Neuropsychopharmacology: official publication of the American College of Neuropsychopharmacology 33: 3058–3068.
45. Roussos P, Giakoumaki SG, Bitsios P (2009) Tolcapone effects on gating, working memory, and mood interact with the synonymous catechol-O-methyltransferase rs4818c/g polymorphism. Biological psychiatry 66: 997–1004.
46. Egan MF, Goldberg TE, Kolachana BS, Callicott JH, Mazzanti CM, et al. (2001) Effect of COMT Val108/158 Met genotype on frontal lobe function and risk for schizophrenia. Proceedings of the National Academy of Sciences of the United States of America 98: 6917–6922.
47. Schmack K, Schlagenhauf F, Sterzer P, Wrase J, Beck A, et al. (2008) Catechol-O-methyltransferase val158met genotype influences neural processing of reward anticipation. NeuroImage 42: 1631–1638.
48. Goldman-Rakic PS (1998) The cortical dopamine system: role in memory and cognition. Advances in pharmacology 42: 707–711.
49. Williams GV, Goldman-Rakic PS (1995) Modulation of memory fields by dopamine D1 receptors in prefrontal cortex. Nature 376: 572–575.
50. Kaptchuk TJ, Kelley JM, Deykin A, Wayne PM, Lasagna LC, et al. (2008) Do "placebo responders" exist? Contemporary clinical trials 29: 587–595.
51. Shapiro AK, Shapiro E (1997) The powerful placebo: from ancient priest to modern physician. Baltimore: Johns Hopkins University Press. xi, 280 p.
52. Whalley B, Hyland ME, Kirsch I (2008) Consistency of the placebo effect. Journal of psychosomatic research 64: 537–541.
53. Kelley JM, Lembo AJ, Ablon JS, Villanueva JJ, Conboy LA, et al. (2009) Patient and practitioner influences on the placebo effect in irritable bowel syndrome. Psychosomatic medicine 71: 789–797.
54. Miller FG, Colloca L, Kaptchuk TJ (2009) The placebo effect: illness and interpersonal healing. Perspectives in biology and medicine 52: 518–539.
55. Wechsler ME, Kelley JM, Boyd IO, Dutile S, Marigowda G, et al. (2011) Active albuterol or placebo, sham acupuncture, or no intervention in asthma. The New England journal of medicine 365: 119–126.
56. Branch WT, Arky RA, Woo B, Stoeckle JD, Levy DB, et al. (1991) Teaching medicine as a human experience: a patient-doctor relationship course for faculty and first-year medical students. Annals of internal medicine 114: 482–489.
57. Egnew TR, Wilson HJ (2011) Role modeling the doctor-patient relationship in the clinical curriculum. Family medicine 43: 99–105.

Infant Safety during and after Maternal Valacyclovir Therapy in Conjunction with Antiretroviral HIV-1 Prophylaxis in a Randomized Clinical Trial

Alison L. Drake[1]*, Alison C. Roxby[2], James Kiarie[7], Barbra A. Richardson[1,3,8], Anna Wald[2,4,5,8], Grace John-Stewart[1,2,4,6], Carey Farquhar[1,2,4]

1 Department of Global Health, University of Washington, Seattle, Washington, United States of America, **2** Department of Medicine, University of Washington, Seattle, Washington, United States of America, **3** Department of Biostatistics, University of Washington, Seattle, Washington, United States of America, **4** Department of Epidemiology, University of Washington, Seattle, Washington, United States of America, **5** Department of Laboratory Medicine, University of Washington, Seattle, Washington, United States of America, **6** Department of Pediatrics, University of Washington, Seattle, Washington, United States of America, **7** Department of Obstetrics and Gynaecology, University of Nairobi, Nairobi, Kenya, **8** Divisions of Vaccine and Infectious Diseases, Fred Hutchinson Cancer Research Center, Seattle, Washington, United States of America

Abstract

Background: Maternal administration of the acyclovir prodrug valacyclovir is compatible with pregnancy and breastfeeding. However, the safety profile of prolonged infant and maternal exposure to acyclovir in the context of antiretrovirals (ARVs) for prevention of mother-to-child HIV-1 transmission (PMTCT) has not been described.

Methods: Pregnant Kenyan women co-infected with HIV-1/HSV-2 with CD4 counts $>$ 250 cells/mm^3 were enrolled at 34 weeks gestation and randomized to twice daily 500 mg valacyclovir or placebo until 12 months postpartum. Women received zidovudine from 28 weeks gestation and single dose nevirapine was given to women and infants at the time of delivery for PMTCT. Infant blood was collected at 6 weeks for creatinine and ALT. Breast milk specimens were collected at 2 weeks postpartum from 71 women in the valacyclovir arm; acyclovir levels were determined for a random sample of 44 (62%) specimens. Fisher's Exact and Wilcoxon rank-sum tests were used for analysis.

Results: One hundred forty-eight women were randomized and 146 mother-infant pairs were followed postpartum. PMTCT ARVs were administered to 98% of infants and all mothers. Valacyclovir was not associated with infant or maternal toxicities or adverse events, and no congenital malformations were observed. Infant creatinine levels were all normal ($<$ 0.83 mg/dl) and median creatinine (median 0.50 mg/dl) and infant growth did not differ between study arms. Acyclovir was detected in 35 (80%) of 44 breast milk samples collected at 2 weeks postpartum. Median and maximum acyclovir levels were 2.62 and 10.15 mg/ml, respectively (interquartile range 0.6–4.19).

Conclusions: Exposure to PMTCT ARVs and acyclovir after maternal administration of valacyclovir during pregnancy and postpartum to women co-infected with HIV-1/HSV-2 was not associated with an increase in infant or maternal toxicities or adverse events.

Trial Registration: ClinicalTrials.gov NCT00530777

Editor: Ravi Jhaveri, Duke University School of Medicine, United States of America

Funding: This work was supported by the National Institutes of Health (NIH) [R03 HD057773, R03 HD057773–02S1, and K24 AI087399 to CF; K24 HD054314 to G.J.S.; K24 AI071113 and PO1 AI30731 to AW; University of Washington CFAR (UW CFAR) P30 AI027757; International AIDS Research and Training Program by the Fogarty International Center (FIC) D43-TW00007; FIC R24 TW007988 to ACR; University of Washington Center for AIDS Research (UW CFAR) core P30 AI027757; UW CFAR T32 AI0714032 to ALD], University of Washington Department of Epidemiology Small Grants Program; Puget Sound Partners for Global Health Research Technology Grant to BAR, and University of Washington Royalty Research Fund Grant [4027] to C.F. GlaxoSmithKline donated study drug (http://www.gsk.com). The funders had no role in study design, data collection and analysis, decision to publish, or preparation of the manuscript.

Competing Interests: ALD, ACR, JK, GJS, BAR, and CF declared that no competing interests exist. AW received grant support from GlaxoSmithKline and has been a consultant for AiCuris.

* E-mail: adrake2@uw.edu

Introduction

Herpes simplex virus type 2 (HSV-2) is the most common cause of genital ulcer disease worldwide. Antiviral treatment for HSV-2 with acyclovir or valacyclovir during pregnancy has been shown to have important clinical benefits, such as reducing genital shedding of HSV-2 and genital ulcers during pregnancy, which are risk factors for mother-to-child HSV-2 transmission. [1] The prevalence of HSV-2 infection among HIV-1 infected women is high, with >75% of women co-infected in some regions. [2,3] Genital ulcers resulting from HSV-2 infection are more common among HIV-1 infected women, [4] and have been associated with a 3–5 times higher risk of mother-to-child HIV-1 transmission. [2,5] Maternal benefits of HSV-2 suppression include reduced frequency and severity of HSV-2 reactivations, which may also improve maternal health or reduce risk of HIV-1 transmission.

Valacyclovir is a prodrug of acyclovir, which is rapidly absorbed and converted to acyclovir and is 3–5 times more bioavailable than acyclovir. [6,7] Both acyclovir and valacyclovir have good safety profiles in pregnant women and infants and have not been associated with congenital malformations or infant toxicity. [8,9,10] However, the safety profile of these drugs has not been previously described in the context of zidovudine (ZDV) and nevirapine (NVP) antiretroviral (ARV) prophylaxis for prevention of mother-to-child HIV-1 transmission (PMTCT) and data on prolonged infant exposure to acyclovir through breast milk is lacking. Acyclovir concentrations are reported to be higher in both amniotic fluid and breast milk than maternal blood, [11,12] and data from animal models suggest the combination of acyclovir and ZDV increases fetal exposure to both drugs. [13] Although previous data suggests the concentration of acyclovir in breast milk is low, equivalent to < 2% of a pediatric dose, [12] PMTCT ARVs may alter the pharmacokinetics of acyclovir in breast milk compartments.

We evaluated infant safety during and after prolonged maternal valacyclovir therapy administered in conjunction with antiretrovirals for PMTCT prophylaxis within a randomized clinical trial of HSV-2 suppression of twice daily 500 mg valacyclovir versus placebo in HIV-1/HSV-2 co-infected pregnant and postpartum Kenyan women. We measured the concentration of acyclovir in breast milk in order to determine the levels of acyclovir infants were exposed to through breast milk when dually exposed to acyclovir and ARV prophylaxis for PMTCT. As a secondary outcome, we also evaluated the safety of valacyclovir in HIV-1 infected pregnant and postpartum women receiving PMTCT prophylaxis.

Methods

The protocol for this trial and supporting CONSORT checklist are available as supporting documentation; see Protocol S1 and Checklist S1.

Ethics Statement

Written informed consent was obtained from study participants and all study procedures were approved by ethical review committees at the University of Washington and the University of Nairobi.

Study Population

At an antenatal clinic in Nairobi, Kenya, we enrolled 148 HIV-1/HSV-2 co-infected pregnant women at 34 weeks gestation who were not eligible for highly active ARV therapy: CD4 > 250 cells/mm^3 and World Health Organization (WHO) stage 1 or 2 between April 2008 and June 2009. [14] The study was completed in August 2010 after the last follow-up visit was completed. At enrollment, women were randomized in a 1:1 allocation scheme to receive twice daily 500 mg valacyclovir or matching placebo for the remainder of their pregnancy and for 12 months postpartum. Women were scheduled for follow-up study visits at 38 weeks gestation and at 2, 6, 10, and 14 weeks and 6, 9, and 12 months postpartum. At each study visit a questionnaire was administered and physical exam conducted, either by a study nurse or by one of two study physicians. Maternal blood samples were collected at enrollment and antenatal follow-up for creatinine assays. A breast milk sample was collected from all women at 2 weeks postpartum and a convenience sample of 44 breast milk specimens collected from women in the valacyclovir arm were tested for acyclovir concentrations (Advion BioSciences, Inc, Ithaca, NY). Advion BioSciences developed a method for use during this study for determining acyclovir concentrations in breast milk using liquid chromatography-mass spectrometry, with a lower limit of quantification of 0.1 ng/mL. Intra- and inter-assay accuracy ranges were −12.12% to 12.87% (mean 0.001%) and 11.51% to −4.83% (mean −7.08%), respectively. The ranges (mean) of intra- and inter-assay precision, measured as percent coefficient of variability, were 0.44% to 14.5% (4.84%) and 3.01% to 5.83% (3.71%), respectively. The sample size calculations for the clinical trial have been previously described [14].

Infants were brought to the clinic at all study visits for physical exams and blood was collected at 6 weeks for ALT and creatinine assays. Women were asked to return to the study clinic for interim visits if they were ill or their infant was ill, and were asked to return at monthly interim visits for pill refills after the 6 month study visit. The clinical trial was regularly reviewed by an external data safety and monitoring board and is registered at http://clinicaltrials.gov (Identification number NCT00530777).

There were no criteria for stopping the trial, other than safety. Sequentially numbered study identifiers were randomly generated by an independent, off-site researcher with block sizes of 20. Study participants were sequentially enrolled. All study investigators and participants were blinded until the end of the study.

Adverse Events and Statistical Analysis

Infants that were stillborn or second-born twins were excluded in the infant analysis. Similarly, women without at least one antenatal study visit or at least one postpartum study visit were excluded in the maternal antenatal and postpartum analyses, respectively. Cause of death and reason for hospitalizations were collected from study participants and medical records, if available. In the event of maternal death, cause of death was obtained from family or community members in addition to available medical records. The 2004 Division of AIDS Table was used to grade the severity of adverse events. [15] The incidence of adverse events, allowing for recurrences, was compared between study arms using the Andersen-Gill method. [16] The 2006 WHO reference population was used to calculate age and gender adjusted Z-scores for infant height and weight. [17] Linear mixed effects models were constructed to evaluate the effect of maternal treatment arm on Z-scores for infant height and weight over 12 months of follow-up. Frequencies of categorical variables were compared using Fisher's Exact tests and distributions of continuous variables were compared using Wilcoxon rank-sum tests. Mean baseline HIV-1 RNA levels were compared between arms using t-tests. Incidence rate ratios (IRR) were calculated to compare incidence of adverse events between study arms. A Cox regression model was constructed to evaluate the effect of maternal study arm on time to infant death. Statistical analyses were conducted using Stata version 11.1 (StataCorp LP, College Station, Texas).

Results

A total of 148 women were enrolled in the study, 74 randomized to valacyclovir and 74 randomized to placebo; 146 (99%) completed at least one study visit after delivery and are included in this analysis. The median age of participants was 25 (interquartile range [IQR], 22–29), 79% were married, and the median CD4 count was 459 cells/mm^3 (IQR, 342–573 cells/mm^3). All women received antenatal ZDV for PMTCT; the median gestational age at initiation was 29 weeks and median duration of antenatal ZDV use was 9.7 weeks. In addition, 140 (98%) women received PMTCT prophylaxis during labor or postpartum: 92% single dose nevirapine (sdNVP) in labor, 4 (3%) postpartum ZDV, 9 (6%) 3TC during labor or postpartum. There were no differences in baseline demographic or clinical characteristics between women randomized to the valacyclovir or placebo arms (Table 1). The CONSORT flow diagram has been previously published [14].

Among the 146 deliveries, 143 infants were live-born infants and 3 were stillborn (1 valacyclovir, 2 placebo). A total of 85 (59%) infants were female and median gestational age at delivery was 39.3 weeks. Risk of cesarean section was higher in the valacyclovir arm (12%) than the placebo arm (7%), but this difference was not statistically significant ($p = 0.40$). Nearly all (98%) infants received PMTCT prophylaxis: 137 (96%) sdNVP at birth, 143 (98%) postnatal ZDV, and 20 (14%) postnatal 3TC. Total infant follow-up time was similar between arms: 64.6 person-years in placebo and 68.2 person-years in valacyclovir. The majority of infants (97%) were breastfed with a median duration of 6.0 months in the placebo arm and 5.3 months in the valacyclovir arm (IQR 3.4–6.5 months, both arms). Comparison of plasma, cervical and breast milk HIV-1 viral levels, the primary outcomes of the randomized clinical trial have been previously described [14].

Infant Safety after Exposure to Acyclovir in Utero and through Breast Milk

The median duration of *in utero* exposure to acyclovir was 5.3 weeks (IQR 3.7 – 6.0 weeks). After *in utero* exposure to maternal ARV prophylaxis, and acyclovir for women in the valacyclovir arm, none of the infants were born with congenital malformations. Median birth weights were similar in infants born to women in the valacyclovir (3.2 kg, IQR 2.9–3.5) and placebo (3.0 kg, IQR 2.9–3.5) arms ($p = 0.09$); the proportion of infants born premature (<37 weeks gestation) was also similar (19% vs. 13%, $p = 0.36$).

During the first year of life, 7 infants in the placebo arm and 2 infants in the valacyclovir arm died (Hazard Ratio (HR) 0.27, 95% CI: 0.06–1.32, $p = 0.11$) (Table 2). Infant hospitalizations and deaths by maternal study arm are summarized in Table 2. The incidence of infant adverse events by study arm is shown in Table 3. The incidence of pneumonia was somewhat higher among infants in the valacyclovir arm than the placebo arm (0.39 vs. 0.22 per 100 person-years, $p = 0.08$). Infants in the valacyclovir arm were less likely to have eczema (IRR 0.29; $p = 0.02$) and oral thrush (IRR 0.67; $p = 0.05$) than infants in the placebo arm. There were no other major differences in the incidence of infant adverse events between study arms. Furthermore, infant growth over time was similar between arms; there were no significant differences in the mean change, or rate of change, in Z-scores for infant weight or height during 12 months of follow-up.

Among the 122 infants with serum collected at 6 weeks, all creatinine levels were normal and the distribution was similar in the valacyclovir and placebo arms (median [range]: 0.49 mg/dl [0.19–0.83] and 0.51 mg/dl [0.30–0.86], respectively). Median ALT levels at 6 weeks were also similar (26.7 U/L [range 12.6–52.4] in placebo, 26.5 U/L [range 10.6–70.1] in valacyclovir) and all levels were within the normal range, with the exception of 1 infant with an ALT level of 70.1 U/L (Grade 1) in the valacyclovir arm [15].

Among women randomized to valacyclovir, 71 had breast milk samples collected at 2 weeks postpartum and 44 of these samples were randomly chosen to test for acyclovir concentrations. Acyclovir was detected in 35 (80%) breast milk samples; the median concentration was 2.62 μg/ml (IQR 0.6–4.19) and range was 0.15 to 10.15 μg/ml. At the 2 week postpartum visit, all women self-reported the number of doses missed in the last 2 days. Women with detectable levels of acyclovir were significantly more likely to report fewer doses missed ($p = 0.03$, Fisher's Exact). Among the 9 women with undetectable levels of acyclovir in breast milk samples, 1 (11%) missed all 4 doses, 2 (22%) missed 2 doses, and 6 (67%) did not miss any doses. In contrast, among the 35 women with detectable levels of acyclovir none missed all doses, 1 (3%) missed 2 doses, 4 (11%) missed 3 doses, and 30 (80%) did not miss any doses.

Table 1. Demographic and clinical characteristics of study participants at baseline, by study arm.

Baseline characteristics	Median (IQR[1]) or n (%)		P
	Valacyclovir (n = 73)	Placebo (n = 73)	
Age (years)	25 (22–30)	25 (22–29)	0.82
Married	57 (78)	58 (79)	1.00
Education (years)	8 (7–12)	8 (7–10)	0.26
Employed	22 (30)	18 (25)	0.58
Monthly rent ($/month)[2,3]	24 (19–33)	21 (13–33)	0.29
History of sexually transmitted diseases	20 (27)	18 (25)	0.85
History of genital ulcer disease	10 (14)	13 (18)	0.65
Syphilis seropositive[4]	0 (0)	0 (0)	-
CD4 count (cells/mm^3)	452 (351–560)	481 (340–598)	0.78
WHO stage[5]			0.18
1	68 (93)	62 (85)	
2	5 (7)	11 (15)	
On ZDV[6] by enrollment	73 (100)	68 (93)	0.06
Plasma HIV-1 RNA (log_{10} copies/mL)[7]	3.89 (3.66–4.11)	3.87 (3.67–4.06)	0.91

Table 2. Infant hospitalizations and deaths, by study arm.

Age	Hospitalizations		Deaths	
	Symptoms and diagnoses		*Cause of death*	
	Placebo (n = 8)	**Valacyclovir (n = 8)**	**Placebo (n = 7)**	**Placebo (n = 2)**
Birth – 2 days	Neonatal asphyxia as a result of obstructed labor	Neonatal distress as a result of nuchal cord	Prematurity	
	Neonatal asphyxia as a result of placenta previa	Hyper-extended leg		
	Mild respiratory distress syndrome	Neonatal sepsis		
> 2 days – 6 weeks	Neonatal sepsis		Respiratory distress, possible neonatal sepsis	Possible neonatal sepsis
> 6 weeks – 6 months	Superficial burns	Vomiting and diarrhea	Malaria, dehydration as a result of gastroenteritis	Complications of tooth extraction, diarrhea
	Pneumonia	Gastroenteritis, dehydration, anemia (2nd hospitalization)	Gastroenteritis and dehydration	
	Gastroenteritis, rickets, malaria, urinary tract infection	Diarrhea	Fever, respiratory distress, abdominal distention	
	Dehydration, malnutrition	Pneumonia, gastroenteritis (3rd hospitalization)	Gastroenteritis, HIV infection	
6–12 months		Gastroenteritis, growth retardation, oral thrush	Meningitis	
		Gastroenteritis, fever		
		Pneumonia, rickets		

Maternal Safety

Maternal safety outcomes were analyzed separately for antenatal and postpartum follow-up. After excluding 43 women who delivered prior to 38 weeks gestation and 3 women without an antenatal follow-up sample, 100 women were included in the pregnancy analysis. Genital ulcers were only found in one woman in the placebo arm during pelvic exam; none were found in the valacyclovir arm. Other adverse events for women during pregnancy were minor and primarily consisted of headache, cough, vomiting, vaginal discharge, urinary tract infection, and weight loss. The only adverse event that was more frequent in women in the valacyclovir group was fever; 5 women reported fevers in the valacyclovir arm for an incidence of 1.02 per 100 person-years and no fevers were reported in the placebo arm ($p = 0.03$) (Table 4). Median serum creatinine at enrollment was the same in both arms (0.74 mg/dL) and all antenatal follow-up levels fell within the normal range; median creatinine change from enrollment to 38 weeks gestation was 0.03 mg/dL in the placebo arm and 0.05 mg/dL in the valacyclovir arm. There were no hospitalizations or maternal deaths during pregnancy; the only severe adverse events that occurred during pregnancy were 3 women with stillbirths (above).

There were 73 women in each study arm included in the postpartum analysis; 1 woman in each arm was lost to follow-up prior to delivery. The median duration of postpartum follow-up was 12 months in both arms and the total follow-up time was 69.3 person-years in the valacyclovir arm and 69.8 person-years in the placebo arm. Overall retention was high with 136 (93%) of women completing the 12 month postpartum visit; median adherence to study drug by pill count was 86% in both arms (IQR 80% to 92%). Three women were hospitalized during postpartum follow-up for the following reasons: severe depression (valacyclovir); gastroenteritis (valacyclovir); and malaria and severe anemia (placebo). Three women also died during postpartum follow-up. One woman in the valacyclovir arm died with peripheral edema and chest pain, which was not considered to be related to the study drug. Two women died in the placebo arm; one died of a hemorrhage at 3 weeks postpartum and may have had undiagnosed tuberculosis, and the other died with abdominal pain with vomiting and diarrhea. The most frequently reported maternal postpartum adverse events included cough, upper respiratory infections, headache, backache, chest pain, and abdominal pain; there were no differences in the incidence of these events between study arms (Table 5). The risk of dizziness ($IRR = 0.50$, $p = 0.03$) and yeast infections (IRR 0.36, $p = 0.04$) were higher in the placebo than valacyclovir arm; incidence of all other reported adverse events was similar between study arms.

Discussion

We did not detect any association between valacyclovir and congenital malformations, infant adverse events, or infant toxicities after exposure *in utero* and through breast milk following administration of maternal valacyclovir and PMTCT ARVs during pregnancy and postpartum. The absence of infant kidney and liver toxicity suggests that valacyclovir exposure does not increase the risk of nevirapine-associated liver toxicity. We also observed that acyclovir was detected in breast milk at low levels at 2 weeks postpartum, demonstrating a low level of infant exposure to acyclovir through breast milk. The median concentration of 2.62 μg/mL was similar to the average breast milk concentration reported in a pharmacokinetic study by Sheffield *et al* conducted in U.S. women who were not HIV-1 infected. [12] Assuming infants ingest 750 mL/day of breast milk, the cumulative exposure to acyclovir for infants in this study over the course of 1 year would be 717 mg (2.62 μg/mL × 750 mL/day × 365 days). For comparison, this is 79% lower than the cumulative exposure from

Table 3. Incidence of infant adverse events, by study arm.

Symptoms and diagnoses	Valacyclovir	Placebo	Incidence rate ratio	P
	Incidence per 100 person-years (n)			
General				
Fever	2.71 (178)	2.90 (181)	0.93	>0.10
Respiratory				
Cough	2.62 (173)	2.87 (178)	0.92	>0.10
Upper respiratory infection	3.10 (204)	3.16 (197)	0.98	>0.10
Bronchitis	0.37 (25)	0.30 (19)	1.25	>0.10
Asthma	0.03 (2)	0.05 (3)	0.63	>0.10
Pneumonia	0.39 (26)	0.22 (14)	1.76	0.08
Tuberculosis	0.01 (1)	0.05 (3)	0.32	>0.10
Wheezing	0.21 (14)	0.14 (9)	1.48	>0.10
Difficulty breathing	0.09 (6)	0.22 (14)	0.40	0.06
Rhinorrhea	1.86 (123)	1.85 (116)	1.00	>0.10
Gastrointestinal				
Vomiting	0.66 (44)	0.87 (55)	0.76	>0.10
Diarrhea	1.60 (106)	1.48 (93)	1.08	>0.10
Behavioral				
Irritability	0.31 (21)	0.42 (27)	0.74	>0.10
Difficulty feeding	0.51 (34)	0.64 (41)	0.79	>0.10
Growth				
Wasting	0.63 (6)	0.14 (9)	0.63	>0.10
Cardiovascular				
Heart murmur	0.13 (9)	0.08 (5)	1.71	>0.10
Hematological				
Anemia[a]	0.04 (3)	0.03 (2)	1.42	>0.10
Malaria	0.08 (5)	0.08 (5)	0.94	>0.10
Sepsis	0.13 (9)	0.17 (11)	0.77	>0.10
Allergic				
Pruritic dermatitis	0.04 (3)	0.08 (5)	0.57	>0.10
Rash	1.62 (107)	1.71 (107)	0.95	>0.10
Skin				
Heat rash	0.49 (33)	0.60 (38)	0.82	>0.10
Eczema	0.06 (4)	0.20 (13)	0.29	0.02
Central nervous system				
Seizures	0.01 (1)	0.01 (1)	0.95	>0.10
Encephalopathy	0.03 (2)	0	-	>0.10
Lymphatic				
Lymphadenopathy	0.06 (4)	0.11 (7)	0.54	>0.10
Head				
Fontanelle sunken	0.10 (7)	0.17 (11)	0.60	>0.10
Conjunctivitis	0.34 (23)	0.42 (27)	0.81	>0.10
Oral thrush	0.67 (42)	0.93 (59)	0.67	0.05
Mouth ulcers	0.07 (5)	0.08 (5)	0.95	>0.10
Otitis media	0.09 (6)	0.08 (5)	1.14	>0.10
Otitis externa	0.09 (6)	0.06 (4)	1.42	>0.10
Liver				
Jaundice	0.01 (1)	0	-	>0.10

[a]Defined as hemoglobin <11 g/dl.

Table 4. Incidence of maternal antenatal adverse events, by study arm.

Symptoms and diagnoses	Valacyclovir	Placebo	Incidence rate ratio	P
	Incidence per 100 person-years (n)			
General				
Fever	1.02 (5)	0	-	0.03
Abdominal pain	1.44 (7)	0.83 (4)	1.73	>0.10
Back pain	0.62 (3)	0.84 (4)	0.74	>0.10
Edema	1.04 (5)	0.64 (3)	1.61	>0.10
Weight loss	2.99 (14)	3.39 (15)	0.88	>0.10
Fatigue	0.20 (1)	0	-	>0.10
Headache	3.34 (15)	2.10 (10)	1.59	>0.10
Respiratory				
Cough	1.69 (8)	2.74 (12)	0.62	>0.10
Cold	0.41 (2)	0.21 (1)	1.97	>0.10
Sneezing	0.41 (2)	0.42 (2)	0.98	>0.10
Nasal congestion	0.41 (2)	0	-	>0.10
Rhinorrhea	0	0.63 (3)	-	>0.10
Gastrointestinal				
Nausea	0.41 (2)	0.63 (3)	0.65	>0.10
Vomiting	2.60 (12)	2.02 (9)	1.29	>0.10
Diarrhea	0.41 (2)	0.20 (1)	1.99	>0.10
Heartburn	0.41 (2)	0.21 (1)	1.97	>0.10
Cardiovascular				
Hypertension	0.20 (1)	0	-	>0.10
Tachycardia	0.20 (1)	0	-	>0.10
Hematological				
Anemia	0.20 (1)	0.21 (1)	0.97	>0.10
Allergic				
Pruritic rash	0	0.21 (1)	-	>0.10
Dizziness	1.01 (5)	0.83 (4)	1.21	>0.10
Obstetrical/Gynecological				
Cervical blood	1.08 (5)	0.21 (1)	5.14	>0.10
Vaginal discharge	4.74 (20)	4.10 (17)	1.16	0.01
Vaginal itching	0.61 (3)	1.27 (6)	0.48	>0.10
Genital ulcer disease	0	0.21 (1)	-	>0.10
Kidney				
Urinary tract infection	10.22 (40)	7.90 (32)	1.29	>0.10
Proteinuria	0.62 (3)	0.63 (3)	0.99	>0.10
Dysuria	1.94 (9)	0.65 (3)	3.00	0.09

intravenous treatment of neonatal herpes administered over only 14–21 days [18].

The incidences of adverse events for pregnant and postpartum women were also similar between study arms, with the exception of fever during pregnancy which was more frequent among women in the valacyclovir arm. However, 3 of 5 fevers were reported only at interim visits and were not measured. Fever has not previously been reported as a side effect of valacyclovir, and is unlikely to be related to valacyclovir suppressive therapy.

Our infant and maternal safety results are consistent with prior studies of HSV-2 antiviral use during pregnancy and breastfeeding. [8,9,19,20] However, safety data on prolonged exposure to acyclovir *in utero* and in breast milk from these studies are limited. Concerns about *in utero* acyclovir exposure stem from pharmacokinetic data that have shown an accumulation of acyclovir in amniotic fluid at levels higher than maternal plasma; however, acyclovir has not been found to accumulate in the fetus. [19,20] The absence of any clinically significant adverse events in dually exposed infants suggests the safety profile is similar to infants exposed to acyclovir or ZDV alone; however, we did not evaluate pharmacokinetics of acyclovir in infants and could not ascertain whether PMTCT ARV prophylaxis with ZDV potentiates infant exposure to acyclovir, as has been suggested in one animal study [13].

Table 5. Incidence of maternal postpartum adverse events, by study arm.

Symptoms and diagnoses	Valacyclovir	Placebo	Incidence rate ratio	P
	Incidence per 100 person-years (n)			
General				
Fever	0.42 (29)	0.55 (38)	0.77	>0.10
Abdominal pain	0.66 (45)	0.64 (44)	1.03	>0.10
Sore mouth	0.06 (10)	0.09 (6)	1.68	>0.10
Back pain	0.39 (27)	0.61 (42)	0.64	0.07
Muscle aches	0.03 (2)	0.03 (2)	1.01	>0.10
Joint pain	0.17 (12)	0.29 (20)	0.60	>0.10
Edema	0	0.01 (1)	-	>0.10
Poor appetite	0.22 (15)	0.23 (16)	0.94	>0.10
Wasting	0.04 (3)	0.04 (3)	1.01	>0.10
Respiratory				
Cough	1.11 (46)	1.26 (50)	0.88	>0.10
Upper respiratory tract infection	1.11 (75)	1.20 (82)	0.92	>0.10
Bronchitis	0.06 (4)	0.06 (4)	1.00	>0.10
Pneumonia	0.04 (3)	0.10 (7)	0.43	>0.10
Sore throat	0.42 (29)	0.49 (34)	0.86	>0.10
Pharyngitis	0.17 (12)	0.08 (6)	2.02	>0.10
Tuberculosis	0.03 (2)	0.01 (1)	2.00	>0.10
Wheezing	0	0.04 (3)	-	>0.10
Rhinorrhea	0.44 (30)	0.33 (23)	1.32	>0.10
Gastrointestinal				
Vomiting	0.13 (9)	0.19 (13)	0.70	>0.10
Diarrhea	0.35 (24)	0.32 (22)	1.10	>0.10
Breast				
Breast pain	0.13 (9)	0.16 (11)	0.82	>0.10
Nipple bleeding/cracking	0.11 (8)	0.22 (15)	0.54	>0.10
Breast engorgement	0.10 (7)	0.09 (6)	1.18	>0.10
Mastitis	0.03 (2)	0.10 (7)	0.29	>0.10
Breast abscess	0.01 (1)	0.03 (2)	0.50	>0.10
Cardiovascular				
Hypertension	0.03 (2)	0	-	>0.10
Heart murmur	0.01 (1)	0.03 (2)	0.50	>0.10
Chest pain	0.45 (31)	0.65 (45)	0.69	>0.10
Hematological				
Anemia	0.06 (4)	0.06 (4)	1.01	>0.10
Malaria	0.17 (11)	0.28 (17)	0.60	>0.10
Allergic				
Pruritic dermatitis	0.32 (22)	0.41 (28)	0.79	>0.10
Dizziness	0.22 (15)	0.43 (30)	0.50	0.03
Skin				
Eczema	0.04 (3)	0.07 (5)	0.60	>0.10
Opportunistic Infection				
Shingles	0.01 (1)	0.04 (3)	0.34	>0.10
Oral thrush	0.03 (2)	0.10 (7)	0.29	>0.10
Mouth ulcers	0.04 (3)	0.01 (1)	3.02	>0.10
Gynecological				
Vaginal discharge	0.04 (3)	0.19 (13)	1.16	0.01
Yeast infection	0.07 (5)	0.2 (15)	0.34	0.03
Genital ulcer disease	0.01 (1)	0.03 (2)	0.50	>0.10

Table 5. Cont.

Symptoms and diagnoses	Valacyclovir	Placebo	Incidence rate ratio	P
	Incidence per 100 person-years (n)			
Lymphatic				
Lymphadenopathy	0.09 (6)	0.04 (3)	2.02	>0.10
Head				
Headache	1.81 (122)	1.56 (106)	1.16	>0.10
Conjunctivitis	0.06 (4)	0	-	0.06

Our study is unique in that it used a combination of laboratory assays and clinical indicators to ascertain infant and maternal safety both during pregnancy and for 1 year postpartum, captured serial infant growth measurements, and evaluated safety exposure to valacyclovir in combination with PMTCT ARVs. However, our study was subject to some limitations. We were unable to determine infant acyclovir concentrations, lacked knowledge regarding the timing between dosing and breast milk sample collection, and did not evaluate infant neutropenia, which has been observed in some neonates with herpes treated with high dose intravenous acyclovir. [21] In addition, we cannot determine whether acyclovir was not detected in breast milk for some women in the valacyclovir arm due to over-reporting adherence, the inability of our assay to detect low concentrations of acyclovir, or because breast milk sample collection occurred too long after the last dose was administered. Although we did not detect any difference in congenital malformations between study arms, valacyclovir suppressive therapy was started late in pregnancy, at 34 weeks gestation, and we are unable to address risk at earlier gestations. Finally, use of block randomization could compromise allocation concealment and lead to selection bias; however we did not detect any statistical differences in maternal baseline characteristics between arms.

Acyclovir and valacyclovir are currently used in developed settings for chronic HSV-2 suppression, including pregnant women with recurrent genital herpes. [22] Our study provides additional safety information on tolerability and safety of acyclovir during late pregnancy, and it includes longer follow-up of than prior studies of valacyclovir in the US (12 months vs. 2 weeks). [23] Antiviral use in resource-limited settings may become more widespread, due to the frequency and severity of HSV-2 reactivations in HIV-1 infected persons coupled with WHO recommendations to use acyclovir for syndromic management of lesions consistent with genital herpes. In addition, HSV-2 suppressive therapy slows HIV-1 disease progression. [24] If antivirals for HSV do become more widely used in HIV-1/HSV-2 co-infected individuals, demonstrating infant and maternal safety of dual exposure to valacyclovir and PMTCT ARVs could help to expand the benefit of HSV-2 suppression in resource-limited settings to pregnant or breastfeeding women.

Maternally administered valacyclovir suppressive therapy used in conjunction with short-course PMTCT ARVs was well tolerated among infants and HIV-1 infected pregnant and postpartum women. Our data suggest PMTCT ARVs do not alter the safety profile of valacyclovir in these women and their perinatally exposed infants; valacyclovir suppression should be considered as a mechanism to reduce HSV-2 recurrences during late pregnancy and breastfeeding among HIV-1 infected women receiving short course ARVs for PMTCT, when clinically indicated.

Supporting Information

Checklist S1 CONSORT Checklist.

Protocol S1 Trial Protocol.

Acknowledgments

We would like to thank our participants and study staff at the Mathare North City Council Clinic for their time and dedication to this study, and our data safety and monitoring committee for their review throughout the study.

Author Contributions

Conceived and designed the experiments: ALD JK BAR AW GJS CF. Performed the experiments: ACR. Analyzed the data: ALD BAR. Contributed reagents/materials/analysis tools: AW. Wrote the paper: ALD ACR AW GJS CF.

References

1. Hollier L, Wendel G (2008) Third trimester antiviral prophylaxis for preventing maternal genital herpes simplex virus (HSV) recurrences and neonatal infection. Cochrane Database Syst Rev. CD004946 p.
2. Drake AL, John-Stewart GC, Wald A, Mbori-Ngacha DA, Bosire R, et al. (2007) Herpes Simplex Virus Type 2 and Risk of Intrapartum Human Immunodeficiency Virus Transmission. Obstet Gynecol 109: 403–409.
3. Mbopi-Keou FX, Gresenguet G, Mayaud P, Weiss HA, Gopal R, et al. (2000) Interactions between herpes simplex virus type 2 and human immunodeficiency virus type 1 infection in African women: opportunities for intervention. J Infect Dis 182: 1090–1096.
4. Hitti J, Watts DH, Burchett SK, Schacker T, Selke S, et al. (1997) Herpes simplex virus seropositivity and reactivation at delivery among pregnant women infected with human immunodeficiency virus-1. Am J Obstet Gynecol 177: 450–454.
5. John GC, Nduati RW, Mbori-Ngacha DA, Richardson BA, Panteleeff D, et al. (2001) Correlates of mother-to-child human immunodeficiency virus type 1 (HIV-1) transmission: association with maternal plasma HIV-1 RNA load, genital HIV-1 DNA shedding, and breast infections. J Infect Dis 183: 206–212.
6. Weller S, Blum MR, Doucette M, Burnette T, Cederberg DM, et al. (1993) Pharmacokinetics of the acyclovir pro-drug valaciclovir after escalating single- and multiple-dose administration to normal volunteers. Clin Pharmacol Ther 54: 595–605.
7. Conant MA, Schacker TW, Murphy RL, Gold J, Crutchfield LT, et al. (2002) Valaciclovir versus aciclovir for herpes simplex virus infection in HIV-infected individuals: two randomized trials. Int J STD AIDS 13: 12–21.
8. Pasternak B, Hviid A (2010) Use of acyclovir, valacyclovir, and famciclovir in the first trimester of pregnancy and the risk of birth defects. JAMA 304: 859–866.

9. Stone KM, Reiff-Eldridge R, White AD, Cordero JF, Brown Z, et al. (2004) Pregnancy outcomes following systemic prenatal acyclovir exposure: Conclusions from the international acyclovir pregnancy registry, 1984–1999. Birth Defects Res A Clin Mol Teratol 70: 201–207.
10. Kimberlin DW, Whitley RJ, Wan W, Powell DA, Storch G, et al. (2011) Oral acyclovir suppression and neurodevelopment after neonatal herpes. N Engl J Med 365: 1284–1292.
11. Jacquemard F, Yamamoto M, Costa JM, Romand S, Jaqz-Aigrain E, et al. (2007) Maternal administration of valaciclovir in symptomatic intrauterine cytomegalovirus infection. BJOG 114: 1113–1121.
12. Sheffield JS, Fish DN, Hollier LM, Cadematori S, Nobles BJ, et al. (2002) Acyclovir concentrations in human breast milk after valaciclovir administration. Am J Obstet Gynecol 186: 100–102.
13. Brown SD, Bartlett MG, White CA (2003) Pharmacokinetics of intravenous acyclovir, zidovudine, and acyclovir-zidovudine in pregnant rats. Antimicrob Agents Chemother 47: 991–996.
14. Drake AL, Roxby AC, Ongecha-Owuor F, Kiarie J, Wald A, et al. (2011) Valacyclovir Suppressive Therapy Reduces Plasma and Breast Milk HIV-1 RNA Levels During Pregnancy and Postpartum: A Randomized Trial. J Infect Dis 205: 366–375.
15. National Institute for Allergy and Infectious Disease (NIAID). Division of AIDS Toxicity Table for Grading the Severity of Adult and Pediatric Adverse Events, Publish Date December (2004) Available at http://www.ucdmc.ucdavis.edu/clinicaltrials/documents/DAIDS_AE_GradingTable_FinalDec2004.pdf. Accessed May 31, 2011.
16. Andersen PK, Gill RD (1982) Cox's Regression Model for Counting Processes: A Large Sample Study. Ann Statist 10: 1100–1120.
17. World Heatlh Organization. (2006) WHO Child Growth Standards.
18. American Academy of Pediatrics (2009) Herpes Simplex. Red Book: 2009 Report of the Committee on Infectious Diseases. 28th ed. Elk Grove Village, IL. pp 363–373.
19. Frenkel LM, Brown ZA, Bryson YJ, Corey L, Unadkat JD, et al. (1991) Pharmacokinetics of acyclovir in the term human pregnancy and neonate. Am J Obstet Gynecol 164: 569–576.
20. Kimberlin DF, Weller S, Whitley RJ, Andrews WW, Hauth JC, et al. (1998) Pharmacokinetics of oral valacyclovir and acyclovir in late pregnancy. Am J Obstet Gynecol 179: 846–851.
21. Kimberlin DW, Lin CY, Jacobs RF, Powell DA, Corey L, et al. (2001) Safety and efficacy of high-dose intravenous acyclovir in the management of neonatal herpes simplex virus infections. Pediatrics 108: 230–238.
22. American College of Obstetrics and Gynecologists (ACOG) (.2007) ACOG Practice Bulletin. Management of herpes in pregnancy. Clinical management guidelines for obstetrician-gynecologists. No. 82 June (2007) Management of herpes in pregnancy. Obstet Gynecol 109: 1489–1498.
23. Andrews WW, Kimberlin DF, Whitley R, Cliver S, Ramsey PS, et al. (2006) Valacyclovir therapy to reduce recurrent genital herpes in pregnant women. Am J Obstet Gynecol 194: 774–781.
24. Lingappa JR, Baeten JM, Wald A, Hughes JP, Thomas KK, et al. (2010) Daily aciclovir for HIV-1 disease progression in people dually infected with HIV-1 and herpes simplex virus type 2: a randomised placebo-controlled trial. Lancet 375: 824–833.

17

Regional Neuroplastic Brain Changes in Patients with Chronic Inflammatory and Non-Inflammatory Visceral Pain

Jui-Yang Hong[1,3,6,8*], Jennifer S. Labus[1,2,3,5,6], Zhiguo Jiang[10,11], Cody Ashe-Mcnalley[1,2,3,6], Ivo Dinov[9], Arpana Gupta[1,2,3,6], Yonggang Shi[12], Jean Stains[1,3,6], Nuwanthi Heendeniya[1,3,6], Suzanne R. Smith[1,3,6], Kirsten Tillisch[1,2,3,6], Emeran A. Mayer[1,2,3,4,5,6,7]

1 Gail and Gerald Oppenheimer Family Center for Neurobiology of Stress, University of California Los Angeles, Los Angeles, California, United States of America, **2** Pain and Interoception Imaging Network (PAIN), University of California Los Angeles, Los Angeles, California, United States of America, **3** Department of Medicine, University of California Los Angeles, Los Angeles, California, United States of America, **4** Department of Psychiatry, University of California Los Angeles, Los Angeles, California, United States of America, **5** Brain Research Institute, University of California Los Angeles, Los Angeles, California, United States of America, **6** Division of Digestive Diseases, University of California Los Angeles, Los Angeles, California, United States of America, **7** Ahmanson Lovelace Brain Mapping Center, David Geffen School of Medicine, University of California, Los Angeles, California, **8** Department of Bioengineering, University of California Los Angeles, Los Angeles, California, United States of America, **9** University of Michigan School of Nursing, Ann Arbor, Michigan, United States of America, **10** Department of Biomedical Engineering, New Jersey Institute of Technology, Newark, New Jersey, United States of America, **11** Human Performance and Engineering Laboratory, Kessler Foundation Research Center, West Orange, New Jersey, United States of America, **12** Laboratory of Neuro-Imaging, University of Southern California, Los Angeles, California United States of America

Abstract

Regional cortical thickness alterations have been reported in many chronic inflammatory and painful conditions, including inflammatory bowel diseases (IBD) and irritable bowel syndrome (IBS), even though the mechanisms underlying such neuroplastic changes remain poorly understood. In order to better understand the mechanisms contributing to grey matter changes, the current study sought to identify the differences in regional alterations in cortical thickness between healthy controls and two chronic visceral pain syndromes, with and without chronic gut inflammation. 41 healthy controls, 11 IBS subjects with diarrhea, and 16 subjects with ulcerative colitis (UC) underwent high-resolution T1-weighted magnetization-prepared rapid acquisition gradient echo scans. Structural image preprocessing and cortical thickness analysis within the region of interests were performed by using the Laboratory of Neuroimaging Pipeline. Group differences were determined using the general linear model and linear contrast analysis. The two disease groups differed significantly in several cortical regions. UC subjects showed greater cortical thickness in anterior cingulate cortical subregions, and in primary somatosensory cortex compared with both IBS and healthy subjects. Compared with healthy subjects, UC subjects showed lower cortical thickness in orbitofrontal cortex and in mid and posterior insula, while IBS subjects showed lower cortical thickness in the anterior insula. Large effects of correlations between symptom duration and thickness in the orbitofrontal cortex and postcentral gyrus were only observed in UC subjects. The findings suggest that the mechanisms underlying the observed gray matter changes in UC subjects represent a consequence of peripheral inflammation, while in IBS subjects central mechanisms may play a primary role.

Editor: André Mouraux, Université catholique de Louvain, Belgium

Funding: This work was funded in part by the National Institutes of Health through Center for Neurobiology (CNS) grants: K08 DK071626, R03 DK084169, K23DK073451, R01 AT007137, P50 DK064539, R01 DK048351, and LONI grants: NIBIB 9P41EB015922-15, NCRR 2-P41-RR-013642-15, NCRR U54 RR021813, U24-RR025736, U24-RR021992. The funders had no role in study design, data collection and analysis, decision to publish, or preparation of the manuscript.

Competing Interests: The authors have declared that no competing interests exist.

* E-mail: usagilberthong@hotmail.com

Introduction

Inflammatory bowel diseases (IBD) such as ulcerative colitis (UC) are characterized by chronically recurring symptoms of abdominal pain associated with flares of mucosal inflammation. In contrast, in irritable bowel syndrome (IBS), chronically recurring symptoms of abdominal pain and discomfort occur in the absence of mucosal inflammation or other identifiable nociceptive triggers (therefore referred to as "functional" pain syndromes), and symptom flares are often triggered by psychosocial stressors. It is generally assumed that abdominal pain in UC results initially from inflammation induced peripheral and central sensitization of visceral afferent pathways [1], while symptoms in IBS may reflect primarily an alteration in central pain modulation, including alterations in endogenous descending pain modulation mechanisms [2]. On the other hand, several pieces of evidence support the concept that IBD patients effectively engage endogenous pain inhibition systems [3], including greater engagement of a cortico limbic-pontine pain modulation network compared to IBS subjects [4]. These differences in the engagement of endogenous pain modulation systems may explain the clinical observation that in uncomplicated UC, abdominal pain is not a prominent symptom even during flares.

Several studies have applied multimodal brain imaging to investigate the presence of grey matter changes in patients with various chronic pain conditions without known nociceptive drive [5–9], with presumed nociceptive drive [10–12], and with known inflammatory drive [13–18]. Reported abnormalities in these studies suggest some similarities in findings (e.g. gray matter reduction in insula [INS] and anterior cingulate cortex [ACC] subregions), and increases in CT in somatosensory regions regardless of pain syndrome, and no clear differences have emerged between the different pain categories, in particular between chronic visceral pain of "functional" and of inflammatory origin. The use of different analysis techniques by different groups, makes interpretive comparisons between studies and between different patient populations more difficult.

In the current study, we used the Laboratory of Neuroimaging (LONI) Pipeline [19,20] for image preprocessing, volumetric analysis and cortical thickness (CT) analysis. We focused on differences of local morphologic brain alterations between UC and healthy control subjects (HCs), and compared them to findings in IBS subjects. Specifically, we aimed to test the following hypotheses: 1) Both IBS and UC patients differ from HCs in terms of regional CT changes. 2) UC patients show CT changes in brain regions involved in somatosensory and viscerosensory processing and modulation. 3) IBS patients show CT changes in brain regions involved in the integration of affective, cognitive and interoceptive signals. 4) In UC patients, there are correlations between CT changes and duration of gut inflammation, reflecting the chronic influence of peripheral inflammation on the brain.

Materials and Methods

Subjects

A total 68 right-handed male and female subjects were recruited through the UCLA Digestive Disease Clinic and advertisements including HCs (n = 41; mean age = 28.2 years old, range = 19–48 years; 16 males), IBS with diarrhea (n = 11; mean age = 31.6 - years old, range = 21–47 years; 2 males), and UC subjects (n = 16; mean age = 28. 6 years old, range 18–48 years; 10 males). 15 HCs and 5 IBS subjects of the respective samples have been included in a previously published gray matter volume analysis [9]. Exclusion criteria for all subjects comprised pregnancy, postpartum or nursing females, current substance abuse or dependence, abdominal surgery, any past or present neurological illness or trauma, claustrophobia or learning disability, and current psychiatric diagnosis. A diagnosis of IBS was made by a gastroenterologist or nurse practitioner with expertise in functional GI disorders based on the ROME II or ROME III symptom criteria during a clinical assessment [21,22]. The diagnostic criteria include recurrent abdominal pain or discomfort associated with two or more of the following: 1) pain/discomfort is relieved/improved by defecation 2) the onset of pain/discomfort is related to a change in frequency of stool 3) the onset of pain/discomfort is related to a change in the form (appearance) of stool. In order to match the predominant bowel habit of UC patients, only IBS patients with diarrhea were used in this study. In addition, IBS subjects with current regular use of analgesic drugs (including narcotics, opioids and alpha2-delta ligands) were excluded. UC patients were diagnosed by a gastroenterologist, which was supported by biopsies obtained by endoscopy. During screening, all subjects completed the modified Mayo UCDAI (disease activity index for Stool frequency, rectal bleeding and physician rating of disease activity) to assess degree of current disease. A score of 0–1 is considered Remission, score of 2–4 mild disease, and >4 is considered active disease [23]. Exclusion criteria specific to the UC population were corticosteroid use within last 6 months, or use of any psychotropic medications. All procedures were approved by the UCLA Medical Institutional Review Board, and all subjects provided written informed consent. Questionnaires were completed before scanning to determine symptom type, severity, duration of symptoms, and abdominal sensation (UCLA Bowel Symptom Questionnaire, BSQ) [24], comorbid affective and mood disorders (Hospital Anxiety Depression Scale, HAD) [25], and IBS-related fears and anxiety (Visceral Sensitivity Index, VSI) [26,27]. Details are shown in Table 1.

Structural MRI Acquisition

All high-resolution T1-weighted brain images were collected at the UCLA Brain Mapping Center using a Siemens 3 Tesla Trio with magnetization prepared rapid gradient echo scanning parameters (TR = 2200 ms, TE = 3.26 ms, flip angle = 9°, duration = 9:03 mins, FOV = 256).

Data analysis

We employed the LONI pipeline for image preprocessing, cortical surface modeling and gray matter thickness analysis [19,20]. Following a de-identification step, the structural neuroimaging data were converted from Digital Imaging and Communications in Medicine to ANALYZE 7.5 format, skull-stripped using the LONI Skull-Stripping Meta Algorithm pipeline workflow [28] and cortical surface models were generated using FreeSurfer 4.0 [29] (http://surfer.nmr.mgh.harvard.edu/fswiki and http://ucla.in/xSQPqT). Cortical grey matter thickness was computed at each point of the surface using the distance from the pial surface to the nearest point on the white matter surface. For numerical implementation, we first built the signed distance function [30,31] of the white matter surface in 3D space and then computed the CT as the value on the signed distance function at those locations. The cortical surfaces and the corresponding CT maps were registered to the International Consortium for Brain Mapping (ICBM) brain surface [32] and then vertex-wise correspondences were established between all cortical surface models using a Conformal Metric Optimization method [33]. An experienced human brain researcher rated each brain surface reconstruction by visually inspecting the surfaces using LONI ShapeViewer (http://www.loni.ucla.edu/Software/ShapeViewer). The quality of surface reconstruction and accuracy of vertex labeling were assessed on the scale of 0 to 1 (0 = completely unacceptable; 1 = perfectly reconstructed and labeled). A threshold of 0.7 was selected as the criterion to reconstruct a subject's surface data to be included in the final analysis.

Region of interest analysis

We examined the CT change in several manually delineated regions of interest (ROIs) in each hemisphere based on previous studies [11,14,34–39]. These ROIs included insular subregions (anterior INS [aINS], mid INS [mINS], and posterior INS [pINS]), cingulate subregions (subgenual ACC [sgACC], pregenual ACC [pgACC], anterior midcingulate cortex [aMCC] and posterior MCC [pMCC]), orbitofrontal gyrus (OFG) (lateral OFG and medial OFG), pre- and postcentral gyri [32]. No subregions of pre- and postcentral gyri were drawn. The subregions of INS and cingulum were manually delineated on the 3D ICBM brain atlas [32] by two well-trained researchers with good command of neuroanatomical knowledge (Figure S1). The 3D ROI masks were transformed back onto the ICBM

Table 1. Clinical and behavioral characteristics.

	HCs			IBS subjects			UC subjects			F	Sig.
	N	Mean	SD	N	Mean	SD	N	Mean	SD		
Sex (Male/Female)	16/25			2/9			10/6				
Age	41	28.17	8.43	11	31.55	9.49	16	28.56	8.95	.66	.52
Anxiety symptoms[1]	41	2.8	2.33	11	6.91	3.67	16	7.31	3.55	18.29	<.01
Depression symptoms[1]	41	.85	1.22	11	2.64	2.73	16	3.44	3.54	7.77	<.01
Visceral Sensitivity Index [2]	40	2.83	5.17	11	37.45	12.94	15	26.13	14.09	61.68	<.01
Overall Bowel Symptoms[3]				11	11.91	2.74	13	4.69	2.46	54.12	<.01
Abdominal Pain[4]				11	10.55	4.3	14	4.14	3.61	18.01	<.01
Abdominal Discomfort[5]				11	11.91	4.21	16	4.06	3.86	49.63	<.01
Duration of symptoms[6]				10	8.5	6.13	16	9.81	9.35	1.67	.69

F = main effect of group from ANOVA and t-tests for four and two group comparisons, respectively.
1. HAD: Hospital Anxiety and Depression [25];
2. VSI: Visceral Sensitivity Index [26,27];
BSQ: Bowel Symptom Questionnaire [24].
3. BSQ Overall Symptoms in the Past week (0–20).
4. BSQ Abdominal Pain in the Past week (0–20).
5. BSQ Discomfort in the Past week (0–20).
6. BSQ Duration in years, derived from onset of symptom.
Statistically significant p<0.05.

surface space by resampling the atlas map based on masks' Euclidean coordinates [33].

Statistical analysis

To determine potential protocol differences in ROIs, a general linear model (GLM) was applied to examine differences in total gray matter volumes within HCs as a function of protocol. Group differences in CT within ROIs as a function of group, sex and group*sex were determined using the GLM and weighted linear contrast analysis controlling for total gray matter volume, and age in SPSS v19. The contrasts testing the interaction between group and sex were weighted to eliminate any bias caused by unbalanced representation of sexes. Although this was a hypothesis driven study, we implemented a conservative procedure to adjust for multiple comparisons in order to control for type I error. Specifically, the false-discovery rate (FDR) for the 66 contrasts (11 bilateral ROIs [n = 22] for each of three independent contrasts) was held at 5% [40–42]. GLM and linear contrast analysis controlling for sex and age were also applied to examine differences in BSQ between IBS and UC subjects as well as group differences in non-BSQ clinical and behavioral characteristics including VSI and HAD. Significance was determined after controlling FDR at 5% [40,41].

Correlation Analysis of Clinic Variables

Within group exploratory partial correlation analyses controlling for total gray matter volume, sex, and age were performed to characterize the association between subjects' clinic characteristics (BSQ, VSI, HAD and Mayo UCDAI) and regions showing significant group differences in CT. However, for the partial correlation between significant ROIs and symptom duration, we did not include age as a covariate, as these explanatory variables were significantly correlated, for IBS group (duration, r = .39, p = .036), and for UC group (duration, r = .67, p = .001) [43]. Significance was determined after controlling FDR at 5% [40,41].

Results

Subject Characteristics

Subjects' clinical data are summarized in Table 1. Compared to the HCs, the two disease groups showed significantly higher measures of symptom related anxiety (VSI scores: IBS>HCs, F = 126.28, p<.001; UC>HCs, F = 71.97, p<.001; IBS>UC, F = 10.61, p = .002), anxiety symptoms (HAD scores: IBS>HCs, F = 17.03, p<.001; UC>HCs, F = 28.02, p<.001), and depression symptoms (HAD scores: IBS>HCs, F = 4.88, p = .031; UC>HCs, F = 15.16, p<.001). IBS subjects had significantly higher overall bowel symptoms scores, more abdominal discomfort and pain than UC subjects. Using the Mayo UCDAI [23], 5 of the UC subjects were in remission, 7 had mild disease and 4 had active disease (mild flare). There were no differences in terms of age of subjects and duration of GI symptoms.

Regional Cortical Thickness Changes Using ROI Analysis

Regional CT differences were observed between UC, IBS and HCs. Mean CT values and statistical significance after FDR correction are shown in Table 2 and Table S1. As depicted in Figure 1A, compared to both IBS and HCs, UC subjects showed greater CT in left cingulate cortical subregions (aMCC, pMCC, pgACC and sgACC), and in left post central gyrus (statistically significant differences following FDR correction for multiple comparisons are shown in Figure 1A and marked with asterisks). As shown in Figure 1B, compared to both IBS and HCs, UC subjects had reduced CT in prefrontal regions (left medial and lateral OFG) and in left INS subregions (most significant in pINS). Following FDR correction for multiple comparisons, the results between HCs and UC remained significant even though some differences (OFG and INS) between IBS and UC groups were no longer significant (significant differences are shown in Figure 1B and marked with asterisks). All results remained significant after controlling for depression. However, after controlling for anxiety, the observed differences between HCs and UC subjects in left pMCC, aINS and mINS were no longer significant after FDR

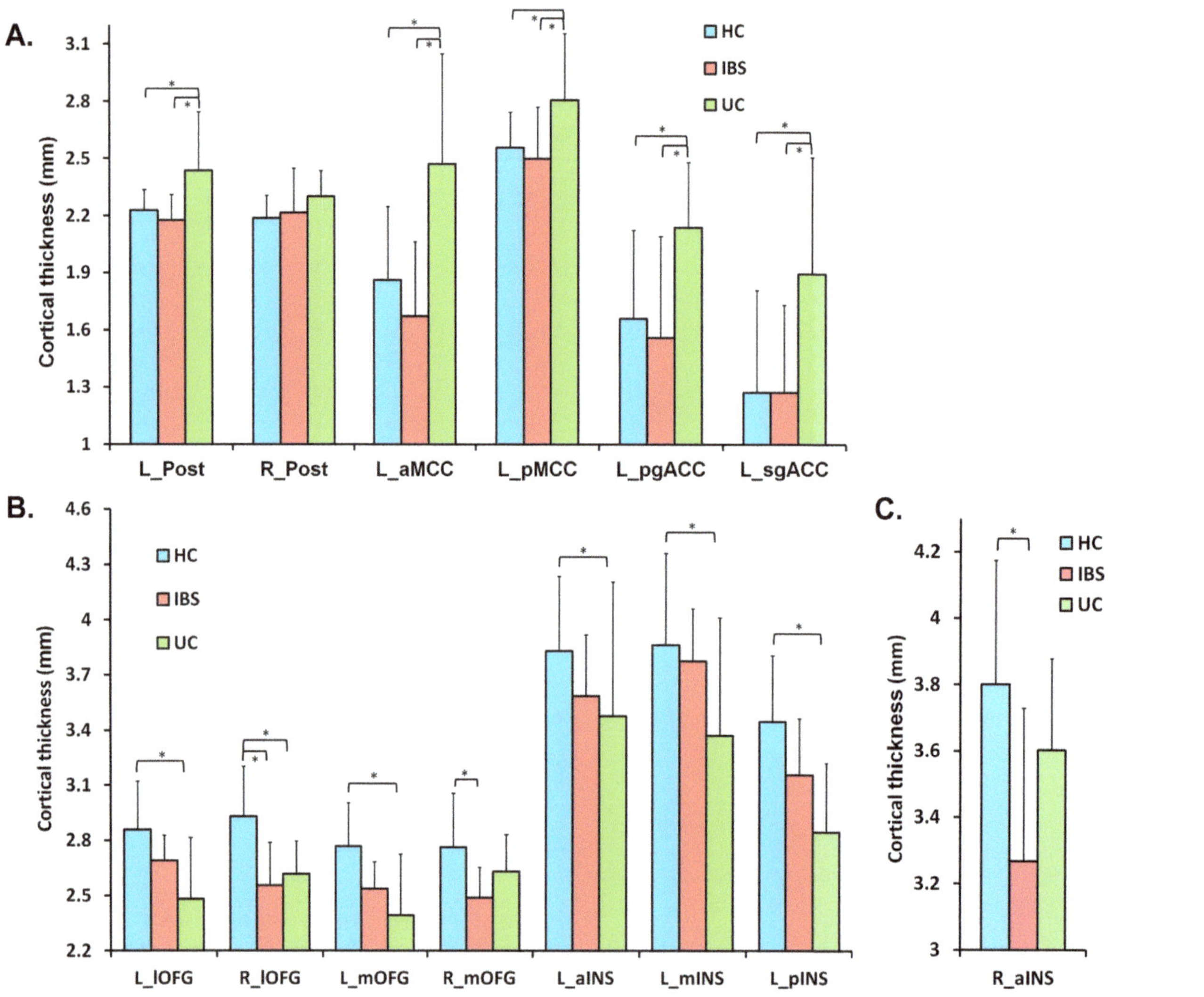

Figure 1. Mean cortical thickness of the ROIs showing significant group differences. (A) UC subjects showed the greatest CT in the regions of somatosensory and cingulate cortex. (B) In the subregions of OFG and INS, UCs had lower CT compared with HCs. (C) IBS subjects had lower CT in right aINS compared to HCs. Error bars reflect standard deviation. Asterisk indicates significant differences between groups ($q<0.05$) after controlling for sex, age, total gray matter volume and FDR correction.

correction (Table 2). As shown in Figure 1C, compared to HCs, IBS subjects showed significantly reduced CT in right aINS after FDR correction, a difference that was not affected by controlling for anxiety and depression.

Correlation of Cortical Thickness with Behavioral and Clinical Variables

In the UC group, symptom duration was *negatively* correlated with CT in left lateral OFG ($r = -.88$, $p = .0002$, $q = .0006$, Figure 2A) and left medial OFG ($r = -.78$, $p = .003$, $q = .003$, Figure 2B) and was *positively* correlated with CT in left postcentral gyrus ($r = .77$, $p = .003$, $q = .003$, Figure 2C). Adding anxiety and depression scores as covariates did not alter the results. No significant correlations with other clinical parameters (including the Mayo UCDAI) were observed.

Discussion

The primary goal of the current study was to assess regional CT differences between subjects with UC, and two comparison groups: a healthy control group and a disease control group without gut inflammation (IBS).The main findings of the study were: 1) Compared to both IBS and HCs, UC subjects showed *greater* CT in left cingulate cortical subregions, and in left primary somatosensory cortex (SI). 2) Compared with HCs, UC subjects showed *lower* CT in left OFG and in primary viscerosensory cortex (pINS). 3) Compared to HCs, IBS subjects showed *lower* CT in the interoceptive association cortex (aINS) in the right hemisphere. 4) There were large significant correlations of CT reductions in left OFG and CT increases in left SI with symptom duration in UC subjects, suggesting a role of chronic inflammation driven afferent input in these changes. The emerging pattern highlights significant differences in CT between patients with chronic gut inflammation, functional GI disorders and HCs, as well as some similarities.

Table 2. Significant cortical thickness differences in the ROIs between HCs, IBS and UC subjects with and without controlling for anxiety and depression scores.

ROI		Difference	F	P value	q value	F(A)	q(A)	F(D)	q(D)
lOFG	L	HC>UC	23.736	<.00001	.00023	15.898	.00411	23.592	.00020
lOFG	R	HC>UC	15.778	.00019	.00160	9.971	.01654	14.000	.00275
		HC>IBS	17.591	.00009	.00086	12.647	.00925	17.184	.00102
mOFG	L	HC>UC	23.124	.00001	.00023	13.904	.00715	26.905	.00009
mOFG	R	HC>IBS	9.052	.00383	.01686	8.744	.02156	9.802	.01304
Post	L	UC>HC	9.895	.00258	.01216	9.397	.01966	17.446	.00102
		UC>IBS	11.701	.00113	.00678	11.859	.01001	15.595	.00155
aINS	L	HC>UC	6.701	.01207	.04193	2.234	.26245	7.698	.02568
aINS	R	HC>IBS	18.098	.00007	.00082	12.384	.00925	16.893	.00102
mINS	L	HC>UC	10.304	.00213	.01173	3.859	.14306	12.453	.00489
pINS	L	HC>UC	30.701	<.00001	.00005	19.658	.00150	29.416	.00008
aMCC	L	UC>HC	18.231	.00007	.00008	11.277	.01137	18.651	.00080
		UC>IBS	19.862	.00004	.00006	19.387	.00150	21.006	.00040
pMCC	L	UC>HC	8.870	.00042	.01724	2.278	.26245	11.277	.00758
		UC>IBS	7.831	.00690	.02677	7.666	.03185	9.082	.01568
pgACC	L	UC>HC	11.713	.00112	.00678	8.839	.02156	8.901	.01607
		UC>IBS	10.127	.00232	.01175	10.014	.01654	9.690	.01304
sgACC	L	UC>HC	11.754	.00110	.00678	8.692	.02156	9.611	.01304
		UC>IBS	7.704	.00734	.02690	7.609	.03185	7.559	.02611

R: right; L: left; lOFG: lateral orbitofrontal gyrus; mOFG: medial orbitofrontal gyrus; Post: postcentral gyrus; aINS: aINSula; mINS: mid insula; pINS: posterior insula; aMCC: anterior mid cingulate cortex; pMCC: posterior mid cingulate cortex; pgACC: pregenual anterior cingulate cortex; sgACC: subgenual anterior cingulate cortex; q value: p value after FDR corrected at 5%, q value <.05 was considered significant; F(A): F score after controlling for anxiety; q(A): corrected p value after controlling for anxiety; F(D): F score after controlling for depression; q(D): corrected p value after controlling for depression.

Greater Regional CT in UC Patients

Somatosensory Cortex. In the current study, greater CT in primary somatosensory cortex (SI) was seen in the UC group. SI is part of the central pain processing network and its thickness is positively correlated with individual experimentally induced acute pain sensitivity in healthy subjects [44,45]. Chronic pain in human patient populations has been shown to be associated with cortical reorganization and changes in SI activity [38,46,47]. For example, SI cortical thickening has been reported in patients with migraine [48] and temporomandibular pain [43]. It has been suggested that the critical factor for S1 to undergo structural reorganization may be the presence of constant sensory input to this brain region [38,43,47]. Additionally, a voxel based morphometry study showed increased left pre- and postcentral gyri in chronic back pain patients [39]. In the current study, CT of left postcentral gyrus in UC groups showed a large positive correlation with symptom duration, consistent with a possible etiologic role of chronically enhanced viscerosensory input to the brain due to sensitization of visceral afferent pathways by chronic mucosal inflammation. However, the degree of somatosensory cortex changes did not correspond to the subjective pain reports, as UC subjects had greater CT in somatosensory cortex, but reported lower abdominal pain and discomfort compared to patients with IBS. Even though the reason(s) for these apparent discrepancies

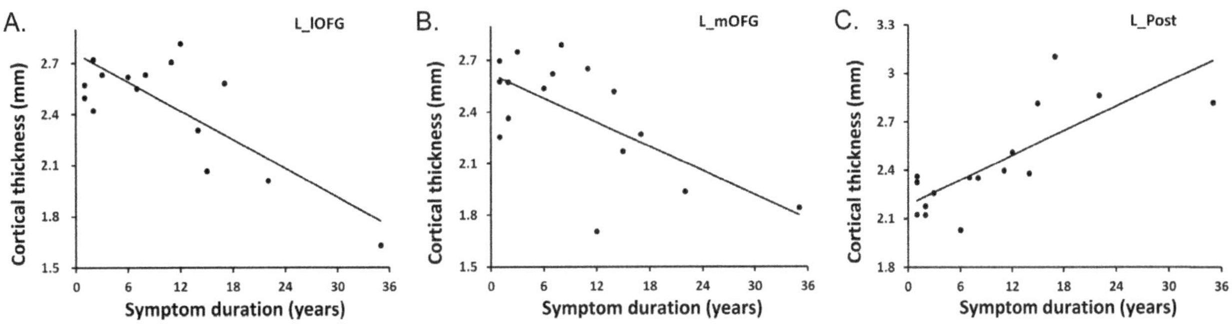

Figure 2. Correlation between cortical thickness and UC symptom duration. (A) Cortical thickness in left lateral orbitofrontal gyrus (L_lOFG) and (B) left medial orbitofrontal gyrus (L_mOFG) were negatively correlated with symptom duration in UC group. (C) Cortical thickness in left postcentral gyrus (L_Post) showed large positive correlation with UC symptom duration.

between CT differences in SI and subjective pain reports are not known, one may speculate that the subjective experience of chronic clinical visceral pain (as opposed to acute experimentally induced pain) is more related to activity and related structural changes in interoceptive association cortex (e.g. the aINS), rather than to primary sensory cortex [4,49].

Midcingulate Cortex. In the current study, compared to HCs and IBS subjects, the UC subjects had greater CT in subregions of the cingulate cortex, e.g. aMCC and pMCC. MCC is involved in emotion processing, skeletomotor regulation, chronic somatic and visceral pain, and along with the aINS (as part of the "salience network") integrating information to form conceptual pain [50–54]. Several studies have reported abnormal MCC activation by acute noxious visceral stimulation in IBS subjects [55–58]. Supporting a possible effect of repeated nociceptive stimuli on MCC structure, repeated application of thermal pain stimuli to healthy subjects over a period of 8 days resulted in gray matter increases in both MCC and SI [59]. Together with the observed greater CT in SI, the findings in UC patients are most consistent with the presence of a constant sensory input from the gut, due to sensitization of visceral afferent pathways by chronic mucosal inflammation. This interpretation is also consistent with the fact that in the current study, the IBS group (e.g. without chronically recurring mucosal inflammation) did not show significant CT change compared to HCs. Further support for differential brain mechanisms underlying chronic visceral pain comes from a recent PET ligand study which showed differences in neurokinin-1 receptor (NK-1R) binding potential (e.g. receptor availability) between patients with IBD (including Crohn's disease and UC) and IBS subjects [60]. Compared to HCs, IBD patients had low NK-1R availability in ACC and MCC, while IBS showed this deficit to a lesser extent. Animal studies have shown that the substance P/NK-1R signaling system is involved in cytogenesis, has neurotrophic and neuroprotective functions and inhibits apoptosis [61–63]. This implies a differential involvement of such neuroplastic mechanisms in the two visceral pain syndromes. Our findings differ from those reported in two other chronic inflammatory conditions, e.g. Crohn's disease [14] and osteoarthritis [64]. In both of these studies lower gray matter in the MCC was observed compared to HCs. Differences in patient populations and analysis methodology make it difficult to directly compare these studies with the current report [14,64].

Reduced Regional CT in IBS and UC Patients

INS Subregions. When compared to HCs, both disease groups showed lower CT in the INS, albeit in different subregions. Several studies in patients with chronic pain including IBS [7,9,12,13,64–68] compared to HCs, have found lower gray matter volumes and CT in the INS, even though subregions were often not specified. In the current study, UC compared to HCs had significantly reduced CT in the left pINS (observed differences in mINS were no longer seen after controlling for anxiety). It is likely that chronically enhanced afferent input from the gut due to recurrent mucosal inflammation is primarily associated with CT changes in the pINS, which represents the primary interoceptive cortex [37,69]. Even though there was no significant correlation between symptom duration or other behavioral measures with CT changes in the pINS, a chronic low back pain study showed that recovery of CT in pINS (and secondary somatosensory cortex) was correlated with reduction of pain intensity after treatment [12], implicating chronic nociceptive and inflammation related signaling as a factor in these CT changes.

In contrast to the UC group, IBS subjects had lower CT in a different subregion of the INS, e.g. the right aINS compared to HCs. The aINS functions as interoceptive association cortex integrates interoceptive input with emotional, salient and cognitive inputs, and provides output to autonomic and pain modulation systems [37,53,69–71]. The aINS also plays a central role in prediction, error processing, and self awareness of sensations [37,71]. Even though both patient groups had greater affective scores compared to HCs, IBS subjects reported more abdominal pain and discomfort compared to the UC group. However, there was no significant correlation of the observed changes with affective measures, symptom scores or duration of symptoms in IBS subjects.

Orbitofrontal Gyrus. UC subjects compared to HCs showed lower CT in the bilateral OFG, a brain region which plays an important role in interoception, emotion evaluation and regulation, and in cognitive reappraisal [43,72,73]. Decreased gray matter in OFG has also been found in other chronic pain disorders with inflammatory/nociceptive drive including hip osteoarthritis [64], low back pain [39] and migraine [74]. A negative correlation between left OFG thickness and symptom duration was observed in UC subjects, suggesting a role of chronic nociceptive input in the observed CT reductions. In contrast, no such correlation between IBS symptom duration and OFG structure were observed.

Limitations

Limitations of the study include the small sample size of the IBS and UC population, the group differences in level of anxiety and depression symptoms, and the heterogeneity of the groups in terms of sex. However, controlling for anxiety and depression, most of the observed results remained significant. In addition, our GLM and linear contrast were weighted to eliminate any bias caused by umbalanced representation of sexes. Furthermore, the fact that large correlations of some structural changes with disease duration were observed in the UC subjects, and the fact that some of the findings were similar to reports in subjects with other chronic inflammatory conditions [13,64], makes it unlikely that the findings are confounded by these limitations. Future, longitudinal studies in larger patient populations, including the correlation of plasma and mucosal inflammatory disease markers with structural brain changes both during disease flares and remissions are needed in order to better understand the role of colonic inflammation in remodeling of the brain. In such larger studies, presence of comorbidities in the IBS group, as well as differences in the impact of the IBS and UC on daily life activities and social interactions should be taken into account.

Conclusions

To our knowledge, this study represents the first comparison of brain structure between UC patients and both HCs and IBS subjects. The findings demonstrate significant differences in CT between UC and HC subjects, and differences between the two disease groups. Based on the correlation of structural changes with symptom duration in IBD, one may speculate that the observed gray matter reorganization of IBD subjects represents a consequence of chronic viscerosensory input to the brain due to sensitization of visceral afferent pathways by recurrent gut inflammation. The mechanisms by which such increased viscerosensory to the brain input can produce both increases and decreases of grey matter in different brain regions remains to be determined.

Supporting Information

Figure S1 Manually delineated subregions of interest on the 3D International Consortium for Brain Mapping brain atlas. (A) Subregions of cingulate cortex: anterior mid cingulate cortex (aMCC), posterior mid cingulate cortex (pMCC), pregenual anterior cingulate cortex (pgACC) and subgenual anterior cingulate cortex (sgACC). (B) Subregions of insula: aINSula (aINS), mid insula (mINS) and posterior insula (pINS).

Table S1 Mean cortical thickness.

Acknowledgments

The authors would like to thank Ahmanson Lovelace Brain Mapping Center for expert technical assistance.

Author Contributions

Conceived and designed the experiments: JL EM. Performed the experiments: JYH ZJ CAM JS NH SS. Analyzed the data: JYH ZJ ID. Contributed reagents/materials/analysis tools: ZJ CAM ID YS KT. Wrote the paper: JYH JL AG EM.

References

1. Bielefeldt K, Davis B, Binion DG (2009) Pain and inflammatory bowel disease. Inflamm Bowel Dis 15: 778–788.
2. Berman SM, Naliboff BD, Suyenobu B, Labus JS, Stains J, et al. (2008) Reduced brainstem inhibition during anticipated pelvic visceral pain correlates with enhanced brain response to the visceral stimulus in women with irritable bowel syndrome. J Neurosci 28: 349–359.
3. Chang L, Munakata J, Mayer EA, Schmulson MJ, Johnson TD, et al. (2000) Perceptual responses in patients with inflammatory and functional bowel disease. Gut 47: 497–505.
4. Mayer EA, Berman S, Suyenobu B, Labus J, Mandelkern MA, et al. (2005) Differences in brain responses to visceral pain between patients with irritable bowel syndrome and ulcerative colitis. Pain 115: 398–409.
5. Schmidt-Wilcke T, Luerding R, Weigand T, Jurgens T, Schuierer G, et al. (2007) Striatal grey matter increase in patients suffering from fibromyalgia – a voxel-based morphometry study. Pain 132 Suppl 1: S109–116.
6. Seminowicz DA, Labus JS, Bueller JA, Tillisch K, Naliboff BD, et al. (2010) Regional gray matter density changes in brains of patients with irritable bowel syndrome. Gastroenterology 139: 48–57 e42.
7. Davis KD, Pope G, Chen J, Kwan CL, Crawley AP, et al. (2008) Cortical thinning in IBS: implications for homeostatic, attention, and pain processing. Neurology 70: 153–154.
8. Hsu MC, Harris RE, Sundgren PC, Welsh RC, Fernandes CR, et al. (2009) No consistent difference in gray matter volume between individuals with fibromyalgia and age-matched healthy subjects when controlling for affective disorder. Pain 143: 262–267.
9. Labus J, Dinov ID, Jiang Z, Ashe-McNalley C, Zamanyan A, et al. (2013) Irritable bowel syndrome in female patients is associated with alterations in structural brain networks. Pain.
10. Apkarian AV, Sosa Y, Sonty S, Levy RM, Harden RN, et al. (2004) Chronic back pain is associated with decreased prefrontal and thalamic gray matter density. J Neurosci 24: 10410–10415.
11. Schmidt-Wilcke T, Leinisch E, Ganssbauer S, Draganski B, Bogdahn U, et al. (2006) Affective components and intensity of pain correlate with structural differences in gray matter in chronic back pain patients. Pain 125: 89–97.
12. Seminowicz DA, Wideman TH, Naso L, Hatami-Khoroushahi Z, Fallatah S, et al. (2011) Effective treatment of chronic low back pain in humans reverses abnormal brain anatomy and function. J Neurosci 31: 7540–7550.
13. Frokjaer JB, Bouwense SA, Olesen SS, Lundager FH, Eskildsen SF, et al. (2012) Reduced cortical thickness of brain areas involved in pain processing in patients with chronic pancreatitis. Clin Gastroenterol Hepatol 10: 434–438 e431.
14. Agostini A, Benuzzi F, Filippini N, Bertani A, Scarcelli A, et al. (2013) New insights into the brain involvement in patients with Crohn's disease: a voxel-based morphometry study. Neurogastroenterol Motil.
15. Farmer MA, Chanda ML, Parks EL, Baliki MN, Apkarian AV, et al. (2011) Brain functional and anatomical changes in chronic prostatitis/chronic pelvic pain syndrome. J Urol 186: 117–124.
16. Wartolowska K, Hough MG, Jenkinson M, Andersson J, Wordsworth BP, et al. (2012) Structural changes of the brain in rheumatoid arthritis. Arthritis Rheum 64: 371–379.
17. Jones AK, Huneke NT, Lloyd DM, Brown CA, Watson A (2012) Role of functional brain imaging in understanding rheumatic pain. Curr Rheumatol Rep 14: 557–567.
18. Gwilym SE, Filippini N, Douaud G, Carr AJ, Tracey I (2010) Thalamic atrophy associated with painful osteoarthritis of the hip is reversible after arthroplasty: a longitudinal voxel-based morphometric study. Arthritis Rheum 62: 2930–2940.
19. Dinov ID, Torri F, Macciardi F, Petrosyan P, Liu Z, et al. (2011) Applications of the pipeline environment for visual informatics and genomics computations. BMC Bioinformatics 12: 304.
20. Dinov I, Lozev K, Petrosyan P, Liu Z, Eggert P, et al. (2010) Neuroimaging study designs, computational analyses and data provenance using the LONI pipeline. PLoS One 5.
21. Drossman DA (2000) Rome II: the functional gastrointestinal disorders: diagnosis, pathophysiology, and treatment: a multinational consensus. McLeanVA: Degnon Associates. xxvii, 764 p.
22. Drossman DA (2006) The functional gastrointestinal disorders and the Rome III process. Gastroenterology 130: 1377–1390.
23. Lewis JD, Chuai S, Nessel L, Lichtenstein GR, Aberra FN, et al. (2008) Use of the noninvasive components of the Mayo score to assess clinical response in ulcerative colitis. Inflamm Bowel Dis 14: 1660–1666.
24. Chang L, Lee OY, Naliboff B, Schmulson M, Mayer EA (2001) Sensation of bloating and visible abdominal distension in patients with irritable bowel syndrome. Am J Gastroenterol 96: 3341–3347.
25. Mykletun A, Stordal E, Dahl AA (2001) Hospital Anxiety and Depression (HAD) scale: factor structure, item analyses and internal consistency in a large population. Br J Psychiatry 179: 540–544.
26. Labus JS, Bolus R, Chang L, Wiklund I, Naesdal J, et al. (2004) The Visceral Sensitivity Index: development and validation of a gastrointestinal symptom-specific anxiety scale. Aliment Pharmacol Ther 20: 89–97.
27. Labus JS, Mayer EA, Chang L, Bolus R, Naliboff BD (2007) The central role of gastrointestinal-specific anxiety in irritable bowel syndrome: further validation of the visceral sensitivity index. Psychosom Med 69: 89–98.
28. Leung KTK (2011) Principal Ranking Meta-Algorithms: UNIVERSITY OF CALIFORNIA, LOS ANGELES.
29. Fischl B, Dale AM (2000) Measuring the thickness of the human cerebral cortex from magnetic resonance images. Proc Natl Acad Sci U S A 97: 11050–11055.
30. Mulder W, Osher S, Sethian JA (1992) Computing interface motion in compressible gas dynamics. Journal of Computational Physics 100: 209–228.
31. Osher S, Sethian JA (1988) Fronts propagating with curvature-dependent speed: algorithms based on Hamilton-Jacobi formulations. Journal of Computational Physics 79: 12–49.
32. Mazziotta J, Toga A, Evans A, Fox P, Lancaster J, et al. (2001) A probabilistic atlas and reference system for the human brain: International Consortium for Brain Mapping (ICBM). Philos Trans R Soc Lond B Biol Sci 356: 1293–1322.
33. Shi Y, Lai R, Gill R, Pelletier D, Mohr D, et al. (2011) Conformal metric optimization on surface (CMOS) for deformation and mapping in Laplace-Beltrami embedding space. Medical image computing and computer-assisted intervention: MICCAI International Conference on Medical Image Computing and Computer-Assisted Intervention 14: 327–334.
34. Tillisch K, Mayer EA, Labus JS (2011) Quantitative meta-analysis identifies brain regions activated during rectal distension in irritable bowel syndrome. Gastroenterology 140: 91–100.
35. Mayer EA, Bushnell MC, International Association for the Study of Pain. (2009) Functional pain syndromes: presentation and pathophysiology. Seattle: IASP Press. xviii, 580 p.
36. Agostini A, Benuzzi F, Filippini N, Bertani A, Scarcelli A, et al. (2012) New insights into the brain involvement in patients with Crohn's disease: a voxel-based morphometry study. Neurogastroenterol Motil.
37. Craig AD (2009) How do you feel – now? The anterior insula and human awareness. Nat Rev Neurosci 10: 59–70.
38. May A (2008) Chronic pain may change the structure of the brain. Pain 137: 7–15.
39. Ung H, Brown JE, Johnson KA, Younger J, Hush J, et al. (2012) Multivariate Classification of Structural MRI Data Detects Chronic Low Back Pain. Cereb Cortex.
40. Benjamini Y, Krieger AM, Yekutieli D (2006) Adaptive linear step-up procedures that control the false discovery rate. Biometrika 93: 491–507.
41. Benjamini Y, Hochberg Y (2000) On the Adaptive Control of the False Discovery Rate in Multiple Testing with Independent Statistics. Journal of Educational and Behavioral Statistics 25: 60–83.
42. Pike N (2011) Using false discovery rates for multiple comparisons in ecology and evolution. Methods in Ecology and Evolution 2: 278–282.
43. Moayedi M, Weissman-Fogel I, Crawley AP, Goldberg MB, Freeman BV, et al. (2011) Contribution of chronic pain and neuroticism to abnormal forebrain gray matter in patients with temporomandibular disorder. Neuroimage 55: 277–286.
44. Apkarian AV, Bushnell MC, Treede RD, Zubieta JK (2005) Human brain mechanisms of pain perception and regulation in health and disease. Eur J Pain 9: 463–484.
45. Erpelding N, Moayedi M, Davis KD (2012) Cortical thickness correlates of pain and temperature sensitivity. Pain 153: 1602–1609.

46. Moseley GL, Flor H (2012) Targeting cortical representations in the treatment of chronic pain: a review. Neurorehabil Neural Repair 26: 646–652.
47. Gustin SM, Peck CC, Cheney LB, Macey PM, Murray GM, et al. (2012) Pain and plasticity: is chronic pain always associated with somatosensory cortex activity and reorganization? J Neurosci 32: 14874–14884.
48. DaSilva AF, Granziera C, Snyder J, Hadjikhani N (2007) Thickening in the somatosensory cortex of patients with migraine. Neurology 69: 1990–1995.
49. Blankstein U, Chen J, Diamant NE, Davis KD (2010) Altered brain structure in irritable bowel syndrome: potential contributions of pre-existing and disease-driven factors. Gastroenterology 138: 1783–1789.
50. Taylor KS, Seminowicz DA, Davis KD (2009) Two systems of resting state connectivity between the insula and cingulate cortex. Hum Brain Mapp 30: 2731–2745.
51. Vogt BA, Berger GR, Derbyshire SW (2003) Structural and functional dichotomy of human midcingulate cortex. Eur J Neurosci 18: 3134–3144.
52. Vogt BA (2005) Pain and emotion interactions in subregions of the cingulate gyrus. Nat Rev Neurosci 6: 533–544.
53. Wiech K, Lin CS, Brodersen KH, Bingel U, Ploner M, et al. (2010) AINSula integrates information about salience into perceptual decisions about pain. J Neurosci 30: 16324–16331.
54. Meier ML, Brugger M, Ettlin DA, Luechinger R, Barlow A, et al. (2012) Brain activation induced by dentine hypersensitivity pain – an fMRI study. J Clin Periodontol 39: 441–447.
55. Labus JS, Naliboff BD, Berman SM, Suyenobu B, Vianna EP, et al. (2009) Brain networks underlying perceptual habituation to repeated aversive visceral stimuli in patients with irritable bowel syndrome. Neuroimage 47: 952–960.
56. Bernstein CN, Frankenstein UN, Rawsthorne P, Pitz M, Summers R, et al. (2002) Cortical mapping of visceral pain in patients with GI disorders using functional magnetic resonance imaging. Am J Gastroenterol 97: 319–327.
57. Verne GN, Himes NC, Robinson ME, Gopinath KS, Briggs RW, et al. (2003) Central representation of visceral and cutaneous hypersensitivity in the irritable bowel syndrome. Pain 103: 99–110.
58. Kwan CL, Diamant NE, Pope G, Mikula K, Mikulis DJ, et al. (2005) Abnormal forebrain activity in functional bowel disorder patients with chronic pain. Neurology 65: 1268–1277.
59. Teutsch S, Herken W, Bingel U, Schoell E, May A (2008) Changes in brain gray matter due to repetitive painful stimulation. Neuroimage 42: 845–849.
60. Jarcho JM, Feier NA, Bert A, Labus JA, Lee M, et al. (2013) Diminished neurokinin-1 receptor availability in patients with two forms of chronic visceral pain. Pain.
61. Lallemend F, Lefebvre PP, Hans G, Rigo JM, Van de Water TR, et al. (2003) Substance P protects spiral ganglion neurons from apoptosis via PKC-Ca2+-MAPK/ERK pathways. J Neurochem 87: 508–521.
62. Tulloch I, Ghazaryan N, Mexhitaj I, Ordonez D, Angulo JA (2011) Role of neurokinin-1 and dopamine receptors on the striatal methamphetamine-induced proliferation of new cells in mice. Brain Res 1399: 33–39.
63. Wang J, Angulo JA (2011) Synergism between methamphetamine and the neuropeptide substance P on the production of nitric oxide in the striatum of mice. Brain Res 1369: 131–139.
64. Rodriguez-Raecke R, Niemeier A, Ihle K, Ruether W, May A (2009) Brain gray matter decrease in chronic pain is the consequence and not the cause of pain. J Neurosci 29: 13746–13750.
65. Valfre W, Rainero I, Bergui M, Pinessi L (2008) Voxel-based morphometry reveals gray matter abnormalities in migraine. Headache 48: 109–117.
66. Kuchinad A, Schweinhardt P, Seminowicz DA, Wood PB, Chizh BA, et al. (2007) Accelerated brain gray matter loss in fibromyalgia patients: premature aging of the brain? J Neurosci 27: 4004–4007.
67. Schmidt-Wilcke T, Leinisch E, Straube A, Kampfe N, Draganski B, et al. (2005) Gray matter decrease in patients with chronic tension type headache. Neurology 65: 1483–1486.
68. Jiang Z, Dinov ID, Labus J, Shi Y, Zamanyan A, et al. (2013) Sex-related differences of cortical thickness in patients with chronic abdominal pain. PLoS One 8: e73932.
69. Farb NA, Segal ZV, Anderson AK (2012) Attentional modulation of primary interoceptive and exteroceptive cortices. Cereb Cortex 23: 114–126.
70. Lewis M, Haviland-Jones JM, Barrett LF (2008) Handbook of emotions. New York: Guilford Press. xvi, 848 p., [844] p. of plates p.
71. Paulus MP, Stein MB (2006) An insular view of anxiety. Biol Psychiatry 60: 383–387.
72. Rolls ET, Grabenhorst F, Parris BA (2008) Warm pleasant feelings in the brain. Neuroimage 41: 1504–1513.
73. Ray RD, Ochsner KN, Cooper JC, Robertson ER, Gabrieli JD, et al. (2005) Individual differences in trait rumination and the neural systems supporting cognitive reappraisal. Cogn Affect Behav Neurosci 5: 156–168.
74. Kim JH, Suh SI, Seol HY, Oh K, Seo WK, et al. (2008) Regional grey matter changes in patients with migraine: a voxel-based morphometry study. Cephalalgia 28: 598–604.

18

Self-Reported Pain Intensity with the Numeric Reporting Scale in Adult Dengue

Joshua G. X. Wong[1]*, Victor C. Gan[1], Ee-Ling Ng[1], Yee-Sin Leo[1,2,3,4], Siew-Pang Chan[1,5,6], Robin Choo[5,7], David C. Lye[1,4]

1 Institute of Infectious Disease and Epidemiology, Tan Tock Seng Hospital, Singapore, Singapore, **2** Saw Swee Hock School of Public Health, National University of Singapore, Singapore, Singapore, **3** Lee Kong Chian School of Medicine, Nanyang Technologicial University, Singapore, Singapore, **4** Yong Loo Lin School of Medicine, National University of Singapore, Singapore, Singapore, **5** Stata Users Group, Singapore, Singapore, **6** Department of Mathematics and Science, La Trobe University, Melbourne, Victoria, Australia, **7** Singapore Institute for Clinical Sciences, Brenner Centre for Molecular Medicine, Singapore, Singapore

Abstract

Background: Pain is a prominent feature of acute dengue as well as a clinical criterion in World Health Organization guidelines in diagnosing dengue. We conducted a prospective cohort study to compare levels of pain during acute dengue between different ethnicities and dengue severity.

Methods: Demographic, clinical and laboratory data were collected. Data on self-reported pain was collected using the 11-point Numerical Rating Scale. Generalized structural equation models were built to predict progression to severe disease.

Results: A total of 499 laboratory confirmed dengue patients were recruited in the Prospective Adult Dengue Study at Tan Tock Seng Hospital, Singapore. We found no statistically significant differences between pain score with age, gender, ethnicity or the presence of co-morbidity. Pain score was not predictive of dengue severity but highly correlated to patients' day of illness. Prevalence of abdominal pain in our cohort was 19%. There was no difference in abdominal pain score between grades of dengue severity.

Conclusion: Dengue is a painful disease. Patients suffer more pain at the earlier phase of illness. However, pain score cannot be used to predict a patient's progression to severe disease.

Editor: Shamala Devi Sekaran, University of Malaya, Malaysia

Funding: This study was funded by a National Medical Research Council (http://www.nmrc.gov.sg) Translational and Clinical Research Flagship Programme Grant NMRC/TCR/005 for Scientific exploration, Translational research, Operational evaluation of disease prevention and Preventative measures through new treatment strategies against Dengue (STOP Dengue). The funders had no role in study design, data collection and analysis, decision to publish, or preparation of the manuscript.

Competing Interests: Y.S.L. received educational grant from Sanofi Pasteur. The authors have read the journal's policy and have the following conflicts.

* E-mail: Joshua_Gx_Wong@ttsh.com.sg

Introduction

The World Health Organization (WHO) reported that over 40% of the global population is at risk of dengue and an estimated 390 million dengue infections happen worldwide every year.

Dengue incidence has increased and its geographic range expanded.[1] Many studies on the clinical features of dengue were pediatric cohorts.[2,3] In Singapore, dengue infections have shifted from a primarily childhood to an adult disease. [4] Today, more than 90% of dengue patients are adults. We previously identified the occurrence of bleeding, lymphopenia, hypoproteinemia and elevated serum urea as independent predictors for dengue hemorrhagic fever (DHF) [5].

Pain is an important component of dengue diagnostic criteria. In WHO 1997 guideline, probable dengue requires the presence of fever with any two of headache, retro-orbital pain, mylagia, arthralgia, rash, positive tourniquet test or or hemarroghic manifestation. [6] In WHO 2009 guideline, the diagnostic criteria were revised to comprise fever and two of nausea/vomiting, rash, aches and pains, positive tourniquet test, leucopenia and any warning sign. Warning signs include abdominal pain or tenderness, persistent vomiting, clinical fluid accumulation, mucosal bleeding, lethargy, hepatomegaly and hematocrit rise with rapid platelet count drop [7].

Higher prevalence of abdominal pain, backache, headache and myalgia was noted in adult dengue patients.[3,8,9] Abdominal pain and myalgia were associated with dengue severity and mortality.[10–12] While these studies identified aches and pains as an important factor for dengue diagnosis and prognosis, we have not found any study assessing the degree of pain reported by dengue patients in predicting progression to severe disease to date. To fill the lacuna in literature, we conducted a prospective cohort study to determine the relationship between pain intensity and disease severity.

Methods

Ethics Statement

Ethical approval was provided by the Domain Specific Review Board of the National Healthcare Group, Singapore (DSRB/E/2009/432). Written informed consent was obtained from all subjects.

Patient Cohort

Acutely febrile patients above the age of 18 were recruited prospectively from January 2010 to September 2012 at the Communicable Disease Center, Tan Tock Seng Hospital, Singapore, a tertiary referral infectious disease centre. All dengue diagnostic testing was performed by the Enviromental Health Institute, a WHO Collaborating Center for Reference and Research on Arbovirus and its Associated Vectors in Singapore. Patients were classified as having laboratory-confirmed dengue according to WHO standards if they were RT-PCR or NS1 positive using the dengue NS1 antigen (Ag) strip (Bio-Rad Laboratories, Marnes-la-Coquette, France).[13] Only laboratory-confirmed dengue patients were included. Detailed daily clinical and laboratory data, including pain score, were collected prospectively until discharge or at the recovery phase of illness. Pain score for all patients, including those who did not return for subsequent follow-ups, were included to increase the sample size.

The Numeric Rating Scale (NRS) is a widely used tool to assess patients' pain level in chronic and acute illnesses with good responsiveness and sensitivity.[14–16]. The NRS was the preferred pain rating scale owing to its ease of use and accurate assessment.[17] The scale ranges from 0 to 10 with 0 being no pain and 10 being the worst possible pain; this is aided with the use of the face pain scale of facial expressions at pain scale of 0,2,4,8 and 10. [18] Separate information on abdominal pain score was captured as a warning sign in the WHO 2009 guideline. On enrolment, patients were asked to rate their pain intensity from day of illness to day of enrolment. Pain scores were then recorded prospectively on subsequent follow-ups.

Outcome Variable

The primary outcome was the severity of dengue: 1: Dengue fever, 2: Dengue hemorrhagic fever (DHF; Grades I–II) [6] and 3: Severe disease, defined as fulfilling dengue shock syndrome (DSS) and severe dengue (SD) [7].

Statistical Analysis

Ordinal logistic regression was used to determine how pain score was associated with age, gender, co-morbidity and ethnicity (1: Chinese 2: Malay 3: Indian 4: Others). Generalized structural equation model (GSEM) was applied as a more confirmatory analysis to analyze the data accounting for temporal data structure and the complex dependence among pain score, fever and the outcome.[19] As the latest development in structural equation modeling which unifies regression models with latent class models, GSEM is deemed to be the most appropriate in the proposed data analysis. It could estimate the direct and indirect effects of pain score and fever on the outcome with a single model set-up. In conventional regression analysis one may have to construct multiple models for dealing with studies involving a final outcome, a set of covariates and some variables that are both predictors for the final outcome and intermediate outcomes.

Two sets of analyses were carried out, with the outcome ascertained on day 2 and day 3 of enrolment. In both analyses, the number of fever days reported by patients preceded fever at presentation which in turn preceded days 2 and 3 of enrolment (see Figures 1 and 2).

The first GSEM model to predict dengue severity on the second day of enrolment (day 2) involved baseline covariates such as age, gender, ethnicity, Charlson's co-morbidity score[20], fever at presentation and number of fever days before day 2 as the direct effects to the outcome. The intermediate variables involved whether patient had fever on day 2, pain score on study days 1 and 2. Fever at presentation and the number of fever days were hypothesized to be associated with pain score on day 1 and fever on day 2. Pain score on day 1 was assumed to be associated with pain score on day 2 (Figure 1). To predict dengue severity on the

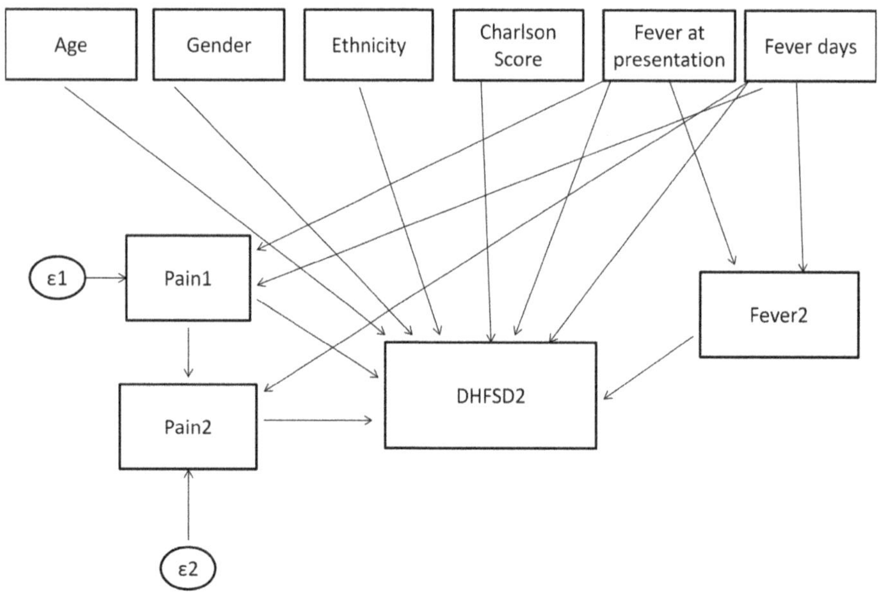

Figure 1. Model specification for study day 2. Feveratpresentation = Fever present at enrolment (Yes/No), Feverdays = Number of fever days up to enrolment, Fever2 = Fever on study day 2, Pain1 = Pain Score at enrolment/presentation, Pain2 = Pain Score on study day 2, DHFSD2 = Outcome on study day 2.

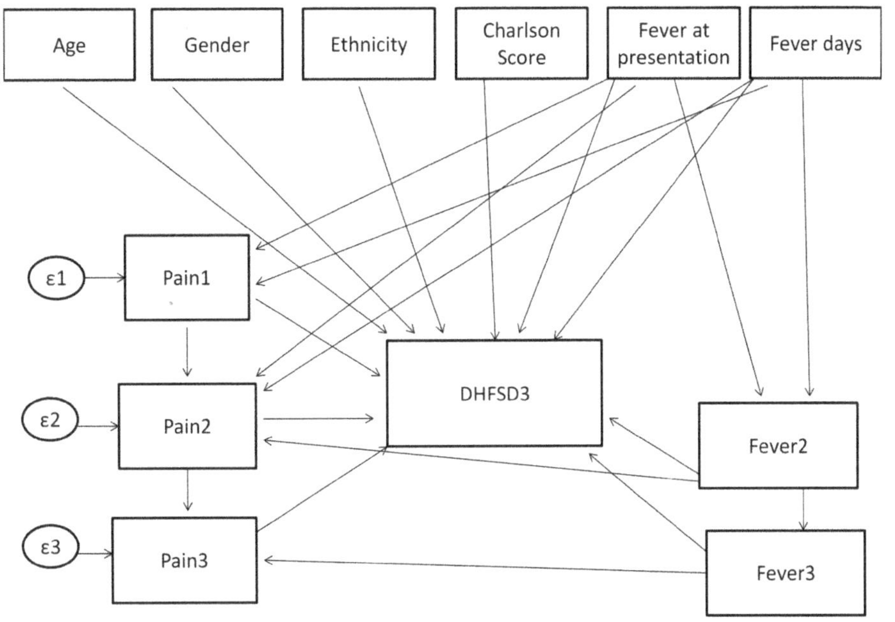

Figure 2. Model specification for study day 3.

third day of enrolment (day 3), the model was extended to accommodate the pain score and fever on day 3 (Figure 2). The GSEM is most appropriate when such data structures with irreversible temporal effects are required in analysis.

Estimated with maximum likelihood, the models were analysed with the multinomial distribution and logit link. Analyzed with Stata MP 13 (Stata Corp, Texas, USA), all statistical tests were conducted with 95% confidence intervals.

Results

Demographic Description of Cohort

Of the 850 patients recruited, 499 tested positive for RT-PCR or NS1 were included in the analysis. There were 111 DHF I–II and 13 DHF III–IV(DSS) cases according to WHO 1997 classification. Twenty were severe dengue cases in accordance with the WHO 2009 classification. The median duration of fever was 6 (3–9) days. One patient died owing to myocarditis. One patient was diagnosed with both DSS and SD. In total, 32 patients fulfilled the severe disease classification.

The median age of the cohort was 34 years (5th–95th percentile, 21–51 years). Male patients comprised 79% and 77.6% of the cohort were Chinese. Medical co-morbidity, mainly myocardial infarction, diabetes and cerebrovascular dieseases was present in 1.8%. The majority (76.3%) of patients had fever on the first visit. The median pain score was similar in DF, DHF I–II and severe disease patients (5 [0–8], p = 0.7). (Table 1) There were no significant statistical association between pain score at first visit and age (p = 0.09), gender (p = 0.32), co-morbidity (p = 0.49) or race (p = 0.19).

Temporal Trend of Overall Pain Score

Figure 3 shows that DF patients generally experienced reduction in pain as they were recovering from dengue infection. Median pain score for patients with DHF I–II or severe disease overlapped. However, pain score diminished to the range of 0–2 on fever day 8. It is visually difficult to draw conclusions on differences between dengue severity from the plots due to the large overlap. (*For detailed sample sizes for each day, refer to Table S1).*

Table 1. Demographic description of study cohort.

	DF (n = 356)	DHF I–II (n = 111)	Severe disease (n = 32)	Overall (n = 499)
Age in years	32 (21–46)	40 (22–58)	36 (23–57)	34 (21–51)
Male gender	289 (81.1%)	89 (80.2%)	18 (56.2%)	396 (79.4%)
Chinese ethnicity	258 (72.5%)	103 (92.8%)	26 (81.2%)	387 (77.6%)
Any co-morbidity	5 (1.4%)	3 (2.7%)	1 (3.1%)	9 (1.8%)
Fever at 1st visit	250 (70.2%)	100 (90.1%)	31 (96.9%)	381 (76.3%)
Fever days at 1st visit	6 (3–9)	6 (3–8)	5 (3–9)	6 (3–8)
Pain score at 1st visit	5 (0–8)	5 (0–8)	5 (0–8)	5 (0–8)

For categorical variables, absolute numbers (and the relative percentage) are being indicated. For continuous variables, medians (and the relative 5th–95th percentile) are being indicated.

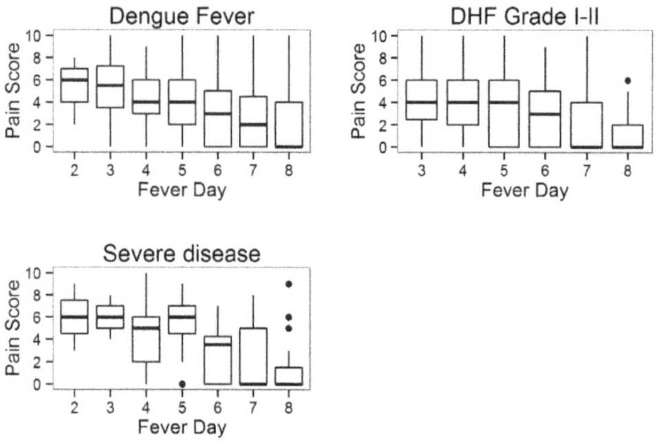

Figure 3. Boxplot of pain scores over fever days by dengue severity. The line inside the box represent the median, box edges represent 25th and 75th percentile and vertical lines represent 1.5 times the interquartile range. Points outside these limits are considered outliers.

Predictive Modeling of Overall Pain Score and Co-variates

Study day 2. Pain score on study days 1 and 2, number of fever days, ethnicity and co-morbidity were not significantly associated with dengue severity (Table 2). The GSEM results showed that age and fever at presentation were predictive of severe disease on study day 2. On average patient's risk of severe disease increased by 3% with every year of increase in age. In addition, fever at presentation increased the risk of developing severe disease (Table 2). Patients experienced less pain as they recovered (odds ratio [OR]: 1.52 [1.33–74]).

Study day 3. Similarly, pain score on study day 2 was not predictive but age and fever on day 3 of study were predictive of dengue severity. The risk of age on severe disease largely remained the same as the day before. In addition, fever on day 3 increased a patient's risk of severe disease. Notably, patients who developed severe disease on day 3 were more likely to report higher pain scores (Table 2).

Abdominal Pain

Ninety five patients (19%) experienced abdominal pain. Four of them had SD while the other 3 had DSS. Of these 7 cases, 3 of them experienced the worst abdominal pain on the same day as they were diagnosed with severe disease or after progressing on to severe disease. The median abdominal pain score for patients with severe disease was 5 (5th–95th percentile, 2–9) and 4 (5th–95th percentile, 1–10) for non-severe disease ($p = 0.38$).

Table 2. GSEM results for likelihood of developing severe dengue disease on days 2 and 3 of enrolment.

Baseline co-variates	Study Day 2 (n = 438) aOR (95% CI)	Study Day 3 (n = 399) aOR (95% CI)
Age	1.03 (1–1.06)*	1.05 (1.00–1.10)*
Gender		
Male	Reference	
Female	1.48 (0.68–3.23)	1.08 (0.32–3.65)
Ethnicity		
Chinese	Reference	
Malay	0.59 (0.07–4.96)	2.14 (0.15–30.07)
Indian	0.14 (0.02–1.06)	0.24 (0.03–1.95)
Others	0.59 (0.07–4.90)	2.70 (0.24–30.73)
Charlson's co-morbidity score		
0	Reference	
≥1	1.51 (0.25–8.91)	1.56 (0.12–21.20)
Fever at presentation		
No	Reference	
Yes	6.76 (1.41–32.4)*	0.77(0.17–3.60)
Fever duration in days	1.29 (0.96–1.73)	1.27 (0.82–1.97)
Fever on Study day 2		
No	Reference	
Yes	1.93 (0.85–4.37)	0.54 (0.18–1.62)
Fever on Study day 3		
No	NA	Reference
Yes	NA	3.97 (1.18–13.34)*
Pain score at presentation	0.96 (0.83–1.10)	1.09 (0.90–1.32)
Study Day 2 pain score	0.96 (0.82–1.13)	1.15 (0.92–1.42)
Study Day 3 pain score	NA	3.97 (1.18–13.34)*

*Statistically significant; equivalent to $p<0.05$.

Discussion

Abdominal pain was identified as one of four warning signs in a retrospective Puerto Rican study on dengue deaths.[21] In Cuba, headache was present in all twelve fatalities.[22] In Singapore abdominal pain was present in half of adult dengue deaths.[23] In Lucknow, India, severe abdominal pain was noted in 18% of children and adults with dengue shock syndrome[24]. In the Philippines, abdominal pain was significantly more common in children with DHF.[25] Abdominal pain was significantly associated with the need for major interventions in the DENCO study [26] while in Brazilian children, abdominal pain was independently associated with severe dengue.[27] Notably, be it dengue shock syndrome or uncomplicated dengue, headache and abdominal pain were significantly more common in adults compared with children [3].

To our knowledge, this is the first study to analyze the utility of a numeric pain score in predicting the progression of dengue severity. We explored the utility of pain score in dengue prognosis accounting for baseline covariates which might affect pain. The results from the GSEM model should not be interpreted as a predictive model for dengue disease severity. We found that pain intensity measured by numeric rating scale experienced by adult dengue patients did not differ by ethnicity, co-morbidity and dengue severity. Additionally abdominal pain intensity did not differ by dengue severity. Age and fever at presentation appeared to correlate with dengue severity. The impact on age on dengue severity was previously studied [28].

There were several limitations in our study. We were unable to monitor patients' parameters before enrolment. Our patient profile at a tertiary center may not reflect those in primary care. Patients were recruited at a median of 6 days of fever. The daily level of pain by recall before enrolment can be unreliable and may be associated with recall bias. Patients who visited the clinic only on enrolment day were included in the analysis for increasing the sample size; we assumed that patients were most painful on enrolment day and subsequent follow-up were missed as they recovered. Our study was conducted in an adult cohort which may not generalize to children with dengue. Further work needs to be done to monitor level of pain in the early course of illness to better understand the relationship between pain and disease progression in dengue.

Conclusion

This study provides evidence for clinicians against using pain score alone in clinical triage or in predicting progression to severe disease.

Supporting Information

Table S1 Sample size at each fever day stratified by outcome (DHF I–II = Dengue hemarroghic fever grades 1–2).

Acknowledgments

We are grateful to all our research assistants and patients who have participated in our study. We are thankful to Dr Tun Linn Thein and Dr Hao Ying for their valuable suggestions.

Author Contributions

Conceived and designed the experiments: YSL DCL. Analyzed the data: SPC RC. Wrote the paper: JGW VCG ELN YSL SPC DCB.

References

1. Bhatt S, Gething PW, Brady OJ, Messina JP, Farlow AW, et al. (2013) The global distribution and burden of dengue. Nature 496: 504–507. doi:10.1038/nature12060.
2. Thein S, Aung MM, Shwe TN, Aye M, Zaw A, et al. (1997) Risk factors in dengue shock syndrome. Am J Trop Med Hyg 56: 566–572.
3. Dinh The T, Le Thi Thu T, Nguyen Minh D, Tran Van N, Tran Tinh H, et al. (2012) Clinical Features of Dengue in a Large Vietnamese Cohort: Intrinsically Lower Platelet Counts and Greater Risk for Bleeding in Adults than Children. PLoS Negl Trop Dis 6. Available: http://www.ncbi.nlm.nih.gov/pmc/articles/PMC3383761/. Accessed 12 March 2014.
4. Ooi E-E, Goh K-T, Gubler DJ (2006) Dengue Prevention and 35 Years of Vector Control in Singapore. Emerg Infect Dis 12: 887–893. doi:10.3201/eid1206.051210.
5. Lee VJ, Lye DCB, Sun Y, Fernandez G, Ong A, et al. (2008) Predictive value of simple clinical and laboratory variables for dengue hemorrhagic fever in adults. J Clin Virol Off Publ Pan Am Soc Clin Virol 42: 34–39. doi:10.1016/j.jcv.2007.12.017.
6. WHO | Dengue guidelines for diagnosis, treatment, prevention and control: new edition (n.d.). WHO. Available: http://www.who.int/rpc/guidelines/9789241547871/en/. Accessed 10 March 2014.
7. WHO | Dengue haemorrhagic fever: diagnosis, treatment, prevention and control. 2nd edition. Geneva: World Health Organization. (n.d.). WHO. Available: http://www.who.int/csr/resources/publications/dengue/Denguepublication/en/. Accessed 10 March 2014.
8. Khan MIH, Anwar E, Agha A, Hassanien NSM, Ullah E, et al. (2013) Factors predicting severe dengue in patients with dengue Fever. Mediterr J Hematol Infect Dis 5: e2013014. doi:10.4084/MJHID.2013.014.
9. Wichmann O, Hongsiriwon S, Bowonwatanuwong C, Chotivanich K, Sukthana Y, et al. (2004) Risk factors and clinical features associated with severe dengue infection in adults and children during the 2001 epidemic in Chonburi, Thailand. Trop Med Int Health 9: 1022–1029. doi:10.1111/j.1365-3156.2004.01295.x.
10. Thein T-L, Leo Y-S, Fisher DA, Low JG, Oh HML, et al. (2013) Risk Factors for Fatality among Confirmed Adult Dengue Inpatients in Singapore: A Matched Case-Control Study. PLoS ONE 8: e81060. doi:10.1371/journal.pone.0081060.
11. Junia J, Garna H, Setiabudi D (2007) Clinical risk factors for dengue shock syndrome in children. Paediatr Indones 47: 7–11.
12. Pongpan S, Wisitwong A, Tawichsari C, Patumanond J (2013) Prognostic Indicators for Dengue Infection Severity. Int J Clin Pediatr. Available: http://ijcp.elmerpress.com/index.php/ijcp/article/view/73. Accessed 10 March 2014.
13. Lai Y-L, Chung Y-K, Tan H-C, Yap H-F, Yap G, et al. (2007) Cost-Effective Real-Time Reverse Transcriptase PCR (RT-PCR) To Screen for Dengue Virus followed by Rapid Single-Tube Multiplex RT-PCR for Serotyping of the Virus. J Clin Microbiol 45: 935–941. doi:10.1128/JCM.01258-06.
14. Bijur PE, Latimer CT, Gallagher EJ (2003) Validation of a Verbally Administered Numerical Rating Scale of Acute Pain for Use in the Emergency Department. Acad Emerg Med 10: 390–392. doi:10.1111/j.1553-2712.2003.tb01355.x.
15. Williamson A, Hoggart B (2005) Pain: a review of three commonly used pain rating scales. J Clin Nurs 14: 798–804. doi:10.1111/j.1365-2702.2005.01121.x.
16. Farrar JT, Young Jr JP, LaMoreaux L, Werth JL, Poole RM (2001) Clinical importance of changes in chronic pain intensity measured on an 11-point numerical pain rating scale. PAIN 94: 149–158. doi:10.1016/S0304-3959(01)00349-9.
17. Chanques G, Viel E, Constantin J-M, Jung B, de Lattre S, et al. (2010) The measurement of pain in intensive care unit: comparison of 5 self-report intensity scales. Pain 151: 711–721. doi:10.1016/j.pain.2010.08.039.
18. Downie WW, Leatham PA, Rhind VM, Wright V, Branco JA, et al. (1978) Studies with pain rating scales. Ann Rheum Dis 37: 378–381. doi:10.1136/ard.37.4.378.
19. Rabe-Hesketh S, Skrondal A, Pickles A (2004) Generalized multilevel structural equation modeling. Psychometrika 69: 167–190. doi:10.1007/BF02295939.
20. Charlson ME, Pompei P, Ales KL, MacKenzie CR (1987) A new method of classifying prognostic comorbidity in longitudinal studies: development and validation. J Chronic Dis 40: 373–383.
21. Rigau-Pérez JG, Laufer MK (2006) Dengue-Related Deaths in Puerto Rico, 1992–1996: Diagnosis and Clinical Alarm Signals. Clin Infect Dis 42: 1241–1246. doi:10.1086/501355.
22. Guzmán MG, Alvarez M, Rodríguez R, Rosario D, Vázquez S, et al. (1999) Fatal dengue hemorrhagic fever in Cuba, 1997. Int J Infect Dis IJID Off Publ Int Soc Infect Dis 3: 130–135.
23. Ong A, Sandar M, Chen MI, Sin LY (2007) Fatal dengue hemorrhagic fever in adults during a dengue epidemic in Singapore. Int J Infect Dis 11: 263–267. doi:10.1016/j.ijid.2006.02.012.

24. Agarwal R, Kapoor S, Nagar R, Misra A, Tandon R, et al. (1999) A clinical study of the patients with dengue hemorrhagic fever during the epidemic of 1996 at Lucknow, India. Southeast Asian J Trop Med Public Health 30: 735–740.
25. Carlos CC, Oishi K, Cinco MTDD, Mapua CA, Inoue S, et al. (2005) Comparison of Clinical Features and Hematologic Abnormalities Between Dengue Fever and Dengue Hemorrhagic Fever Among Children in the Philippines. Am J Trop Med Hyg 73: 435–440.
26. Alexander N, Balmaseda A, Coelho ICB, Dimaano E, Hien TT, et al. (2011) Multicentre prospective study on dengue classification in four Southeast Asian and three Latin American countries. Trop Med Int Health 16: 936–948. doi:10.1111/j.1365-3156.2011.02793.x.
27. Giraldo D, Sant'Anna C, Périssé ARS, March M de FP, Souza AP, et al. (2011) Characteristics of children hospitalized with dengue fever in an outbreak in Rio de Janeiro, Brazil. Trans R Soc Trop Med Hyg 105: 601–603. doi:10.1016/j.trstmh.2011.07.007.
28. García-Rivera EJ, Rigau-Pérez JG (2003) Dengue severity in the elderly in Puerto Rico. Rev Panam Salud Pública Pan Am J Public Health 13: 362–368.

19

Increased Diagnostic Yield of Capsule Endoscopy in Patients with Chronic Abdominal Pain

Liping Yang, Yu Chen, Bingling Zhang, Chunxiao Chen, Min Yue, Juan Du, Chaohui Yu, Youming Li*

Department of Gastroenterology, the First Affiliated Hospital, College of Medicine, Zhejiang University, Hangzhou, China

Abstract

Background and Study Aims: Chronic abdominal pain is one of the most common chief complaints, but the underlying pathophysiology often remains unknown after routine clinical evaluation. Capsule endoscopy (CE) is a new technique for the visualization of the entire small bowel. The aim of this study was to evaluate the diagnostic efficacy of CE in patients with chronic abdominal pain of obscure origin.

Patients and Methods: Two hundred forty three patients with chronic abdominal pain with no significant lesions were enrolled in this study. CE was performed in all patients.

Results: A diagnosis was made in 23.0% of patients screened with CE. Of the 243 patients, 19 (7.8%) were diagnosed with Crohn's disease, 15 (6.2%) with enteritis, 11 (4.5%) with idiopathic intestinal lymphangiectasia, 5 (2.1%) with uncinariasis, and a number of other diagnoses including small bowel tumor, ascariasis, and anaphylactoid purpura. Five patients had abnormal transit time, and capsule retention occurred in two patients.

Conclusions: In contrast to other previous studies, we found that CE is an effective diagnostic tool for patients with abdominal pain.

Editor: Erica Villa, University of Modena & Reggio Emilia, Italy

Funding: The authors have no support or funding to report.

Competing Interests: The authors have declared that no competing interests exist.

* E-mail: zlym@zju.edu.cn

Introduction

Chronic abdominal pain (CAP) that persists either continuously or intermittently for more than three months is one of the most common chief complaints in clinical medicine. The causes of abdominal pain are varied and complex, and include both functional and structural gastrointestinal abnormalities. Unfortunately, in many patients with CAP, the underlying cause of the disease remains unknown even after routine laboratory testing.

Capsule endoscopy (CE) is a new technology for painless endoscopic imaging of the entire small bowel [1,2]. To date, several studies have demonstrated that CE is superior to barium follow-through, push enteroscopy, and computed tomography (CT) for the diagnosis of small bowel disease [3–5], and more specifically for the evaluation of patients with obscure gastrointestinal bleeding [6–10] and Crohn's disease [11–14]. However, there is a paucity of data regarding the diagnostic yield of CE in patients with CAP, and in previously published studies, CE was not informative in these patients [15,16]. The primary objective of our study was to determine the diagnostic efficacy of CE in patients with CAP of obscure origin.

Methods

Ethics statement

After informed of the benefits and potential risks of capsule endoscopy examination, all the patients signed an informed consent form prior to their enrollment for capsule endoscopy examination. In addition, all the patients agreed that their clinical examination results could be used for non-commercial teaching or scientific research purposes and these verbal consents were recorded in the patient file. All the patient information was anonymized prior to analysis. The Ethical Review Committee (the First Affiliated Hospital, College of Medicine, Zhejiang University) approved this retrospective study and stated that "This study appears to be in accordance with the scientific principles generally accepted and to the ethical standards of research. The study was led in the respect of the Chinese law and regulation".

Patients and controls

Inpatients and outpatients who complained of either continuous or intermittent abdominal pain for at least three months at the First Affiliated Hospital, College of Medicine, Zhejiang University between January 2006 and December 2012 were screened for enrollment in this study. Patients were excluded if they presented with any of the following conditions: pregnancy, symptoms/signs of bowel obstruction, presence of implanted pacemaker, swallowing disorders, and any abdominal surgery except appendicectomy. Two hundred forty three patients (136 male and 107 female, with mean age of 44.1 years) were enrolled in this study.

Out of 243 patients, 112 patients complained of mid-epigastric pain, 37 of lower abdominal pain, and 94 of diffuse abdominal pain. All patients underwent routine clinical examinations and

Table 1. Demographic data and clinical characteristics of the study population.

Characteristics	OMOM	PillCam SB	Total
No. of patients	144	99	243
Sex			
Male	75	61	136
Female	69	38	107
Median age (range), years	44.9(15–76)	44.0(9–79)	44.1(9–79)
Positive findings	32	24	56
Yield, %	22.2%	24.2%	23.0%

laboratory tests (including blood tests, urine tests, and stool examinations), ultrasound examinations or computed tomography (CT), esophagogastroduodenoscopy, and colonoscopy. We did not perform any barium studies as they are rarely used in our hospital. The studies did not reveal any obvious lesions that could contribute to clinical manifestations of disease.

Capsule endoscopy

For CE, 144 patients were examined by OMOM CE system (JinShan Science & Technology Co, Ltd, ChongQing, China) and 99 patients were examined by Given PillCam SB Diagnostic System (Given Imaging Ltd., Yoqneam, Israel).

Table 2. CE findings in 243 patients with chronic abdominal pain.

	OMOM	PillCam SB	Total
No. of patients	144	99	243
Specific capsule endoscopy findings			
Ileal and jejuna ulcers	23	19	42
Ileal occupation	1	0	1
Jejunal occupation	0	1	1
Intestinal lymphandiectasia	9	2	11
Erythema and edema in jejuna and ileum	4	3	7
Ileal and jejuna polyps	1	0	1
Uncinariasis	5	0	5
Ascariasis	0	2	2
Diverticulum	1	0	1
Fistula	0	1	1
Follicular hyperplasia	1	2	3
Presumed diagnosis after capsule endoscopy			
Crohn's disease	9	10	19
Enteritis	8	7	15
Idiopathic intestinal lymphangiectasia	9	2	11
Uncinariasis	5	0	5
Ascariasis	0	2	2
Small bowel occupying lesion	1	2	3
Anaphylactoid purpura	0	1	1

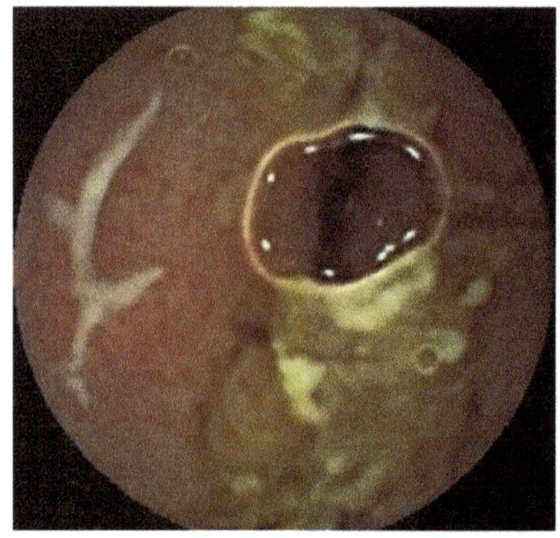

Figure 1. Ulcers and stenosis found by CE. Ulcers and stenosis in the upper part of the small intestine were found by CE in a 56-year-old woman with abdominal pain. The diagnosis of Crohn's disease was confirmed both surgically and pathologically.

The patients were maintained on a liquid diet for one day and fasted for at least 10 hours prior to the examination. When the capsule was activated, the patient ingested it with one glass of water. Two hours after swallowing the capsule patients were allowed to drink water and in another two hours could have a light snack. The examination lasted approximately eight hours, and during this time the patient avoided any physical activity that involved sweating and abstained from bending. At the end of the procedure, the sensor belt and data recorder were removed by the physician.

Statistical analysis

All the data recorded were analyzed by professional gastroenterologists.

Results

Demographic data and clinical characteristics of the study population are listed in Table 1. Of the 243 patients evaluated, 56 patients were diagnosed with abnormalities in the small intestine (yield 23.0%). Forty four of these patients presented with periumbilial pain as the primary symptom (yield 78.6%). Specific CE findings included ulcers, erythema and edema, occupation,

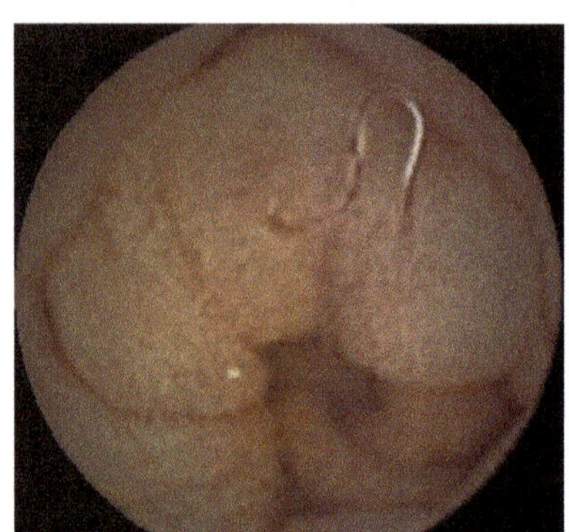

Figure 2. Hookworms identified by CE. Hookworms throughout the small bowel were identified by CE in a 42-year-old woman with lower abdominal pain for three years.

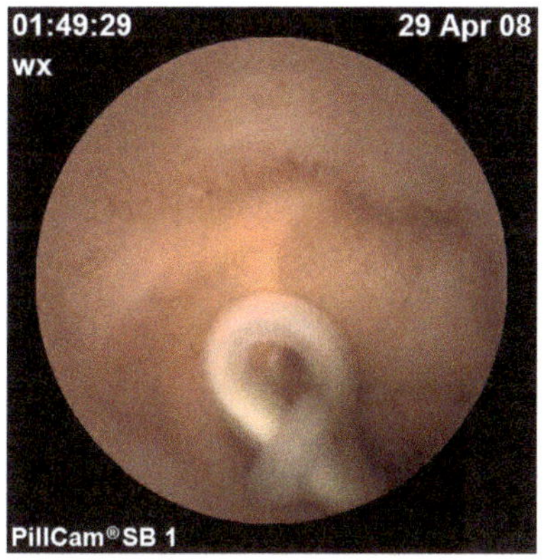

Figure 3. Roundworm detected by CE. Roundworm was detected by CE in the small bowel in a 49-year-old woman with periumbilial pain for more than one year.

lymphangiectasia, diverticulum, fistula, uncinariasis, and ascariasis. The presumed diagnoses included Crohn's disease (19 patients), enteritis (15), idiopathic intestinal lymphangiectasia (11), uncinariasis (five), small bowel occupying lesion (three), ascariasis (two), and anaphylactoid purpura (one) (Table 2).

The diagnosis of Crohn's disease was based on the following criteria: ulcers, mucosal erosion, ileal ulcerated stenosis, and featureless small bowel [11,17,18]. CE detected roundworms (*Ascaris lumbricoides*) and hookworms (*ancylostome*) in patients with ascariasis and uncinariasis, which was previously undetected in the stool examination. The patient with occupation in the proximal jejunum was diagnosed with adenocarcinoma by pathological findings. The patient with small bowel occupying lesion was diagnosed surgically with gastrointestinal stromal tumor. The patient with anaphylactoid purpura had multiple congestion and ulcers in the small bowel (Figures 1, 2, 3, 4, 5, and 6).

Five patients exhibited abnormal transit time of the capsule. One had a prolonged transit time (1 hour 22 minutes to leave the stomach and 9 hours to reach the colon) and four had a rapid transit time (on average, 1 hour 15 minutes to reach the colon). Capsule retention occurred in two patients (0.82%), and localization was confirmed by X-ray KUB in the stomach and pelvic cavity.

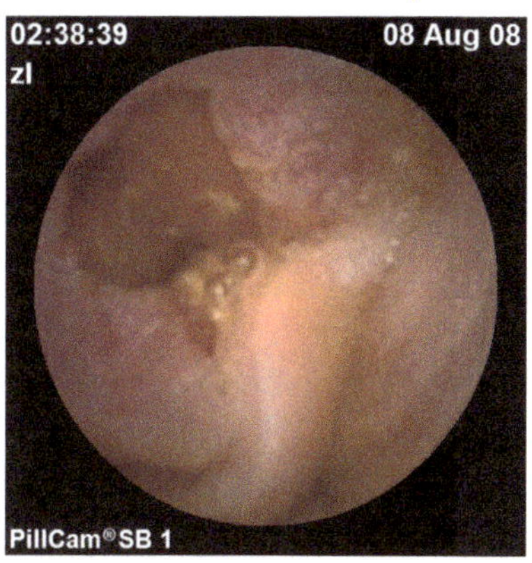

Figure 4. An occupying lesion identified by CE. An occupying lesion was identified by CE in the jejunum of a 52-year-old woman with abdominal pain for more than three months. With subsequent pathology evaluation, a diagnosis of adenocarcinoma was confirmed.

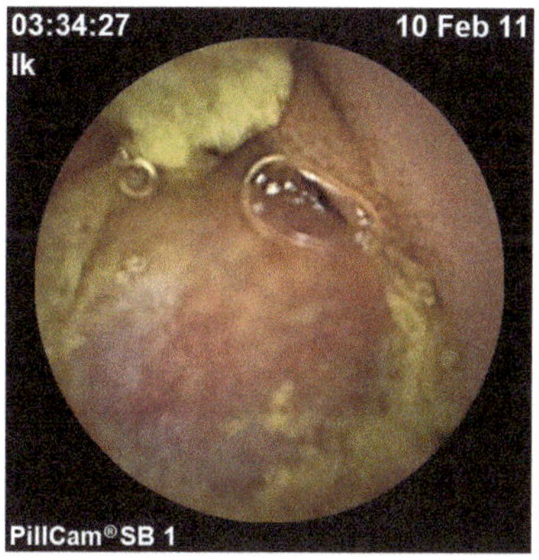

Figure 5. An eminence lesion identified by CE. An eminence lesion was identified by CE in the small bowel of a 30-year-old man with periumbilial pain. The lesion was surgically diagnosed as gastrointestinal stromal tumor.

Discussion

For gastroenterologists, the small intestine is known as the "Dark Continent" because of the inherent difficultly to visualize this organ enteroscopically. In particular, small-bowel endoscopy is constrained by procedural discomfort and limits on the advancement of enteroscopes into the small bowel [1]. CE, which allows painless endoscopic imaging of the whole small bowel, has become a very important tool for the diagnosis of many small-bowel disorders [1,19]. For example, gastrointestinal bleeding is the primary and most frequent indication for CE. As reported by various studies, the overall diagnostic yield for obscure gastrointestinal bleeding is in the range of 55%–70%, which is much higher than that for other diagnostic tests [5–10,19]. CE was also efficacious for the diagnosis of small bowel lesions in Crohn's disease, suggesting it may be useful for early disease management [11–14,19]. Moreover, CE can be used to diagnose patients with celiac disease and hereditary polyposis syndromes [20–22]. More recently, small bowel tumors have been detected with CE, where 6–9% of patients were diagnosed small bowel tumors [23–25]. Some studies revealed that CE could help to identify the intensity and extent of the gastrointestinal involvement in patients with anaphylactoid purpura [26–28].

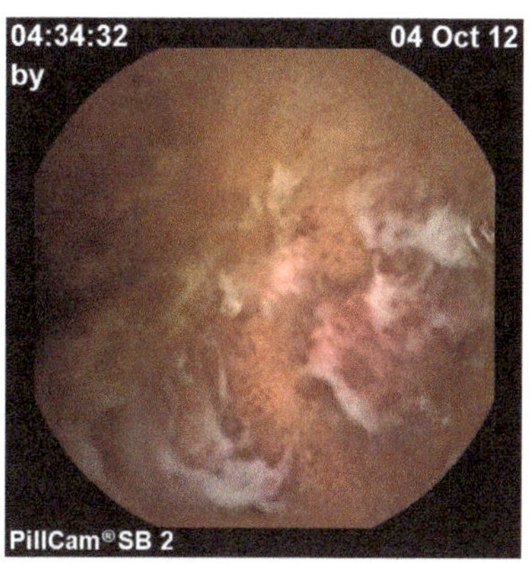

Figure 6. Multiple congestion and ulcers identified by CE. Multiple congestion and ulcers in the small bowel were identified by CE in a 17-year-old man with recurrent abdominal pain.

In contrast to findings of other investigators, we demonstrated that CE increased diagnostic yield (23.0%) for patients with chronic abdominal pain of previously undetermined origin [15,16]. We enrolled patients in our study who complained of continuous or intermittent abdominal pain for at least three months. Our findings made presumed diagnoses of Crohn's disease, enteritis, idiopathic intestinal lymphangiectasia, uncinariasis, small bowel occupying lesion, ascariasis, and anaphylactoid purpura in patients who presented with negative routine clinical examination. Therefore, our data suggest that CE is an effective diagnostic tool for the evaluation of patients with CAP.

The main advantage of our study over others is the enrollment of a large number of patients who had a previous negative clinical workup (including routine laboratory tests, esophagogastroduodenoscopy, and colonoscopy). There are some limitations, primarily the inherent defects of any retrospective study. Although data collection regarding details of every patient was a priority, tiny omissions were inevitable. Also, we used two kinds of CE, but we believe the intensive and elaborate analyses by our expert gastroenterologists make this potential limitation unlikely.

In conclusion, we found that visualization of the small bowel with CE is a diagnostically effective tool for patients with chronic abdominal pain of obscure origin. Our results have important implications for the diagnosis of multiple disorders of the small bowel and the development and refinement of appropriate treatment regimens clinically.

Author Contributions

Conceived and designed the experiments: CY YL. Performed the experiments: LY BZ CC MY JD. Analyzed the data: LY YC. Wrote the paper: LY BZ CC MY JD.

References

1. Iddan G, Meron G, Glukhovsky A, Swain P (2000) Wireless capsule endoscopy. Nature 405: 417.
2. Ginsberg GG, Barkun AN, Bosco JJ, Isenberg GA, Nguyen CC, et al. (2002) Wireless capsule endoscopy: August 2002. Gastrointest Endosc 56(5): 621–4.
3. Appleyard M, Fireman Z, Glukhovsky A, Jacob H, Shreiver R, et al. (2000) A randomized trial comparing wireless capsule endoscopy with push enteroscopy for the detection of small-bowel lesions. Gastroenterology 119(6): 1431–8.
4. Costamagna G, Shah SK, Riccioni ME, Foschia F, Mutignani M, et al. (2002) A prospective trial comparing radiographs and video capsule endoscopy for suspected small bowel disease. Gastroenterology 123(4): 999–1005.
5. Hara AK, Leighton JA, Sharma VK, Fleischer DE (2004) Small bowel: preliminary comparison of capsule endoscopy with barium study and CT. Radiology 230: 260–265.
6. Ell C, Remke S, May A, Helou L, Henrich R, et al. (2002) The first prospective controlled trial comparing wireless capsule endoscopy with push enteroscopy in chronic gastrointestinal bleeding. Endoscopy 34(9): 685–9.
7. Lewis BS, Swain P (2002) Capsule endoscopy in the evaluation of patients with suspected small intestinal bleeding: Results of a pilot study. Gastrointest Endosc 56(3): 349–53
8. Mylonaki M, Fritscher-Ravens A, Swain P (2003) Wireless capsule endoscopy: a comparison with push enteroscopy in patients with gastroscopy and colonoscopy negative gastrointestinal bleeding. Gut 52(8): 1122–6.
9. Adler DG, Knipschield M, Gostout C (2004) A prospective comparison of capsule endoscopy and push enteroscopy in patients with GI bleeding of obscure origin. Gastrointest Endosc 59(4): 492–8.
10. Nakamura M, Niwa Y, Ohmiya N, Miyahara R, Ohashi A, et al. (2006) Preliminary comparison of capsule endoscopy and double-ballon enteroscopy in patients with suspected small-bowel bleeding. Endoscopy 38(1): 59–66.
11. Fireman Z, Mahajna E, Broide E, Shapiro M, Fich L, et al. (2003) Diagnosing small bowel Crohn's disease with wireless capsule endoscopy. Gut 52(3): 390–2.
12. Herrarías JM, Caunedo A, Rodríquez-Téllez M, Pellicer F, Herrerías JM JR (2003) Capsule endoscopy in patients with suspected Crohn's disease and negative endoscopy. Endoscopy 35(7): 564–8.
13. Chong AK, Taylor A, Miller A, Hennessy O, Connell W, et al. (2005) Capsule endoscopy vs. push enteroscopy and enteroclysis in suspected small-bowel Crohn's disease. Gastrointest Endosc 61(2): 255–61.
14. Voderholzer WA, Beinhoelzl J, Rogalla P, Murrer S, Schachschal G, et al. (2005) Small bowel involvement in Crohn's disease: a prospective comparison of wireless capsule endoscopy and computed tomography enteroclysis. Gut 54(3):369–73.
15. Bardan E, Nadler M, Chowers Y, Fidder H, Bar-Meir S (2003) Capsule endoscopy for the evaluation of patients with chronic abdominal pain. Endoscopy 35(8):688–9.
16. Fry LC, Carey EJ, Shiff AD, Heigh RI, Sharma VK, et al. (2006) The yield of capsule endoscopy in patients with abdominal pain or diarrhea. Endoscopy 38(5):498–502.
17. Dubcenco E, Jeejeebhoy KN, Petroniene R, Tang SJ, Zalev AH, et al. (2005) Capsule endoscopy findings in patients with established and suspected small-bowel Crohn's disease: correlation with radiologic, endoscopic, and histologic findings. Gastrointest endosc 62: 538–544.
18. De Bona M, Bellumat A, Cian E, Valiante F, Moschini A, et al. (2006) Capsule endoscopy findings in patients with suspected Crohn's disease and biochemical markers of inflammation. Dig Liver Dis 38(5): 331–5.
19. Rey JF, Ladas S, Alhassano A, Kuznetsov K; ESGE Guidelines Committee (2006) European society of gastrointeastinal endoscopy (ESGE). Video capsule endoscopy: update to guidelines (May 2006). Endoscopy 38(10):1047–53.
20. Petroniene R, Dubcenco E, Baker JP, Ottaway CA, Tang SJ, et al. (2005) Given capsule endoscopy in celiac disease: evaluation of diagnostic accuracy and interobserver agreement. Am J Gastroenterol 100:685–694.
21. Culliford A, Daly J, Diamond B, Rubin M, Green PH (2005) The value of wireless capsule endoscopy in patients with complicated celiac disease. Gastrointest Endosc 62:55–60.
22. Mata A, Liac J, Castell A, Rovira JM, Pellisé M, et al. (2005) A prospective trial comparing wireless capsule endoscopy and barium contrast series for small bowel surveillance in hereditary GI polyposis syndrome. Gastruintest Endosc 61:721–725.
23. Cobrin GM, Pittman RH, Lewis BS (2004) Diagnosing small bowel tumors with capsule endoscopy. Gastrenterology 26 (Suppl.2): AB1322.
24. Bailey AA, Debinski HS, Appleyard MN, Remedios ML, Hooper JE, et al. (2006) Diagnosis and outcome of small bowel tumors by capsule endoscopy: a three-center Australian experience. Am J Gastroenterol 101(10):2237–43.
25. Cobrin GM, Pittman RH, Lewis BS (2006) Increased diagnostic yield of small bowel tumors with capsule endoscopy. Cancer 107(1):22–7.
26. Skogestad E (2005) Capsule endoscopy in Henoch-Schonlein purpura. Endoscopy 37(2):189.
27. Preud'Homme DL, Michail S, Hodges C, Milliken T, Mezoff AG (2006) Use of wireless capsule endoscopy in the management of severe Henoch-Schonlein purpura. Pediatrics 118(3):e904–6.
28. Ichikawa R, Hosoe N, Imaeda H, Takabayashi K, Bessho R, et al. (2011) Evaluation of small-intestinal abnormalities in adult patients with Henoch-Schonlein purpura using video capsule. Endoscopy 43:E162–3.

The Analysis of Factors Associated with Progression of Isolated Terminal Ileal Lesions

Zhang Fangbin[1]*, Hao Weiwei[1], Zhao Wugan[2], Zheng Cong[1], Chu Yanjun[1], Xu Feng[1]

1 Department of Gastroenterology, The First Affiliated Hospital of Zhengzhou University, Zhengzhou, People's Republic of China, **2** Department of Pathology, The First Affiliated Hospital of Zhengzhou University, Zhengzhou, People's Republic of China

Abstract

Objective: To assess the factors associated with the progression of isolated terminal ileal lesions (ITILs) at colonoscopy in Chinese patients.

Methods: Patients diagnosed with ITILs were enrolled. The ileoscopy was performed by two experienced gastroenterologists every 52 weeks. A logistic regression analysis was used to elucidate the factors associated with Crohn's disease (CD) and mucosal healing. A log rank test was used to assess the differences of the cumulative proportion of CD and mucosal healing in different groups at different times.

Results: (1) A total of 34 patients were included and no patient had taken nonsteroidal anti-inflammatory drug in the last 6 months; eight (23.5%) patients had a clinical diagnosis of CD, 14 (41.2%) patients achieved mucosal healing, and 12 (35.3%) patients showed no significant changes in the lesions at last follow-up. (2) The logistic regression analysis showed that only abdominal pain was a factor in the ITIL disease outcomes. (3) The cumulative proportion of CD in the abdominal pain group after 3 years was statistically higher than that in the non-abdominal pain group (42.7% *vs.* 6.2%, $\chi^2=10.129$, $P=0.001$). However, the cumulative proportion of mucosal healing in the non-abdominal pain group was statistically higher than that in the abdominal pain group (73.3% *vs.* 5.6%, $\chi^2=5.225$, $P=0.022$). (4) The numbers of lesions observed on the initial colonoscopy exams and the initial histologic findings were not related to the ITIL disease outcomes.

Conclusions: Clinical symptoms may be related to ITIL disease outcomes. Patients with abdominal pain had a high likelihood of CD, whereas those without abdominal pain had a high likelihood of mucosal healing.

Editor: John Green, University Hospital Llandough, United Kingdom

Funding: This study was sponsored by research funding for the doctoral program of higher education of China and the Youth Innovation Fund of the First Affiliated Hospital of Zhengzhou University. The funders had no role in study design, data collection and analysis, decision to publish, or preparation of the manuscript.

Competing Interests: The authors have declared that no competing interests exist.

* E-mail: dr_mingren@163.com

Introduction

Ileal intubation is increasingly recognized as being valuable in patients with abdominal pain, diarrhea or bloody stools—particularly where inflammatory bowel disease is a consideration. [1–3] This has led to an increased identification of patients (about 0.1–0.3%) who are not easily classified—those with Isolated ileal abnormalities, which we have coined isolated terminal ileal lesions (ITILs). [4,5] It is likely that a proportion of these patients are suffering from a restricted form or so-called forme fruste of Crohn's disease (CD). Currently, the clinical significance of this entity is unclear. [2,6,7].

The present study evaluated the clinical course of patients with ITILs to determine the clinical significance of these lesions.

Materials and Methods

Subjects

Patients diagnosed with ITILs at the Gastroenterology clinic of the First Affiliated Hospital of Zhengzhou University Hospital from 2005 to 2010 were actively recruited to this study with the goal of evaluating the natural history of terminal ileal lesions. All patients underwent gastroscopy and double contrast small bowel radiography to evaluate their upper gastrointestinal and small intestinal mucosa.

Subjects were excluded if they fulfilled any of the following criteria: (1) a follow-up of less than 2 years; (2) a history of nonsteroidal anti-inflammatory drug or glucocorticoid use within the 6 months before the study; (3) erosions in other parts of the colon in addition to the terminal ileum; (4) oral or genital ulcerations suggestive of Behçet disease; (5) infectious colitis (except tuberculosis); (6) a prior history of CD or ulcerative colitis; (7) a history of colorectal cancer or surgery; (8) a history of systemic lupus erythematosus or vasculitis; or (9) poor adherence to the study: rejection of colonoscopies during the follow-up.

Study Design

Clinical data, including sex, age, clinical symptoms and medical records were recorded. The patient information was collected by a clinician. All patients were asked to ingest 2 L of polyethylene glycol solution in the evening before the ileoscopy. The ileoscopy was performed by two experienced gastroenterologists at weeks 0, 52, 104, 156, 208, 260, 312, 364, 416, 468, and 520. Two biopsy specimens were obtained from the most severe area of the lesion in each subject. All of the biopsy specimens were evaluated separately by two experienced pathologists. In cases in which they did not agree on an evaluation, a discussion with a senior gastrointestinal pathologist was employed.

Drug therapy was directed toward the dominant symptoms: a selective smooth-muscle relaxant for abdominal pain, loperamide for diarrhea, and lactulose syrup or polyethylene glycol for constipation. (Table 1) The treatments were withdrawn when the clinical symptoms resolved and reintroduced when the clinical symptoms recurred. Patients with positive occult blood test, mild abdominal discomfort, or surveillance after colorectal polypectomy underwent no any treatment during the total duration of follow-up.

The symptoms were assessed daily by asking the patient to complete a diary regarding the following: abdominal pain, discomfort, stool frequency, and stool consistency.

Assessment of overall symptom relief was measured weekly. (Table 2) Patients were assessed for symptom recurrence weekly by telephone interview and monthly at a clinic visit.

The patients recorded the overall clinical symptom relief in a diary by answering 'yes' or 'no' to the following question: 'Do you consider that over the past week you have had satisfactory relief from your symptoms?' 'Satisfactory' meant that compared with their typical experience of the disorder in the past, the patient felt that during the past week their clinical symptoms had been alleviated to the extent that they would take medication to maintain that state.

At scheduled doctor visits, response to initial treatment was designated when patients' overall satisfactory relief from symptoms for at least 2 of the 4 previous weeks; those whose overall satisfactory relief from symptoms for less than 2 weeks in the 4 previous weeks were considered nonresponders.

Patients requesting urgent restoration of medication treatment because of recurring/worsening symptoms before or at a scheduled telephone contact during the withdrawal period were considered to have relapsed.

Statistical Analyses

Statistical analysis was performed using SPSS software, version 16.0 (SPSS Inc., Chicago, Ill, USA). To elucidate the factors associated with developing CD and mucosal healing, a logistic regression analysis was used and results were expressed as odds ratios (OR) with 95% confidence intervals (CI). A Kaplan–Meier plot and a log-rank test were used to visualize and to test differences between CD and mucosal healing in probability of remaining in the study. A χ^2 test was used to compare the endoscopic findings, pathologic findings on the initial colonoscopy exams and disease outcomes of ITILs. A *P*-value less than 0.05 was considered to be significant.

Ethical Considerations

The ethics committee of the participating center approved the study (reference numbers: 20050401GS-7 (University of Zhengzhou)). The study was conducted according to the principles expressed in the Declaration of Helsinki. Written informed consent was obtained from all participants at recruitment.

Results

Subject Characteristics

During the study period, 32,197 patients underwent colonoscopic examinations at the Gastrointestinal Endoscopy Center. Of these, 43 were assigned an endoscopic diagnostic code for ITILs. Of these 43 patients, seven patients (16.3%) with a follow-up of less than 2 years and two patients (4.7%) with poor compliance were excluded, the data of these 9 patients wasn't analyzed in this study; the remaining 34 patients (79.1%) met the study criteria. These 34 patients including in this study have no a history of nonsteroidal anti-inflammatory drug (such as aspirin) or glucocorticoid use within the 6 months before the study. These 34 patients including in this study have no family history of IBD.

The patient sample consisted of 19 men and 15 women with a mean age of 33.3±11.1 years (range 22–62 years), and the mean follow-up was 3 years (range 2–5 years). The indications for colonoscopy included abdominal pain in 10 (29.4%) patients, stools >3 times daily in nine patients (26.5%), abdominal pain and diarrhea in four patients (11.8%), abdominal pain and constipation in two patients (5.9%), positive occult blood test in two patients (5.9%), mild abdominal discomfort in two patients (5.9%), constipation in one patient (2.9%), diarrhea in one patient (2.9%), and surveillance after colorectal polypectomy in three patients (8.8%). Table 3 shows the demographic characteristics of the 34 patients.

According to the Rome III criteria, [9] two of the 34 patients (5.9%) with abdominal pain and diarrhea and two of the 34 patients (5.9%) with abdominal pain and constipation met criteria for irritable bowel syndrome (IBS), two of the 34 patients (5.9%) with abdominal discomfort were considered functional bloating,

Table 1. Possible Drugs for a Dominant Symptom in Patients.

Symptom	Drug	Dose
Abdominal Pain	Pinaverium bromide	50 mg qd to qid ac
	Amitriptyline	Start 25–50 mg hs, then adjust
	Paroxetine hydrochloride	Start 20 mg hs, then adjust
Diarrhea	Loperamide	2–4 mg when necessary/maximum 12 mg/d
	Pinaverium bromide	50 mg qd to qid ac
Constipation	Lactulose syrup	10–20 g bid
	Polyethylene glycol	17 g in 8 oz water qd
	Mosapride	5 mg tid ac

qd, quaque die; bid, bis in die; qid, quater in die; hs, hora somni; ac, ante cibum; oz, ounce.

Table 2. Overall Relief Assessment.

Abdominal pain
0 = none (no symptoms)
1 = mild (presence of symptoms but well-tolerated)
2 = moderate (symptoms interfere with but do not prevent normal daily activities such as work and/or sleep)
3 = severe (symptoms prevent normal daily activities such as work and/or sleep)
Stool frequency
the daily number of bowel movements was recorded
Stool consistency [8]
1 = separate hard lumps, like nuts
2 = sausage-like, but lumpy
3 = like a sausage but with cracks in the surface
4 = like a sausage, smooth and soft
5 = soft blobs with clear-cut edges
6 = fluffy pieces with ragged edges, a mushy stool
7 = watery, no solid pieces

one of the 34 patients (2.9%) with constipation was considered functional constipation, one of the 34 patients (2.9%) with diarrhea was considered functional diarrhea, two of the 34 patients (5.9%) with abdominal pain and diarrhea were considered unspecified functional bowel disorder.

Clinical Findings

Of the 34 patients, eight (23.5%) were eventually diagnosed with CD on follow-up, 14 (41.2%) achieved mucosal healing, and 12 (35.3%) showed no significant changes in the lesions. Of the 31 patients categorized as symptomatic (symptom onset at least 3 days per month in the last 3 months), eight (26%) had a clinical diagnosis of CD during the follow-up; the mean interval between the first visit and the appearance of typical CD symptoms was 2.0 years (range 1.0–4.0 years). Of the three patients categorized as asymptomatic (without symptom or symptom onset less than 3 days per month in the last 3 months), 2 (66.7%) achieved mucosal healing, and one (33.3%) showed no significant changes in the lesions.

Table 3. The Demographic Characteristics of the 34 Patients.

Sex (male:female)	19:15
Mean age at diagnosis (y)	33±11 (22–62)
Duration of follow-up (y)	3 (2–5)
Symptoms	
Abdominal pain	10 (29%)
Stools >3 times daily	9 (26%)
Abdominal pain and diarrhea	4 (12%)
Abdominal pain and constipation	2 (6%)
Positive occult blood test	2 (6%)
Mild abdominal discomfort	2 (6%)
Constipation	1 (3%)
Diarrhea	1 (3%)
Surveillance after colorectal polypectomy	3 (9%)
Colonoscopy	3±1 (2–5)

Of the 31 symptomatic patients, 29 (93.5%, 29/31) underwent drug therapy based on their dominant symptoms, 26 (89.7%, 26/29) attained recovery during the initial treatment period, 23 (88.5%, 23/26) experienced symptoms relapse during the withdrawal period, and 20 (87.0%, 20/23) attained recovery during the retreatment period.

Of the 12 patients who showed no significant changes in the lesions, all attained recovery during the initial treatment period, 10 (83.3%, 10/12) experienced symptom relapse during the withdrawal period, and nine (90.0%, 9/10) attained recovery during the retreatment period.

Endoscopic and Pathologic Findings

Normal mucosa was observed on the gastroscopies and radiological exams in the 34 patients.

All of the 34 patients underwent ileoscopy. On the initial colonoscopy exams, each case demonstrated one to several discrete, focal erosions within an otherwise normal small bowel mucosa. The erosions were located less than 5 cm proximal to the ileocecal valve. Most of the erosions were surrounded by normal or edematous mucosa and were covered by thin or faint exudates. (Fig. 1a, 1b, and 1c) The size of the erosions was estimated to be 2 to 3 mm. Of the 34 patients, 10 patients (29.4%) had a single erosion, and 24 patients (70.6%) had several erosions.

Of the eight patients with a clinical diagnosis of CD, typical longitudinal ulcerations existed in seven patients, irregular ulcerations existed in one patient (Fig. 2a and 2b), narrowing or stricture on imaging in four patients, perianal disease in one patient, and multiple episodes of small bowel obstruction in one patient.

The initial histologic findings in the patients included mucosal edema (7), erosions (8), acute or chronic inflammatory cells (11) and architectural alterations (3). The 8 patients with a final diagnosis of CD had non-caseating granulomas (3), architectural alterations (9) cryptitis (3), or focal chronic (lymphocytes and plasma cells) inflammation (7).

All of the patients responded to inflammatory bowel disease (IBD) treatments (1 patient was treated with infliximab and

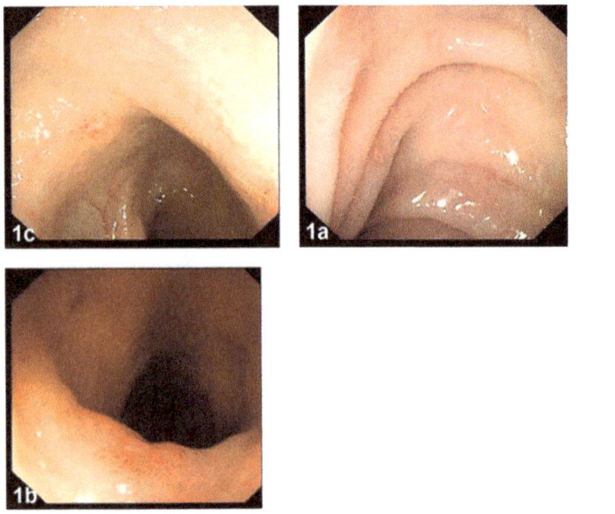

Figure 1. Initial colonoscopic images in the 34 patients. Erosions surrounded by normal mucosa (1a), edematous mucosa (1b), and covered by thin or faint exudates (1a, 1b, and 1c).

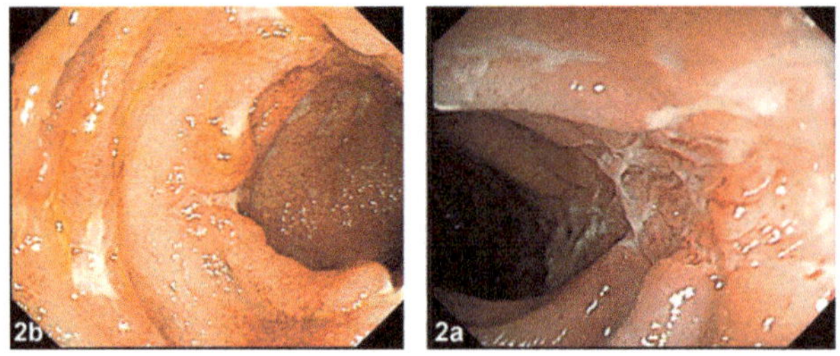

Figure 2. Colonoscopic images in the patients who developed CD. Typical longitudinal ulcerations of CD covered with mucous exudates (2a), and irregular ulcerations existed of CD covered with mucous exudates (2b). CD, Crohn's disease.

azathioprine, two patients were treated with azathioprine, and five patients were treated with 5-amino salicylic acid) and were still on maintenance therapy for CD at the most recent follow-up.

Clinical Symptoms and Outcomes

We conducted a logistic regression analysis to assess the factors associated with progression of isolated terminal ileal lesions in the 34 patients. The independent variables were age, sex, clinical symptoms, and duration of follow-up; the dependent variables were developing CD and mucosal healing. In this regression model, only abdominal pain was significantly associated with developing CD and mucosal healing (developing CD: OR 13.1 95% CI, 1.4–124.5, $P = 0.025$; mucosal healing OR = 38.1 95% CI, 3.5–414.0, $P = 0.003$).

The 34 patients were divided into an abdominal pain group and an non-abdominal pain group based on their clinical symptoms; the abdominal pain group contained 16 patients (10 patients with abdominal pain, four patients with abdominal pain and diarrhea, and two patients with abdominal pain and constipation), and the non-abdominal pain group contained 18 patients (nine patients with stools >3 times daily, two patients with positive occult blood tests, two patients with mild abdominal discomfort, three patients with surveillance after colorectal polypectomy, one patient with constipation, and one patient with diarrhea). In the abdominal pain group, seven patients were eventually diagnosed with CD on follow-up, Including two patients with IBS. The median interval between the first visit and the presentation of typical CD symptoms was 2 years (range 1–4 years). In the remaining nine patients with abdominal pain, eight showed no significant changes compared with their initial colonoscopic findings, and one patient achieved mucosal healing after anti-tuberculosis therapy for 9 months. In the non-abdominal pain group, 13 patients achieved mucosal healing. The median interval between the first visit and mucosal healing was 3 years (range 1–5 years). In the remaining five patients without abdominal pain, four showed no significant changes, and one patient with a positive occult blood test developed CD in the 3rd year of follow-up.

Of the 34 patients, sex and age were not significantly different between the abdominal pain and non-abdominal pain groups. The Kaplan–Meier method showed that the cumulative proportions of CD in the abdominal pain group in the 1st, 2nd, and 3rd years of follow-up were 6.2%, 31.2% and 42.7%, respectively, whereas in the non-abdominal pain group, the proportions were 0, 0, and 6.2%, respectively. The log-rank test showed that the cumulative proportion of CD in the abdominal pain group after 3 years was statistically higher than that in the non-abdominal pain group (42.7% *vs.* 6.2%, $\chi^2 = 10.129$, $P = 0.001$). (Fig. 3) The cumulative proportions of mucosal healing in the non-abdominal pain group in the 1st, 2nd, 3rd, and 4th years of follow-up were 6.2%, 27.8%, 55.6% and 73.3%, respectively, whereas the proportions in the abdominal pain group were 5.6%, 5.6%, 5.6% and 5.6%, respectively. The cumulative proportion of mucosal healing in the non-abdominal pain group after 4 years was statistically higher

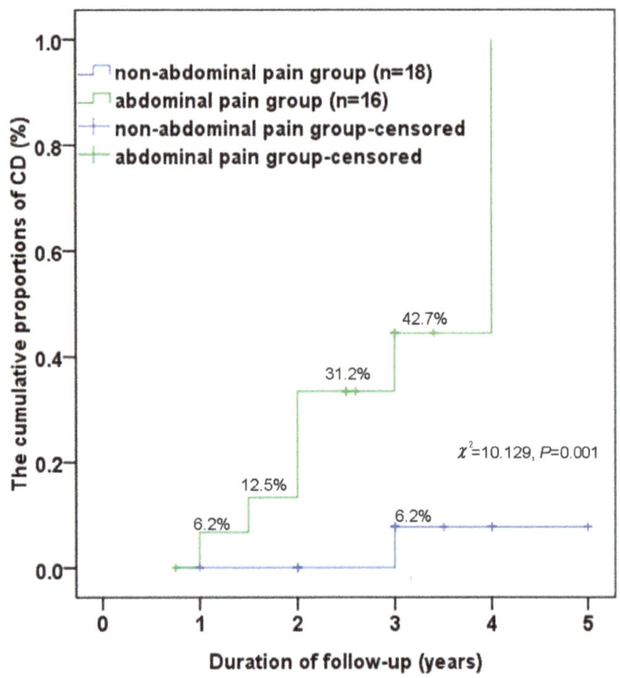

Figure 3. The cumulative proportions of CD in the 34 patients. The cumulative proportions of CD in the abdominal pain group in the 1st, 2nd, and 3rd years of follow-up were 6%, 31% and 43%, respectively, and the proportions in the non-abdominal pain group were 0, 0, and 6%, respectively. Moreover, the cumulative proportion of CD in the abdominal pain group after 3 years was statistically higher than that in the non-abdominal pain group (43% *vs.* 6%, $\chi^2 = 10.129$, $P = 0.001$). CD, Crohn's disease.

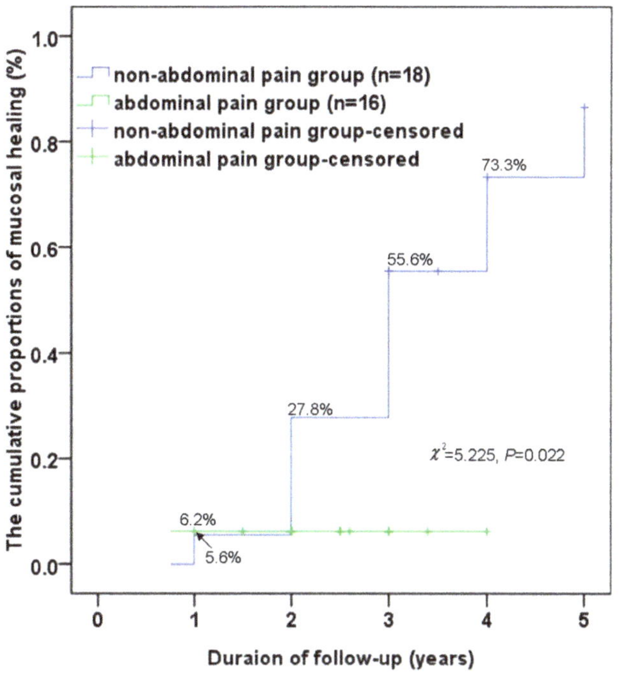

Figure 4. The cumulative proportions of mucosal healing in the 34 patients. The cumulative proportions of mucosal healing in the non-abdominal pain group in the 1st, 2nd, 3rd, and 4th years of follow-up were 6%, 28%, 56% and 73%, respectively, and the proportions in the abdominal pain group were 6%, 6%, 6% and 6%, respectively. Moreover, the cumulative proportion of mucosal healing in the non-abdominal pain group after 4 years was statistically higher than that in the abdominal pain group (73% *vs.* 6%, $\chi^2 = 5.225$, $P = 0.022$).

than that in the abdominal pain group (73% *vs.* 6%, $\chi^2 = 5.225$, $P = 0.022$). (Fig. 4)

Endoscopic Findings, Pathologic Findings and Outcomes

Next, we analyzed the association between the initial endoscopic findings and ITIL disease outcomes. We found that the numbers of lesions on the initial colonoscopy exams did not differ in the patients who were eventually diagnosed with CD on follow-up, achieved mucosal healing, and showed no significant changes in the lesions (2 (1–3) *vs.* 2.5 (1–3) *vs.* 2.5 (1–3), $\chi^2 = 1.252$, $P = 0.535$). Similarly, the initial histologic findings did not differ in these three groups (the proportion of patients with mucosal edema 25.0% (2/8) *vs.* 21.4% (3/14) *vs.*16.7% (2/12), $\chi^2 = 0.427$, $P = 1.000$; the proportion of patients with erosions 12.5% (1/8) *vs.* 21.4% (3/14) *vs.* 33.3% (4/12), $\chi^2 = 1.144$, $P = 0.678$; the proportion of patients with acute or chronic inflammatory cells 25.0% (2/8) *vs.* 50.0% (7/14) *vs.*16.7% (2/12), $\chi^2 = 3.304$, $P = 0.207$; and the proportion of patients with architectural alterations 12.5% (1/8) *vs.* 0 (0/14) *vs.* 16.7% (2/12), $\chi^2 = 2.543$, $P = 0.317$).

Discussion

Through a prospective study, we aimed to assess the factors associated with progression of ITILs in 34 Chinese patients.

ITILs are not uncommonly seen during routine screening colonoscopy, the frequency was about 0.1–0.3% and 0.1% (34/32,197) in this study. [4,5] The clinical significance of the ITILs is unclear. Goldstein et al. reported that eight of 28 patients (28.6%) developed typical CD at an average interval of 3.6 years. [7] Then, Courville et al. reported that 10 of 29 patients (34.5%) developed typical CD at an average interval of 2.2 to 12.6 years. [10] A recent study by Chang et al. reported that 1 of 93 patients (1.1%) developed typical CD at an average interval of 29.9 months. [4] Conversely, Lengeling et al. reported that 40 patients identified with "ulcerative ileitis" at ileocolonoscopy had no specific disease process development in a median follow-up of 3.2 years. [5] In this study, 23.5% of the patients were eventually diagnosed with CD on follow-up, and 41.2% of the patients achieved mucosal healing. The lower probability of achieving mucosal healing in this study could have been the result of the patients with different clinical symptoms, different follow-up lengths, and racial differences.

Aphthoid or small erosions have been considered one of the earliest manifestations of CD. Two previous studies showed that 44% (4/9) and 50% (5/10) of patients with aphthous-type CD later developed typical CD. [11,12] More recent studies have shown that the disease outcomes of ITILs are related to the clinical symptoms of patients. A study by Goldstein et al. reported that all 8 patients (29%) with ITILs who had developed CD on follow-up presented with abdominal pain, mucus-rich, blood-tinged stools; irregular bowel function with intermittent constipation and diarrhea; and low-level systemic malaise. [7] Recently, a study by Courville et al. reported that 10 of 15 (66.7%) symptomatic patients, and 0 of 14 asymptomatic patients had developed CD at the most recent follow-up. [10] Our findings are similar in those patients undergoing colonoscopy for symptoms; eight of 31 (26%) symptomatic patients and zero of three asymptomatic patients had developed CD during the follow-up. We conducted a logistic regression analysis and found that only abdominal pain was significantly associated with developing CD. Further analysis showed that the cumulative proportion of CD in the abdominal pain group after 3 years was statistically higher than that in the non-abdominal pain group.

Should patients with ITILs be treated? Two studies reported that isolated terminal ileal ulcerations completely resolved without any treatment on follow-up colonoscopy in 66.7% of asymptomatic patients (four of six patients and 62 of 93 patients, respectively). [4,10] In this present study, two of the three (66.7%) asymptomatic patients completely resolved without inflammatory bowel disease-related treatment. We conducted a logistic regression analysis and found that only abdominal pain was significantly associated with mucosal healing. Further analysis showed that the cumulative proportion of mucosal healing in the non-abdominal pain group was statistically higher than that in the abdominal pain group. Our findings suggest that these patients in the non-abdominal pain group do not warrant any inflammatory bowel disease-related treatment, and a wait and watch approach seems to be the most prudent at the present time.

A study by Courville et al. reported that the endoscopic and histopathological findings in patients with asymptomatic ileitis closely mimicked those observed in CD, but these patients did not progress to overt CD on long-term follow-up. [10] A recent study by Chang et al. reported that the proportion of patients with ulcerations <5 mm in diameter was not significantly different between the 60 patients showing isolated terminal ileal ulcerations resolution without treatment and the 31 patients with continued isolated terminal ileal ulcerations on follow-up. [4] Similar to these reports, we found that the numbers of lesions on the initial colonoscopy exams were not related to the ITIL disease outcomes. Similarly, the initial histologic findings were not related to the ITIL disease outcomes. Thus, the endoscopic or histopathological findings may not be useful in predicting the disease outcomes in patients with ITILs.

Irregular bowel movements, pain or bloating may coexist in a considerable number of IBD patients, which were present in 35.4–46% of CD patients and 37.5% (3/8) in this study. [13,14] There is uncertainty as to the aetiology of these apparent functional symptoms in IBD patients. Genetic factors, disordered gut permeability, psychosocial stress, or a persistent increase in TNF-α or mucosal pain receptor in colonic mucosa may contribute to these symptoms. [14–21] A previous study by Keohane et al. found that faecal calprotectin levels were helpful to identify CD patients with IBS-type symptoms. [22] Then, a study by Berrill et al. found a conflicting result. [23] However, a systematic diagnostic approach is required to assess IBD patients with IBS-type symptoms as sub-clinical inflammation may play a role in a proportion of cases. [23]

Calprotectin is an abundant calcium-binding protein that is derived predominantly from neutrophils and, to a lesser extent, from monocytes and reactive macrophages. [24] The presence of calprotectin in faeces is directly proportional to neutrophil migration towards the intestinal tract. [25–27] Two studies by Tibble and Carroccio et al. found that approximately half of patients with active celiac disease had elevated fecal calprotectin concentrations. [28,29] Another study by Berni et al examined a total of 38 children with celiac disease. They found that those patients with active celiac disease had elevated fecal calprotectin concentrations compared with healthy control subjects and that there was a trend toward normal values after 4 weeks of an exclusion diet. [30] However, the specificity for the diagnosis of ITILs should be low, as several diseases such IBD, microscopic colitis, allergic colitis, colorectal neoplasia, gastrointestinal infection and chronic diarrhea can also increase faecal calprotectin. [29,31–34] High concentration of calprotectin in faeces is a strong argument to carry out a colonoscopy in order to rule out the presence of IBD or other organic pathologies. Maybe faecal calprotectin is useful during the follow-up on ITILs.

In conclusion, the results of this study suggest that the ITIL disease outcomes are related to the clinical symptoms. ITILs are likely to develop into CD in patients with abdominal pain but are likely to resolve in patients without abdominal pain. It should be noted that all patients underwent gastroscopy and double contrast small bowel radiography instead of MRI, or videocapsule to evaluate their upper gastrointestinal and small intestinal mucosa, so subtle small bowel lesions may be missed diagnosis in these patients. Our study is limited by the small number of patients. Larger prospective studies are needed to confirm these initial findings. It remains unclear whether ITILs should be treated with 5-aminosalicylates or corticosteroids in patients with abdominal pain. Thus, further randomized, double-blind, placebo-controlled studies in large cohorts of subjects are needed to verify this question.

Author Contributions

Conceived and designed the experiments: ZF HW CY. Performed the experiments: ZF ZW XF. Analyzed the data: ZF HW. Contributed reagents/materials/analysis tools: ZF ZC CY. Wrote the paper: ZF ZC.

References

1. McHugh JB, Appelman HD, McKenna BJ (2007) The diagnostic value of endoscopic terminal ileum biopsies. Am J Gastroenterol 102:1084–1089.
2. Geboes K, Ectors N, D'Haens G, Rutgeerts P (1998) Is ileoscopy with biopsy worthwhile in patients presenting with symptoms of inflammatory bowel disease? Am J Gastroenterol 93:201–206.
3. Geboes K (2007) The strategy for biopsies of the terminal ileum should be evidence based. Am J Gastroenterol 102:1090–1092.
4. Chang HS, Lee D, Kim JC, Song HK, Lee HJ, et al. (2010) Isolated terminal ileal ulcerations in asymptomatic individuals: natural course and clinical significance. Gastrointest Endosc 72:1226–1232.
5. Lengeling RW, Mitros FA, Brennan JA, Schulze KS (2003) Ulcerative ileitis encountered at ileo-colonoscopy: likely role of nonsteroidal agents. Clin Gastroenterol Hepatol 1:160–169.
6. Greaves ML, Pochapin M (2006) Asymptomatic ileitis: past, present, and future. J Clin Gastroenterol 40:281–285.
7. Goldstein NS (2006) Isolated ileal erosions in patients with mildly altered bowel habits. A follow-up study of 28 patients. Am J Clin Pathol 125:838–846.
8. O'Donnell LJD, Virjee J, Heaton KW (1990) Detection of pseudodiarrhea by simple clinical assessment of intestinal transit rate. BMJ 300: 439–440.
9. Longstreth GF, Thompson WG, Chey WD, Houghton LA, Mearin F, Spiller RC (2006) Functional bowel disorders. Gastroenterology 130:1480–1491.
10. Courville EL, Siegel CA, Vay T, Wilcox AR, Suriawinata AA, Srivastava A (2009) Isolated asymptomatic ileitis does not progress to overt Crohn disease on long-term follow-up despite features of chronicity in ileal biopsies. Am J Surg Pathol 33:1341–1347.
11. Hizawa K, Iida M, Kohrogi N, Kuroki F, Yao T, et al. (1994) Crohn disease: early recognition and progress of aphthous lesions. Radiology 190:451–454.
12. Matsumoto T, Iida M, Nakamura S, Hizawa K, Yao T, Fujishima M (2000) Crohn's disease of aphthous type: serial changes in intestinal lesions. Br J Radiol 73:1046–1051.
13. Halpin SJ, Ford AC (2012) Prevalence of symptoms meeting criteria for irritable bowel syndrome in inflammatory bowel disease: systematic review and meta-analysis. Am J Gastroenterol 107:1474–1482.
14. Vivinus-Nébot M, Frin-Mathy G, Bzioueche H, Dainese R, Bernard G, et al. (2013) Functional bowel symptoms in quiescent inflammatory bowel diseases: role of epithelial barrier disruption and low-grade inflammation. Gut [Epub ahead of print]
15. Zucchelli M, Camilleri M, Andreasson AN, Bresso F, Dlugosz A, et al. (2011) Association of TNFSF15 polymorphism with irritable bowel syndrome. Gut 60:1671–1677.
16. Villani AC, Lemire M, Thabane M, Belisle A, Geneau G, et al. (2010) Genetic risk factors for post-infectious irritable bowel syndrome following a waterborne outbreak of gastroenteritis. Gastroenterology 138:1502–1513.
17. Porter CK, Gloor K, Cash BD, Riddle MS (2011) Risk of functional gastrointestinal disorders in U.S. military following self-reported diarrhea and vomiting during deployment. Dig Dis Sci 56:3262–3269.
18. Zhou Q, Zhang B, Verne GN (2009) Intestinal membrane permeability and hypersensitivity in the irritable bowel syndrome. Pain 146:41–46.
19. Singh S, Graff LA, Bernstein CN (2009) Do NSAIDs, antibiotics, infections, or stress trigger flares in IBD? Am J Gastroenterol 104:1298–1313.
20. Spiller R, Garsed K (2009) Postinfectious irritable bowel syndrome. Gastroenterology 136:1979–1988.
21. Akbar A, Yiangou Y, Facer P, Brydon WG, Walters JR, et al. (2010) Expression of the TRPV1 receptor differs in quiescent inflammatory bowel disease with or without abdominal pain. Gut 59:767–774.
22. Keohane J, O'Mahony C, O'Mahony L, O'Mahony S, Quigley EM, Shanahan F (2010) Irritable bowel syndrome-type symptoms in patients with inflammatory bowel disease: a real association or reflection of occult inflammation? Am J Gastroenterol 105:1788, 1789–1794.
23. Berrill JW, Green JT, Hood K, Campbell AK (2013) Symptoms of irritable bowel syndrome in patients with inflammatory bowel disease: examining the role of sub-clinical inflammation and the impact on clinical assessment of disease activity. Aliment Pharmacol Ther 38:44–51.
24. Bjerke K, Halstensen TS, Jahnsen F, Pulford K, Brandtzaeg P (1993) Distribution of macrophages and granulocytes expressing L1 protein (calprotectin) in human Peyer's patches compared with normal ileal lamina propria and mesenteric lymph nodes. Gut 34:1357–1363.
25. Vermeire S, Van Assche G, Rutgeerts P (2006) Laboratory markers in IBD: useful, magic, or unnecessary toys? Gut 55:426–431.
26. Vermeire S, Van Assche G, Rutgeerts P (2004) C-reactive protein as a marker for inflammatory bowel disease. Inflamm Bowel Dis 10:661–665.
27. Vermeire S, Van Assche G, Rutgeerts P (2005) The role of C-reactive protein as an inflammatory marker in gastrointestinal diseases. Nat Clin Pract Gastroenterol Hepatol 2:580–586.
28. Tibble JA, Sigthorsson G, Foster R, Forgacs I, Bjarnason I (2002) Use of surrogate markers of inflammation and Rome criteria to distinguish organic from nonorganic intestinal disease. Gastroenterology 123:450–460.
29. Carroccio A, Iacono G, Cottone M, Di Prima L, Cartabellotta Fe, et al. (2003) Diagnostic accuracy of fecal calprotectin assay in distinguishing organic causes of chronic diarrhea from irritable bowel syndrome: a prospective study in adults and children. Clin Chem 49(6 Pt 1):861–867.
30. Berni Canani R, Rapacciuolo L, Romano MT, Tanturri de Horatio L, Terrin G, et al. (2004) Diagnostic value of faecal calprotectin in paediatric gastroenterology clinical practice. Dig Liver Dis 36:467–470.
31. Tibble J, Teahon K, Thjodleifsson B, Roseth A, Sigthorsson G, et al. (2000) A simple method for assessing intestinal inflammation in Crohn's disease. Gut 47:506–513.

32. Stavlo PL, Libsch KD, Rodeberg DA, Moir CR (2003) Pediatric ileal pouch-anal anastomosis: functional outcomes and quality of life. J Pediatr Surg 38:935–939.
33. Limburg PJ, Ahlquist DA, Sandborn WJ, Mahoney DW, Devens ME, et al. (2000) Fecal calprotectin levels predict colorectal inflammation among patients with chronic diarrhea referred for colonoscopy. Am J Gastroenterol 95:2831–2837.
34. Gisbert JP, McNicholl AG (2009) Questions and answers on the role of faecal calprotectin as a biological marker in inflammatory bowel disease. Dig Liver Dis 41:56–66.

21

Gastro-Esophageal Reflux Disease Symptoms and Demographic Factors as a Pre-Screening Tool for Barrett's Esophagus

Xinxue Liu[1], Angela Wong[1], Sudarshan R. Kadri[1], Andrej Corovic[1], Maria O'Donovan[2], Pierre Lao-Sirieix[1], Laurence B. Lovat[4], Rodney W. Burnham[3], Rebecca C. Fitzgerald[1]*

1 MRC Cancer Unit, University of Cambridge, Cambridge, United Kingdom, **2** Department of Histopathology, Addenbrooke's Hospital, Cambridge, United Kingdom, **3** Queen's Hospital, Romford, Essex, United Kingdom, **4** University College London Hospital (UCLH), London, United Kingdom

Abstract

Background: Barrett's esophagus (BE) occurs as consequence of reflux and is a risk factor for esophageal adenocarcinoma. The current "gold-standard" for diagnosing BE is endoscopy which remains prohibitively expensive and impractical as a population screening tool. We aimed to develop a pre-screening tool to aid decision making for diagnostic referrals.

Methodology/Principal Findings: A prospective (training) cohort of 1603 patients attending for endoscopy was used for identification of risk factors to develop a risk prediction model. Factors associated with BE in the univariate analysis were selected to develop prediction models that were validated in an independent, external cohort of 477 non-BE patients referred for endoscopy with symptoms of reflux or dyspepsia. Two prediction models were developed separately for columnar lined epithelium (CLE) of any length and using a stricter definition of intestinal metaplasia (IM) with segments ≥2 cm with areas under the ROC curves (AUC) of 0.72 (95%CI: 0.67–0.77) and 0.81 (95%CI: 0.76–0.86), respectively. The two prediction models included demographics (age, sex), symptoms (heartburn, acid reflux, chest pain, abdominal pain) and medication for "stomach" symptoms. These two models were validated in the independent cohort with AUCs of 0.61 (95%CI: 0.54–0.68) and 0.64 (95%CI: 0.52–0.77) for CLE and IM≥2 cm, respectively.

Conclusions: We have identified and validated two prediction models for CLE and IM≥2 cm. Both models have fair prediction accuracies and can select out around 20% of individuals unlikely to benefit from investigation for Barrett's esophagus. Such prediction models have the potential to generate useful cost-savings for BE screening among the symptomatic population.

Editor: Wayne A. Phillips, Peter MacCallum Cancer Centre, Australia

Funding: This study was supported by a Medical Research Council grant to Rebecca Fitzgerald, a grant from Barking and Havering R&D Department and by the Cambridge Biomedical Research Centre and Experimental Cancer Research Centre. The BEST2 study used for validation was funded by Cancer Research UK. The funders had no role in study design, data collection and analysis, decision to publish, or preparation of the manuscript.

Competing Interests: Rebecca Fitzgerald has developed the Cytosponge technology which has been licensed to Covidien since this study was completed.

* E-mail: rcf@hutchison-mrc.cam.ac.uk

Introduction

Barrett's esophagus (BE) is a recognized pre-malignant condition in the pathogenesis of esophageal adenocarcinoma (EAC), a malignancy whose incidence in the Western world has increased six-fold over the past 30 years[1] and which carries a five-year mortality in excess of 80% [2–4]. The squamous-to-columnar metaplasia that is the hallmark of BE is thought to confer a survival advantage on cells exposed to chronic gastro-esophageal reflux [5], yet at the expense of an increased risk of progression to esophageal adenocarcinoma [6]. In view of this malignant potential, current endoscopic surveillance programs in patients with known BE aim to identify patients with dysplasia at risk for adenocarcinoma, yet prevalence data would suggest that the vast majority of individuals with this condition remain undiagnosed [7,8]. Several studies have reported risk factors associated with BE including older age [9,10], male gender [9,11,12], Caucasian race [13–15], gastro-esophageal reflux disease (GERD) [10,16,17], smoking [18–20] and central obesity [21,22].

The current "gold-standard" for diagnosing BE is endoscopy, which remains prohibitively expensive and impractical for widespread use. In recent years, novel screening modalities, including trans-nasal endoscopy and a non-endoscopic cell collection device (Cytosponge) coupled with an immuno-marker TFF3, have been suggested as alternatives to standard endoscopy in the diagnosis of BE and have shown promise in early phase studies [23–26]. The Cytosponge comprises a gelatin capsule containing a compressed sponge material attached to a string. The capsule is swallowed and after a few minutes the compressed sponge is released from the capsule which when retrieved, by pulling on the string, collects a large cell sample which can then be processed for a BE specific biomarker TFF3. In a study conducted in primary care the sensitivity and specificity of this approach was 90.0% and 93.5% for detection of intestinal metaplasia (IM) within segments of 2 cm or more [26]. Even if these methods prove highly sensitive and specific for the detection of BE, however, it is unlikely that one would want to screen the entire targeted population. Regardless of the method employed, the "pre-selection" of individuals for further investigation may be one way of maximizing the cost-effectiveness and detection rate of any putative screening program. To achieve the goal of maximizing cost-effectiveness, the "pre-selection" tool needs to have at least three characteristics: 1) low cost; 2) be easy to administer; 3) excellent sensitivity with fair specificity. Therefore, previous studies have investigated the application of a prediction model based on a questionnaire collecting clinical and demographic characteristics to identify those individuals most likely to have BE, thus warranting further endoscopic investigation [27–30]. However, none of the studies have validated their model in another independent prospective cohort study.

In view of recent advances in the development of novel non-endoscopic BE screening modalities, we sought in this study to re-appraise the feasibility of using a prediction model based on demographic characteristics and GERD symptoms as a selection tool to help clinicians decide who should be offered screening. To this end, the primary aim of our prospective study was to investigate the epidemiological factors and symptoms that may predict the presence of BE in a large UK cohort of patients attending upper GI endoscopy. The secondary aim was to develop a pre-screening tool to exclude a subgroup of patients at extremely low risk of having BE from requiring a screening intervention and thus improve the cost-effectiveness of screening.

Materials and Methods

This study was approved by the local ethics committees of Addenbrooke's Hospital, Barking Havering and Redbridge Hospitals, and University College London Hospitals. In the validation cohort, after written informed consent had been obtained, the participants completed a socio-demographic and clinical questionnaire which had an assessment of symptoms, and were then given a Cytosponge screening test.

Study population

Training Cohort. The training cohort was a cross sectional multicentre survey of epidemiological factors predictive of BE in unselected patients between the ages of 18–75, attending an upper gastrointestinal endoscopic examination on clinical grounds between 2001 and 2004. 2171 patients were recruited from Addenbrooke's Hospital, Barking Havering and Redbridge Hospitals, and University College London Hospitals during the study period after approval from the local ethics committee. Informed consent was obtained from each study participant. Exclusion criteria included those with a prior diagnosis of BE or a previous gastrointestinal malignancy. Among the 2171 participants, 252 individuals did not complete the questionnaire and 11 people had missing information on endoscopy results leading to 263 excluded. Furthermore, we excluded 277 participants with known BE undergoing surveillance and 28 patients with a history of cancer as their responses to the questionnaire may be biased by awareness of their health condition. Hence, 1603 were included in the training cohort for analysis.

Validation Cohort. The validation cohort was obtained from a prospective study, called BEST2 whose primary aim is to evaluate the Cytosponge diagnostic device. The study has a case-control design in which cases are patients with known Barrett's oesophagus and controls are unselected patients between the ages of 18–75, with symptoms of reflux or dyspepsia attending an upper gastrointestinal endoscopic examination on clinical grounds. Hence, the control arm is very similar to the training cohort described above. In total, there were 477 participants recruited after approval from the local ethics committee. Informed consent was obtained from each study participant.

Definition of Barrett's esophagus

There is no uniform consensus regarding the definition of BE. The American Gastroenterological Association recommends that IM is required for the diagnosis [31], while the British Society of Gastroenterology does not require IM[32]. There have also been variations in the length of columnar lined segment required in different countries and over time; and it is recognized that with short lengths the reliability coefficients for diagnostic agreement diminish considerably [33]. Therefore, in the current study, two definitions of BE were used. The first one was defined as columnar lined epithelium of esophagus (CLE) of any length reported in the endoscopy report with columnar epithelium on biopsy regardless of whether it was gastric or intestinal in type. The second definition was stricter to minimize any misclassification, and comprised a maximal endoscopic length of BE ≥2 cm with IM confirmed on histopathological assessment (IM≥2 cm). We reported the maximal length of BE in line with the Prague classification. All endoscopists were trained in how to identify the landmarks and the top of the gastric folds was used to identify the gastroesophageal junction.

Questionnaires

The data collected in the training and validation cohorts was broadly similar though they used different questionnaires to collect the information. The questionnaire in the training cohort included 65 questions and was developed based on two validated questionnaires, the gastro-esophageal reflux questionnaire of 80 items[28] and another 27-item GERD symptom questionnaire [27]. In the validation cohort, the GERD symptoms were collected by a questionnaire adapted from the GERD Impact Scale [34]. The last question in the GERD Impact Scale, "How often did you take additional medication other than what the physician told you to take (such as Tums, Rolaids, Maalox)" was adapted to "Are you taking medication for your stomach symptoms". The demographic information was collected at the endoscopy appointment in a semi-structured interview. All the information was captured by an online database specially designed for the study.

Statistical Methods

Fifteen candidate variables which were collected in both cohorts were used to build the prediction model, including 1) demographic factors: age, sex, BMI, ethnic group, education, smoking status, and alcohol consumption; 2) family history: BE and EAC; 3) symptoms: heartburn, acid reflux, chest pain, upper stomach pain, and being woken at night by symptoms; 4) medication for "stomach" symptoms. The associations between the fifteen variables and a diagnosis of BE were tested using the chi-square test for categorical variables, trend test for ordinal variable and t-test for continuous variables. Only those reaching the significance level of 0.05 or borderline significant level of 0.10 were included as potential predictors for model training. A backward logistic regression model was developed based on all the potential predictors to select the final panel for validation. Each predictor in the panel was weighted based on the coefficients from the backward logistic regression model in the training cohort. A risk score was calculated using the weights of each predictor for each patient in the validation cohort. Receiver operating characteristic (ROC) curve was created using the risk scores in the validation

Table 1. Demographic characteristics according to endoscopic BE and pathological BE in the training cohort*.

	CLE			IM≥2 cm		
	BE	**Normal**	**P**	**BE**	**Normal**	**P**
N	182	1421		69	1534	
Age (yrs)	58.1 (12.7)	51.7 (14.2)	<0.001	60.9 (11.9)	52.0 (14.1)	<0.001
BMI (kg/m²)	27.1 (4.2)	26.6 (5.1)	0.21	27.5 (4.5)	26.6 (5.1)	0.16
Ethnic						
Caucasian	128 (11.4%)	996 (88.6%)	0.19	51 (4.5%)	1,073 (95.5%)	0.30
Bangladeshi	32 (13.9%)	198 (86.1%)		11 (4.8%)	219 (95.2%)	
Other	6 (6.7%)	83 (93.3%)		1 (1.1%)	88 (98.9%)	
Sex						
Male	118 (15.1%)	665 (84.9%)	<0.001	46 (5.9%)	737 (94.1%)	0.003
Female	62 (7.6%)	756 (92.4%)		23 (2.8%)	795 (97.2%)	
Education						
High school or less	128 (12.2%)	917 (87.8%)	0.21	50 (4.8%)	995 (95.2%)	0.51
College	29 (11.4%)	225 (88.6%)		10 (3.9%)	244 (96.1%)	
University or higher	16 (7.3%)	203 (92.7%)		8 (3.7%)	211 (96.3%)	
Other	3 (9.4%)	30 (90.6%)		0 (0%)	33 (100.0%)	
Smoking						
Never	59 (10.6%)	500 (89.4%)	0.05	18 (3.2%)	541 (96.8%)	0.05
Former	57 (12.9%)	385 (87.1%)		25 (5.7%)	417 (94.3%)	
Current	26 (7.5%)	322 (92.5%)		9 (2.6%)	339 (97.4%)	
Alcohol drinking						
Non-drinker	18 (8.8%)	186 (91.2%)	0.35	9 (4.4%)	195 (95.6%)	0.74
Drinker	127 (11.0%)	1,024 (89.0%)		45 (3.9%)	1,106 (96.1%)	
Family history of BE						
Yes	3 (16.7%)	15 (83.3%)	0.45	2 (11.1%)	16 (88.9%)	0.18
No	179 (11.3%)	1,406 (88.7%)		67 (4.2%)	1,518 (95.8%)	
Family history of EAC						
Yes	8 (12.7%)	55 (87.3%)	0.73	2 (3.2%)	61 (96.8%)	1.0
No	174 (11.3%)	1366 (88.7%)		67 (4.4%)	1,473 (95.6%)	
Heartburn						
Never	25 (8.4%)	271 (91.6%)	0.007†	9 (3.0%)	287 (97.0%)	0.04†
Sometimes	14 (8.1%)	159 (91.9%)		3 (1.7%)	170 (98.3%)	
Often	46 (10.1%)	410 (89.9%)		18 (3.9%)	438 (96.1%)	
Daily	60 (14.6%)	351 (85.4%)		23 (5.6%)	388 (94.4%)	
Acid flux						
Never	37 (9.1%)	371(90.9%)	0.009†	12 (2.9%)	396 (97.1%)	0.07†
Sometimes	17 (6.3%)	253 (93.7%)		8 (3.0%)	262 (97.0%)	
Often	57 (13.1%)	378 (86.9%)		20 (4.6%)	415 (95.4%)	
Daily	31 (14.0%)	190 (86.0%)		12 (5.4%)	209 (94.6%)	
Chest Pain						
Never	70 (13.0%)	467 (87.0%)	0.03†	29 (5.4%)	508 (94.6%)	0.07†
Mild	31 (9.4%)	299 (90.6%)		10 (3.0%)	320 (97.0%)	
Moderate	35 (10.3%)	305 (89.7%)		10 (2.9%)	330 (97.1%)	
Severe	8 (6.3%)	120 (93.8%)		4 (3.1%)	124 (96.9%)	
Being woken at night by symptoms						
No	86 (11.6%)	654 (88.4%)	0.75	32 (4.3%)	708 (95.7%)	0.97
Yes	96 (11.1%)	767 (88.9%)		37 (4.3%)	826 (95.7%)	
Abdominal pain						
No	59 (16.4%)	301 (83.6%)	<0.001	28 (7.8%)	332 (92.2%)	<0.001

Table 1. Cont.

	CLE			IM≥2 cm		
	BE	Normal	P	BE	Normal	P
Yes	85 (8.7%)	895 (91.3%)		25 (2.6%)	955 (97.4%)	
Anti-reflux medication						
No	47 (7.3%)	597 (92.7%)	<0.001	14 (2.2%)	630 (97.8%)	<0.001
Yes	88 (14.3%)	528 (85.7%)		38 (6.2%)	578 (93.8%)	

*Data shown are mean (SD) for continuous variables and number (percentage) for categorical variables
†P for trend test.

cohort to evaluate the sensitivity and specificity of the prediction model.

All the analyses were performed using SPSS version 19.0 (SPSS Inc, Chicago, IL, USA) and R version 2.15.0.

Results

Demographic factors and GERD symptoms are associated with presence of BE

Among the 1,603 patients in the training cohort analysis, the average age of the cohort was 52.4 years, and the male to female sex ratio was 0.96:1. The prevalence of CLE was 11.4% (182/1603) whereas the prevalence of IM≥2 cm was 4.3% (69/1603). Among the 113 patents not fulfilling the criteria of IM≥2 cm, there were 95 (84.1%) patents without IM and 18 (15.9%) patients with IM<2 cm. Table 1 shows the demographic and clinical characteristics of the study population according to the two different definitions of BE. The associations of all these factors with CLE and IM≥2 cm were similar, except that the associations with acid reflux and chest pain for IM≥2 cm were borderline significant ($p = 0.07$) while both associations were significant for CLE.

Prediction model for BE

All eight factors that reached the significance level of 0.1 (age, sex, smoking, heartburn, acid reflux, chest pain, abdominal pain, medicine for symptoms) in the training cohort were used to build a statistical model by backward logistic regression. To simplify the model for clinical usage, we dichotomized the symptoms that have four categories based on the univariate analysis, including heartburn (Never & Sometimes vs. Often & Daily), acid reflux (Never & Sometimes vs. Often & Daily) and chest pain (No chest pain vs chest pain). Table 2 shows the predictors selected for both

Table 2. The coefficients, weights and odds ratios of selected predictors for BE.

	CLE			IM≥2 cm		
	β	Weight	OR (95%CI)	β	Weight	OR (95%CI)
Age (per 1 yr)	0.025	1	1.03 (1.01–1.04)	0.037	1	1.04 (1.01–1.06)
Sex						
Female	0	0	Ref	0	0	Ref
Male	0.725	29	2.06 (1.37–3.11)	0.679	18	1.97 (1.03–3.79)
Heartburn*						
Never & Sometimes	n/a	n/a	n/a	0	0	Ref
Often & Daily	n/a	n/a	n/a	0.594	16	1.81 (0.87–3.79)
Acid flux*						
Never & Sometimes	0	0	Ref	n/a	n/a	n/a
Often & Daily	0.663	27	1.94 (1.28–2.94)	n/a	n/a	n/a
Chest Pain						
No	0	0	Ref	0	0	Ref
Yes	−0.483	−19	0.62 (0.41–0.93)	−0.552	−15	0.58 (0.30–1.09)
Abdominal pain						
No	0	0	Ref	0	0	Ref
Yes	−0.579	−23	0.56 (0.37–0.85)	−1.125	−30	0.33 (0.17–0.61)
Anti-reflux medication						
No	0	0	Ref	0	0	Ref
Yes	0.784	31	2.19 (1.45–3.32)	1.308	35	3.70 (1.82–7.53)

*n/a: not applicable.

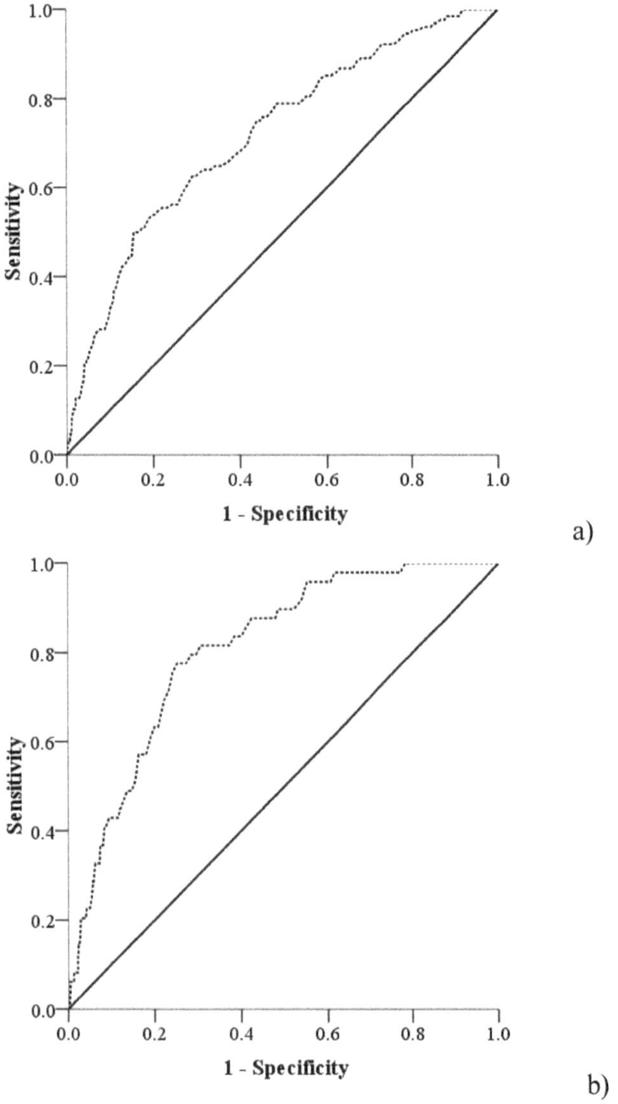

Figure 1. ROC curve for a) endoscopically visible CLE of any length independent of histology (AUC: 0.72), b) segment containing IM≥2 cm (AUC: 0.81) in the training cohort (N = 1603). ROCs curve were developed using the risk scores which are calculated using the weights of different predictors. The weights were developed based on the coefficients of predictors in the backward logistic regression model in the training cohort.

definitions of BE by backward logistic regression models and the weight for each predictor based on the coefficients of the models. The odds ratio and 95%CI for each predictor was also reported. Age, sex, chest pain, abdominal pain and medication for "stomach" symptoms were selected as predictors for both CLE and IM≥2 cm. Heartburn was selected as a predictor for IM≥2 cm only, while acid reflux was selected only for CLE. Internal validation was carried out based on the weights given in Table 2. Risk scores for CLE and IM≥2 cm were calculated separately. For example, the CLE risk score of a 60-year male with symptoms of heartburn, acid reflux, chest pain who has used medications for "stomach" symptoms is: $60\times1+29+27-19+31=128$, while the risk score for IM≥2 cm for that patient is: $60\times1+18+16-15+35=114$. The medians and inter quartile ranges for the risk scores of CLE and IM≥2 cm in the training cohort were 65 (45–87) and 57 (34–79), respectively. The AUCs generated using the risk scores were 0.72 (95%CI: 0.67–0.77) for CLE, and 0.81 (95%CI: 0.76–0.86) for IM≥2 cm (Figure 1).

Table 3. Summary of the predictors for BE in the external validation cohort*.

External validation cohort	
N	477
CLE	67 (14.0%)
IM≥2 cm	21 (4.4%)
Age (yrs)	54.7 (14.7)
Sex(male)	217 (45.5%)
Heartburn	
Never & Sometimes	314 (66.4%)
Often & Daily	159 (33.6%)
Acid reflux	
Never & Sometimes	329 (69.6%)
Often & Daily	144 (30.4%)
Chest Pain	
No	184 (38.9%)
Yes	289 (61.1%)
Abdominal pain	
No	159 (33.6%)
Yes	314 (66.4%)
Anti-reflux medication	
No	188 (39.7%)
Yes	285 (60.3%)

*Data shown are mean (SD) for continuous variables and number (percentage) for categorical variables.

Demographic characteristics of the external validation cohort

Table 3 shows the summary of the predictors for BE in the validation cohort. Among the 477 participants in the external validation cohort, the prevalence of CLE and IM≥2 cm were 13.8% (66/477) and 4.4% (21/477), respectively. There were 45 CLE patients not fulfilling the criteria of IM≥2 cm, including 26 (57.8%) CLE patients without IM and 19 (42.2%) CLE patients with IM but having a segment of BE less than 2 cm. The mean age of the validation cohort was 54.7 years and 45.5% of the patients were male. There was no significant difference in the prevalence of CLE and IM≥2 cm between the training cohort and the validation cohort ($p=0.17$ and $p=1.0$, respectively), while people in the external validation cohort were older than those in the training cohort (mean age: 54.7 yrs vs. 52.4 yrs, $p=0.002$). The sex ratio of male to female in the validation cohort was 0.83:1, which is not significantly different from the training cohort ($p=0.18$).

External validation of the eight factor panel

The risk scores for both CLE and IM≥2 cm were then calculated by the weights of the predictors in each panel for CLE and IM≥2 cm from the training cohort. The median and inter quartile ranges for CLE and IM≥2 cm were 67 (46–89.5) and 60 (40–79.5), respectively. Figure 2 shows the ROC curves for the two BE definitions in the validation cohort. The AUCs were 0.61

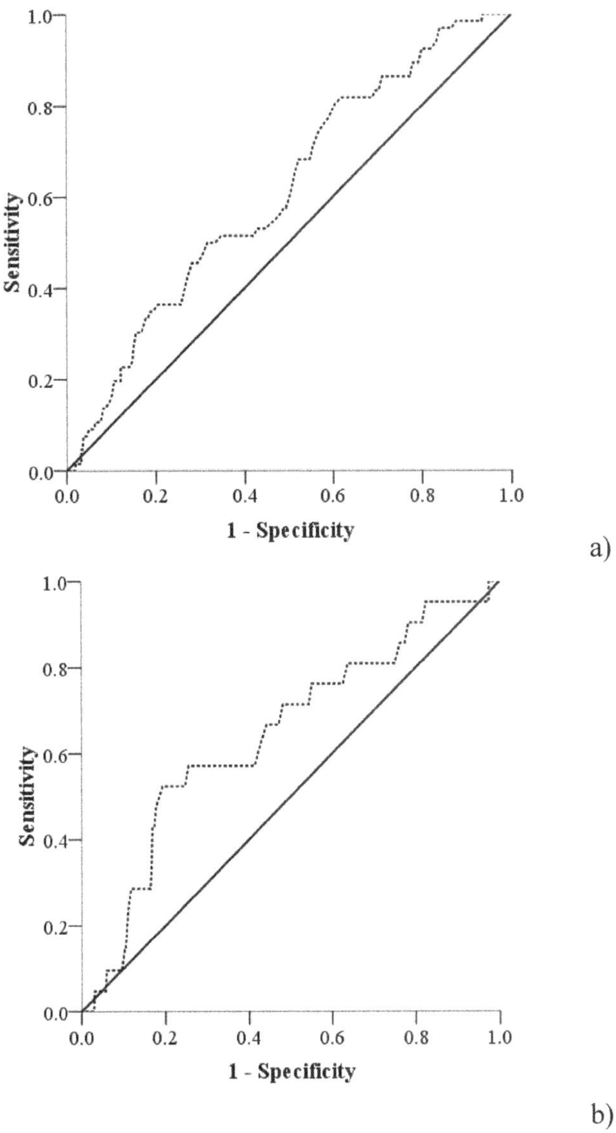

Figure 2. ROC curve for a) endoscopically visible CLE of any length independent of histology (AUC: 0.61), b) segment containing IM≥2 cm (AUC: 0.64) in the external validation cohort (N = 477). ROCs curve were developed using the risk scores which are calculated by the weights of different predictors. The weights were developed based on the coefficients of predictors in the backward logistic regression model in the training cohort.

(95%CI: 0.54–0.68) and 0.64 (95%CI: 0.52–0.77) for CLE and IM≥2 cm, respectively. We used 2000 bootstraps to estimate the specificities of the ROCs in the validation cohort at sensitivities of 90% and 95%. The median specificities were 21% (95%CI: 15%–37%) and 22% (95%CI: 2%–53%) for CLE and IM≥2 cm at sensitivity of 90%, respectively, while at sensitivity of 95%, the median specificities were 17% (95%CI: 11%–25%) and 19% (2%–41%), respectively.

Discussion

In the current study, we set out to develop a pre-screening tool to improve the cost-effectiveness and logistics of screening for BE. We did this by evaluating the associations of demographic factors, symptoms and medication with the presence of BE in a prospective cohort study including 1603 patients. Two different panels were developed in the training cohort for endoscopically identified CLE (any length and with or without IM) and IM≥2 cm, respectively. The panel for CLE included age, sex, chest pain, abdominal pain, medication for "stomach" symptoms and acid reflux, while the panel for IM≥2 cm included the same factors except acid reflux was replaced by heartburn and the weightings given to these factors varied as summarized in Table 2. We then validated the two panels in another independent cohort comprising 477 patients and found that both panels have a fair diagnostic accuracy.

Previous studies have reported a number of risk factors associated with BE, including age [9,10], gender [9,11,12], ethnicity [13–15], GERD [10,16,17], smoking[18–20] and central obesity [9,21,22]. The results in the current study were consistent with previous studies except for smoking, ethnicity and central obesity. Although smoking was significantly associated with BE in the univariate analysis, the association was no longer significant after controlling for other variables and thus the association is very likely confounded by other factors. Since the current study did not collect the information on waist and hip circumference, we cannot evaluate the association with central obesity. We did not find a significant association with ethnicity. The possible explanation is that there were only a small percentage of patients with self-reported ethnicities other than Caucasian and Bangladeshi. In this study, we found Bangladeshi patients living in the UK have a similar prevalence of BE compared to Caucasian patients, which was about twice as much as the prevalence seen in other ethnic patients. To our best knowledge, this is the first study reporting a high prevalence of BE in Bangladeshi patients.

Table S1 shows a summary of four previous studies which aimed to use a questionnaire to predict BE [27–30]. Although the target populations, BE definitions and hence the prevalence of BE were different between the current study and previous studies, the prediction panel was similar, and included a combination of demographic factors, GERD symptoms and anti-reflux medication. In addition, the accuracy of the prediction panels in the training cohort of our current study is similar to the previous studies, in which the AUCs were between 0.70–0.76 (Table S1). However, neither Gerson *et al.* nor Locke *et al.* nor Rubenstein *et al.* validated their panel in another independent cohort. It is likely that the diagnostic accuracy will drop significantly in validation cohorts because of over-fitting of the model in the training dataset. Although Thrift *et al.* validated their panel in another independent study, both the training and the validation datasets in their study used a retrospective case-control design. Moreover, in this study, all patients were interviewed after the endoscopy examination, which may have introduced recall bias [29]. The strengths of the current study are that we developed the prediction panels based on a prospective unselected cohort referred for endoscopy, and further validated the panels in another similar prospective cohort referred for endoscopy. In addition, we collected all the information before the endoscopy in both training and validation cohorts.

Whether or not to screen for BE has been a subject of intense debate. Currently, both the British Society of Gastroenterology (BSG) and the American Gastroenterological Association (AGA) guidelines recommend against routine endoscopic screening of individuals with GERD due to the low incidence of esophageal cancer in BE and the high cost and side effect of endoscopy [31,32,35]. In addition, several studies have concluded that identification and surveillance for BE patients has minimal public health impact on esophageal adenocarcinoma, and this is at least in part because the vast majority of esophageal adenocarcinomas are diagnosed in patients who did not have a prior diagnosis of BE [36,37]. On the other hand, surveillance-detected cancers and cancers with a previous diagnosis of BE are associated with earlier stage and have a better prognosis compared to those presenting *de novo*, although evidence from randomized trials is lacking [35,38,39]. It is likely that a large group of BE patients are undiagnosed because they do not meet the indications for endoscopy. Furthermore, the possibility of using lower cost non-endoscopic screening tools [26] and the advent of endoscopic techniques to treat early cancer means that the time is ripe to reconsider screening [40].

Whilst far from perfect the panels developed in our study have a similar accuracy to those reported in previous studies (Table S1). As a pre-screening tool, the panels are low cost and easy to perform. Most importantly, the panels can identify 95% of BE patients for further investigation while saving unnecessary screening for around 20% of patients who at endoscopy are subsequently found not to have BE. Figure S1 shows a flowchart outlining the proposed use of the panel as a pre-screening tool before screening. To give some idea of the implications of such a pre-screening tool, we built cost-effective models based on the following assumptions: 1) the population size is 100,000; 2) the starting age for screening is 40 years and life expectancy is 85 years; 3) surveillance is conducted every three years in BE patients diagnosed by screening [31]; and 4) the progression rate from BE to high grade dysplasia (HGD) or EAC is taken to be 0.38% per year [41]. Table S2 shows the comparison of the number of procedures required before and after the introduction of the panels in populations with a hypothetical prevalence of BE of 1%, 5% and 10%. For example, in the population with the prevalence of BE of 1%, 100,000 screening tests and another 14,229 surveillance tests are needed to diagnose all 157 EACs predicted to occur in the 45 years of follow-up; in contrast by using our panels as a pre-screening tool, only 80,150 screening tests and another 13,584 surveillance tests are needed to detect 95% EAC patients (8 patients missed). The pre-screening tool can be designed as an online tool and the cost of the pre-screening process will be significantly less than the cost of saved procedures. Hence, at 95% sensitivity the introduction of the panel saves 20,565 tests per 100,000 screening population overall or 101 tests to detect one EAC patient. We believe that our panel can be further improved by including central adiposity measurement since it has been reported as a risk factor of BE in several other studies [30,42,43]. In addition, Thrift *et al.* reported that biomarkers, such as circulating serum levels of inflammatory cytokines and leptin can improve the model performance in predicting BE [42]. However, we believe that it may be impractical to add biomarkers to a pre-screening panel given the cost and logistical considerations for biomarker measurement.

There are several limitations to the current study. First of all, the questionnaire used in the training cohort was developed based on two previous published studies and was not independently validated, but the effect on our study results was limited as the previous studies have validated the questionnaires. Secondly, in the current study, we used a slightly different questionnaire in the training cohort compared with the validation cohort. However, to minimize any effect on the validation and simplify the clinical usage of the panels, we dichotomized the symptoms.

In conclusion, we have demonstrated that prediction models which incorporate demographics, symptoms and medication for "stomach" symptoms can predict the prevalence of BE with high sensitivity and fair specificity to a range within the intended aims of this study. Hence, the models have the potential to be used as a pre-screening tool to avoid around 20% of patients having unnecessary investigations and thus pre-select a more relevant population of patients to have a diagnostic test for BE such as trans-nasal endoscopy or the Cytosponge.

Supporting Information

Figure S1 Application of our panels as a pre-screening tool before endoscopy or other screening test.

Table S1 Summary of all the studies aiming to predict the presence of BE by questionnaire.

Table S2 Comparison of the cost-effectiveness before and after the application of a prediction model as a pre-screening tool in three simulated populations.

Acknowledgments

We would like to thank staff and participants from Addenbrooke's Hospital, Barking Havering and Redbridge Hospitals, and University College London Hospitals for making this study possible. We would also like to thank all the participants of BEST2 study.

Author Contributions

Conceived and designed the experiments: XL AW RCF. Performed the experiments: AW. Analyzed the data: XL. Wrote the paper: XL AC RCF. Inputted data: AW PLS SRK AC. Provided expert histopathological diagnosis: MO. Managed patient recruitment: AW SRK RWB. Oversaw patient recruitment: LL.

References

1. Pohl H, Sirovich B, Welch HG (2010) Esophageal Adenocarcinoma Incidence: Are We Reaching the Peak? Cancer Epidem Biomar 19: 1468–1470.
2. Cancer Research UK. Oesophageal cancer survival statistics.
3. Natinal Cancer Institute. Surveillance Epidemiology and End Results Stat Fact Sheets: Esophagus.
4. Eloubeidi MA, Mason AC, Desmond RA, El-Serag HB (2003) Temporal trends (1973–1997) in survival of patients with esophageal adenocarcinoma in the United States: a glimmer of hope? Am J Gastroenterol 98: 1627–1633.
5. Quante M, Bhagat G, Abrams JA, Marache F, Good P, et al. (2012) Bile acid and inflammation activate gastric cardia stem cells in a mouse model of Barrett-like metaplasia. Cancer Cell 21: 36–51.
6. Lagergren J (2005) Adenocarcinoma of oesophagus: what exactly is the size of the problem and who is at risk? Gut 54 Suppl 1: i1–5.
7. Ronkainen J, Aro P, Storskrubb T, Johansson SE, Lind T, et al. (2005) Prevalence of Barrett's esophagus in the general population: an endoscopic study. Gastroenterology 129: 1825–1831.
8. Zagari RM, Fuccio L, Wallander MA, Johansson S, Fiocca R, et al. (2008) Gastro-oesophageal reflux symptoms, oesophagitis and Barrett's oesophagus in the general population: the Loiano-Monghidoro study. Gut 57: 1354–1359.
9. Edelstein ZR, Bronner MP, Rosen SN, Vaughan TL (2009) Risk factors for Barrett's esophagus among patients with gastroesophageal reflux disease: a community clinic-based case-control study. Am J Gastroenterol 104: 834–842.
10. Eloubeidi MA, Provenzale D (2001) Clinical and demographic predictors of Barrett's esophagus among patients with gastroesophageal reflux disease - A multivariable analysis in veterans. Journal of Clinical Gastroenterology 33: 306–309.
11. Ford AC, Forman D, Reynolds PD, Cooper BT, Moayyedi P (2005) Ethnicity, gender, and socioeconomic status as risk factors for esophagitis and Barrett's esophagus. Am J Epidemiol 162: 454–460.
12. Ward EM, Wolfsen HC, Achem SR, Loeb DS, Krishna M, et al. (2006) Barrett's esophagus is common in older men and women undergoing screening colonoscopy regardless of reflux symptoms. Am J Gastroenterol 101: 12–17.

13. Spechler SJ, Jain SK, Tendler DA, Parker RA (2002) Racial differences in the frequency of symptoms and complications of gastro-oesophageal reflux disease. Aliment Pharmacol Ther 16: 1795–1800.
14. Thukkani N, Sonnenberg A (2010) The influence of environmental risk factors in hospitalization for gastro-oesophageal reflux disease-related diagnoses in the United States. Aliment Pharmacol Ther 31: 852–861.
15. Wang A, Mattek NC, Holub JL, Lieberman DA, Eisen GM (2009) Prevalence of complicated gastroesophageal reflux disease and Barrett's esophagus among racial groups in a multi-center consortium. Dig Dis Sci 54: 964–971.
16. Anderson LA, Watson RG, Murphy SJ, Johnston BT, Comber H, et al. (2007) Risk factors for Barrett's oesophagus and oesophageal adenocarcinoma: results from the FINBAR study. World J Gastroenterol 13: 1585–1594.
17. Abrams JA, Fields S, Lightdale CJ, Neugut AI (2008) Racial and ethnic disparities in the prevalence of Barrett's esophagus among patients who undergo upper endoscopy. Clin Gastroenterol Hepatol 6: 30–34.
18. Johansson J, Hakansson HO, Mellblom L, Kempas A, Johansson KE, et al. (2007) Risk factors for Barrett's oesophagus: a population-based approach. Scand J Gastroenterol 42: 148–156.
19. Smith KJ, O'Brien SM, Green AC, Webb PM, Whiteman DC (2009) Current and past smoking significantly increase risk for Barrett's esophagus. Clin Gastroenterol Hepatol 7: 840–848.
20. Steevens J, Schouten LJ, Driessen AL, Huysentruyt CJ, Keulemans YC, et al. (2011) A prospective cohort study on overweight, smoking, alcohol consumption, and risk of Barrett's esophagus. Cancer Epidemiol Biomarkers Prev 20: 345–358.
21. Corley DA, Kubo A, Levin TR, Block G, Habel L, et al. (2007) Abdominal obesity and body mass index as risk factors for Barrett's esophagus. Gastroenterology 133: 34–41.
22. Edelstein ZR, Farrow DC, Bronner MP, Rosen SN, Vaughan TL (2007) Central adiposity and risk of Barrett's esophagus. Gastroenterology 133: 403–411.
23. Peery AF, Hoppo T, Garman KS, Dellon ES, Daugherty N, et al. (2012) Feasibility, safety, acceptability, and yield of office-based, screening transnasal esophagoscopy (with video). Gastrointest Endosc 75: 945–953 e942.
24. Shariff MK, Bird-Lieberman EL, O'Donovan M, Abdullahi Z, Liu X, et al. (2012) Randomized crossover study comparing efficacy of transnasal endoscopy with that of standard endoscopy to detect Barrett's esophagus. Gastrointest Endosc 75: 954–961.
25. Lao-Sirieix P, Boussioutas A, Kadri SR, O'Donovan M, Debiram I, et al. (2009) Non-endoscopic screening biomarkers for Barrett's oesophagus: from micro-array analysis to the clinic. Gut 58: 1451–1459.
26. Kadri SR, Lao-Sirieix P, O'Donovan M, Debiram I, Das M, et al. (2010) Acceptability and accuracy of a non-endoscopic screening test for Barrett's oesophagus in primary care: cohort study. BMJ 341: c4372.
27. Gerson LB, Edson R, Lavori PW, Triadafilopoulos G (2001) Use of a simple symptom questionnaire to predict Barrett's esophagus in patients with symptoms of gastroesophageal reflux. Am J Gastroenterol 96: 2005–2012.
28. Locke GR, Zinsmeister AR, Talley NJ (2003) Can symptoms predict endoscopic findings in GERD? Gastrointest Endosc 58: 661–670.
29. Thrift AP, Kendall BJ, Pandeya N, Vaughan TL, Whiteman DC (2012) A Clinical Risk Prediction Model for Barrett Esophagus. Cancer Prev Res (Phila).
30. Rubenstein JH, Morgenstern H, Appelman H, Scheiman J, Schoenfeld P, et al. (2012) Prediction of Barrett's Esophagus Among Men. Am J Gastroenterol 108: 353–362.
31. Spechler SJ, Sharma P, Souza RF, Inadomi JM, Shaheen NJ (2011) American Gastroenterological Association medical position statement on the management of Barrett's esophagus. Gastroenterology 140: 1084–1091.
32. Fitzgerald RC, di Pietro M, Ragunath K, Ang Y, Kang JY, et al. (2014) British Society of Gastroenterology guidelines on the diagnosis and management of Barrett's oesophagus. Gut 63: 7–42.
33. Vahabzadeh B, Seetharam AB, Cook MB, Wani S, Rastogi A, et al. (2012) Validation of the Prague C & M criteria for the endoscopic grading of Barrett's esophagus by gastroenterology trainees: a multicenter study. Gastrointest Endosc 75: 236–241.
34. Jones R, Coyne K, Wiklund I (2007) The gastro-oesophageal reflux disease impact scale: a patient management tool for primary care. Aliment Pharm Therap 25: 1451–1459.
35. Spechler SJ, Sharma P, Souza RF, Inadomi JM, Shaheen NJ (2011) American Gastroenterological Association Technical Review on the Management of Barrett's Esophagus. Gastroenterology 140: E18–E52.
36. Dulai GS, Guha S, Kahn KL, Gornbein J, Weinstein WM (2002) Preoperative prevalence of Barrett's esophagus in esophageal adenocarcinoma: a systematic review. Gastroenterology 122: 26–33.
37. Reid BJ, Li X, Galipeau PC, Vaughan TL (2010) Barrett's oesophagus and oesophageal adenocarcinoma: time for a new synthesis. Nat Rev Cancer 10: 87–101.
38. Wang KK, Sampliner RE (2008) Updated guidelines 2008 for the diagnosis, surveillance and therapy of Barrett's esophagus. Am J Gastroenterol 103: 788–797.
39. Cooper GS, Kou TD, Chak A (2009) Receipt of Previous Diagnoses and Endoscopy and Outcome From Esophageal Adenocarcinoma: A Population-Based Study With Temporal Trends. American Journal of Gastroenterology 104: 1356–1362.
40. Lao-Sirieix P, Fitzgerald RC (2012) Screening for oesophageal cancer. Nat Rev Clin Oncol 9: 278–287.
41. Bhat S, Coleman HG, Yousef F, Johnston BT, McManus DT, et al. (2011) Risk of malignant progression in Barrett's esophagus patients: results from a large population-based study. J Natl Cancer Inst 103: 1049–1057.
42. Thrift AP, Garcia JM, El-Serag HB (2013) A Multibiomarker Risk Score Helps Predict Risk for Barrett's Esophagus. Clin Gastroenterol Hepatol.
43. Thrift AP, Kramer JR, Alsarraj A, El-Serag HB (2014) Fat Mass by Bioelectrical Impedance Analysis is not Associated With Increased Risk of Barrett Esophagus. J Clin Gastroenterol 48: 218–223.

22

The Duration of Gastrointestinal and Joint Symptoms after a Large Waterborne Outbreak of Gastroenteritis in Finland in 2007 – A Questionnaire-Based 15-Month Follow-Up Study

Janne Laine[1,2*¶], Jukka Lumio[3], Salla Toikkanen[2], Mikko J. Virtanen[2], Terhi Uotila[1], Markku Korpela[1,3], Eila Kujansuu[4¤], Markku Kuusi[2]

1 Tampere University Hospital, Department of Internal Medicine, Tampere, Finland, **2** National Institute of Health and Welfare, Epidemiologic Surveillance and Response Unit, Helsinki, Finland, **3** University of Tampere, School of Medicine, Tampere, Finland, **4** Nokia Health Centre, Nokia, Finland

Abstract

An extensive drinking water-associated gastroenteritis outbreak took place in the town of Nokia in Southern Finland in 2007. 53% of the exposed came down with gastroenteritis and 7% had arthritis-like symptoms (joint swelling, redness, warmth or pain in movement) according to a population-based questionnaire study at 8 weeks after the incident. *Campylobacter* and norovirus were the main pathogens. A follow-up questionnaire study was carried out 15 months after the outbreak to evaluate the duration of gastrointestinal and joint symptoms. 323 residents of the original contaminated area were included. The response rate was 53%. Participants were inquired about having gastroenteritis during the outbreak and the duration of symptoms. Of those with gastroenteritis, 43% reported loose stools and abdominal pain or distension after the acute disease. The prevalence of symptoms declined promptly during the first 3 months but at 15 months, 11% reported continuing symptoms. 32% of the respondents with gastroenteritis reported subsequent arthritis-like symptoms. The disappearance of arthritis-like symptoms was more gradual and they levelled off only after 5 months. 19% showed symptoms at 15 months. Prolonged gastrointestinal symptoms correlated to prolonged arthritis-like symptoms. High proportion of respondents continued to have arthritis-like symptoms at 15 months after the epidemic. The gastrointestinal symptoms, instead, had declined to a low level.

Editor: Oliver Schildgen, Kliniken der Stadt Köln gGmbH, Germany

Funding: This study was financially supported by the Competitive Research Funding of the Tampere University Hospital (Grants 9E129 and 9M124). The funders had no role in study design, data collection and analysis, decision to publish, or preparation of the manuscript.

Competing Interests: The authors have declared that no competing interests exist.

* E-mail: janne.laine@pshp.fi

¤ Current address: Department of Social Services and Health Care, Tampere, Finland

¶ The Pirkanmaa Waterborne Outbreak Study Group: Jaakko Antonen[1,3], Pekka Collin[1,3], Tina Katto[1], Anna-Leena Kuusela [1,3], Sami Mustajoki[1], Jukka Mustonen[1,3], Heikki Oksa[1,3], Petri Ruutu[2] and Sirpa Räsänen[1]

Introduction

Although acute gastroenteritis is a common disease, little is known about its consequences after passing the acute phase of the disease. As nearly everyone meets episodes of acute gastroenteritis occasionally, the possible connection with later health problems is easily missed. Food- and waterborne epidemics give special opportunity to study this connection prospectively as a cohort of people is infected in a relatively short period, often with identified pathogens. Epidemics large enough to conduct a study are, however, uncommon in developed countries with a good level of investigation capabilities.

Reactive arthritis (ReA) and milder forms of joint complaints are well known and fairly common acute complications of bacterial gastroenteritis [1]. There is also growing evidence of increased incidence of irritable bowel syndrome (IBS) after bacterial [2,3] and possibly viral [4] gastroenteritis. The most intensively studied waterborne outbreak is the Walkerton epidemic in Ontario, Canada. According to the Walkerton Health Study, increased risk of reactive arthritis, irritable bowel syndrome, pregnancy-related hypertension, hypertension, kidney disease, and even cardiovascular events has been observed after the epidemic [5,6,7,8,9,10].

A large drinking-waterborne epidemic occurred in a Finnish town Nokia in November–December 2007. Shortly after the incident, a comprehensive outbreak investigation of short- and long-term health effects was initiated. Details on the epidemiology, microbial findings, and early arthritic complaints have been published previously [11,12,13,14,15]. We performed a questionnaire study at 15 months after the exposure to contaminated water to observe the duration of symptoms and the remaining health complaints at 15 months after the incident. Here, we present data on the persistence of gastrointestinal and joint symptoms after the outbreak.

Methods

Setting

The town of Nokia is located in Southern Finland and has a population of 30 000. At the end of November 2007, maintenance work was carried out in the town's wastewater plant. During the work, a valve connecting the wastewater plant's effluent line and household water distribution line was opened and it was accidentally left open for two days. Approximately 450 m^3 of plant's effluent water contaminated the drinking water of 9 500 residents. This resulted in a large gastroenteritis outbreak in the contaminated area of the town. Some excess morbidity was also detected in the uncontaminated area [11]. The epidemic peaked four days after the incident, and most gastroenteritis cases occurred within two weeks.

Seven pathogens were found from the patients' stools. Six of those were also detected from tap water or water-distribution network samples. *Campylobacter* was the most common pathogen found in 27% (N = 148) of stool samples. In addition, norovirus was also considered as a major pathogen [16]. Non-typhoidal *Salmonellae* and *Giardiae* [13] were detected in less number of samples. In a study focusing on children with gastroenteritis, other viruses and infections with mixed pathogens were also observed [12].

According to a population-based questionnaire survey performed eight weeks after the incident 53% of the population in the contaminated area reported falling ill with gastroenteritis and 6.7% reported having arthritis-like joint symptoms [15]. In spite of active encouragement to refer new cases of probable arthritis to a rheumatologist at the local university hospital, only 21 confirmed cases of ReA were detected [14].

Questionnaire studies

Two consecutive questionnaires were mailed 13 months apart. The first was mailed eight weeks after the incident to detect the immediate morbidity [15]. The second, a follow-up study, was performed fifteen months after the outbreak in order to study the persistence of gastrointestinal and joint symptoms.

Details of the first questionnaire at 8 weeks were presented in previous articles [11,15]. In brief, two target populations were defined from Nokia; those residing in the part of town with contaminated water supply ("contaminated group") and those residing in the uncontaminated area ("uncontaminated group"). A third group ("control group") was chosen among the citizens of another municipality in the same district. Approximately, 1000 participants were randomly picked from the national population registry for each group (Table 1). All the ages were included and the groups were matched for age and gender. Only one participant per household was allowed.

The second questionnaire at 15 months ("follow-up") was mailed to persons who had participated in the first survey and given their consent for being contacted again. Therefore, the groups became smaller (Table 1.). No reminder was mailed to those who did not respond. Participants were asked whether they had gastroenteritis during the outbreak period (from November 28 to December 31 2007). They were also asked for how long (weeks or months) abdominal or joint symptoms persisted after the acute gastroenteritis.

Gastrointestinal symptoms, such as the presence of loose stools, constipation, nausea, abdominal pain, and abdominal distension were recorded. After analyzing these symptoms separately, a combination of gastrointestinal symptoms was created to observe IBS-like symptoms, such as loose stools and abdominal pain or distension. This combination is close to the Manning 3 and/or Rome I IBS-criteria [17].

Of joint symptoms, joint pain, pain in joint movement and the presence of swelling, redness, or warmth of the joint were recorded. The condition was classified as arthritis-like if pain in joint movement or any of the symptoms of joint swelling, redness, or warmth was present as defined in our previous study of early joint symptoms [15].

The persistence of gastrointestinal and arthritis-like symptoms was then analyzed as the remaining prevalence of a symptom in the course of time among those who had declared as having had gastroenteritis during the epidemic.

Use of microbiological data

Data of the stool specimens sent for microbiological analysis were obtained from the database of the Fimlab laboratories. This institution is a district-wide and public-run clinical laboratory serving the entire public health-care sector in the district. From year 2005 to 2009, the quantity, dates, and microbiological findings among the residents of Nokia and the control municipality were collected for comparison.

Statistical methods

Completed forms were stored in a database and analysed in the National Institute of Health and Welfare. Estimation of the effect of selection was done in two steps. First, the probability to be included in the study (i.e., those who gave permission to be contacted again) within all the initial study subjects was estimated by using univariate logistic regression. Secondly, the probability of returning the questionnaire within the included subjects was estimated in a similar manner. Confidence intervals for the proportion of subjects continuing to have symptoms at each time point were calculated by using ordinary bootstrap. All analyses were done with R version 2.15.2.

Ethical considerations

When answering the first questionnaire, participants were asked whether they would accept a follow-up contact. An informed consent was attached in the second questionnaire. The follow-up study was approved by the ethical committee of the Tampere University Hospital.

Results

Response rates and selection

Answer on the first questionnaire was received from 808 (79%) persons of the contaminated group, 717 (73%) of the uncontaminated group and 598 (60%) of the control group (Table 1). Taking all groups together, 667 (31.4%) of those responding declined the request for further contact. Response rates to the follow-up questionnaire were 53% (323/615), 46% (230/498), and 54% (186/343), respectively.

The odds ratios (ORs) for probability to be included in the follow-up questionnaire (i.e., giving permission to be contacted again) were 1.2 (95% CI 1.0–1.5) for the female gender, 1.7 (1.3–2.1) for those who had reported gastroenteritis and 1.7 (1.3–2.2) for those reporting joint symptoms in the first questionnaire. For these features the ORs for responding to the follow-up questionnaire were 1.1 (0.9–1.3), 1.0 (0.8–1.2) and 1.03 (0.8–1.3), respectively.

Of those participating in the follow-up study, 54% (174/323) in the contaminated group, 13% (31/230) in the uncontaminated group, and 3% (6/186) in the control group reported that they had gastroenteritis during the outbreak.

Table 1. Evolution of the study groups in the follow-up study.

	Nokia, contaminated	Nokia, uncontaminated	Control population
Population 2007	9 538	20 478	27 259
Size of the study groups in the first study	1 021	979	1 000
Responded to the first study	808	717	598
Sample size in the follow-up study (i.e., those who gave permission to be contacted again)	615	498	343
Responded to the follow-up study	323	230	186
Gastroenteritis during the epidemic, according to the follow-up study	174		

Study groups were based on the original population samples that were used in the first survey. The study groups became step-wise smaller because of lack of response to the first survey, denying further contact, and lack of response to the follow-up survey.

Gastrointestinal symptoms

Of the 174 persons in the contaminated group who had gastroenteritis, 53.6% (93) reported continuing loose stools, 47.9% (83) abdominal pain, and 32.7% (57) abdominal distension after the acute disease. 42.7% (74) experienced loose stools and abdominal pain or distension in the beginning of the follow-up (Figure 1). After a rapid decrease in the proportion of symptomatic persons in one month, the decline started to level off. At 15 months, 10.9% (19) of the respondents continued to have loose stools and abdominal pain or distension. This figure was 11.5% for adults 16 years of age or older and 8.9% for children.

Arthritis-like symptoms

Among the 174 participants in the contaminated group who had experienced gastroenteritis, 31.8% (55/174) reported arthritis-like symptoms after acute gastroenteritis. The proportion of persons with arthritis-like symptoms declined more slowly over time than the corresponding proportion with gastrointestinal symptoms (Figure 1). At 15 months, 19.0% (33/174) reported as continuing to have arthritis-like symptoms. The persistence of gastrointestinal symptoms (loose stools and abdominal pain or distension) predicted the presence of arthritis-like symptoms at 3 and 15 months (Table 2).

Use of microbiological tests

In Nokia, a sharp peak in the number of microbiological stool specimens was observed during the outbreak. Thereafter, the number of specimens diminished gradually and reached the pre-outbreak level in six months. In Nokia, the incidence of positive findings was high during the outbreak and for two months thereafter, but no difference was observed compared to the control municipality after one month (Figure 2).

Discussion

The faecal contamination of household water and the subsequent large epidemic of gastroenteritis was an exceptional accident [11]. The contamination was extensive as over half of the exposed population became ill. A remarkable proportion of the population suffered also from joint symptoms within the following eight weeks [15]. Two questionnaire surveys done thirteen months apart, based on representative population samples, focused on short- and long-term health effects of the epidemic. The 15-month follow-up questionnaire study reported here describes the duration of gastrointestinal and arthritis-like symptoms after the epidemic.

53.6% of those having had gastroenteritis during the epidemic reported loose stools and abdominal pain after the acute disease and 42.7% loose stools and abdominal pain or distension. Although the prevalence decreased rapidly within five months, 10.9% was still having symptoms resembling IBS (loose stools and abdominal pain or distension) at 15 months.

Irritable bowel syndrome (IBS) is a condition characterized by altered bowel function and abdominal pain or discomfort. The studies on the prevalence of symptoms compatible with IBS in the general population have given widely variable figures depending on the definition used. For example, in a population-based Finnish study, the prevalence of IBS ranged from 5.1% to 16.2%, depending on diagnostic criteria [17]. According to a recent systematic review of worldwide IBS-studies, the pooled prevalence of IBS was 11.2% among adult subjects [18].

IBS occurring after an episode of infective gastroenteritis has been referred as post-infectious irritable bowel syndrome (PI-IBS). Generally about 10% of IBS-patients regard that their symptoms began after an infective gastroenteritis [3]. According to a meta-analysis of eight studies published until December 2005, the median prevalence of IBS was 9.8% in the infective gastroenteritis groups and 1.2% in the control groups [19]. The observed frequency of PI-IBS is likely to depend on the pathogen(s) involved. In Walkerton, Canada, the prevalence of IBS was 27.5% among adult subjects who had had gastroenteritis during the epidemic while the prevalence among those without gastroenteritis was 10.1% at 2–3 years after the outbreak [9]. Diarrhoea was found to be a more prominent feature in gastroenteritis-associated IBS than in the case of sporadic IBS. The prognosis of PI-IBS is thought to be better than IBS without infectious onset [3]; however, the condition can still take more than 8 years to resolve as was observed by the Walkerton group [3,20]. If PI-IBS occurs after viral gastroenteritis, it is short lived and rarely lasts for 6 months or longer [4,21].

Commonly used diagnostic criteria for IBS were not utilized in this study. However, abdominal pain or discomfort or distension and loose stools are the principal parts of these criteria. Analyzing these symptoms in such a combination makes it reasonably close to Manning 3 and/or Rome I criteria for IBS. The high prevalence of gastrointestinal symptoms within the first five months after the epidemic in our study may therefore indicate PI-IBS. However, at the end of the follow-up, the prevalence of these symptoms was 11.5% among adults ≥16 years of age. In the population-based study among adults in Finland, the prevalence of IBS was 9.7% according to the Manning 3 criteria [17]. Therefore, the

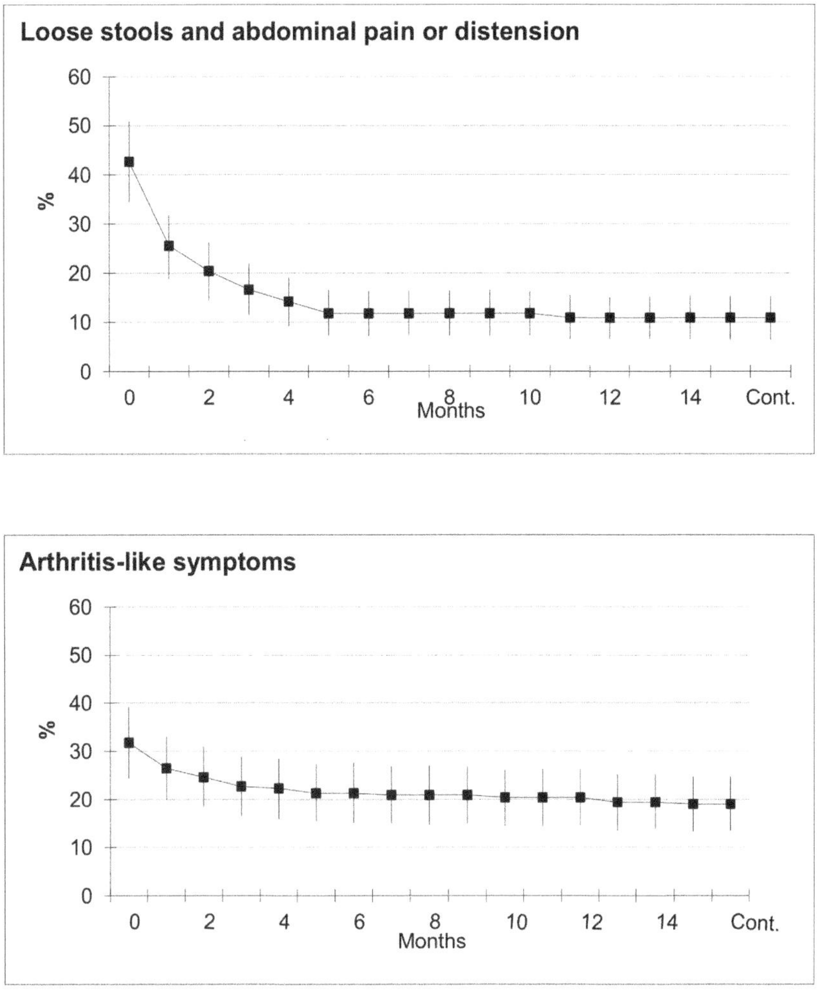

Figure 1. The prevalence of gastrointestinal and arthritis-like symptoms in the contaminated group within fifteen months from the outbreak. The proportions were counted as dividing the number of subjects with symptoms by the number of subjects having fallen ill with gastroenteritis at the time of the outbreak (N = 174). The curves represent the proportion of subjects with symptoms and the vertical lines are the 95% confident intervals.

remaining prevalence of gastrointestinal symptoms in the present study may be close to the natural occurrence of these symptoms.

Other reasons for long-lasting symptoms than PI-IBS must be considered in an epidemic where more than half of the exposed residents fell ill with gastroenteritis caused by mixed pathogens. There may have been prolonged circulation of the pathogens in the population leading to secondary infections. Bacterial stool cultures were extensively examined during the following months in the affected town. No excess frequency of positive findings could be noticed after the peak of the epidemic (Figure 2). This evidence does not support the prolonged circulation of bacterial pathogens in the population. Viral pathogens (especially, norovirus), are highly contagious and could well have started to spread horizontally after the outbreak. Such a possibility could not be excluded reliably because samples for viral diagnostics were not routinely taken during the study period. Giardiasis often causes long-lasting gastrointestinal symptoms. This epidemic was the first domestic *Giardia*-cluster in Finland [13]. The whole population was informed about the possibility of giardiasis and individuals were called for parasitological investigation if they suffered from prolonged symptoms. In spite of that, only 55 cases were found out of the 872 persons tested, a number that is probably too low to solely explain the magnitude of prolonged gastrointestinal symptoms.

As the data relies on self-reported symptoms, psychological factors like anger, anxiety or distress may have influenced the participants' expressions. The connection of psychological factors on the duration of IBS has been observed in epidemics caused by drinking water [20]. The public anger and anxiety in the town of Nokia was considerable for several months after the epidemic.

Table 2. The prevalence of arthritis-like symptoms among participants with and without gastrointestinal symptoms (loose stools and abdominal pain or distension) at 3 and 15 months after the water contamination.

	At 3 months	At 15 months
With gastrointestinal symptoms	54.3% (19/35)	52.2% (12/23)
Without gastrointestinal symptoms	10.9% (6/55)	10.4% (7/67)
p-value	<0.0001	<0.0001

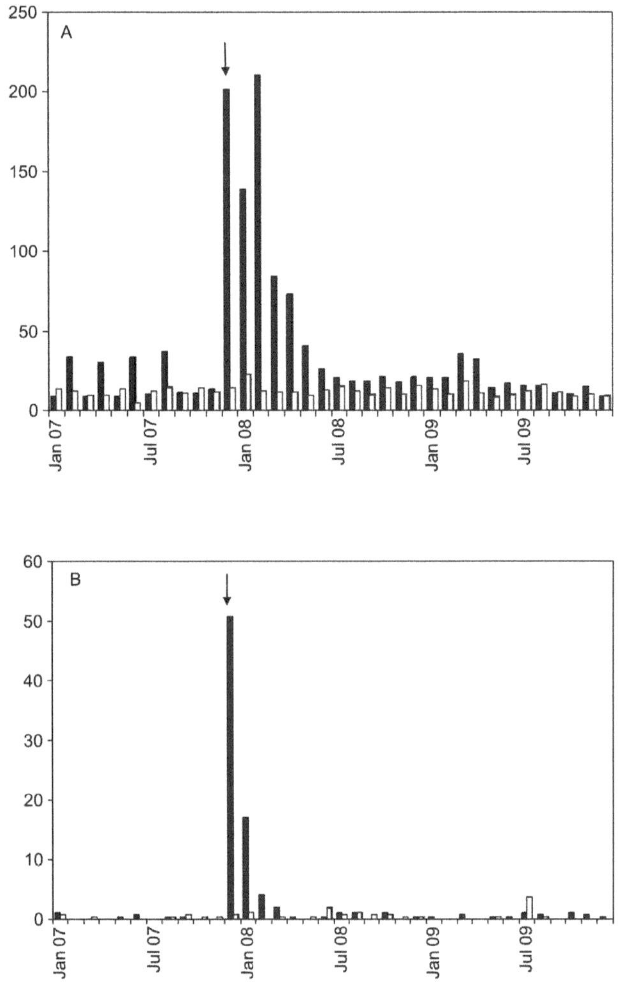

Figure 2. a–b. Monthly incidence (/10 000 inhabitants) of microbiological stool specimens (Fig. 2a) and positive findings (Fig. 2b). Black bars represent the town of Nokia and white bars the control municipality. The arrows indicate the outbreak month, December 2007. Only findings of *Campylobacter* and *Giardia* from January 2007 to December 2009 were counted.

Psychological influences of the incident on health experience will be investigated in another project and reported later.

Previously, we have reported a frequency of 6.7% of arthritis-like symptoms among the participants of the contaminated group within eight weeks from the incident [15]. According to the follow-up study, 31.8% of those who reported having had gastroenteritis during the epidemic announced subsequent arthritis-like symptoms. The explanation for the difference lies in the fact that joint symptoms in the follow-up study were asked for only from those with gastroenteritis and through a selection bias towards those with joint symptoms in the first study.

The arthritis-like symptoms were fairly longstanding. About a third of the symptoms were resolved within five months. Thereafter, the decline was slow and 19% of the respondents were still experiencing arthritis-like symptoms 15 months after the epidemic. In a previously published population-based study of verified ReA cases related to this outbreak, 21 cases of ReA were observed [14], mostly relatively mild cases. According to a follow-up study (one year) of this cohort, over a half of all the patients were still taking analgesics because of ReA symptoms and 33% was on antirheumatic medication [22]. This proportion of residual symptoms among verified ReA-cases is quite well in line with the findings of the present study.

ReA is a well-known complication of bacterial gastroenteritis [1]. *Giardia* has also been associated rarely with ReA [23]. To our knowledge, there are hardly any observations possibly linking rotavirus or norovirus to ReA. Considering this and the microbiological findings, we regard that campylobacter infections probably have been the major trigger of joint symptoms in this epidemic.

There are few population-based studies on the duration of self-reported joint symptoms following gastroenteritis epidemics. The previous literature deals with those fulfilling the criteria for ReA, either according to self-reporting or clinical judgement. In studies done in Finland, the average duration of ReA symptoms has been 3–5 months [1]. Symptoms persisting over six months have often been considered as a sign of chronic disorder. Development to the chronic condition has been reported in 12–16% of the cases [1]. The proportion of subjects with arthritis-like symptoms (19%), after 15 months in this study, is therefore, reasonably well in line with previous observations, especially, since this was a questionnaire study with no clinical verification of the symptoms.

The persistence of gastrointestinal symptoms correlated with the presence of arthritis-like symptoms (Table 2.). As PI-IBS and ReA are inflammatory disorders, pathogenesis of both gastrointestinal and arthritis-like symptoms may have common immunological mechanisms, although the genetic predisposition for these two conditions seems to be different [24].

There are some limitations of this study. First, although the initial sample for the first questionnaire was carefully randomized, there were three subsequent steps in which a selection bias could have taken place. They are responding to the first questionnaire, giving permission to be re-contacted, and finally responding to the follow-up survey (Table 1). The response rates of the first survey were good and the authors concluded that the survey was representative. For the follow-up survey, some selection in sample formation took place, but not any more in responding to the follow-up survey. Those with joint symptoms in the original cohort were more prone (OR 1.7, 95% CI 1.3–2.2) to participate in the 15-month follow-up. As the aim of the present study was to observe the duration of symptoms, selection towards participants who experienced symptoms during the outbreak does not seriously hamper the conclusions. Secondly, prolonged symptoms were asked only from those who fell ill with gastroenteritis during the outbreak. As one could assume, there were hardly any such cases in the control group and this made meaningful comparisons impossible. Thirdly, as the follow-up survey was done 15 months after the exposure, recalling the symptoms by those surveyed may have been difficult, thereby, creating a recall-bias of some degree. Fourthly, the outbreak and the faults causing it were widely discussed in the public media and several claims for compensation were made. Therefore, it is possible that some subjects with a disease that may have been potentially connected to the water contamination were prone to overweigh their symptoms.

The contamination of drinking water and the subsequent epidemic in the town of Nokia was a potentially dangerous situation. Large amounts of pathogens were distributed through household water and thousands of people fell ill. Given these circumstances, consequences could have been much more serious. In addition, more virulent bacterial strains, such as *Escherichia coli* O157:H7 were avoided. Despite the relatively favourable outcome of this epidemic, however, there were cases of people who suffered from consequences, especially, joint symptoms up to one year or more. In addition, individual patients have suffered from serious, prolonged, or permanent damages caused by joint destruction [22], IBS, or chronic fatigue syndrome.

In conclusion, prolonged gastrointestinal and joint symptoms were common among those who fell ill with gastroenteritis during the epidemic. The frequency of gastrointestinal symptoms declined during the follow-up period of 15 months. However, over half of the subjects with arthritis-like symptoms after the outbreak were still symptomatic at the end of the follow-up.

Acknowledgments

We thank Anneli Keinonen for providing the register data of microbiological specimens.

Author Contributions

Conceived and designed the experiments: JLaine JLumio MJV MKuusi. Performed the experiments: JLaine JLumio MJV MKuusi. Analyzed the data: JLaine JLumio ST MJV TU MKorpela EK MKuusi. Wrote the paper: JLaine JLumio ST MJV TU MKKorpela EK MKuusi.

References

1. Leirisalo-Repo M (2005) Reactive arthritis. Scand J Rheumatol 34: 251–259.
2. DuPont AW (2008) Postinfectious irritable bowel syndrome. Clin Infect Dis 46: 594–599.
3. Spiller R, Garsed K (2009) Postinfectious irritable bowel syndrome. Gastroenterology 136: 1979–1988.
4. Marshall JK, Thabane M, Borgaonkar MR, James C (2007) Postinfectious irritable bowel syndrome after a food-borne outbreak of acute gastroenteritis attributed to a viral pathogen. Clin Gastroenterol Hepatol 5: 457–460.
5. Clark WF, Sontrop JM, Macnab JJ, Salvadori M, Moist L, et al. (2010) Long term risk for hypertension, renal impairment, and cardiovascular disease after gastroenteritis from drinking water contaminated with Escherichia coli O157:H7: a prospective cohort study. Bmj 341: c6020.
6. Garg AX, Moist L, Matsell D, Thiessen-Philbrook HR, Haynes RB, et al. (2005) Risk of hypertension and reduced kidney function after acute gastroenteritis from bacteria-contaminated drinking water. Cmaj 173: 261–268.
7. Garg AX, Pope JE, Thiessen-Philbrook H, Clark WF, Ouimet J (2008) Arthritis risk after acute bacterial gastroenteritis. Rheumatology (Oxford) 47: 200–204.
8. Marshall JK (2009) Post-infectious irritable bowel syndrome following water contamination. Kidney Int Suppl: S42–43.
9. Marshall JK, Thabane M, Garg AX, Clark WF, Salvadori M, et al. (2006) Incidence and epidemiology of irritable bowel syndrome after a large waterborne outbreak of bacterial dysentery. Gastroenterology 131: 445–450; quiz 660.
10. Moist LM, Sontrop JM, Garg AX, Clark WF, Suri RS, et al. (2009) Risk of pregnancy-related hypertension within five years of exposure to bacteria-contaminated drinking water. Kidney Int Suppl: S47–49.
11. Laine J, Huovinen E, Virtanen MJ, Snellman M, Lumio J, et al. (2011) An extensive gastroenteritis outbreak after drinking-water contamination by sewage effluent, Finland. Epidemiol Infect: 1–9.
12. Rasanen S, Lappalainen S, Kaikkonen S, Hamalainen M, Salminen M, et al. (2010) Mixed viral infections causing acute gastroenteritis in children in a waterborne outbreak. Epidemiol Infect 138: 1227–1234.
13. Rimhanen-Finne R, Hanninen ML, Vuento R, Laine J, Jokiranta TS, et al. (2010) Contaminated water caused the first outbreak of giardiasis in Finland, 2007: a descriptive study. Scand J Infect Dis 42: 613–619.
14. Uotila T, Antonen J, Laine J, Kujansuu E, Haapala AM, et al. (2011) Reactive arthritis in a population exposed to an extensive waterborne gastroenteritis outbreak after sewage contamination in Pirkanmaa, Finland. Scand J Rheumatol 40: 358–362.
15. Laine J, Uotila T, Antonen J, Korpela M, Kujansuu E, et al. (2012) Joint symptoms after a large waterborne gastroenteritis outbreak–a controlled, population-based questionnaire study. Rheumatology (Oxford) 51: 513–518.
16. Maunula L, Kllemola P, Kauppinen A, Söderberg K, Nguyen T, et al. (2009) Enteritic viruses in a large waterborne outbreak of acute gastroenteritis in Finland. Food Environ Virol 1: 31–36.
17. Hillila MT, Farkkila MA (2004) Prevalence of irritable bowel syndrome according to different diagnostic criteria in a non-selected adult population. Aliment Pharmacol Ther 20: 339–345.
18. Lovell RM, Ford AC (2012) Global Prevalence of, and Risk Factors for, Irritable Bowel Syndrome: a Meta-analysis. Clin Gastroenterol Hepatol.
19. Halvorson HA, Schlett CD, Riddle MS (2006) Postinfectious irritable bowel syndrome–a meta-analysis. Am J Gastroenterol 101: 1894–1899; quiz 1942.
20. Marshall JK, Thabane M, Garg AX, Clark WF, Moayyedi P, et al. (2010) Eight year prognosis of postinfectious irritable bowel syndrome following waterborne bacterial dysentery. Gut 59: 605–611.
21. Porter CK, Faix DJ, Shiau D, Espiritu J, Espinosa BJ, et al. (2012) Postinfectious gastrointestinal disorders following norovirus outbreaks. Clin Infect Dis 55: 915–922.
22. Uotila TM, Antonen JA, Paakkala AS, Mustonen JT, Korpela MM (2013) Outcome of reactive arthritis after an extensive Finnish waterborne gastroenteritis outbreak: a 1-year prospective follow-up study. Clin Rheumatol.
23. Morris D, Inman RD (2012) Reactive arthritis: developments and challenges in diagnosis and treatment. Curr Rheumatol Rep 14: 390–394.
24. Nielsen H, Steffensen R, Ejlertsen T (2012) Risk and prognosis of campylobacteriosis in relation to polymorphisms of host inflammatory cytokine genes. Scand J Immunol 75: 449–454.

23

Excitability of the Motor Cortex in *De Novo* Patients with Celiac Disease

Giovanni Pennisi[1]*, Giuseppe Lanza[2], Salvatore Giuffrida[1], Luisa Vinciguerra[1], Valentina Puglisi[1], Mariagiovanna Cantone[3], Manuela Pennisi[3], Carmela Cinzia D'Agate[4], Pietro Naso[4], Giuseppe Aprile[4], Giulia Malaguarnera[5], Raffaele Ferri[2], Rita Bella[1]

1 Department "G.F. Ingrassia", Section of Neurosciences, University of Catania, Catania, Italy, **2** Department of Neurology I.C., Oasi Institute for Research on Mental Retardation and Brain Aging (I.R.C.C.S.), Troina (Enna), Italy, **3** Department of Chemistry, University of Catania, Catania, Italy, **4** Gastroenterology and Endoscopy Unit, University of Catania, Catania, Italy, **5** Department of Biomedical Sciences, University of Catania, Catania, Italy

Abstract

Introduction: Celiac disease (CD) may initially present as a neurological disorder or may be complicated by neurological changes. To date, neurophysiological studies aiming to an objective evaluation of the potential central nervous system involvement in CD are lacking.

Objective: To assess the profile of cortical excitability to Transcranial Magnetic Stimulation (TMS) in a group of *de novo* CD patients.

Materials and methods: Twenty CD patients underwent a screening for cognitive and neuropsychiatric symptoms by means of the Mini Mental State Examination and the Structured Clinical Interview for DSM-IV Axis I Disorders, respectively. Instrumental exams, including electroencephalography and brain computed tomography, were also performed. Corticospinal excitability was assessed by means of single and paired-pulse TMS using the first dorsal interosseus muscle of the dominant hand. TMS measures consisted of resting motor threshold, motor evoked potentials, cortical silent period (CSP), intracortical inhibition (ICI) and facilitation (ICF). None of the CD was on gluten-free diet. A group of 20 age-matched healthy controls was used for comparisons.

Results: CD showed a significantly shorter CSP (78.0 *vs* 125.0 ms, $p<0.025$), a reduced ICI (0.3 *vs* 0.2, $p<0.045$) and an enhanced ICF (1.1 *vs* 0.7, $p<0.042$) compared to controls. A dysthymic disorder was identified in five patients. The effect size between dysthymic and non-dysthymic CD patients indicated a low probability of interference with the CSP (Cohen's *d* -0.414), ICI (-0.278) and ICF (-0.292) measurements.

Conclusion: A pattern of cortical excitability characterized by "disinhibition" and "hyperfacilitation" was found in CD patients. Immune system dysregulation might play a central role in triggering changes of the motor cortex excitability.

Editor: François Tremblay, University of Ottawa, Canada

Funding: The authors have no support or funding to report.

Competing Interests: The authors have declared that no competing interests exist.

* Email: pennigi@unict.it

Introduction

Celiac disease (CD) is a systemic autoimmune disorder triggered by gliadin ingestion in genetically susceptible individuals [1–3]. Genetic factors strongly contribute to CD, especially regarding HLA-DQ2 and DQ8, but also involving other non-HLA regions [1,4,5].

Although the main target in CD is the proximal small bowel, the clinical presentation is highly heterogeneous, ranging from asymptomatic to dramatically symptomatic forms and affecting several organs, such as skin, joints, bones, blood cells, endocrine glands, the reproductive system and the nervous system. In this context, approximately 50% of CD patients manifest extraintestinal dysfunctions and up to 22.5% have otherwise unexplained neurological symptoms [6]. Furthermore, neurological disorders may complicate the course or represent the onset of CD. Ataxia, peripheral neuropathy and seizures (with or without cerebral calcifications) are the most common neurological complications, with cerebellar ataxia being the most frequent, often associated with cerebellar atrophy at neuroimaging [7]. A possible association between CD and progressive cognitive impairment can be particularly observed, at neuropsychological tests evaluating verbal memory and executive functions [8,9]. Different neuropsychiatric disorders, such as schizophrenia, depression, and anxiety, have also been reported to be associated with CD [10]. Therefore, CD should be considered in patients with unexplained neurological

Table 1. Clinical-serological features and diagnostic work-up of CD patients.

Patient	Symptoms at onset	Co-morbidities	Antibodies	Endoscopy	Histopathology
1	Dyspepsia, tiredness	-	tTG, EMA	Scalloped duodenal folds	3b
2	Tiredness	-	tTG, EMA	Reduced duodenal folds	3b
3	Abdominal pain	Thyroiditis	tTG, EMA	Scalloped duodenal folds	3b
4	Diarrhea, abdominal pain	-	tTG, EMA	Reduced duodenal folds	3c
5	Constipation	-	tTG	Mucosal fissures	3b
6	Diarrhea	Asthma	tTG, EMA	Mosaic pattern	3c
7	Poliabortivity, tiredness	-	tTG, EMA	Mucosal fissures	3c
8	Abdominal pain	Thyroiditis	tTG, EMA	Reduced duodenal folds	3c
9	Dyspepsia, tiredness	Thyroiditis	tTG, EMA	Mosaic pattern	3c
10	None (screening, family history for CD)	-	tTG	Mosaic pattern	3c
11	Diarrhea, abdominal pain	Asthma	tTG, EMA	Absent duodenal folds	3c
12	Weight loss	Thyroiditis	tTG, EMA	Mosaic pattern	3c
13	Abdominal pain	-	tTG	Mucosal fissures	3b
14	Weight loss, diarrhea	Vitiligo	tTG, EMA	Scalloped duodenal folds	3a
15	Infertility, tiredness	Thyroiditis	tTG, EMA	Reduced duodenal folds	3c
16	Diarrhea	-	negative	Scalloped duodenal folds	3a
17	Weight loss	-	tTG, EMA	Mosaic pattern	3c
18	Weight loss, abdominal pain,	-	tTG, EMA	Mosaic pattern	3c
19	Dyspepsia, abdominal pain, diarrhea	-	tTG, EMA	Mosaic pattern	3c
20	Tiredness	Thyroiditis	tTG, EMA	Mosaic pattern	3c

CD = celiac disease; tTG = tissue transglutaminase antibodies; EMA = endomysial antibodies.
Histopathological classification is based on the Marsh–Oberhuber grading system [51]. 3a: mild villous flattening; 3b: marked villous flattening; 3c: total villous flattening.

disorders and a neurological screening might disclose valuable information in these patients.

Nevertheless, although there is a relevant impact of CD and its complications on health and social life, to date techniques allowing an objective evaluation of the potential central nervous system involvement in CD are lacking.

In the last years, several investigators have used transcranial magnetic stimulation (TMS) to define the electrophysiological profile of several neuropsychiatric disorders [11,12], physiological brain aging [13], different models of cognitive decline [14,15] and some systemic diseases with a neurological involvement [16,17]. TMS is a safe and non-invasive neurophysiological technique specifically able to evaluate the excitability and functioning of the primary motor cortex and the cortico-spinal tract [18]. TMS studies have provided findings that, although not disease specific, shed light on the cortical pathophysiology and the neurochemical basis underlying disease processes and represent a rationale for the plasticity-based interventions [18,19]. More recently, TMS-derived parameters have allowed to explore the regulatory mechanisms of cortical excitability, supporting the concept of a cortical motor network whose output is also influenced by non-primary motor areas, including ventral and dorsal premotor cortex, supplementary motor area and cingulate cortex [20]. In particular, it is known that the cingulate cortex, together with the dorsolateral prefrontal cortex, is crucial for cognition and mood regulation [21].

Converging evidences suggest that gluten-mediated immune response in CD is associated with neuropsychiatric manifestations. Given that glutamic acid decarboxylase (GAD) antibodies may interfere with the GABAergic synaptic transmission, thus affecting inhibitory interneurons activity, in the present paper we first aimed to explore the potential involvement of inhibitory and facilitatory intracortical circuits to single- and paired-pulse TMS in *de novo* CD patients. We hypothesized that gluten intolerance might be associated with changes of specific TMS measures of excitation and inhibition.

Materials and methods

Ethics Statement

The study was approved by the ethics committee of the Azienda Ospedaliero-Universitaria "Policlinico-Vittorio Emanuele", Catania (Italy). Written informed consent was obtained from all participants prior to participation in accordance with the Declaration of Helsinki. All assessments were performed in a controlled laboratory environment.

Subjects

Twenty *de novo* CD patients (4 males and 16 females; median age 33.0 years, interquartile range 24.0–45.0), according to the European Society for Paediatric Gastroenterology Hepatology and Nutrition (ESPGHAN) guidelines for the diagnosis of CD [22], were consecutively recruited from the Regional Center for Celiac Disease of the University of Catania, Italy. The clinical-serological features and the main findings from the diagnostic work-up of CD patients are summarized in Table 1. Twenty age-matched healthy volunteers (8 males and 14 females; median age 29.5 years, interquartile range 26.0–45.5) were used as a control group. At the time of the examination, none of the patients was on gluten-free diet. Exclusion criteria were: major neurological disorder (i.e.

Parkinson's disease, stroke, Alzheimer's disease, etc.); head trauma or epilepsy; acute, chronic or not compensated medical illness (i.e. myocardial infarction, kidney or liver failure, heart failure, etc.); Mini Mental State Examination score <24 [23], alcohol or drug abuse; age <18 years; use of drugs affecting cortical excitability (i.e. mood stabilizers, benzodiazepines, antipsychotics); any condition precluding TMS execution. On a total sample of 23 consecutive CD patients, 2 were excluded because of current intake of benzodiazepines and one refused the TMS protocol.

Assessment

The clinical-demographic evaluation included: age, gender, education, handedness, social and living conditions, general and neurological examinations, and co-morbidities. Neuropsychological tests included a screening of overall cognitive functions (Mini Mental State Examination), evaluation of neuropsychiatric symptoms diagnosed by the Structured Clinical Interview for DSM-IV Axis I Disorders (SCID-I) and the 17-items Hamilton Depression Rating Scale [24], for the quantification of any depressive symptom. Cognitive assessment was performed by a physician blind to the aim of the study. Instrumental exams included standard electroencephalogram (EEG), brain computed tomography (CT) scan and both single- and paired-pulse TMS.

EEG was recorded by means of a Micromed Brain Quick (System Plus), with a standard montage according to the 10-20 International System and with a pre-cabled EEG head cap. Brain CT was acquired with a helical 64-slices General Electric Scanning, with 2.5 mm slice thickness. Only the clinical, neuropsychological and TMS studies were carried out in controls.

Transcranial magnetic stimulation

TMS was performed using a High-power Magstim 200 magnetic stimulator (Magstim Co., Whitland, Dyfed, UK). A 70 mm figure-of-eight coil was held over the motor cortex at the optimum scalp position to elicit Motor Evoked Potentials (MEPs) in the contralateral First Dorsal Interosseous (FDI) muscle of the dominant hand, according to the Edinburgh Handedness Inventory [25]. Resting motor threshold (rMT) was defined as the lowest stimulus intensity able to elicit MEPs at rest of an amplitude >50 μV in at least 5 of 10 trials, according to the IFCN recommendation [26]. Central motor conduction time was calculated by subtracting the conduction time in peripheral nerves, estimated by F wave techniques, from MEP latency obtained during moderate active muscle contraction, with a stimulus intensity set at 130% of the rMT. M and F waves are elicited by giving supramaximal electrical stimulation to the ulnar nerve at wrist. The size of the MEPs was expressed as a percentage of supramaximal M wave amplitude (A ratio). The cortical silent period (CSP) was determined with an approximately 50% of maximum tonic voluntary contraction of the FDI muscles, induced by single TMS pulses delivered at 130% of rMT. The mean CSP duration of 10 rectified trials was calculated. Intracortical inhibition (ICI) and Intracortical facilitation (ICF) were studied using the conditioning-test paradigm applying two magnetic stimuli in rapid succession [27]. The conditioning stimulus was set at 80% of the subjects rMT whereas the test stimulus at 130% of the rMT. The interstimulus intervals (ISIs) tested were 2, 3, 10 and 15 ms. Ten trials for each ISI were recorded in a random way with an 8-s interval between each trial. The responses were expressed as the ratio between the MEP amplitude produced by paired stimulation and that produced by TS alone. Paired-pulse TMS curves of intracortical excitability were obtained with a 70-mm figure-of-eight coil deriving pulses from a couple of Magstim 200 Stimulators, connected each other through a BiStim module (The Magstim Company, Whitland, Dyfed). The BiStim was connected to a CED Micro 1401 interface (Cambridge Electronic Design, Cambridge, UK) allowing stimulus generation and data capture. Electromyographic (EMG) activity was recorded with silver/silver-chloride disposable self-adhesive and self-conductive surface electrodes. The active electrode was placed over the muscular belly of the target muscle (FDI), the reference distally at the metacarpo-phalangeal joint of the index finger and the ground on the dorsal face of the wrist. For the motor nerve conduction study (M and F waves from the FDI muscle), a bipolar nerve stimulation electrode with 6-mm diameter felt pads and an interelectrode separation of 25 mm was used and applied to the ulnar nerve at wrist, bilaterally. All measurements were conducted while subjects were seated in a comfortable chair with continuous EMG monitoring to ensure either a constant level of EMG activity during tonic contraction or complete relaxation at rest. Data were collected and stored on a computer with an *ad-hoc* software, allowing data acquisition, processing and analysis [28]. To minimize the inter-subjects variability, all TMS procedures were performed in the same laboratory and situation, by the same operators and at the same time during the day.

Statistical analysis

The comparison of the frequency of observation of some features in the CD group and in the control group was carried out by means of the Chi-square test. Because of the relatively low number of subjects in both groups and the non normal distribution of data (as determined by the Shapiro-Wilk's test of normality), all the other comparisons were performed by means of the non-parametric Mann-Whitney test for unpaired datasets. Differences were considered significant when they were below the $p<0.05$ level. However, because of the relatively limited number of subjects available and to rule out possible type II errors, we also calculated effect sizes using the Cohen's d value [29]. Cohen's d is defined as the difference between two means divided by their pooled standard deviation. According to Cohen, 0.2 is indicative of a small effect, 0.5 of a medium and 0.8 of a large effect size.

Results

Demographic, clinical and neuropsychological characteristics of the participants are summarized in Table 2. The general examination of the CD group was unremarkable except for one overweight patient. The neurological examination of all patients was essentially normal. Nine patients had autoimmune co-morbidities, the most common being positive antithyroid peroxidase autoantibodies (six, altough euthyroid), followed by asthma (two) and vitiligo (one). Patients and controls were similar in terms of age, gender, handedness and educational level. The 17 item-HDRS scores were significantly worse in patients (7.0 *vs* 2.0, $p< 0.0058$), whereas the SCID-I disclosed a dysthymic disorder in five CD patients; anxiety was also found in two of them. EEG and CT scan ruled out epileptic changes as well as intracranial calcifications or other clear neuroradiological abnormalities.

As shown in Table 3, CSP duration was significantly shorter in CD subjects with respect to controls (78.0 *vs* 125.0 ms, $p<0.025$), whereas no statistically significant differences were found for rMT. Fig. 1 shows curves of intracortical excitability at the different ISIs obtained in the two groups of participants. Conditioned MEPs amplitudes at ISI of 2 (0.3 *vs* 0.2, $p<0.045$) and 10 ms (1.1 *vs* 0.7, $p<0.042$) were significantly higher in CD patients than controls, indicating a reduced ICI and enhanced ICF in celiac individuals, respectively.

Table 2. Clinical features of the subjects included in this study.

	Celiac disease (n = 20)		Controls (n = 20)		Mann-Whitney		Effect size
	median	(25th-75th quartile)	median	(25th-75th quartile)	U	p<	Cohen's d
Age, years	33.0	(24.0–45.0)	29.5	(26.0–45.5)	180	NS	−0.123
Education, years	13.0	(9.0–13.0)	14.0	(13.5–14.0)	133	NS	−0.402
MMSE	30.0	(29.0–30.0)	30.0	(28.8–30.0)	182	NS	0.183
17 item-HDRS	7.0	(2.0–9.0)	2.0	(0.0–4.0)	98	0.0058	1.451
					Chi^2	**p<**	
Sex, males/females	4/16		8/12		1.90	NS	
Handedness, right/left	18/2		18/2		0.00	NS	
Neurological signs, yes/no	3/17		0/20		3.24	NS	
Comorbidity, yes/no	9/11		0/20		11.60	0.001	
SCID-I, yes/no	5/15		0/20		5.71	0.017	

MMSE = Mini Mental State Examination; HDRS = Hamilton Depression Rating Scale; SCID-I = Structured Clinical Interview for DSM-IV Axis I.

Table 3. Comparison of electrophysiological data in patients with celiac disease and controls.

	Celiac disease (n = 20)		Controls (n = 20)		Mann-Whitney		Effect size
	median	(25th-75th quartile)	median	(25th-75th quartile)	U	p<	Cohen's d
rMT	35.0	(34.0–41.5)	37.0	(32.0–40.0)	194.5	NS	0.070
CSP, ms	78.0	(61.5–100.0)	125.0	(69.5–160.0)	117	0.025	−0.872
MEP latency, ms	18.6	(18.2–19.7)	19.3	(18.5–20.2)	151	NS	−0.428
CMCT	5.9	(4.5–6.3)	5.8	(5.6–6.6)	168	NS	−0.368
CMCTF	4.8	(4.5–5.6)	5.3	(4.2–5.7)	175	NS	−0.148
A ratio	0.2	(0.2–0.5)	0.5	(0.3–0.7)	88.5	0.0026	−0.653
F amplitude, μV	0.1	(0.1–0.2)	0.1	(0.1–0.2)	179.5	NS	0.627

rMT = resting motor threshold; CSP = cortical silent period; MEP = Motor Evoked Potentials; CMCT = central motor conduction time; CMCTF = central motor conduction time estimated by F wave; A ratio = amplitude ratio.

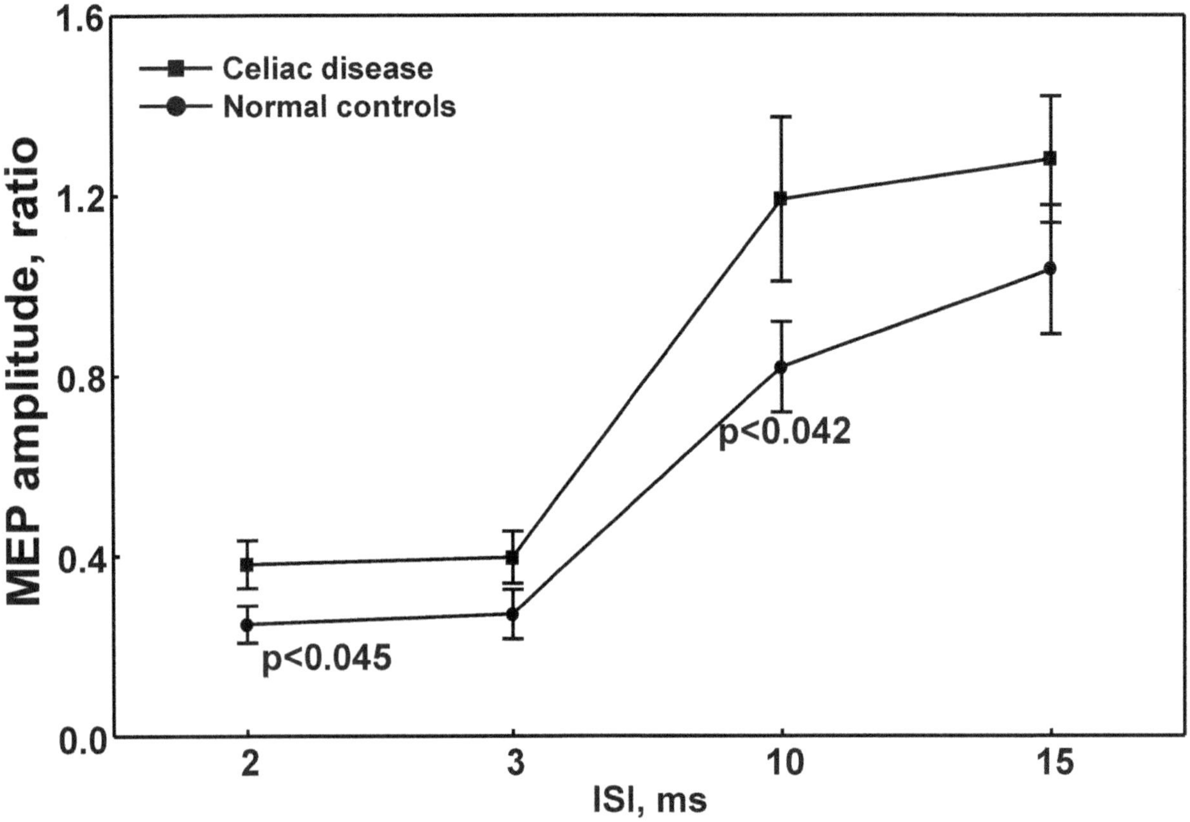

Figure 1. Intracortical excitability at different interstimuls intervals obtained from patients and controls. ISI = interstimuls interval; MEP = Motor Evoked Potential.

Additionally, in order to evaluate the eventual influence of the five dysthymic CD patients on the TMS data, we have estimated the effect size between dysthymic and non-dysthymic CD patients, which was very low in all instances indicating a low probability of interference with the CSP (Cohen's d -0.414), ICI (-0.278) and ICF (-0.292) measurements.

Discussion

This is the first multi-disciplinary investigation examining the impact of CD on motor cortex excitability. The main finding is the observation of electrophysiological changes within the motor cortex of these patients. In particular, we observed a significant reduction of the intracortical inhibitory amount indicated by shortened CSP and reduced ICI, together with a significant enhancement of ICF, in patients with CD compared to controls. This pattern, basically characterized by a "disinhibition" and "hyperfacilitation", was observed in the absence of substantial changes of rMT. On the other hand, changes of different TMS measures without modification of rMT has already been reported and is likely due to the different electrophysiological and neurochemical basis that these measures have and explore [30,31]. Resting MT represents a global parameter of cortical excitability and reflects the neuronal membrane excitability, as well as the local density of the excitatory interneurons and the cortico-spinal neurons within the motor cortex [18]. CSP, defined as the interval of suppressed voluntary EMG activity following a single-pulse TMS stimulus, is an index of motor cortical inhibition, basically due to the activation of GABA-B cortical inhibitory interneurons [32,33]. ICI is probably mediated by GABA-A receptors [34], whereas ICF may represent an activating phenomenon arising from intracortical glutamatergic neurons [18,35], but also tempered by GABAergic inhibition and modulated by serotoninergic, adrenergic, cholinergic and dopaminergic neurotransmission [36].

The mechanisms underlying this cortical disinhibition in CD patients are rather complex to explain, also because of the lack of similar studies. The pathophysiology of CD and the most accepted hypothesis explaining its neurological involvement may help understanding our results. Vitamins and trace elements deficiency is unlikely to explain the subtle neurophysiological changes to TMS, because it usually occurs in the most affected CD patients, in whom a wide intestinal damage is already evident, resulting in severe malabsorption and related consequences [7,37].

An autoimmune-mediated pathogenesis for CD is supported by increasingly convincing evidence. Molecular mimicry between gliadin and nervous system proteins could lead to a cross-reaction of anti-gliadin antibodies (Abs) with nervous system antigens. Abs can react with Purkinje cells and peripheral nerve epitopes [10,38]. Furthermore, anti-gliadin Abs have a immunoreactivity to synapsin I, which is very similar to gliadin because of the high frequency of proline and glutamine regions. Synapsin I is a neuronal phosphoprotein of the central and peripheral nervous system involved in forming and maintaining the reserve pool of synaptic vesicles and in managing neurotransmitter release [39,40]. In CD patients, anti-gliadin Abs might possibly interfere with the normal balance between excitatory and inhibitory neural circuits as a consequence of the interaction with synapsin I.

Another interesting hypothesis regards a possible involvement of GABA, which is the main inhibitory neurotransmitter synthesized in the central nervous system from glutamate by GAD. Since GABA and GAD are also synthesized by neurons of the enteric plexus [41], anti-GAD Abs may arise in CD patients and concentrate in the Purkinje cells and peripheral nerves [42,43] and may interfere with GABAergic synaptic transmission, thus affecting inhibitory interneurons activity [10].

Within humoral autoimmunity to neuronal antigens, anti-transglutaminase 2- or transglutaminase 6-related immunoglobulin depositions have been identified not only in the gut but also in the cerebellum, pons, medulla and around brain blood vessels [38,44]. Additional findings show diffuse T-lymphocytic infiltration within the perivascular cuffing with inflammatory cells that could possibly damage the blood-brain barrier and expose the cerebral tissues to Abs [7], driving altered ion levels. Taken together, this may lead to a vicious circle resulting in a imbalance between inhibitory and facilitatory neuronal excitability.

Finally, growing evidence indicates that immune system dysregulation might play a central role in triggering neurological impairment in CD, leading not only to the neurophysiological alterations but also to neurobehavioral changes. In this context, another finding of our study is the evidence of a degree of depressive and anxiety symptoms in CD patients, adding further support to the relationship between psychiatric disorders and CD [45,46]. Major depression has been widely studied by TMS, which has confirmed the key role of the GABAergic dysfunction in the neurochemical pattern of depressed mood, as indexed by a reduction of both CSP and ICI [11,47-50]. In this view, it can be argued that our TMS findings might be explained as a result of depressive mood in five of the CD patients. However, to our knowledge no study assessing cortical excitability to TMS in dysthimia is available. Besides, in this series of patients, TMS modifications do not seem to be significantly influenced by the depressive disorder. Therefore, it can be hypothesized that the observed TMS changes of inhibitory circuits might be related to the synaptic disruption due to the gluten-mediated immune response and that an imbalance between inhibitory and facilitatory intracortical circuits occurs even at a subclinical neurological stage of CD.

This study has some limitations. First, TMS-related measures of cortical excitability do not provide specific pathophysiological information although they are sensitive to the "global weight" of several neurotransmitters, as well as to subcortical and cortical motor inputs. Second, the observed findings obtained from a relatively small number of patients do not allow to draw conclusions on the eventual causal relationship between CD and a specific pattern of cortical excitability to TMS. Therefore, these results need to be confirmed by further independent investigations with larger group sizes and to be correlated to the clinical presentation and course of CD, even after an adequate course of gluten-free dietary regimen. In this context, a "normalization" of the TMS parameters after the gluten-free diet might add support to the hypothesis of a direct correlation between TMS profile and CD.

In conclusion, this study reveals that CD patients seem to exhibit a relatively distinct pattern of cortical excitability to TMS, suggesting that even asymptomatic patients might disclose a subclinical neurological involvement. The identification of potential neuromarkers might be useful in the diagnosis, follow-up and prognosis of these patients, such as in the monitoring of any change of clinical, neuropsychological and neurophysiological data over time or after a gluten-free dietary regimen. TMS, together with clinical-cognitive, immunological and imaging data, can be considered to be an additional tool able to capture subtle changes in the pathophysiological and neurochemical mechanisms underlying the exciting connections between gut and brain.

Author Contributions

Conceived and designed the experiments: GP SG RB. Performed the experiments: GL LV VP. Analyzed the data: MP RF. Contributed reagents/materials/analysis tools: PN GA. Contributed to the writing of the manuscript: MC CCD GM.

References

1. Di Sabatino A, Corazza GR (2009) Coeliac disease. Lancet 25;373(9673):1480–93.
2. Volta U, De Giorgio R (2010) Gluten sensitivity: an emerging issue behind neurological impairment? Lancet Neurol 9(3):233–5.
3. Volta U, De Giorgio R (2012) New understanding of gluten sensitivity. Nat Rev Gastroenterol Hepatol 28;9(5):295–9.
4. Sollid LM, Jabri B (2005) Is celiac disease an autoimmune disorder? Curr Opin Immunol 17(6):595–600.
5. Greco L, Romino R, Coto I, Di Cosmo N, Percopo S, et al. (2002) The first large population based twin study of coeliac disease. Gut 50(5):624–8
6. Briani C, Zara G, Alaedini A, Grassivaro F, Ruggero S, et al. (2008) Neurological complications of celiac disease and autoimmune mechanisms: a prospective study. J Neuroimmunol 195(1-2):171–5.
7. Hadjivassiliou M, Sanders DS, Grünewald RA, Woodroofe N, Boscolo S, et al. (2010) Gluten sensitivity: from gut to brain. Lancet Neurol 9(3):318–30.
8. Bürk K, Bösch S, Müller CA, Melms A, Zühlke C, et al. (2001) Sporadic cerebellar ataxia associated with gluten sensitivity. Brain 124(Pt 5):1013–9.
9. Hu WT, Murray JA, Greenaway MC, Parisi JE, Josephs KA (2006) Cognitive impairment and celiac disease. Arch Neurol 63(10):1440–6.
10. Jackson JR, Eaton WW, Cascella NG, Fasano A, Kelly DL (2012) Neurologic and psychiatric manifestations of celiac disease and gluten sensitivity. Psychiatr Q 83(1):91–102.
11. Radhu N, De Jesus DR, Ravindran LN, Zanjani A, Fitzgerald PB, et al. (2013) A meta-analysis of cortical inhibition and excitability using transcranial magnetic stimulation in psychiatric disorders. Clin Neurophysiol 124(7):1309–20.
12. Bella R, Ferri R, Cantone M, Pennisi M, Lanza G, et al. (2011) Motor cortex excitability in vascular depression. Int J Psychophysiol 82(3):248–53.
13. Rossini PM, Rossi S, Babiloni C, Polich J (2007) Clinical neurophysiology of aging brain: from normal aging to neurodegeneration. Prog Neurobiol 83(6):375–400.
14. Pennisi G, Ferri R, Cantone M, Lanza G, Pennisi M, et al. (2011) A review of transcranial magnetic stimulation in vascular dementia. Dement Geriatr Cogn Disord 31(1):71–80.
15. Pennisi G, Ferri R, Lanza G, Cantone M, Pennisi M, et al. (2011) Transcranial magnetic stimulation in Alzheimer's disease: a neurophysiological marker of cortical hyperexcitability. J Neural Transm 118(4):587–98.
16. Andersen H, Nielsen S, Nielsen JF (2006) Motor cortical excitability remains unaffected of short-term hyperglycemia in Type 1 diabetic patients. J Diabetes Complications 20(1):51–5.
17. Oliviero A, Gaspari R, Tonali PA, Pennisi MA, Mercurio G, et al. (2002) Changes in excitability of motor cortex in severe hepatic failure. J Neurol Neurosurg Psychiatry 72(3):414–6.
18. Kobayashi M, Pascual-Leone A (2003) Transcranial magnetic stimulation in neurology. Lancet Neurol 2(3):145–56.
19. Rossini PM, Rossi S (2007) Transcranial magnetic stimulation: diagnostic, therapeutic, and research potential. Neurology 68(7):484–8.
20. Reis J, Swayne OB, Vandermeeren Y, Camus M, Dimyan MA, et al. (2008) Contribution of transcranial magnetic stimulation to the understanding of cortical mechanisms involved in motor control. J Physiol 586(2):325–51.
21. Leech R, Sharp DJ (2014) The role of the posterior cingulate cortex in cognition and disease. Brain 137(Pt 1):12–32.
22. Husby S (2012) European Society for Pediatric Gastroenterology, Hepatology, and Nutrition guidelines for the diagnosis of coeliac disease. J Pediatr Gastroenterol Nutr 54:136–160.
23. Folstein MF, Folstein SE, McHugh PR (1975). Mini-Mental State. A practical method for grading the cognitive state of patients for the clinician. J Psychiatr Res 12(3):189–98.
24. Hamilton M (1960) A rating scale for depression. J Neurol Neurosurg Psychiatry. 23:56–62.
25. Oldfield RC (1971) The assessment and analysis of handedness: the Edinburgh Inventory. Neuropsychologia 9(1):97–113.

26. Rossini PM, Barker AT, Berardelli A, Caramia MD, Caruso G, et al. (1994) Non-invasive electrical and magnetic stimulation of the brain, spinal cord and roots: basic principles and procedures for routine clinical application. Report of an IFCN committee. Electroencephalogr Clin Neurophysiol 91(2):79–92.
27. Kujirai T, Caramia MD, Rothwell JC, Day BL, Thompson PD, et al. (1993) Corticocortical inhibition in human motor cortex. J Physiol 471:501–19.
28. Giordano D, Kavasidis I, Spampinato C, Bella R, Pennisi G, et al. (2012) An integrated computer-controlled system for assisting researchers in cortical excitability studies by using transcranial magnetic stimulation. Comput Methods Progr Biomed 107(1):4–15.
29. Cohen J (1988) Statistical power analysis for the behavioural sciences (2nd ed.). Erlbaum. Hillsdale, NJ.
30. Bella R, Ferri R, Pennisi M, Cantone M, Lanza G, et al. (2011) Enhanced motor cortex facilitation in patients with vascular cognitive impairment no-dementia. Neurosci Lett 10;503(3):171–5.
31. Paulus W, Classen J, Cohen LG, Large CH, Di Lazzaro V, et al. (2008) State of the art: pharmacologic effects on cortical excitability measures tested by transcranial magnetic stimulation, Brain Stimul 1(3):151–63.
32. Werhahn KJ, Kunesch E, Noachtar S, Benecke R, Classen J (1999) J Physiol. Differential effects on motorcortical inhibition induced by blockade of GABA uptake in humans. J Physiol 1;517(Pt 2):591–7.
33. Chen R, Lozano AM, Ashby P (1999) Mechanism of the silent period following transcranial magnetic stimulation: evidence from epidural recordings. Exp Brain Res 128: 539–42.
34. Di Lazzaro V, Oliviero A, Meglio M, Cioni B, Tamburrini G, et al. (2000) Direct demonstration of the effect of lorazepam on the excitability of the human motor cortex. Clin Neurophysiol 111(5):794–9.
35. Ziemann U, Rothwell JC, Ridding MC (1996) Interaction between intracortical inhibition and facilitation in human motor cortex. J Physiol 1;496(Pt 3):873–81.
36. Ziemann U (2004) TMS and drugs. Clin Neurophysiol 115(8):1717–29.
37. Freeman HJ (2008) Pearls and pitfalls in the diagnosis of adult celiac disease. Can J Gastroenterol 22(3):273–80.
38. Hadjivassiliou M, Aeschlimann P, Strigun A, Sanders DS, Woodroofe N, et al. (2008) Autoantibodies in gluten ataxia recognize a novel neuronal transglutaminase. Ann Neurol 64(3):332–43.
39. Alaedini A, Okamoto H, Briani C, Wollenberg K, Shill HA, et al. (2007) Immune cross-reactivity in celiac disease: anti-gliadin antibodies bind to neuronal synapsin I. J Immunol 15;178(10):6590–5.
40. Humeau Y, Doussau F, Vitiello F, Greengard P, Benfenati F, et al. (2001) Synapsin Controls Both Reserve and Releasable Synaptic Vesicle Pools during Neuronal Activity and Short-Term Plasticity in Aplysia. J Neurosci 21(12):4195–206.
41. Williamson S, Faulkner-Jones BE, Cram DS, Furness JB, Harrison LC (1995) Transcription and translation of two glutamate decarboxylase genes in the ileum of rat, mouse and guinea pig. J Auton Nerv Syst 5;55(1-2):18–28.
42. Takenoshita H, Shizuka-Ikeda M, Mitoma H, Song S, Harigaya Y, et al. (2001) Presynaptic inhibition of cerebellar GABAergic transmission by glutamate decarboxylase autoantibodies in progressive cerebellar ataxia. J Neurol Neurosurg Psychiatry 70(3):386–9.
43. Hadjivassiliou M (2004) Glutamic acid decarboxylase as a target antigen in gluten sensitivity: the link to neurological manifestation? Proceedings of the 11th International Symposium on Celiac Disease. Belfast.
44. Hadjivassiliou M, Mäki M, Sanders DS, Williamson CA, Grünewald RA, et al. (2006) Autoantibody targeting of brain and intestinal transglutaminase in gluten ataxia. Neurology 14;66(3):373–7.
45. Hallert C, Derefeldt T (1982) Psychic disturbances in adult coeliac disease. Scand J Gastroenterol 17(1):17–9.
46. Ciacci C, Iavarone A, Mazzacca G, De Rosa A (1998) Depressive symptoms in adult coeliac disease. Scand J Gastroenterol 33(3):247–50.
47. Spampinato C, Aguglia E, Concerto C, Pennisi M, Lanza G, et al. (2013) Transcranial magnetic stimulation in the assessment of motor cortex excitability and treatment of drug-resistant major depression. IEEE Trans Neural Syst Rehabil Eng 21(3):391–403.
48. Bajbouj M, Lisanby SH, Lang UE, Danker-Hopfe H, Heuser I, et al. (2006) Evidence for impaired cortical inhibition in patients with unipolar major depression. Biol Psychiatry 1;59(5):395–400.
49. Fitzgerald PB, Brown TL, Marston NA, Daskalakis ZJ, de Castella A, et al. (2004) Motor cortical excitability and clinical response to rTMS in depression. J Affect Disord 82(1):71–6.
50. Brambilla P, Perez J, Barale F, Schettini G, Soares JC (2003) GABAergic dysfunction in mood disorders. Mol Psychiatry 8(8):721–37,715.
51. Oberhuber G (2000) Histopathology of celiac disease. Biomed Pharmacother. 54(7):368–72.

24

How and When Should NSAIDs Be Used for Preventing Post-ERCP Pancreatitis?

Ignasi Puig[1,2,3*], Xavier Calvet[3,4,5], Mireia Baylina[3,6], Álvaro Isava[1,2], Pau Sort[1,2], Jordina Llaó[1,2], Francesc Porta[1,2], Francesc Vida[1,2]

1 Digestive Diseases Department, Althaia Xarxa Assistencial Universitària de Manresa, Barcelona, Spain, **2** Universitat Internacional de Catalunya, Barcelona, Spain, **3** Departament de Medicina, Universitat Autònoma de Barcelona, Barcelona, Spain, **4** Digestive Diseases Department, Corporació Sanitària Parc Taulí, Sabadell, Barcelona, Spain, **5** Centro de Investigación Biomédica en Red de enfermedades hepáticas y digestivas (CIBERehd), Madrid, Spain, **6** Internal Medicine Department, Corporació Sanitària Parc Taulí, Sabadell, Barcelona, Spain

Abstract

Background: Non-steroidal anti-inflammatory drugs (NSAIDs) have been shown to be efficacious to prevent pancreatitis after endoscopic retrograde cholangiopancreatography (ERCP). However, the target patients, the type of NSAID, the route of administration and the time of drug delivery remain unclear, as well as the potential efficacy in reducing the severity of pancreatitis, length of hospital stay and mortality. The objective of the study was to evaluate these questions by performing a systematic review and meta-analysis.

Methods: Multiple searches were performed in the main databases. Randomized controlled trials (RCTs) comparing NSAIDs vs. placebo in the prevention of post-ERCP pancreatitis were included. Primary endpoint of the study was the efficacy for pancreatitis prevention. Sub-analyses were performed to determine the risk reduction in high and low risk patients, and to define optimal time, route of administration, and type of NSAID. Secondary endpoints were safety, moderate to severe pancreatitis prevention and reduction of hospital stay and mortality.

Results: Nine RCTs enrolling 2133 patients were included. The risk of pancreatitis was lower in the NSAID group than in the placebo group (RR 0.51; 95%CI 0.39–0.66). The number needed to treat was 14. The risk of moderate to severe pancreatitis was also lower in the NSAID group. (RR 0.46; 95%CI 0.28–0.76). No adverse events related to NSAID use were reported. NSAIDs were effective in both high-risk and unselected patients (RR 0.53; 95%CI 0.30–0.93 and RR 0.57; 95%CI 0.37–0.88). In the subanalyses, only rectal administration of either indomethacin (RR 0.54; 95%CI 0.38–0.75) or diclofenac (RR 0.42; 95%CI 0.21–0.84) was shown to be effective. There were not enough data to perform a meta-analysis in hospital stay reduction. No deaths occurred.

Conclusion: A single rectal dose of indomethacin or diclofenac before or immediately after ERCP is safe and prevents procedure-related pancreatitis both in high risk and in unselected patients.

Editor: Juan Sastre, University of Valencia, Spain

Funding: The Centro de Investigación Biomédica en Red de enfermedades hepáticas y digestivas (CIBERehd) is funded by the Instituto de Salud Carlos III. The funders had no role in study design, data collection and analysis, decision to publish, or preparation of the manuscript.

Competing Interests: Ignasi Puig, Mireia Baylina, Álvaro Isava, Jordina Llaó, Pau Sort, Francesc Porta and Francesc Vida have no relevant conflicts of interest to report. Xavier Calvet: Astra-Zeneca, Pfizzer, MSD, Abbvie: advisory boards, research grants, fees for educational activities. Janssen-Cilag: Research grants. Almirall SA: advisor, fees for educational activities.

* E-mail: ignasipuig@gmail.com

Introduction

Endoscopic retrograde cholangiopancreatography (ERCP) is a widely used procedure that combines upper gastrointestinal endoscopy and radiography to diagnose and treat bile- and pancreas-related diseases such as choledocholithiasis, benign and malignant strictures, and so on. It is estimated that 500,000 procedures are performed annually in the United States [1]. The most common complication of ERCP is pancreatitis, occurring in 2–9% of patients in unselected prospective series [1]. It is associated with substantial morbidity and long hospitalization, although mortality is rare [2,3]. Diagnostic criteria for post-ERCP pancreatitis (PEP) are new onset of pancreatic-type abdominal pain and amylase or lipase at least three times the normal rate more than 24 hours after the procedure requiring hospital admission or a prolongation of planned admission [4].

It is widely accepted that the local and systemic inflammatory response induced by ERCP is the physiopathological event that triggers PEP [5–7]. It has been proposed that phospholipase A2 (PLA2) plays an important role in the pathogenesis of this inflammatory response [5]. In vitro assays show that non-steroidal anti-inflammatory drugs (NSAIDs) are potent inhibitors of PLA2 activity in the serum in patients with severe acute pancreatitis and indomethacin and diclofenac are the most effective PLA2 inhibitors [8].

The fact that the initial triggering event of PEP is well defined has prompted researchers to seek out measures for its prevention. Pancreatic stent is not performed by all endoscopists because stent insertion may be difficult in patients with small or tortuous ducts, and there is a risk of pancreatic ductal injury [9]. Furthermore, a follow-up endoscopy is necessary for stent removal. For all these reasons, this procedure is not widely applied and an effective protective pharmacological agent would be of great benefit. The results of RCTs using nitroglycerine, ceftazidime, somatostatin, octreotide, antiprotease drugs, glucocorticoids, drugs reducing sphincter of Oddi pressure, antioxidant drugs, heparin, and Interleukin-10 have been disappointing [4]. Some studies have shown a benefit with NSAIDs [10–18], but a practice survey study performed some years ago showed that they were not widely used [19]. The main reason quoted was insufficient supporting evidence, but the authors speculate that clinicians' scepticism related to the failure of many other large studies with other pharmacological agents also played an important role.

Previous meta-analyses have suggested that NSAIDs are effective in preventing post-ERCP pancreatitis [20–22], and the ESGE guidelines [4], based on four RCTs, recommend routine rectal administration of 100 mg of diclofenac or indomethacin immediately before or after ERCP. For this reason, NSAID use is increasing rapidly. However, after the publication of more recent studies, certain clinically relevant issues regarding the drug administration and the target patients remain unresolved. The rectal route is uncomfortable and drugs' absorption may be erratic. For this reason, it may be useful to determine whether the parenteral route is also effective. In addition, whether NSAIDs should be given only to selected patients at high risk of developing PEP, or to all patient who undergo ERCP, is still a matter of debate. We conducted a systematic review and meta-analysis in order to determine the effectiveness of non-rectal and rectal NSAIDs, to establish the optimal moment of drug delivery and the most appropriate type of NSAID, and to assess their efficacy according to risk factors for developing pancreatitis. We also evaluated their safety and the efficacy for reducing pancreatitis severity, length of hospital stay, and mortality.

Methods

The study was performed in accordance with the PRISMA recommendations for systematic reviews and meta-analyses [23]. The PRISMA 2009 checklist is shown in Checklist S1 and the PRISMA 2009 flow diagram in Figure 1. We did not register the protocol.

Search strategy

Multiple searches were performed in Scopus, Medline, the Cochrane Library database and the ISI Web of Knowledge from 1980 to November 2013. Details of the search are shown in Appendix S1. In addition, the references of the selected articles and those of significant reviews on the topic were also examined for articles missed in the previous searches.

Inclusion criteria

Published studies were included if: a) they evaluated the efficacy of NSAIDs for prevention of post-ERCP pancreatitis; b) they were randomized controlled trials with a placebo arm; 3) they reported the incidence of post-ERCP pancreatitis in each arm.

Definitions

Post-ERCP pancreatitis (PEP) was defined according to previous consensus as: "clinical pancreatitis with amylase at least three times the normal rate more than 24 hours after the procedure, requiring hospital admission or a prolongation of planned admission" [24]. However, subsequent modified definitions that specified the meaning of "clinical pancreatitis" were also accepted [4]: "new or worsened abdominal pain" [25], "typical pain and symptoms" [26] or "abdominal pain and tenderness" [27].

Risk factors for developing PEP were extracted from previous reviews and meta-analyses [4,28]: female sex, young age, suspected SOH, prior post-ERCP pancreatitis, recurrent pancreatitis, pancreatic duct injection, pancreatic sphincterotomy, balloon dilatation, difficult or failed cannulation, precut sphincterotomy and ampullectomy.

Regarding the inclusion criteria, a study was considered to involve high-risk patients when all patients included presented at least one risk factor. On the other hand, a study was considered to include unselected patients if the presence of risk factors was not a criterion for inclusion in the study. In this case, studies could include either all patients who underwent ERCP or patients with suspected bile obstruction, which is not considered an independent risk factor for PEP.

Endpoints of the study

The primary endpoint of the study was the efficacy of NSAIDs for preventing PEP. This was evaluated by comparing the number of patients presenting PEP in the NSAIDs group *vs.* the placebo group.

Sub-analyses of the primary endpoint were planned to compare the incidence of PEP according to: a) the type of NSAID (indomethacin or diclofenac); b) route of administration (rectal or non-rectal); c) time of administration (before or after ERCP); d) risk of pancreatitis according to inclusion criteria (high risk or unselected patients); e) presence of each individual risk factor (female sex, young age, suspected SOH, prior post-ERCP pancreatitis, recurrent pancreatitis, pancreatic duct injection, pancreatic sphincterotomy, balloon dilatation, difficult or failed cannulation, pre-cut sphincterotomy and ampullectomy); f) the placement of a pancreatic stent.

Most subanalyses were performed separating the studies in the subgroup in question according to study design, but the two last subanalyses (each individual risk factor and the placement of a pancreatic stent) were based on the data extracted from the stratified results of each study (i.e. the number of PEP in females receiving NSAIDs *vs.* the number of PEP in females receiving placebo). Studies reporting only the baseline characteristics of patients (not the incidence of PEP in each subgroup) were not included.

Secondary endpoints were the efficacy of NSAIDs for reducing the number of moderate and severe pancreatitis, number of adverse events related to NSAIDs, length of hospital stay, and mortality. They were summarized through a quantitative meta-analysis when feasible, or described otherwise.

Data extraction

Data extraction was performed in duplicate by two observers (MB & AI). Discordances were resolved by consensus with a third observer (IP). For each study we extracted the following variables: first author, year of publication, country, inclusion criteria, exclusion criteria, the definition of pancreatitis, differences in baseline risk factors between the groups, the use of pancreatic stent for PEP prophylaxis, the type, schedule and route of administra-

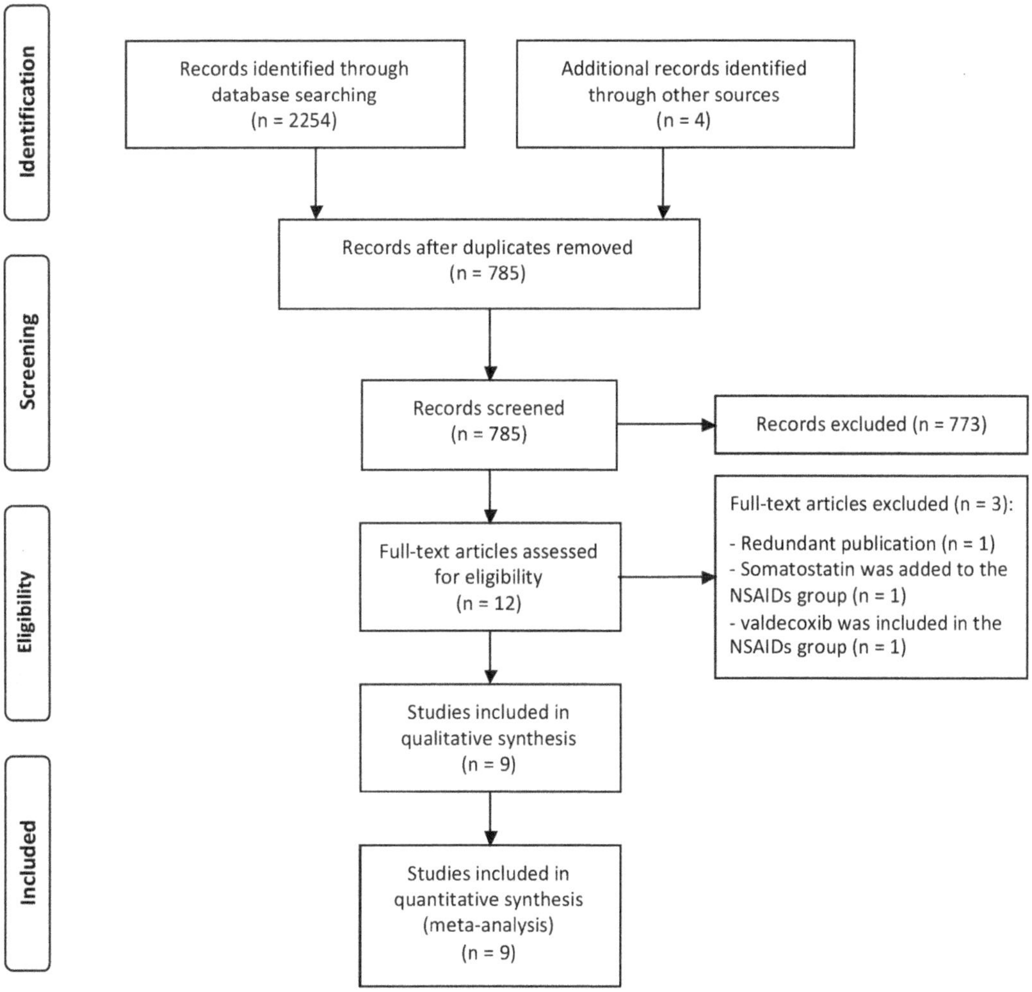

Figure 1. Flow diagram of included and excluded trials.

tion of the NSAID, the incidence of PEP in all groups, the incidence of PEP in the subgroup of patients with risk factors (when stratified results were reported), the incidence of moderate to severe PEP, adverse events related to NSAID administration, mortality, and length of hospital stay.

Quality assessment of the studies

Two independent reviewers assessed the quality of trials with the Jadad scale (AI & IP). In the case of one article published in Hungarian [11], we contacted the authors who helped us to assess the Jadad scale. Disagreements were discussed by the reviewers and resolved through consensus. According to this scale, low-quality studies had a score of ≤2 and high-quality studies had a score of ≥3 [29].

Statistical analysis

Differences observed between the groups were expressed as risk ratios (RR) with their 95% confidence intervals (CI). In the case of primary and secondary endpoints, numbers needed to treat (NNT) were also calculated. Heterogeneity was measured using the I^2 test and was considered significant when the I^2 value was above 50% [30,31]. A fixed-effects model weighted by the Mantel-Haenszel method was used for pooling the RR's because of the low heterogeneity between studies. Funnel plot was used to estimate the risk of publication bias. All calculations were performed using the freeware Review Manager 5.1 (Cochrane Foundation, McMaster University, Ontario, Canada) [32].

Results

Original searches retrieved more than 1000 articles. After review of the abstracts, 12 studies met the inclusion criteria. After careful evaluation, nine were included in the systematic review and the meta-analysis (Figure 1).

Studies excluded

Three studies were finally excluded from the meta-analysis: 1) Montaño Loza et al [33] reported the preliminary results of another study which was already included; 2) Katsinelos et al [34] administered somatostatin along with NSAIDs and found a significantly lower incidence of PEP in this treatment group (4.7% vs 10.4%, p = 0.015); 3) Bhatia et al [35] did not find statistically significant differences when comparing valdecoxib iv vs. placebo (9.9% vs 10.3%, p = 0.99). This study was excluded because valdecoxib is a selective COX2 inhibitor. The effect of coxibs in reducing PLA2 activity is unknown, and therefore they may not be as effective as conventional NSAID for PEP prevention.

Table 1. Basic characteristics of included studies in the meta-analysis.

Author, year, country	N	Inclusion criteria	Does the study include patients with a pancreatic stent for PEP prophylaxis?	Intervention	Definition of PEP	Jadad score
Murray, 2003, Scotland [15]	220	High risk patients (Pancreatography or cholangiogaphy with SOH)	Yes[a, b]	100 mg rectal diclofenac in recovery area	Amylase >x4 ULN and epigastric pain, back pain and abdominal rebound tenderness	5
Sotoudehmanesh, 2007, Iran [18]	442	Unselected patients (ERCP, all-comers)	No	100 mg rectal indomethacin immediately prior to ERCP	Amylase >x3 ULN and epigastric or back pain and epigastric tenderness	5
Khoshbaten, 2008, Iran [13]	200	High risk patients (Pancreatography ± cholangiography)	Yes[a, b]	100 mg rectal diclofenac on arrival in recovery area	Amylase >x4 ULN and epigastric and back pain and epigastric rebound tenderness	5
Montaño Loza, 2007, Mexico [14]	150	Unselected patients (ERCP, suspected bile duct obstruction)	No	100 mg rectal indomethacin immediately prior to ERCP	Amylase >x3 ULN + sharp pain radiating to back + nausea or vomiting	2
Cheon, 2007, USA [10]	207	Unselected patients (ERCP, all-comers)	Yes[b]	50 mg diclofenac before and after ERCP by mouth	Amylase >x3 ULN 18h after ERCp + abdominal pain that prolonged hospital stay	5
Senol, 2009, Turkey [17]	80	Unselected patients (ERCP, cholestasis)	No	75 mg diclofenac im and i.v. isotonic after ERCP	Amylase >x3 ULN + epigastric pain or back pain + epigastric tenderness	2
Otsuka, 2012, Japan [16]	104	Unselected patients (ERCP, all-comers)	No	50 mg rectal diclofenac 30 mins before ERCP	Amylase >x3 ULN + abdominal pain within 24h after ERCP	2
Elmunzer, 2012, USA [12]	602	High risk patients (1 major or 2 minor previously defined risk factors)	Yes[b]	100 mg rectal indomethacin after ERCP	Amylase >x3 ULN +upper abdominal pain 24 h after ERCP + hospitalization for ≥ 2 nights	5
Döbrönte, 2012, Hungary [11]	228	Unselected patients (ERCP, all-comers)	No	100 mg rectal indomethacin 10 mins before ERCP	Amylase >x3 ULN, abdominal pancreatic pain within 24h after ERCP and extension of hospitalization	5

[a]A pancreatic stent was placed only in 25 and 5 patients in these studies.
[b]Not statistically significant differences between placebo and NSAIDs group.
ERCP: endoscopic retrograde cholangiopancreatography; *NSAIDs:* non-steroidal anti-inflammatory drugs; *PEP:* post-ERCP pancreatitis; *SOH:* sphincter of Oddi hypertension; *ULN:* upper limit of normal.

Studies included

Nine studies, all published as full text articles, were included [10–18]. The characteristics and quality of the studies are shown in table 1. Six studies were scored as high-quality (Jadad score 5) [10–13,15,18] and three as low-quality (Jadad score 2) [14,16,17].

According to the inclusion criteria (table 1), three studies included only high risk patients for PEP: Murray et al [15] included only patients with pancreatography or cholangiography and manometrically documented SOH; Khoshbaten et al [13] included patients with pancreatography with or without cholangiography; Elmunzer et al [12] included selected high risk patients having at least one major or two minor criteria which had been previously defined. The remaining six studies [10,11,14,16–18] included unselected patients.

Risk factors for PEP were similar for both the treatment and the placebo arms in all studies. Only one study [16] reported a statistically significant difference in sex distribution: 31 women were included in the diclofenac group *vs.* 20 in the placebo group; p value was 0.019.

Pancreatic stent for PEP prophylaxis was placed in selected patients in four studies [10,12,13,15]. The rate of stent placement was similar in the NSAID and the placebo groups. Five studies reported that they did not use pancreatic stent for PEP prophylaxis [11,14,16–18].

Main exclusion criteria were the same for all the studies: NSAID use immediately before inclusion in the study, the presence of active pancreatitis before ERCP and the existence of contraindications for NSAID administration.

Four studies [10,12,16,18] graded the severity of post-ERCP pancreatitis according to the criteria proposed by Cotton et al. [24] and accepted in the current guidelines [4]: mild PEP was defined as the need for hospital admission or prolongation of planned admission up to three days; moderate PEP is defined by the need for hospitalization lasting 4 – 10 days, and severe PEP by hospitalization for more than 10 days, or necrosis or pseudocyst, or need for percutaneous drainage or surgical intervention. Montaño Loza et al [14] graded the severity of pancreatitis according to Ranson's criteria, while Murray et al [15] graded it according to CT findings.

Length of hospital stay was reported in different ways. Murray et al [15] and Elmunzer et al [12] reported the median length of hospital stay only for the patients who developed PEP in each arm.

Cheon et al [10] reported the median length of hospital stay for all the patients included in each arm, not those with pancreatitis. Finally, in four additional studies [10,12,16,18] the number of patients with pancreatitis needing hospitalization for more than three days could be extracted because they reported the number of moderate and severe pancreatitis, which had previously been defined according to hospital stay.

Post-ERCP pancreatitis incidence

Nine studies including 2133 patients reported the number of cases of pancreatitis in the NSAID and the placebo arms. Heterogeneity between these studies was low ($I^2 = 22\%$). PEP occurred in 80 out of 1077 patients (7.4%) in the NSAID group vs. 154 out of 1056 patients (14.6%) in the placebo group (RR 0.51; 95% CI 0.39–0.66; $p < 0.00001$) (Figure 2). NNT was 14. The funnel plot showed a visual trend suggesting that small studies reported the highest risk reductions, inducing a publication bias (Figure 3). However, even though the reduction was lower, large studies also found a significant reduction in the risk of pancreatitis.

Risk of moderate to severe pancreatitis, adverse events and mortality and length of hospital stay

Six studies [10,12,14–16,18] reported pancreatitis severity. NSAIDs were effective in reducing the incidence of moderate to severe pancreatitis compared with placebo (RR 0.46; 95% CI 0.28–0.76, $p = 0.003$; I^2: 0%) (Figure 4). NNT was 33.

Regarding adverse events, Elmunzer et al [12] reported four cases of gastrointestinal bleeding in the NSAID group compared to seven in the placebo group. Cheon et al. [10] reported six cases of post endoscopic sphincterotomy (ES) bleeding during the procedure in the placebo group and eight cases in the diclofenac group ($P = 0.921$). Two cases (one in each group) required epinephrine injection. No cases of delayed bleeding were observed. Senol et al [17] also reported two cases of post ES bleeding in the control group and one case in the diclofenac group: all of them were self-limited and stopped during endoscopy, without intervention. The remaining studies did not report any NSAID-related adverse event. No deaths occurred in any study.

A reduced median length hospital stay in patients with pancreatitis was reported by Murray et al [15] (three days in the seven patients with pancreatitis in the experimental group *vs.* five days in the 17 patients with pancreatitis in the control group, P not reported) and by Elmunzer et al [12] (3.5 days in the 27 patients with pancreatitis in the indomethacin group vs. four days in the 52 patients with pancreatitis in the control group, $P < 0.001$). Cheon et al [10] reported a non-significant reduction in the median length of hospital stay for all patients in the diclofenac arm. Hospital stay was 0.73 days in the 105 patients in the diclofenac group vs. 1.3 days in the 102 patients in the placebo group. Finally, the number of patients with pancreatitis requiring a hospital stay of more than three days was reported in four studies [10,12,16,18]. Meta-analyses considering the number of patients with hospital stay of more than three days also showed a trend towards a reduced hospital stay in the experimental group, but the differences were not significant (RR 0.80; 95% CI 0.53–1.21, $p = 0.3$; I^2: 0%).

Type of NSAIDs, route and time of administration and risk factors for PEP

The results of the different sub-analyses are summarized in Figure 5. Both indomethacin and diclofenac induced statistically significant reductions in the risk of pancreatitis (RR 0.54; 95% CI 0.38–0.75, $p = 0.0002$; I^2: 0% and RR 0.42; 95% CI 0.21–0.84, $p = 0.01$; I^2: 54%). Rectal administration was the only effective route (RR 0.45; 95% CI 0.34–0.61, $p < 0.0001$; I^2: 0%), while other routes – oral in one study and intramuscular in another – showed a non-significant benefit (RR 0.81; 95% CI 0.47–1.41, $p = 0.46$; I^2: 22%). NSAIDs were effective when administered either before or after the ERCP (RR 0.46; 95% CI 0.28–0.74, $p = 0.001$; I^2: 0% and RR 0.45; 95% CI 0.32–0.64, $p < 0.0001$; I^2: 0%), and in both high risk patients and non-selected patients (RR 0.53; 95% CI 0.30–0.93, $p = 0.03$; I^2: 58% and RR 0.57; 95% CI 0.37–0.88; I^2: 23%, $p = 0.01$).

Few studies reported the incidence of PEP according to each risk factor. In order to avoid misleading results, studies that administered NSAIDs through non-rectal routes (which did not prove effective) were not considered. Rectal administration of NSAIDs was effective in young people and females and did not depend on whether a sphincterotomy or pancreatography was performed. NSAIDs were also equally effective in patients with and without suspected or confirmed sphincter of Oddi hypertension (table 2). NSAIDs showed a benefit regardless of the placement or non-placement of a prophylactic stent. By contrast, they were not effective in old patients and in men. The data available for other risk factors were insufficient to perform a meta-analysis.

	Experimental		Control			Risk Ratio
Study or Subgroup	Events	Total	Events	Total	Weight	M-H, Fixed, 95% CI
Cheon et al [10]	17	105	17	102	11.2%	0.97 [0.53, 1.80]
Döbrönte et al [11]	11	130	11	98	8.1%	0.75 [0.34, 1.67]
Elmunzer et al [12]	27	295	52	307	33.0%	0.54 [0.35, 0.84]
Khosbaten et al [13]	2	50	13	50	8.4%	0.15 [0.04, 0.65]
Montaño Loza et al [14]	4	75	12	75	7.8%	0.33 [0.11, 0.99]
Murray et al [15]	7	110	17	110	11.0%	0.41 [0.18, 0.95]
Otsuka et al [16]	2	51	10	53	6.3%	0.21 [0.05, 0.90]
Senol et al [17]	3	40	7	40	4.5%	0.43 [0.12, 1.54]
Sotoudehmanesh et al [18]	7	221	15	221	9.7%	0.47 [0.19, 1.12]
Total (95% CI)		**1077**		**1056**	**100.0%**	**0.51 [0.39, 0.66]**
Total events	80		154			

Heterogeneity: Chi² = 10.28, df = 8 (P = 0.25); I² = 22%
Test for overall effect: Z = 5.14 (P < 0.00001)

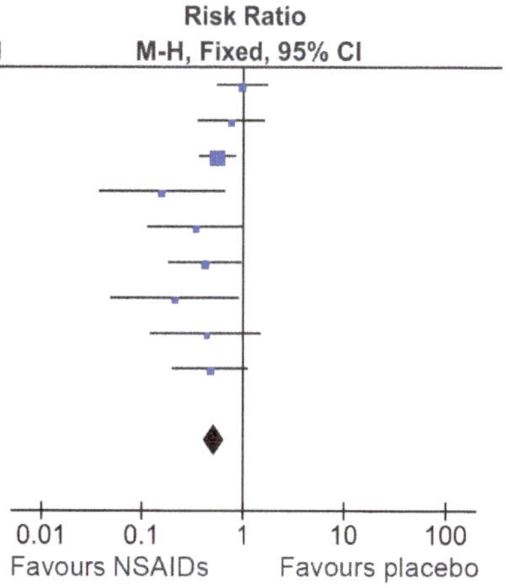

Figure 2. Meta-analysis comparing NSAIDs vs. placebo in reducing the number of patients with PEP. *CI*, confidence interval; *M-H*, Mantel-Haenszel; *NSAIDs*, non-steroidal anti-inflammatory drugs.

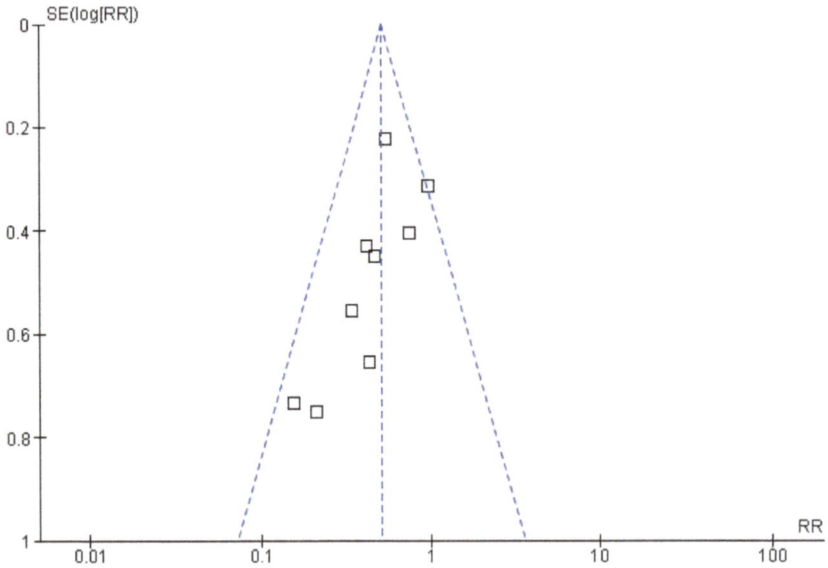

Figure 3. Funnel plot of the meta-analysis.

Discussion

The present study showed that rectal administration of indomethacin or diclofenac, before or after ERCP, is an efficacious and safe measure for reducing the incidence and the severity of post-ERCP pancreatitis. According to the current data, either diclofenac or indomethacin can be used interchangeably. A single rectal dose administered either before or immediately after ERCP seems the most suitable schedule. The sub-analysis showed that rectal NSAIDs were beneficial in both high-risk patients (including those with sphincterotomy, pancreatography and suspected or confirmed SOH) and in unselected patients. Finally, rectal NSAIDs appear to be effective whether or not a prophylactic pancreatic stent was inserted.

Two previous meta-analyses with few studies conclude that NSAIDs are effective in preventing PEP [20,21]. The recent meta-analysis published by Ding et al [22] includes additional studies, but one was reported only in abstract form and is as yet unpublished as a full text, and another evaluated the use of the Cox2 inhibitor valdecoxib. The authors conclude that NSAIDs reduce the incidence and severity of PEP. However, our meta-analysis, including an additional randomized controlled trial [11], determines that the evidence is conclusive only for rectal NSAIDs. In addition, our study highlights some clinically relevant issues: rectal NSAIDs may be administered either before or after ERCP, both indomethacin and diclofenac seem effective, and NSAIDs are effective in both selected and unselected patients. These data agree with previous sub-analyses published by Zheng et al [36]. Although a trend towards reducing length of hospital stay was observed, few data were reported in the studies and so this cannot be confirmed.

A first limitation of the meta-analysis is a possible overestimation of the risk reduction because of the high prevalence of PEP in the control group of the included studies (7–26%). This high incidence contrasts with the rates reported in previous series that range from 1% to 10% [25,28,37]. A reasonable explanation for this high complication rate is that many studies include high-risk patients. Another possible limitation is that a proportion of the studies [14,16,17] were rated as low-quality (Jadad = 2) [38]. However, the risk reduction observed when low-quality studies were excluded was very similar to those of the main analysis (RR 0.55; 95% CI 0.42–0.73, I^2: 33%, data not shown). In addition,

Study or Subgroup	Experimental Events	Experimental Total	Control Events	Control Total	Weight	Risk Ratio M-H, Fixed, 95% CI
Cheon et al [10]	6	105	7	102	15.8%	0.83 [0.29, 2.39]
Elmunzer et al [12]	13	295	27	307	58.8%	0.50 [0.26, 0.95]
Montaño Loza et al [14]	0	75	0	75		Not estimable
Murray et al [15]	0	110	2	110	5.6%	0.20 [0.01, 4.12]
Otsuka et al [16]	0	51	3	53	7.6%	0.15 [0.01, 2.80]
Sotoudehmanesh et al [18]	0	221	5	221	12.2%	0.09 [0.01, 1.63]
Total (95% CI)		**857**		**868**	**100.0%**	**0.46 [0.28, 0.76]**
Total events	19		44			

Heterogeneity: Chi² = 3.35, df = 4 (P = 0.50); I² = 0%
Test for overall effect: Z = 2.99 (P = 0.003)

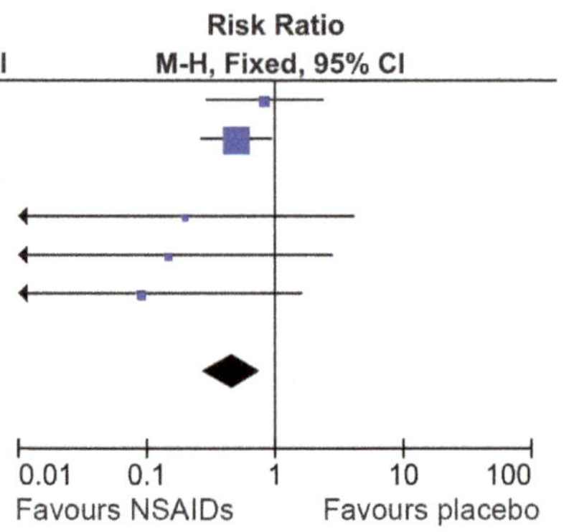

Figure 4. Meta-analysis comparing NSAIDs vs. placebo in reducing the number of moderate to severe pancreatitis. *CI*, confidence interval; *M-H*, Mantel-Haenszel; *NSAIDs*, non-steroidal anti-inflammatory drugs.

Subanalysis	Studies (ref.)	Patients	Risk Ratio (M-H-Fixed-95% CI)	I2	I^2
Type of NSAIDs					
Indomethacin	4 [10,11,13,17]	1422	0.54 (0.38-0.75)	0%	0%
Diclofenac	5 [9,12,14-16]	711	0.42 (0.21-0.84)	55%	55%
Route administration					
Rectal route	7 [10-15,17]	1846	0.45 (0.34-0.61)	0%	0%
Non rectal route	2 [9,16]	287	0.81 (0.47-1.41)	22%	22%
Time of administration					
Before ERCP	4 [10,13,15,17]	924	0.46 (0.28-0.74)	0%	0%
After ERCP	4 [11,12,14,16]	1002	0.45 (0.32-0.64)	0%	0%
Patients inclusion criteria					
ERCP, all comers or cholestasis	6 [9,10,13,15-17]	1211	0.57 (0.37-0.88)	23%	23%
ERCP, high risk patients	4 [9,11,12,14]	1101	0.53 (0.30-0.93)	58%	58%
ERCP, low risk patients	1 [9]	28	1.15 (0.08-16.67)		

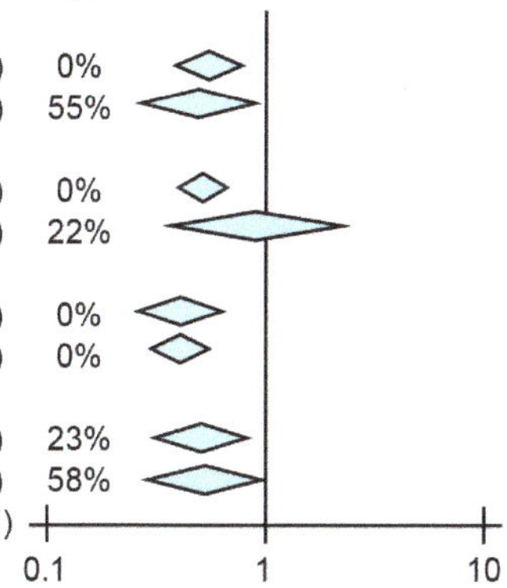

Figure 5. Summary of subanalyses comparing NSAIDs vs. placebo in reducing the number of patients with PEP according to: type of NSAID, route and time of administration and patients inclusion criteria.

severity of pancreatitis was assessed by Ranson's criteria in one study [14] and by CT findings in another [15], rather than using the currently accepted consensus definition proposed by Cotton [4]. However the risk reduction of moderate and severe pancreatitis when these studies were excluded was also very similar to the main group analysis (RR 0.47; 95% CI 0.28–0.80, data not shown). Finally, some of the sub-analyses should be interpreted with great caution because they include few studies and a low number of patients. The reduced power of some of the comparisons may explain the non-significant results in males and older age.

Our findings suggest that rectal NSAIDs are also effective when a pancreatic stent is placed. Elmunzer et al. [39] concludes in a post hoc analysis that rectal indomethacin could replace the placement of pancreatic stents. However, no RCTs comparing rectal NSAIDs alone vs. NSAIDs plus pancreatic stent placement have been carried out to date. Combinations of these agents, which act on different steps in the pathogenesis of post-ERCP pancreatitis, may reduce PEP even more in selected high risk patients, but adequately performed RCTs are needed to confirm this point.

In conclusion, there is evidence supporting the rectal administration of indomethacin or diclofenac, either before or immediately after ERCP. There is no evidence to recommend oral or

Table 2. Subanalysis: rectal NSAIDs *vs.* placebo in reducing the number of pancreatitis in subgroup of patients with a risk factor.

Subanalysis	Studies [ref.]	Patients	Risk Ratio (M-H-Fixed-95% CI)	I^2
Age				
Young patients	2 [12,18]	527	0.50 (0.30–0.83)	0%
Old patients[a]	2 [12,18]	570	0.57 (0.32, 1.05)	0%
Sex				
Females	2 [12,18]	513	0.54 (0.34–0.85)	0%
Males	2 [12,18]	327	0.54 (0.23, 1.24)	8%
Sphincterotomy				
Yes	4 [12,15,16,18]	786	0.53 (0.35–0.83)	0%
No	4 [12,15,16,18]	572	0.41 (0.23–0.72)	0%
Suspected or confirmed SOH				
Yes	2 [12,15]	662	0.50 (0.31–0.83)	10%
No	2 [12,15]	274	0.36 (0.17–0.77)	0%
Pancreatic duct injection				
Yes	3 [13,15,18]	454	0.29 (0.13–0.63)	0%
No	1 [18]	348	0.62 (0.21–1.80)	-
Prophylactic pancreatic stent[b]				
Yes	1 [12]	496	0.61 (0.38–0.98)	-
No	5 [11,12,16–18]	960	0.45 (0.28–0.70)	0%

SOH: sphincter of Oddi hypertension; *ERCP:* endoscopic retrograde cholangiopancreatography; *NSAIDs:* non-steroidal anti-inflammatory drugs.
[a]The two different studies used different cut-off values to separate young and old patients, one using 45 years and the other 60 years.
[b]Prophylactic measure, not risk factor.

parenteral administration. Rectal NSAID seem to be safe and effective in reducing the incidence and the severity of post-ERCP pancreatitis, both in high risk patients and unselected patients.

Supporting Information

Appendix S1 Search strategy used in Scopus, Pubmed, ISI Web of Knowledge and the Cochrane Library.

Checklist S1 PRISMA 2009 checklist.

Acknowledgments

Our thanks to Dr. Döbrönte for his help in the translation of some points of his article published in Hungarian and to Michael Maudsley for his help with the English.

Author Contributions

Conceived and designed the experiments: FV XC FP IP. Performed the experiments: IP AI JL PS. Analyzed the data: IP MB AI. Contributed reagents/materials/analysis tools: MB JL PS. Wrote the paper: IP XC FP FV.

References

1. Freeman ML, Guda NM (2004) Prevention of post-ERCP pancreatitis: a comprehensive review. Gastrointest Endosc 59: 845–64.
2. Masci E, Toti G, Mariani A, Curioni S, Lomazzi A, et al. (2001) Complications of diagnostic and therapeutic ERCP: a prospective multicenter study. Am J Gastroenterol 96: 417–23.
3. Cheng CL, Sherman S, Watkins JL, Barnett J, Freeman M, et al. (2006) Risk factors for post-ERCP pancreatitis: a prospective multicenter study. Am J Gastroenterol 101: 139–47.
4. Dumonceau JM, Andriulli A, Deviere J, Mariani A, Rigaux J, et al. (2010) European Society of Gastrointestinal Endoscopy (ESGE) Guideline: prophylaxis of post-ERCP pancreatitis. Endoscopy 42: 503–15.
5. Gross V, Leser HG, Heinisch A, Scholmerich J (1993) Inflammatory mediators and cytokines—new aspects of the pathophysiology and assessment of severity of acute pancreatitis? Hepatogastroenterol 40: 522–30.
6. Bhatia M, Brady M, Shokuhi S, Christmas S, Neoptolemos JP, et al. (2000) Inflammatory mediators in acute pancreatitis. J Pathol 190: 117–25.
7. Karne S, Gorelick FS (1999) Etiopathogenesis of acute pancreatitis. Surg Clin North Am 79: 699–710.
8. Makela A, Kuusi T, Schroder T (1997) Inhibition of serum phospholipase-A2 in acute pancreatitis by pharmacological agents in vitro. Scand J Clin Lab Invest 57: 401–7.
9. Kozarek RA (1990) Pancreatic stents can induce ductal changes consistent with chronic pancreatitis. Gastrointest Endosc 36: 93–5.
10. Cheon YK, Cho KB, Watkins JL, McHenry L, Fogel EL, et al. (2007) Efficacy of diclofenac in the prevention of post-ERCP pancreatitis in predominantly high-risk patients: a randomized double-blind prospective trial. Gastrointest Endosc 66: 1126–32.
11. Dobronte Z, Toldy E, Mark L, Sarang K, Lakner L (2012) Effects of rectal indomethacin in the prevention of post-ERCP acute pancreatitis. Orvosi hetilap 153: 990–6.
12. Elmunzer BJ, Scheiman JM, Lehman GA, Chak A, Mosler P, et al. (2012) A randomized trial of rectal indomethacin to prevent post-ERCP pancreatitis. N Engl J Med 366: 1414–22.
13. Khoshbaten M, Khorram H, Madad L, Ehsani Ardakani MJ, Farzin H, et al. (2008) Role of diclofenac in reducing post-endoscopic retrograde cholangiopancreatography pancreatitis. J Gastroenterol Hepatol 23: 11–6.
14. Montano Loza A, Rodriguez Lomeli X, Garcia Correa JE, Davalos Cobian C, Cervantes Guevara G, et al. (2007) Effect of the administration of rectal indomethacin on amylase serum levels after endoscopic retrograde cholangio-pancreatography, and its impact on the development of secondary pancreatitis episodes. Rev Esp Enferm Dig 99: 330–6.
15. Murray B, Carter R, Imrie C, Evans S, O'Suilleabhain C (2003) Diclofenac reduces the incidence of acute pancreatitis after endoscopic retrograde cholangiopancreatography. Gastroenterology 124: 1786–91.
16. Otsuka T, Kawazoe S, Nakashita S, Kamachi S, Oeda S, et al. (2012) Low-dose rectal diclofenac for prevention of post-endoscopic retrograde cholangiopancreatography pancreatitis: a randomized controlled trial. J Gastroenterol 47: 912–7.
17. Senol A, Saritas U, Demirkan H (2009) Efficacy of intramuscular diclofenac and fluid replacement in prevention of post-ERCP pancreatitis. World J Gastroenterol 15: 3999–4004.
18. Sotoudehmanesh R, Khatibian M, Kolahdoozan S, Ainechi S, Malboosbaf R, et al. (2007) Indomethacin may reduce the incidence and severity of acute pancreatitis after ERCP. Am J Gastroenterol 102: 978–83.
19. Dumonceau JM, Rigaux J, Kahaleh M, Gomez CM, Vandermeeren A, et al. (2010) Prophylaxis of post-ERCP pancreatitis: a practice survey. Gastrointest Endosc 71: 934–9.
20. Elmunzer BJ, Waljee AK, Elta GH, Taylor JR, Fehmi SM, et al. (2008) A meta-analysis of rectal NSAIDs in the prevention of post-ERCP pancreatitis. Gut 57: 1262–7.
21. Dai HF, Wang XW, Zhao K (2009) Role of nonsteroidal anti-inflammatory drugs in the prevention of post-ERCP pancreatitis: a meta-analysis. Hepatobiliary Pancreat Dis Int 8: 11–6.
22. Ding X, Chen M, Huang S, Zhang S, Zou X (2012) Nonsteroidal anti-inflammatory drugs for prevention of post-ERCP pancreatitis: a meta-analysis. Gastrointest Endosc 76: 1152–9.
23. Liberati A, Altman DG, Tetzlaff J, Mulrow C, Gotzsche PC, et al. (2009) The PRISMA statement for reporting systematic reviews and meta-analyses of studies that evaluate health care interventions: explanation and elaboration. PLoS Medicine 6: e1000100
24. Cotton PB, Lehman G, Vennes J, Geenen JE, Russell RC, et al. (1991) Endoscopic sphincterotomy complications and their management: an attempt at consensus. Gastrointest Endosc 37: 383–93.
25. Freeman ML, Nelson DB, Sherman S, Haber GB, Herman ME, et al. (1996) Complications of endoscopic biliary sphincterotomy. N Engl J Med 335: 909–18.
26. Choi CW, Kang DH, Kim GH, Eum JS, Lee SM, et al. (2009) Nafamostat mesylate in the prevention of post-ERCP pancreatitis and risk factors for post-ERCP pancreatitis. Gastrointest Endosc 69: 11–8.
27. Lee KT, Lee DH, Yoo BM (2008). The prophylactic effect of somatostatin on post-therapeutic endoscopic retrograde cholangiopancreatography pancreatitis: a randomized, multicenter controlled trial. Pancreas 37: 445–8.
28. Masci E, Mariani A, Curioni S, Testoni PA (2003) Risk factors for pancreatitis following endoscopic retrograde cholangiopancreatography: a meta-analysis. Endoscopy 35: 830–4.
29. Kjaergard LL, Villumsen J, Gluud C (2001) Reported methodologic quality and discrepancies between large and small randomized trials in meta-analyses. Ann Intern Med 135: 982–9.
30. Higgins JP, Thompson SG (2002) Quantifying heterogeneity in a meta-analysis. Stat Med 21: 1539–58.
31. Higgins JP, Thompson SG, Deeks JJ, Altman DG (2003) Measuring inconsistency in meta-analyses. BMJ 327: 557–60.
32. Review Manager (RevMan) (2011) Version 5.1 ed: Copenhagen: The Nordic Cochrane Centre, The Cochrane Collaboration.
33. Montano Loza A, Garcia Correa J, Gonzalez Ojeda A, Fuentes Orozco C, Davalos Cobian C, et al. (2006) Prevention of hyperamilasemia and pancreatitis after endoscopic retrograde cholangiopancreatography with rectal administration of indomethacin. Rev Gastroenterol Mex 71: 262–8.
34. Katsinelos P, Fasoulas K, Paroutoglou G, Chatzimavroudis G, Beltsis A, et al. (2012) Combination of diclofenac plus somatostatin in the prevention of post-ERCP pancreatitis: a randomized, double-blind, placebo-controlled trial. Endoscopy 44: 53–9.
35. Bhatia V, Ahuja V, Acharya SK, Garg PK (2011) A randomized controlled trial of valdecoxib and glyceryl trinitrate for the prevention of post-ERCP pancreatitis. J Clin Gastroenterol 45: 170–6.
36. Zheng MH, Xia HH and Chen YP (2008) Rectal administration of NSAIDs in the prevention of post-ERCP pancreatitis: a complementary meta-analysis. Gut 57: 1632–3.
37. Cheon YK, Cho KB, Watkins JL, McHenry L, Fogel EL, et al. (2007) Frequency and severity of post-ERCP pancreatitis correlated with extent of pancreatic ductal opacification. Gastrointest Endosc 65: 385–93.
38. Moher D, Pham B, Jones A, Cook DJ, Jadad AR, et al. (1998) Does quality of reports of randomised trials affect estimates of intervention efficacy reported in meta-analyses? Lancet 352: 609–13.
39. Elmunzer BJ, Higgins PDR, Saini SD, Scheiman JM, Parker RA, et al. (2013) Does rectal indomethacin eliminate the need for prophylactic pancreatic stent placement in patients undergoing high-risk ercp post hoc efficacy and cost-benefit analyses using prospective clinical trial data. Am J Gastroenterol 108: 410–415.

The Association between GP Consultations for Non-Specific Physical Symptoms in Children and Parents

Mujahed Shraim[1,2,3], Milisa Blagojevic-Bucknall[1], Christian D. Mallen[1], Kate M. Dunn[1]*

1 Arthritis Research UK Primary Care Centre, Keele University, Keele, United Kingdom, **2** Work Environment Department, University of Massachusetts Lowell, Lowell, Massachusetts, United States of America, **3** Center for Disability Research, Liberty Mutual Research Institute for Safety, Hopkinton, Massachusetts, United States of America

Abstract

Background: Non-specific physical symptoms (NSPS) such as abdominal pain, headache and musculoskeletal pain are widespread in the community, and are common reasons for visiting a general practitioner (GP). Causes of NSPS are multifactorial, but may include parental influences.

Objective: To investigate associations between GP consultations for NSPS in parents and their children.

Methods: Matched case-control study using GP consultation data from 12 GP practices in the United Kingdom. Participants were 1328 children who consulted a GP for NSPS in 2009 (cases), 3980 controls who consulted a GP in 2009 but not for NSPS, plus parents of cases and controls (n = 8354). Primary outcome measure: child consultation status for NSPS.

Results: Maternal consultation for NSPS was associated with significantly increased odds of their child consulting for NSPS (odds ratio (OR) 1.51, 95% confidence intervals (CI) 1.33, 1.73); there was no significant association with paternal consultations (OR 0.87, 95% CI 0.71, 1.08). Each additional maternal consultation for NSPS was associated with an increase in the rate ratio for number of consultations for NSPS in the child by 1.03 (95% CI 1.01, 1.05). This overall association was clearest in maternal-child consultations for painful NSPS and for specific bodily systems including gastrointestinal, musculoskeletal and neurologic symptoms.

Conclusions: Maternal GP consultation for NSPS is associated with increased odds of GP consultations for NSPS in children. This study included a large sample of children and parents and used medical records data which is not subject to recall bias. However, analysis was based on medical records, thus the presence of NSPS not leading to consultations is unknown. Medical practitioners managing children with NSPS need to be aware of this association.

Editor: Martin Chalumeau, Université Paris Descartes; AP-HP, Groupe Hospitalier Cochin-Saint-Vincent-de-Paul, France

Funding: MS was funded by NHS Research and Development Support for New Medical Schools. CDM is funded by a Clinician Scientist Fellowship (19634) from Arthritis Research UK. KMD is funded through a Research Career Development Fellowship from the Wellcome Trust (083572). MB is supported by a NIHR National School for Primary Care Research Fellowship. CiPCA is funded by the North Staffordshire Primary Care Research Consortium and Keele University Research Institute for Primary Care and Health Sciences. The funders had no role in study design, data collection and analysis, decision to publish, or preparation of the manuscript.

Competing Interests: The authors have declared that no competing interests exist.

* Email: k.m.dunn@keele.ac.uk

Introduction

Non-specific physical symptoms (NSPS), such as musculoskeletal pain, abdominal pain, and headache are common in children [1,2]. Annually, about one third of children consult a general practitioner (GP) for NSPS [3,4]. NSPS among children are associated with functional impairment and negative impact on quality of life [5,6]. This represents a significant burden on health care services through frequent general practitioner (GP) consultations, diagnostic testing, and referrals to secondary care services [7–9]. The causes of NSPS in children are yet to be fully explained, but are likely to be multifactorial, including genetic and psychosocial factors, such as parental influence on childhood illness and health-seeking behavior [3,10,11].

A recent systematic review found evidence of an association between GP consultations for NSPS in parents and children, but its findings were limited by the methodology used in the empirical studies, including the use of cross-sectional designs, reliance on self-reported data by either parents or children, and including children from specific age groups only [12]. Further research using documented GP consultation data may provide more precise information about the impact of parental NSPS on the child's health and GP consulting behavior for NSPS.

The objective of this study was to investigate the association between GP consultations for NSPS in parents and their children, assess whether this is different for mothers and fathers, and identify gradients of association for any observed associations.

Methods

Ethics statement

Ethical approval for the Consultations in Primary Care Archive (CiPCA) database was given by the North Staffordshire and Staffordshire Research Ethics Committees (UK), who gave permission to download and store anonymised medical record information for research use from participating general practices. All general practices participating in CiPCA inform their patient populations that their anonymised records will be used in this way and all patients are offered the opportunity to withdraw their records from inclusion in CiPCA.

Study design and setting

This was a matched case-control study of children and their parents registered with UK GP practices. The setting was GP practices contributing to CiPCA, a primary care research database containing all recorded primary care consultations occurring at a subset of GP practices in Staffordshire, UK. In 2007, 12 GP practices contributed to the CiPCA database. The total population registered with these practices at mid-year 2009 was 104,911. CiPCA is a high quality, anonymized, and validated database, and the contributing practices have regular cycles of training, assessment and feedback with respect to the quality of coded clinical data [13]. Data from CiPCA on the annual consultation prevalence for musculoskeletal conditions are comparable to data from larger national primary care databases [14].

Participants

Eligible participants were children and their parents registered with CiPCA practices between January 2007 and December 2009. We randomly selected only one child per household for inclusion in the study, because the main exposure of interest was parental consultation for NSPS, which would be the same for siblings; this thereby avoids over representing families with more than one child. Cases were defined as children, aged 2 to 16 years in 2009, who had at least one recorded GP consultation for NSPS between 1 January and 31 December 2009 (inclusive). We used the same criteria to define controls except that controls had at least one GP consultation, but not for NSPS.

We matched controls to cases on sex, maternal age group, and GP practice. We included between one to four controls per case (depending on the availability of suitable controls). If more than four controls per case were available, four were randomly selected. The sample size was calculated for 80% study power and 95% confidence using EpiCalc 2000 [15]. Sample size calculations showed that 535 children were required (107 cases and 428 controls) for each analysis (within mothers and children, and within fathers and children) to be able to detect an association between GP consultation for NSPS in parents and children with an odds ratio (OR) of 2, assuming the proportion exposed in the control group is 20%, and with 1:4 ratio of cases to controls.

Study variables

Outcome measures were the child's GP consultation status for NSPS and stratified by type of NSPS (painful and not-painful), different body systems, and single NSPS (see table 1), number of GP consultations for NSPS, and number of different NSPS consulted for.

Ascertainment of child GP consultations for NSPS

We identified GP consultations for NSPS by using a comprehensive list of standardized diagnostic Read codes referring to the list of NSPS presented in table 1. This list includes 33 NSPS from the diagnostic criteria in the third revision of Diagnostic and Statistical Manual of Mental Disorders for Somatization Disorder [16] and nine NSPS from the somatization factor of the Hopkins Symptom Checklist [17]. These NSPS were included in previous studies of Children's Somatization Inventory [18,19] and other epidemiological studies investigating NSPS in children and adolescents [1,20].

Read codes are a hierarchy of morbidity, symptoms and process codes that are used to record all electronic morbidity data in primary care in the UK [21]. We developed this list of Read codes by reviewing all Read codes referring to signs and symptoms in Read coding system. The full list of Read codes for included NSPS is available upon request from the authors. We classified GP consultations for NSPS as such if the reason for encounter was coded by the GP using any Read codes from our list. Also, one reviewer (MS) reviewed all free-text records for these consultations to ensure that the cause of symptoms (in the opinion of the GP) was not-specific: (a) not due to trauma or pregnancy (in mothers) (b) no recorded abnormalities on physical examination and/or diagnostic testing. If no information indicating (a) or (b) was available in the free-text records, we classified such consultations as consultations for NSPS.

Assessment of exposure to parental consultations for NSPS

Within the CiPCA database, household identification codes were used to link household members, then date of birth was used to determine parents of included children. A mother/father of a randomly selected child within each household was defined as being a female/male aged 17 to 45 years at the birth of the child. All GP consultations made by parents between 1 January 2007 and 31 December 2008 were extracted from the CiPCA database. Maternal and paternal GP consultation status for NSPS between 2007 and 2008 were identified using the same method as described above for children. In children with GP consultation data on both parents, parental GP consultation status for NSPS was grouped into four categories. These comprised: both parents consulted for NSPS, only mother consulted for NSPS, only father consulted for NSPS, and neither parent consulted for NSPS. We also measured the total number of GP consultations for NSPS, and number of different NSPS in consulting parents during 2007-8. We also measured NSPS in parents sorted by painful and not-painful NSPS, body system, and single NSPS (table 1).

Measurement of other independent variables

Besides variables used for case-control matching, we also obtained child's age, paternal age group, child birth order, household member count, index of multiple deprivation (IMD) 2007 scores for residential area level deprivation for included children, and parental history of anxiety or depressive disorders.

Children's age was split into tertiles (2–6, 7–11 and 12–16) and parents' age into quartiles (19–28, 29–39, 40–50 and 51–61 for mothers and 22–29, 30–40, 41–51 and 52–62 for fathers). Parents' age in 2009 rather than 2007 was used to reflect their age at the time of children's consultation. For example, mothers in the age group 19–28 years were two years younger at the time of their consultation in 2007.

Younger siblings for index children were defined as persons from the same household born after the index child, whereas older siblings were defined as persons from the same household and aged 16 or less at the birth of the index child. The birth order of the child was classified as "first" if the child had no siblings or if the child was the oldest child in the household (with no other household members' meeting the definition for a sibling).

Table 1. List of NSPS and their distribution in children and parents.

Non-specific physical symptoms	Case-children (n = 1328)	All mothers (n = 5308)	All fathers (n = 3058)
Musculoskeletal symptoms			
Pain in extremities	99 (7.5)	253 (4.8)	124 (4.1)
Back pain	59 (4.4)	460 (8.6)	237 (7.8)
Joint pain	209 (15.7)	627 (11.8)	148 (4.8)
Muscle soreness	5 (0.4)	15 (0.3)	7 (0.2)
Gastrointestinal symptoms			
Abdominal pain	346 (26.1)	547 (10.3)	130 (4.3)
Vomiting	146 (11.0)	39 (0.7)	13 (0.4)
Nausea	20 (1.5)	60 (1.1)	9 (0.3)
Bloating	3 (0.2)	37 (0.7)	6 (0.2)
Diarrhea	83 (6.3)	56 (1.1)	28 (0.9)
Constipation	132 (9.9)	59 (1.1)	10 (0.3)
Multiple food intolerance	0	0	0
Globus (lump in the throat)	0	7 (0.1)	0
Dysphagia (difficulty swallowing)	0	0	0
Cardiopulmonary symptoms			
Palpitations	9 (0.7)	17 (0.3)	34 (1.1)
Chest pain	62 (4.7)	211 (4.0)	119 (3.9)
Hyperventilation or Dyspnea	44 (3.3)	63 (1.2)	12 (0.4)
Hot or cold spells	1 (0.1)	17 (0.3)	4 (0.1)
Urogenital symptoms			
Pain during urination	1 (0.1)	0	0
Difficulty urinating (Dysuria)	77 (5.8)	4 (0.1)	3 (0.1)
Burning sensation in sexual organs or rectum	0	0	0
Dysmenorrhea (painful menstruation)	0	28 (0.5)	**
Metrorrhagia (irregular menstrual periods)	0	99 (1.9)	**
Menorrhagia (heavy menstrual bleeding)	0	210 (4.0)	**
Sexual indifference (decreased libido)*	*	16 (0.3)	16 (0.5)
Dyspareunia (pain during intercourse)*	*	26 (0.5)	**
Neurologic symptoms			
Dizziness/fainting (syncope)	22 (1.7)	168 (3.2)	43 (1.4)
Transient Amnesia (loss of memory)	0	4 (0.1)	1 (0.0)
Transient Aphonia (loss of voice)	0	0	0
Transient deafness	0	0	0
Transient Diplopia (double vision)	0	0	0
Transient blurred vision	1 (0.1)	4 (0.1)	0
Transient blindness	0	0	0
Transient seizure or convulsion	11 (0.8)	0	0
Transient Ataxia (trouble walking)	0	0	0
Transient Paresis (paralysis)	0	0	0
Headache	167 (12.6)	454 (8.6)	90 (2.9)
Paresthesia (numbness or tingling sensation)	4 (0.3)	58 (1.1)	33 (1.1)
Weakness in parts of the body	0	0	0
Heavy feelings in arms or legs	1 (0.1)	0	0
General symptoms			
Fatigue	68 (5.1)	225 (4.2)	58 (1.9)

NSPS = non-specific physical symptoms; values are numbers (%); * = Symptoms were excluded from analysis for children;** = Not Applicable.

Table 2. Baseline characteristics of children.

	Cases (n = 1328) n(%)[a]	Controls (n = 3980) n(%)[a]	*p*-value
Child gender (Female)[b]	739 (55.6)	2073 (52.1)	0.99
Child age[c]	10 (9)	8 (8)	<0.01
Child age group [b]			
2–6 years	428 (32.2)	1688 (42.4)	
7–11 years	325 (24.5)	1114 (28.0)	
12–16 years	575 (43.3)	1178 (29.6)	
Child birth order [b]			
First	63 (57.5)	2083 (52.3)	<0.01
Not first	565 (42.5)	1897 (47.7)	
Household members' count	4 (1)	4 (1)	0.02
Household member count [b]			
≤3	691 (52.0)	1908 (47.9)	
>3	637 (48.0)	2072 (52.1)	
IMD 2007 score[c]	22.4 (22.9)	23.1 (22.9)	0.93
IMD 2007quartiles [b]			
I	272 (20.5)	819 (20.6)	
II	262 (19.7)	785 (19.7)	
III	263 (19.8)	792 (19.9)	
IV	280 (21.1)	809 (20.3)	
V	244 (18.4)	759 (19.1)	
Missing IMD score [b]	7 (0.5)	16 (0.4)	
Mother age[c]	39 (11)	38 (9)	<0.01
Mother age group [b]			
19–29 years	216 (16.3)	722 (18.1)	
30–40 years	604 (45.5)	1972 (49.5)	
41–51 years	475 (35.8)	1227 (30.8)	
52–62 years	33 (2.5)	59 (1.5)	
Father age[c]	41 (10)	40 (9)	<0.01
Father age group[b]			
22–32 years	101 (13.2)	378 (16.6)	
33–43 years	381 (49.9)	1241 (54.4)	
44–54 years	246 (32.2)	590 (25.9)	
55–65 years	36 (4.7)	73 (3.2)	
Mother history of anxiety or depressive disorder 2007–2008 [b]			
No	993 (74.8)	3188 (80.1)	<0.01
Yes	335 (25.2)	792 (19.9)	
Father history of anxiety or depressive disorder 2007–2008[b,d]			
No	699 (91.4)	2110 (92.4)	0.39
Yes	65 (8.5)	172 (7.5)	

[a]Percentages may not total 100 due to rounding; [b]Number (%); [c]Median (Interquartile range) Index of Multiple Deprivation 2007; [d]564 (42.5%) of cases and 1698 (42.7%) of controls had no paternal records. Controls were matched to cases on sex, maternal age group, and GP practice.

The child household member count was dichotomized into households with three members or less and households with more than three households. Households with 13 or more members were excluded to prevent including families living in shared households. The IMD 2007 scores were constructed by the Department of Communities and Local Government, and conceptualized as a weighted area level aggregation of scores for seven domains of deprivation including income; employment; health deprivation and disability; education, skills and training; barriers to housing and services; crime; living environment [22]. IMD 2007 scores range from 0% to 100% where higher scores indicate greater deprivation [22]. IMD 2007 scores were also presented as quintiles with "1" representing the most affluent and "5" representing the most deprived. Maternal and paternal history of anxiety or depressive disorders status (yes, no) was identified by searching parental electronic primary care records between 2007 and 2008 using a list of symptom and diagnostic Read codes referring to anxiety and depressive disorders (this list is available on request from the authors).

Statistical methods

Chi-squared tests and Mann-Whitney U tests were performed to test for significant baseline differences between cases and controls. We performed univariable analyses to examine crude associations between the independent variables and the child GP consultation status for NSPS using Cox regression. Effect size estimates were summarised using odds ratios (OR) with 95% confidence intervals (CI). We included all independent variables in the multivariable Cox regression to obtain adjusted associations between parental and child consultation for NSPS. In separate multivariable analyses, we also tested for any interaction effects between parental GP consultations for NSPS and other independent variables on the child GP consultation for NSPS.

In order to test for any potential gradient in associations, logistic regression was used to model effect of increasing number of paternal GP consultations for NSPS, and increasing number of different NSPS a parent consults for, on whether a child consults for NSPS. Similar analyses tested the relationship between consultation for multiple NSPS in parents and children. Furthermore, using Poisson regression we investigated whether there was a relationship between number of maternal consultations for NSPS and number of NSPS consultations in children.

In analyses for associations for painful and not-painful NSPS, body system, and single NSPS we adopted an unmatched case-control approach using logistic regression because relatively small number of cases have consulted for these symptoms categories. All analyses were carried out using SPSS (version 20.0) [23] and STATA (version 12) [24].

Results

Characteristics of cases and controls

5308 children were included (1328 cases and 3980 controls). The mothers of all children were identified. The fathers of 42.5% of cases and 42.7% of controls were unknown based on GP registration data, leaving 766 cases and 2292 controls with identifiable fathers. This may be because fathers were registered with other GP practices or were not registered with any practice at all, or because children were living with single-mothers. The baseline characteristics of all study participants are shown in table 2. Cases and controls differed significantly on all variables except for IMD 2007 scores and father history of anxiety or depressive disorders. Median age for cases was 10 years (Interquartile range 9) and 8 (8) years for controls (table 2). Maternal age was significantly different in cases and controls despite matching them on maternal age group. The most common single NSPS in children were abdominal pain, joint pain and headache. Abdominal pain, joint pain and back pain were the most common symptoms in parents (table 1).

The association between GP consultations for NSPS in parents and children

Overall, 52% of cases and 41% of controls had a maternal history of consultation for NSPS, and 30% of cases and controls (with available paternal records) had paternal history of consultation for NSPS.

Initially, analyses included all children, irrespective of whether both parents were identified. Univariable analysis revealed that cases were more likely than controls to have a history of maternal GP consultation for NSPS (crude OR 1.55, 95% CI 1.37, 1.76), a finding which persisted in multivariable analysis (adjusted OR 1.51, 95% CI 1.33, 1.73) after adjustment for child age group, father age group, child birth order, household members' count, and maternal history of anxiety and depressive disorders. We found no significant association between GP consultation for NSPS in fathers and children (table 3). Subsequently, analyses included only those children who had both parents identified in the study sample (764 cases and 2183 controls).

We found that in instances where only a mother consulted for NSPS, the odds of a child having a GP consultation for NSPS was 1.38 (95% CI 1.14, 1.69) as compared to a child with neither parent consulting for NSPS. We found no significant association between GP consultations for NSPS in fathers and children (see Table 4). However, GP consultation for NSPS in both parents was associated with increased odds of child consulting for NSPS (adjusted OR 1.57, 95% CI 1.23, 2.01).

No significant interaction effects were identified between parental consultation for NSPS and other independent variables on the child GP consultation status for NSPS.

Gradients association between GP consultations for NSPS in parents and children

Analyses for gradients association were restricted to mother-child pairs because we found no significant associations between GP consultations for NSPS in fathers and children. Logistic regression analysis showed a significant increase in the odds of child consulting for NSPS with increasing number of GP consultations for NSPS and number of different NSPS consulted for in the mother (see table 5). Children whose mother consulted only once had odds of consulting almost 1.4 times higher than children whose mother didn't consult. These odds increased to 2.14 (95% CI 1.68, 2.72) for those children whose mother consulted more than three times.

Restricting the analysis only to cases, Poisson regression showed that each additional one maternal GP consultation for NSPS was associated with increase in the rate ratio for number of consultations for NSPS in the child by 1.03 (95% CI 1.01, 1.05). Additionally, using logistic regression, we found that cases whose mothers consulted with multiple NSPS (two or more NSPS) had increased odds of consulting with multiple NSPS as compared to cases whose mothers did not consult for NSPS (adjusted OR 2.24, 95% CI 1.68, 2.99).

The association between GP consultations for NSPS groups and single NSPS in parents and children

As shown in table 6, we found significant associations between consultations for painful NSPS in mothers and children (OR 1.49, 95% CI 1.28, 1.74), but not for not-painful NSPS (OR 1.11, 95% CI 0.88, 1.40). Logistic regression analysis showed significant associations between maternal and child consultations for musculoskeletal, gastrointestinal, and neurologic symptoms, but not for cardiopulmonary and urogenital symptoms (table 6). Additionally, the association between maternal and child consultations for single NSPS was statistically significant for abdominal pain, joint pain, extremities pain, headache, and vomiting (table 6)

Discussion

This study found statistically significant associations between GP consultations for NSPS in mothers (but not fathers) and their children. The association between parental and child consultation was stronger when both parents consulted for NSPS. We also found a statistically significant gradient of association between the number of GP consultations for NSPS and the number of NSPS in mothers and children. Additionally, we found significant associ-

Table 3. Associations between consultations for NSPS in either parant and children.

	Cases (n = 1328) n(%)	Controls (n = 3980) n(%)	Crude OR (95% CI)	Adjusted OR (95% CI)
Maternal consultation history for NSPS 2007–2008				
Yes	695 (52.3)	1642 (41.3)	1.55 (1.37, 1.76)	1.51 (1.33, 1.73)
No	633 (47.7)	2338 (58.7)	1	1
Paternal consultation history for NSPS 2007–2008				
Yes	228 (29.9)	692 (30.4)	0.89 (0.73, 1.09)	0.87 (0.71, 1.08)
No	536 (70.1)	1590 (69.6)	1	1

NSPS = non-specific physical symptoms; OR = odds ratio; CI = confidence intervals; 564 (42.5%) of cases and 1698 (42.7%) of controls had no paternal records. ORs were adjusted for child age, father age, child birth order; household members' count, Index of Multiple Deprivation 2007 scores; maternal and paternal anxiety or depressive disorder.

ations between maternal and child consultation for painful symptoms, specific body systems, and single NSPS.

The observed associations between GP consultations for NSPS in mothers and children are consistent with the findings of a systematic review which found evidence of an association between GP consultations for NSPS in parents and children [12]. However, that review found only eight studies, and the majority of studies used self-reported data by either parents or children and used cross-sectional designs. One study reported that the associations between GP consultations for abdominal pain or headache were greater for mother-child pairs than father-child pairs [3]. Another study found maternal GP consultations NSPS more predictive of the child consultations for gastrointestinal NSPS than those of fathers [25].

With respect to the significant association between maternal and child consultation for painful NSPS, but not for not-painful symptoms, it may be that consulting behavior is influenced by level of pain severity and perceived seriousness of the symptoms [26,27]. For example, parents may perceive painful NSPS in themselves and in their children as more serious than not-painful NSPS, which influences their GP consultation rates for these NSPS.

One possible explanation for these associations is an inherited genetic predisposition to NSPS. There is some evidence that genetic effects contribute to the onset of some NSPS and syndromes, such as headache and irritable bowel syndrome [28,29]. However, it is seems unlikely for genetic factors to fully explain this, because only maternal (and not paternal) consultations for NSPS were associated with the child consulting for NSPS. Another explanation is shared exposure of family members to certain social and environmental factors (e.g. stressful events, lack of social support, socioeconomic circumstances, and poor family functioning) which have been found to be associated with greater reporting of NSPS [30,31] and GP consultations for NSPS in parents and children [7]. One plausible explanation is the childhood social learning of illness behavior, which has been hypothesised to play an important role in the development of illness and healthcare seeking behavior among children [32–34]. A number of studies have suggested that parental responses and attitudes toward the child illness (reinforcement) and parental coping mechanisms with their own illness (role modelling) may influence symptom frequency, disability days, and healthcare consultations in their children [35,36]. We would expect social learning and role modeling to increase with child's age. However, we found no significant interaction effects between the child age group (or other independent variables) and maternal consultations for NSPS on the child GP consultation status for NSPS. This suggests that the maternal effect on child consultations for NSPS through "reinforcement" is present at all ages and represent a more important influence.

Strengths and limitations

The main limitations of the previous few studies that examined the association between GP consultations for NSPS in parents and children were the use of self-reported data which is prone to recall bias, including children from specific age groups, and the use of cross-sectional designs that are unable to distinguish the direction of associations. Strengths of our study therefore include the fact that we used documented GP consultations, which are more precise source of information on attendance in primary care than relying on self-reported data by children or their parents that may be prone to recall bias [37]. Additionally, we included a large sample (n = 5308) and relied on documented GP attendance from

Table 4. Associations between consultations for NSPS in both parents and children.

	Cases (n = 764) n(%)	Controls (n = 2183) n(%)	Crude OR (95% CI)	Adjusted OR (95% CI)
Both parents did not consult for NSPS	276 (36.1)	989 (45.3)	1	1
Only father consulted for NSPS	78 (10.2)	335 (15.3)	0.82 (0.63, 1.08)	0.83 (0.63, 1.10)
Only mother consulted for NSPS	260 (34.0)	568 (26.0)	1.44 (1.20, 1.74)	1.38 (1.14, 1.69)
Both parents consulted for NSPS	150 (19.6)	291 (13.3)	1.63 (1.29, 2.06)	1.57 (1.23, 2.01)

NSPS = non-specific physical symptoms; OR = odds ratio; CI = confidence intervals. ORs were adjusted for child age, father age, child birth order; household members' count, Index of Multiple Deprivation 2007 scores; maternal and paternal anxiety or depressive disorder.

Table 5. Associations between number of consultations for NSPS and number of different NSPS in mother and child consultation for NSPS.

NSPS	Cases n = 1328 n(%)	Controls n = 3980 n(%)	Crude OR (95% CI)	Adjusted OR (95% CI)
Maternal number of consultations for NSPS				
0	633 (47.7)	2338 (58.7)	1	1
1	300 (22.6)	809 (20.3)	1.37 (1.17, 1.61)	1.38 (1.17, 1.63)
2	156 (11.7)	406 (10.2)	1.41 (1.14, 1.73)	1.36 (1.10, 1.68)
3	96 (7.2)	198 (5)	1.77 (1.36, 2.31)	1.69 (1.28, 2.22)
>3	143 (10.8)	229 (5.8)	2.24 (1.78, 2.82)	2.14 (1.68, 2.72)
Maternal number of different NSPS				
0	663 (47.7)	2338 (58.7)	1	1
1–2	601 (45.3)	1494 (37.5)	1.47 (1.29, 1.68)	1.45 (1.27, 1.66)
>2	94 (7.1)	148 (3.7)	2.37 (1.79, 3.12)	2.24 (1.68, 2.99)

OR = odds ratio; CI = confidence intervals. ORs were adjusted for child age, child birth order; household members' count, Index of Multiple Deprivation 2007 scores; maternal anxiety or depressive disorder.

12 practices which increases the internal and external validity of our findings. Also, as described in the methods section, CiPCA is a high quality validated database, which enhances the validity of our findings. For example, 97% of all GP consultations that occurred in the CiPCA practices in 2006 were given a morbidity code [38]. Another important strength is that parental consultation status for NSPS was ascertained using parental consultations data in the two years preceding the child consultation, which provides a clear temporal relationship. Additionally, the observed associations were supported by evidence of gradients of association.

One limitation is the potential for diagnostic misclassification, which is a common problem in primary care [39]. However, diagnostic misclassification is unlikely to completely explain the associations found in this study due to the high quality of coded clinical data within CiPCA practices. Additionally, the current classification system used in primary care allows for coding definitive diagnoses (e.g. urinary tract infection) as well as symptoms' diagnoses (e.g. abdominal pain) when a definitive diagnosis is not established, which reduces the potential for diagnostic misclassification. One potential limitation is the lack of blinding of GPs to symptoms in parents and children at time of consultation. However, we believe that this is minimal and not systematic because it does not explain differences in associations between mothers and fathers, and that our findings were based on association between parents' consultations in 2007–2008 and the child's consultations in 2009. Another limitation is that, based on GP practice registered population data, we were not able to examine whether our findings are different for children living or not living in the same house as their mother and father. Also, paternal consultations status for NSPS was unknown for 43% of children. However, this was distributed equally between cases and controls. Additionally, it is unlikely that the lack of significant associations between GP consultations for NSPS in fathers and children is entirely attributed to low study power as the numbers of children with paternal consultation data were more than those needed based on sample size calculations. Although we matched controls and cases on maternal age group, they differed significantly on maternal age. However, it is unlikely for this to lead to significant changes in our ORs estimates because we also found statistically significant associations for single NSPS in mother and children after adjustment for maternal age in unmatched analyses.

Although this study set out to examine the association between consultation patterns for NSPS in parents and children, GP consultation data only provides a measure of health problems for which practice registered populations have consulted. Thus, the presence of other NSPS which did not result in GP consultation remains unknown.

Generalizability

In the UK over 97% of the population is registered with a GP practice, which usually provides first point access to non-emergency healthcare [40]. We used a large population-based sample of families registered with GP practices from Staffordshire. This area is more deprived than England as a whole, but we found no significant associations between child GP consultation for NSPS and area level deprivation in either univariable or multivariable analyses. Although the healthcare setting in UK may be different from other healthcare settings, similar associations for specific symptoms between parents and children were reported in different countries [3,25,41].

Implications for clinical practice and future research

These findings indicate that GPs and other medical practitioners managing children with NSPS in secondary care settings should be aware of the association between consultations for NSPS in parents and children, as such insights might direct medical practitioners toward alternative management approaches. For example, a recent randomized controlled trial has demonstrated that cognitive behavioral therapy (CBT) targeting children's coping responses to recurrent abdominal pain and parents' responses to pain in their children was associated with significant reduction in pain and gastrointestinal symptoms severity in children at six month follow-up [42]. It is not clear whether CBT had an impact on the consultation behavior of children for NSPS. There is some evidence from literature on adults that CBT, pharmacological therapy, and aerobic exercise for patients presenting with NSPS in primary care and general outpatient clinics are effective in reducing frequency of symptoms, the number of consultations, and related psychological distress [43–46]. Potentially, such interventions for parents could impact on the illness and healthcare seeking behavior of both parents and their children, but no studies exist to confirm or refute this. This provides a rationale for future research to focus on development of

Table 6. Associations between consultation for specific symptoms in mothers & children.

	NSPS in the child			
NSPS in the mother	**Yes**	**No**	**Crude OR (95% CI)**	**Adjusted OR (95% CI)**
Painful NSPS				
Yes	376	1441	1.53 (1.32, 1.77)	1.49 (1.28, 1.74)
No	509	2982	1	1
Not-painful NSPS				
Yes	111	843	1.21 (0.97, 1.50)	1.11 (0.88, 1.40)
No	429	3925	1	1
Musculoskeletal NSPS				
Yes	130	1128	1.53 (1.23, 1.90)	1.41 (1.22, 1.75)
No	284	3766	1	1
Gastrointestinal NSPS				
Yes	112	576	1.51 (1.21, 1.89)	1.40 (1.12, 1.76)
No	527	493	1	1
Neurological NSPS				
Yes	44	558	1.92 (1.36, 2.69)	2.10 (1.46, 3.02)
No	186	4520	1	1
Cardiopulmonary NSPS				
Yes	5	210	1.62 (0.65, 4.04)	1.27 (0.50, 3.25)
No	74	5019	1	1
Urogenital NSPS				
Yes	5	352	0.96 (0.39, 2.40)	0.90 (0.36, 2.26)
No	72	4879	1	1
Abdominal pain				
Yes	59	488	1.89 (1.40, 2.53)	1.81 (1.34, 2.44)
No	287	4474	1	1
Joint pain				
Yes	37	590	1.64 (1.14, 2.37)	1.55 (1.07, 2.25)
No	172	4509	1	1
Headache				
Yes	23	431	1.75 (1.11, 2.74)	2.02 (1.26, 3.24)
No	144	4710	1	1
Vomiting				
Yes	6	33	6.67 (2.75, 16.15)	4.98 (2.00, 12.40)
No	140	5129	1	1
Constipation				
Yes	1	58	0.67 (0.09, 4.90)	0.60 (0.08, 4.40)
No	131	5118	1	1
Pain in extremities				
Yes	10	243	2.30 (1.18, 4.47)	2.12 (1.08, 4.16)
No	89	4966	1	1
Diarrhea				
Yes	2	54	2.36 (0.57, 9.86)	2.17 (0.51, 9.36)
No	81	5171	1	1
Fatigue				
Yes	2	223	0.68 (0.17, 2.80)	0.70 (0.17, 2.89)
No	66	5017	1	1
Back pain				
Yes	8	452	1.67 (0.79, 3.53)	1.42 (0.66, 3.05)
No	51	4797	1	1

Table 6. Cont.

	NSPS in the child			
NSPS in the mother	**Yes**	**No**	**Crude OR (95% CI)**	**Adjusted OR (95% CI)**
Fainting/dizziness				
Yes	1	167	0.54 (0.08, 3.95)	0.52 (0.07, 3.86)
No	56	5084	1	1

OR = odds ratio; CI = confidence intervals. ORs were adjusted for child age, child sex, mother age, child birth order; household members' count, Index of Multiple Deprivation 2007 scores; maternal anxiety or depressive disorder, and GP practice.

appropriate clinical guidelines on management of parents and children with consultations for NSPS. Additionally, more prospective and qualitative research is required to fully explain the exact mechanisms underlying the association between GP consultations for NSPS in mothers and children. Such research may shed light on interventions that may help in preventing the development or recurrence of consultations for NSPS in children.

Conclusions

This study suggests that exposure to maternal GP consultations for NSPS is a significant risk factor for similar consultations in the child. This finding was strengthened by evidence of gradients of association between number of GP consultations for NSPS and number of NSPS in mothers and children as well as associations for specific type symptom groups and single NSPS especially painful NSPS. This study adds further evidence that children may learn their illness and consultation behavior from their mothers, and that recurrent consultation for NSPS in children should be viewed within a family context.

Acknowledgments

The Keele GP Research Partnership and the Informatics team at the Arthritis Research UK Primary Care Centre.

MS is funded by NHS Research and Development Support for New Medical Schools. MB is supported by a NIHR National School for Primary Care Research Fellowship. CDM is funded by a Clinician Scientist Fellowship (19634) from Arthritis Research UK. KMD is funded through a Research Career Development Fellowship from the Wellcome Trust [083572]. CiPCA is funded by the North Staffordshire Primary Care Research Consortium and Keele University Institute for Primary Care and Health.

Author Contributions

Conceived and designed the experiments: MS CDM KMD. Analyzed the data: MS MB. Contributed reagents/materials/analysis tools: MS MB CDM KMD. Wrote the paper: MS MB CDM KMD.

References

1. Eminson M, Benjamin S, Shortall A, Woods T, Faragher B (1996) Physical symptoms and illness attitudes in adolescents: An epidemiological study. J Child Psychol Psychiatry 37: 519–528.
2. Perquin CW, Hazebroek-Kampschreur AA, Hunfeld JA, Bohnen AM, van Suijlekom-Smit LW, et al. (2000) Pain in children and adolescents: A common experience. Pain 87: 51–58.
3. Cardol M, van den Bosch WJ, Spreeuwenberg P, Groenewegen PP, van Dijk L, et al. (2006) All in the family: Headaches and abdominal pain as indicators for consultation patterns in families. Ann Fam Med 4: 506–511.
4. van Eekelen FC, Perquin CW, Hunfeld JA, Hazebroek-Kampschreur AA, van Suijlekom-Smit LW, et al. (2002) Comparison between children and adolescents with and without chronic benign pain: Consultation rate and pain characteristics. Br J Gen Pract 52: 211–213.
5. Roth-Isigkeit A, Thyen U, Raspe HH, Stoven H, Schmucker P (2004) Reports of pain among German children and adolescents: An epidemiological study. Acta Paediatr 93: 258–263.
6. Domenech-Llaberia E, Jane C, Canals J, Ballespi S, Esparo G, et al. (2004) Parental reports of somatic symptoms in preschool children: Prevalence and associations in a Spanish sample. J Am Acad Child Adolesc Psychiatry 43: 598–604.
7. Little P, Somerville J, Williamson I, Warner G, Moore M, et al. (2001) Family influences in a cross-sectional survey of higher child attendance. Br J Gen Pract 51: 977–81, 984.
8. Jackson JL, Kroenke K (2008) Prevalence, impact, and prognosis of multi-somatoform disorder in primary care: A 5-year follow-up study. Psychosom Med 70: 430–434.
9. Reid S, Wessely S, Crayford T, Hotopf M (2001) Medically unexplained symptoms in frequent attenders of secondary health care: Retrospective cohort study. BMJ 322: 767.
10. El-Metwally A, Mikkelsson M, Stahl M, Macfarlane GJ, Jones GT, et al. (2008) Genetic and environmental influences on non-specific low back pain in children: A twin study. Eur Spine J 17: 502–508.
11. Levy RL, Jones KR, Whitehead WE, Feld SI, Talley NJ, et al. (2001) Irritable bowel syndrome in twins: Heredity and social learning both contribute to etiology. Gastroenterology 121: 799–804.
12. Shraim M, Mallen CD, Dunn KM (2013) GP consultations for medically unexplained physical symptoms in parents and their children: A systematic review. Br J Gen Pract 63: e318–25.
13. Porcheret M, Hughes R, Evans D, Jordan K, Whitehurst T, et al. (2004) Data quality of general practice electronic health records: The impact of a program of assessments, feedback, and training. J Am Med Inform Assoc 11: 78–86.
14. Jordan K, Clarke AM, Symmons DP, Fleming D, Porcheret M, et al. (2007) Measuring disease prevalence: A comparison of musculoskeletal disease using four general practice consultation databases. Br J Gen Pract 57: 7–14.
15. Gilman J, Myatt M (1998) EpiCalc 2000. 1.02.
16. American Psychiatric Association (1987) Diagnostic and statistical manual of mental disorders. Washington, DC: American Psychiatric Association.
17. Derogatis LR, Lipman RS, Rickels K, Uhlenhuth EH, Covi L (1974) The Hopkins symptom checklist (HSCL): A self-report symptom inventory. Behav Sci 19: 1–15.
18. Walker LS, Beck JE, Garber J, Lambert W (2009) Children's somatization inventory: Psychometric properties of the revised form (CSI-24). J Pediatr Psychol 34: 430–440.
19. Garber J, Walker LS, Zeman J (1991) Somatization symptoms in a community sample of children and adolescents: Further validation of the children's somatization inventory. Psychological Assessment 3: 588–595.
20. Rask CU, Olsen EM, Elberling H, Christensen MF, Ornbol E, et al. (2009) Functional somatic symptoms and associated impairment in 5-7-year-old children: The Copenhagen child cohort 2000. Eur J Epidemiol 24: 625–634.
21. Chisholm J (1990) The Read clinical classification. BMJ 300: 1092.
22. Department for Communities and Local Government (2007) The English indices of deprivation 2007. London: Department for Communities and Local Government.
23. IBM Corp (2011) IBM SPSS statistics for windows. 20.0.
24. Stata Corp (2011) Stata statistical software. 12.
25. Levy RL, Whitehead WE, Von Korff MR, Feld AD (2000) Intergenerational transmission of gastrointestinal illness behavior. Am J Gastroenterol 95: 451–456.
26. Perquin CW, Hunfeld JA, Hazebroek-Kampschreur AA, van Suijlekom-Smit LW, Passchier J, et al. (2001) Insights in the use of health care services in chronic benign pain in childhood and adolescence. Pain 94: 205–213.

27. Masiero S, Carraro E, Sarto D, Bonaldo L, Ferraro C (2010) Healthcare service use in adolescents with non-specific musculoskeletal pain. Acta Paediatr 99: 1224–1228.
28. Larsson B, Bille B, Pedersen NL (1995) Genetic influence in headaches: A Swedish twin study. Headache 35: 513–519.
29. Morris-Yates A, Talley NJ, Boyce PM, Nandurkar S, Andrews G (1998) Evidence of a genetic contribution to functional bowel disorder. Am J Gastroenterol 93: 1311–1317.
30. Kashikar-Zuck S, Lynch AM, Slater S, Graham TB, Swain NF, et al. (2008) Family factors, emotional functioning, and functional impairment in juvenile fibromyalgia syndrome. Arthritis Rheum 59: 1392–1398.
31. Groholt EK, Stigum H, Nordhagen R, Kohler L (2003) Recurrent pain in children, socio-economic factors and accumulation in families. Eur J Epidemiol 18: 965–975.
32. Levy RL, Langer SL, Whitehead WE (2007) Social learning contributions to the etiology and treatment of functional abdominal pain and inflammatory bowel disease in children and adults. World J Gastroenterol 13: 2397–2403.
33. Cardol M, van Dijk L, van den Bosch WJ, Spreeuwenberg P, de Bakker DH, et al. (2007) Striking variations in consultation rates with general practice reveal family influence. BMC Fam Pract 8: 4.
34. Craig TK, Cox AD, Klein K (2002) Intergenerational transmission of somatization behaviour: A study of chronic somatizers and their children. Psychol Med 32: 805–816.
35. Whitehead WE, Crowell MD, Heller BR, Robinson JC, Schuster MM, et al. (1994) Modeling and reinforcement of the sick role during childhood predicts adult illness behavior. Psychosom Med 56: 541–550.
36. Walker LS, Zeman JL (1992) Parental response to child illness behavior. J Pediatr Psychol 17: 49–71.
37. Jordan K, Jinks C, Croft P (2006) Health care utilization: Measurement using primary care records and patient recall both showed bias. J Clin Epidemiol 59: 791–797.
38. Jordan KP, Kadam UT, Hayward R, Porcheret M, Young C, et al. (2010) Annual consultation prevalence of regional musculoskeletal problems in primary care: An observational study. BMC Musculoskelet Disord 11: 144-2474-11-144.
39. de Lusignan S (2005) The barriers to clinical coding in general practice: A literature review. Med Inform Internet Med 30: 89–97.
40. Department of Health (2011) Andrew Lansley: Moving forward on modernising the NHS. Available: http://www.dh.gov.uk/en/MediaCentre/Pressreleases/DH_128162. Accessed 2012 April 24.
41. Campo JV, Bridge J, Lucas A, Savorelli S, Walker L, et al. (2007) Physical and emotional health of mothers of youth with functional abdominal pain. Arch Pediatr Adolesc Med 161: 131–137.
42. Levy RL, Langer SL, Walker LS, Romano JM, Christie DL, et al. (2010) Cognitive-behavioral therapy for children with functional abdominal pain and their parents decreases pain and other symptoms. Am J Gastroenterol 105: 946–956.
43. Husain K, Browne T, Chalder T (2007) A review of psychological models and interventions for medically unexplained somatic symptoms in children. Child & Adolescent Mental Health 12: 2–8.
44. Sumathipala A, Hewege S, Hanwella R, Mann AH (2000) Randomized controlled trial of cognitive behaviour therapy for repeated consultations for medically unexplained complaints: A feasibility study in sri lanka. Psychol Med 30: 747–757.
45. Speckens AE, van Hemert AM, Spinhoven P, Hawton KE, Bolk JH, et al. (1995) Cognitive behavioural therapy for medically unexplained physical symptoms: A randomised controlled trial. BMJ 311: 1328–1332.
46. Peters S, Stanley I, Rose M, Kaney S, Salmon P (2002) A randomized controlled trial of group aerobic exercise in primary care patients with persistent, unexplained physical symptoms. Fam Pract 19: 665–674.

26

A School-Based Cross-Sectional Survey of Adverse Events following Co-Administration of Albendazole and Praziquantel for Preventive Chemotherapy against Urogenital Schistosomiasis and Soil-Transmitted Helminthiasis in Kwale County, Kenya

Sammy M. Njenga[1]*, Paul M. Ng'ang'a[2], Mariam T. Mwanje[2], Fatuma S. Bendera[3], Moses J. Bockarie[4]

1 Eastern and Southern Africa Centre of International Parasite Control (ESACIPAC), Kenya Medical Research Institute (KEMRI), Mbagathi Road, Nairobi, Kenya, **2** Division of Vector-Borne Diseases & Neglected Tropical Diseases (DVBD-NTD), Ministry of Health, Nairobi, Kenya, **3** Environmental Health Department, Kwale County, Kenya, **4** Centre for Neglected Tropical Diseases, Liverpool School of Tropical Medicine, Liverpool, United Kingdom

Abstract

Background: Soil-transmitted helminths and schistosomiasis are mostly prevalent in developing countries due to poor sanitation and lack of adequate clean water. School-age children tend to be the target of chemotherapy-based control programmes because they carry the heaviest worm and egg burdens. The present study examines adverse events (AEs) experienced following co-administration of albendazole and praziquantel to school-age children in a rural area in Kwale County, Kenya.

Methods: Children were treated with single doses of albendazole and praziquantel tablets and then interviewed using a questionnaire for post treatment AEs.

Results: Overall, 752 children, 47.6% boys, participated in the study. Their median (interquartile range) age was 12.0 (10.0–14.0) years. A total of 190 (25.3%) children reportedly experienced at least one AE. In total, 239 cases of AEs were reported with the most frequent being abdominal pains (46.3%), dizziness (33.2%) and nausea (21.1%). Majority of the reported AEs (80.8%) resolved themselves while 12.1% and 6.3% were countered by, respectively, self-medication and visiting a nearby health facility. More girls (60.5%) than boys (39.5%) reported AEs ($P = 0.027$).

Conclusions: The AEs were mild and transient, and were no worse than those expected following monotherapy. The current study adds to the evidence base that dual administration of albendazole and praziquantel in school-based mass drug administration is safe with only mild adverse events noted.

Editor: Thomas Eisele, Tulane University School of Public Health and Tropical Medicine, United States of America

Funding: Financial support for this study was provided by the European Foundations Initiative of Neglected Tropical Diseases (EFINTD) through a postdoctoral fellowship (Grant No. I/84000) awarded to Prof. Njenga (http://www.europeanfoundations.eu/content/Pages/European-Foundations-Initiative-for-African-Research-into-Neglected-Tropical-Diseases-(EFINTD).aspx). The funders had no role in study design, data collection and analysis, decision to publish, or preparation of the manuscript.

Competing Interests: The authors have declared that no competing interests exist.

* E-mail: snjenga@kemri.org

Introduction

Soil-transmitted helminths (STH) and schistosomiasis are mostly prevalent in developing countries where poor sanitation and lack of adequate clean water are commonplace. STH infections are among the most prevalent infections in the world with around 1.4 billion individuals infected by *Ascaris lumbricoides*, 1.0 billion by *Trichuris trichiura*, and 1.3 billion by hookworms [1]. About 200 million people are estimated to be infected with schistosomiasis with 170 million living in sub-Saharan Africa while the remaining 30 million live in North Africa, Asia and South America [2]. The coastal areas of Kenya are highly endemic for urogenital schistosomiasis and STH [3,4]. Children have the highest prevalence and intensity of STH and schistosomiasis infections, but the consequences of chronic infection, such as growth stunting, anaemia, hepatic/urinary fibrosis, and impaired cognitive development, continue to have an effect throughout adulthood [5].

In 2001, during the 54th WHA, the WHO urged its member states to ensure provision for the regular antihelminthic treatment of all school-age children living in areas of schistosomiasis and STH endemicity [2]. Presently, schistosomiasis and STH control strategies focus on mass administration of praziquantel and albendazole, with special emphasis on treating school age children [6]. An integrated approach, against urogenital schistosomiasis and STH using praziquantel and albendazole, respectively, has been shown to be effective at reducing prevalence and intensity of infections in several countries in sub-Saharan Africa in various programmes [7,8]. These orally administered drugs are affordable, efficacious and safe for the large-scale treatment of human populations [9,10]. Further, they are given as single dose tablets and are therefore expected to ensure greater compliance [11]. School-aged children tend to be the target of chemotherapy-based control programmes because they carry the heaviest worm and egg burdens. This is due, in part, to their hygiene and behavioural practices, determining higher exposures and rates of acquisition of infection [12].Treatment of children is also likely to be more successful in averting the development of subsequent, more serious disease sequelae because earlier stages of infection-induced pathology may be reversible if treated promptly [13].

In 2009, a research project to evaluate a pilot schistosomiasis/ STH control programme and its integration with the national LF elimination programme was established in Kwale District, Kwale County, Kenya. Kwale has previously been shown to be highly endemic for urogenital schistosomiasis and STH [14–16]. The aim of the present study was to determine the safety of co-administration of albendazole and praziquantel to school-age children for control of STH and urogenital schistosomiasis.

Methods

Ethical Statement

Permission to conduct the current study, including review and approval by the Scientific Steering and Ethical Review Committees, was obtained from Kenya Medical Research Institute (KEMRI). The district education office, district health office, local leaders, teachers and parents were informed about the study in the area. Written informed consent was obtained, from a guardian, caretaker or a parent, for each of the participants in the study. Besides, oral informed consent was obtained from the study participants. No respondent's identifiers were included in the dataset used for these analyses. The dataset is available, for free, upon making a written request to the corresponding author.

Study Site

The study was conducted in Mwaluphamba Location, Matuga District, Kwale County, Kenya. The district covers an area of 1,043 km^{2}and has an estimated population of 151,978 residents [17]. The study area was previously described in a related publication by Njenga et al [14]. Mwaluphamba Location is situated in a rural setting of Matuga District bordering a drier Kinango District in the West. The district experiences a bimodal rainfall pattern with long rains occurring between mid-March and June while the short rains occur between October and December. The majority of the residents of the study area practice subsistence farming.

Study Design and Population

The population involved in the present cross-sectional study included 752 school-age children from five sentinel schools, namely; Maponda (161), Miatsani (140), Mirihini (155), Kajiweni (167) and Mlafyeni (129).

Treatment

In the month of July, 2010, children from the five schools received the first round of combination therapy. They were treated with a single dose of praziquantel (Prazitel®, Cosmos Ltd) using the dose pole method to determine the number of tablets to be administered to each child [9]. Additionally, the children were treated for soil-transmitted helminths using a single dose of albendazole 400 mg tablets (Unibazole®, Universal Pharmacy (K) Ltd). The programme, through the teachers, requested parents/ guardians to provide a morning meal to the children on the day the MDA took place. Further, schoolteachers, who participated in the distribution of study drugs, were given a one day training facilitated by district health and education officers who were assisted by a national team from the Ministries of Health and Education and the research team from KEMRI.

Data Collection and Statistical Analysis

One week after the administration of the medications, the children were interviewed for AEs using an interviewer-administered structured questionnaire. Details of the AEs experienced 48 hours post treatments, if any, were recorded. The reported AEs were classified as defined in the WHO guidelines whereby mild AEs were defined as undesirable experiences associated with use of the antihelmithics but not affecting daily activities (e.g. playing) whereas moderate AEs were defined as those affecting performance of daily activities. Severe AEs were defined as those requiring total rest and/or medication while serious AEs were defined as those that were life-threatening requiring admission to hospital [18,19].

Data were entered into a computer using Microsoft Excel and then exported to IBM SPSS Statistics 19.0 for analyses. Appropriate descriptive statistics were computed. Chi-square (χ^2) test was used to compare proportions. Statistical significance was set at $p < 0.05$.

Results

A total of 752 school-aged children, 47.6% of whom were boys, were interviewed for AEs experienced following administration of albendazole and praziquantel tablets. Their median age was 12.0 years (interquartile range: 10.0 to 14.0 years) with a majority of them (70.7%) being in the age category of 10–14 years as shown in Table 1.

After taking the medications, 190 (25.3%) children reported experiencing at least one AE as shown in Figure 1. The number of respondents who experienced one and two AEs were 146 (19.4%) and 36 (4.8%), respectively. Only eight respondents (1.0%) experienced more than two AEs.

Table 2 presents the description and frequencies of AEs reported by the school children interviewed. Overall, 239 cases of AEs were reported with abdominal pain being the most commonly reported AE. The other commonly reported AEs

Table 1. Characteristics of the respondents.

Variable	Number (n = 752)	%
Gender		
Male	358	47.7
Female	393	52.3
No response	1	0.1
Age category (years)		
< 10	76	10.1
10 - 14	532	70.7
>14	144	19.1

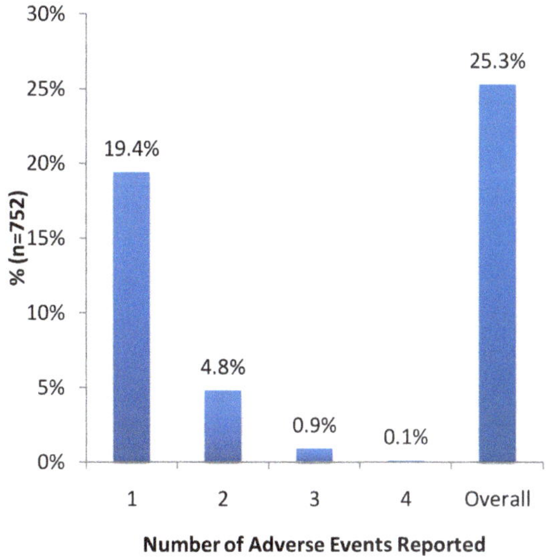

Figure 1. Distribution of the number of adverse events experienced.

included dizziness, nausea, head ache and vomiting. Of the 239 AEs reported, majority (84.0%) lasted a day or less.

The majority of the reported AEs were mild (166, 69.5%) while moderate and severe AEs constituted 23.8% (57) and 6.3% (15) of the total AEs reported respectively (Table 3). All the respondents who reported having experienced one or more AEs opined that the AEs were related to the study medications except for one respondent whose response was unavailable. Majority of the reported AEs (193, 80.8%) did not involve any intervention measures to mitigate those undesired events. Only 6.3% cases were reported to have involved seeking medical attention in a nearby hospital while 12.1% were countered by self-medication involving taking painkillers and anti-allergy drugs available in kiosks as Panadol® (paracetamol) and Piriton® (chlorpheniramine), respectively.

Table 2. Description and frequency of reported adverse events.

Description	Number (n = 239)	%
Nature of adverse event		
Abdominal pain	89	37.2
Dizziness	44	18.4
Nausea	40	16.7
Headache	33	13.8
Vomiting	10	4.2
Drowsiness	13	5.4
Urination*	5	2.1
Itching	5	2.1
Duration of adverse events		
1 day or less	199	83.3
More than a day	38	15.9
No response	2	0.8

*Polyuria (3) and dysuria (2).

Table 3. Characteristics of the children who experienced adverse reactions.

Variable	No. (n = 190)	%	*p*-value
Age (years)			
<10	17	8.9	0.117
10 - 14	127	66.8	
>14	46	24.2	
Sex			
Male	75	39.5	0.027
Female	115	60.5	

Gender was significantly associated with AEs with more girls than boys reporting to have experienced AEs to the study drugs (60.5% versus 39.5%, $P = 0.027$). Investigations into the age categories showed that more children in the 10 to 14 years age category (66.8%) had had adverse reactions as compared to those in other age categories though this was not statistically significant (Table 3).

Overall, no AE was rated by the respondents as serious while only a few AEs were rated as severe (23, 6.5%) as shown in Figure 2. The 23 cases of AEs were reportedly taken to hospital for treatment though no admissions were done. These severe AEs were constituted by vomiting (21.1%), stomachaches (11.9%) and headaches (8.9%).

Table 4 presents the relationship between gender and the type of AEs. Generally, more AEs were reported by girls than boys except for drowsiness. Nevertheless, this trend was not significant, statistically, but for dizziness (30.6% for boys versus 69.4% for girls, $\chi 2 = 6.114$, df = 1, p = 0.013).

Discussion

A substantial proportion of children (25%) reported having experienced one or more AEs following co-administration of

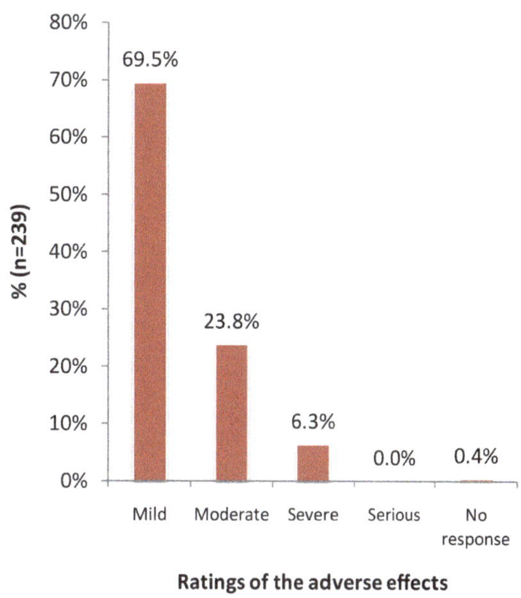

Figure 2. Severity of the adverse events.

Table 4. Association between adverse events and gender.

Adverse Event	Total(n = 752)	Male (n = 358)	Female (n = 393)	χ^2	df	*P*-value
Stomachache						
Yes	88	41(46.6%)	47(53.4%)	0.047	1	0.829
No	663	317(47.8%)	346(52.2%)			
Headache						
Yes	33	13(39.4%)	20(60.6%)	0.948	1	0.330
No	718	345(48.1%)	373(51.9%)			
Dizziness						
Yes	49	15(30.6%)	34(69.4%)	6.114	1	0.013
No	702	343(48.9%)	359(51.1%)			
Vomiting						
Yes	10	3(30.0%)	7(70.0%)	1.268	1	0.260
No	741	355(47.9%)	386(52.1%)			
Drowsiness						
Yes	13	9(69.2%)	4(30.8%)	2.465	1	0.116
No	738	349(47.3%)	389(52.7%)			

albendazole and praziquantel tablets. However, most of these AEs were mild and resolved within a day or two. The AEs reported in the current study included gastrointestinal disturbances such as abdominal pain, nausea and vomiting. Headaches, drowsiness and dizziness were also reported as AEs. Adoubryn et al [20] conducted a similar study in Biankouma, Côte d'Ivoire and found the frequency of AEs to be 40.8%, which is higher than in the current study. In another study, N'Goran et al found 33.3% of school children treated with praziquantel alone experienced one side effect AE or more which is also much higher compared to the present study [21]. A study on the side effects of praziquantel in a community of western Côte d'Ivoire, however, found a lower prevalence of side effects compared to the current study with only 12.5% of the individuals reporting one or more side effects 24 hours post-treatment [22]. The results of the current study are discordant with those from a study done in Southern Ethiopia where 83% of children treated with praziquantel alone complained that they experienced two or more treatment-related symptoms suggestive of side effects of the drug [23]. The reasons for the variations in proportions of AEs experienced after antihelminthic treatment could probably be due to dissimilar intensities of parasites as well as differences in socio-economic status, types of foods and environmental conditions associated with the diverse populations. Nevertheless, all the studies were in agreement with the current study by rating the side effects as mild.

By and large, the proportion of children who reportedly experienced AEs is comparable to what has been observed in other studies involving praziquantel whereby a higher proportion of respondents are reported to experience AEs as compared to albendazole. Indeed, a review by Horton (2000), reported that incidences of side effects associated with albendazole at the doses used for the treatment of intestinal helminths are very low, mild and self-limiting with only gastrointestinal side effects occurring with an overall frequency of just greater than 1% [24]. Side effects due to praziquantel, however, have been reported to occur in 30–60% of the patients, but, just like for albendazole, they are also mild and transient and disappear within 24 hours [21,25,26]. The most prevalent AE in the present study was abdominal pain (37.2%), followed by dizziness (18.4%) and nausea (16.7%). Other researchers have also found abdominal pain to be the most common AE reported after administration of praziquantel and/or albendazole. Studies conducted among school children in different parts of Kenya where intestinal schistosomiasis is endemic also found abdominal pain to be the most frequently reported AE following treatment [26,27]. Further, a double-blind placebo-controlled study involving 11500 children from China, Kenya and Philippines concluded that AEs due to co-administrations of both albendazole and praziquantel are no worse than those observed with praziquantel alone and the main side effects are abdominal pain and headache [28].

The current study reported no serious life-threatening AEs. In fact, only 15(6.3%) respondents reported severe AEs while the rest were either were mild (69.5%) or moderate AEs (23.8%). The frequencies of side effects and also severity have been loosely linked to the proportion of the dying parasites and the subsequent release of their products [27,29]. The abdominal pain may be related to a direct pharmacologic effect on the parasite, and possibly to a massive shift or death of worms in the mesenteric veins, which may lead to congestion and ultimately acute intestinal colic [29].

Significantly more girls than boys experienced AEs in the current study. A study by Raso et al using praziquantel alone reported abdominal pain to occur more frequently in women than men [17]. The reasons for differences in occurrence of AEs between males and females is unclear but could be due to physiological differences.

The current study's limitations include the unavailability parasitological data which would have enriched the discussion since adverse effects are usually related to infection intensity. Moreover, having such data would allow comparisons with other published studies in the field. The delay before administering the interview seems too long, particularly given the age of the children and this may have lead to recall bias.

Conclusions

Generally, a range of AEs were associated with the current drugs used in the treatment of schistosomiasis and STH, i.e., praziquantel and albendazole. This study, however, confirms that the safety of the two drugs even when co-administered. Approximately 6% of the children interviewed reported experiencing severe AEs related to the medications. Therefore, it is imperative that preventive chemotherapy intervention programmes put in place surveillance measures in order to ensure timely detection, management and reporting of potential life-threatening AEs. The current study adds to the evidence base that dual administration of albendazole and praziquantel in school-based MDA is safe with only mild adverse events (AEs) noted.

Acknowledgments

The Matuga District Health Management Team (DHMT) is thanked for its support of the research project. The teachers, parents and pupils of the study schools are thanked for their cooperation. We are grateful to the Director, KEMRI, for granting us the permission to publish this paper.

Author Contributions

Conceived and designed the experiments: SMN MJB. Performed the experiments: SMN FSB. Analyzed the data: SMN PMN. Wrote the paper: SMN PMN. Critically revised the manuscript for intellectual content: MTM MJB.

References

1. World Health Organization (2002) Prevention and control of schistosomiasis and soil-transmitted helminthiasis: report of a WHO expert committee. In: WHO Technical Report Series No 912. Geneva. 349 p.
2. World Health Organization (2005) Programme Report no. 17 - Seventeenth Programme Report of the UNICEF/UNDP/World Bank/WHO Special Programme for Research & Training in Tropical Diseases. Geneva: WHO, 433 p.
3. Muchiri EM, Ouma JH, King CH (1996) Dynamics and control of *Schistosoma haematobium* transmission in Kenya: an overview of the Msambweni Project. Am J Trop Med Hyg. 55(5 Suppl): 127–134.
4. Brooker S, Peshu N, Warn PA, Mosobo M, Guyatt HL, et al (1999) The epidemiology of hookworm infection and its contribution to anaemia among pre-school children on the Kenyan coast. Trans R Soc Trop Med Hyg. 93(3): 240–246.
5. Wiest PM (1996) The epidemiology of morbidity of schistosomiasis. Parasitol Today. 12(6): 215–220.
6. Fenwick A, Savioli L, Engels D, Bergquist RN, Todd HM (2003) Drugs for the control of parasitic diseases: current status and development in schistosomiasis. Trends Parasitol. 19(11): 509–515.
7. Kabatereine NB, Brooker S, Koukounar A, Kazibwe F, Tukahebwa E, et al (2007) Impact of a national helminth control programme on infection and morbidity in Ugandan schoolchildren. Bull World Health Organ. 85: 91–99.
8. Koukounari A, Gabrielli AF, Toure S, Bosque-Oliva E, Zhang Y, et al (2007) *Schistosoma haematobium* infection and morbidity before and after large-scale administration of praziquantel in Burkina Faso. J Infect Dis 196: 659–669.
9. Montresor A, Crompton DW, Gyorkos TW, Savioli L (2002) Helminth control in school age children: a guide for managers of control programmes Geneva: World Health Organization.238 p.
10. Southgate VR, Tchuem R, Tchuem LA, Rollinson D, Hagan P (2005) Towards control of schistosomiasis in sub-Saharan Africa. J Helminthol. 79: 181–185.
11. Kabatereine NB, Tukahebwa EM, Kazibwe F, Namwanje H, Zaramba S, et al (2006) Progress towards country-wide control of schistosomiasis and soil-transmitted helminthiasis in Uganda. Trans R Soc Trop Med Hyg 100: 208–15.
12. Anderson RM, May RM (1985) Helminth infections of humans: mathematical models, population dynamics, and control. Adv Parasitol. 24: 1–11.
13. Stothard JR, French MD, Khamis S, Basánez M, Rollinson D (2009) The epidemiology and control of urogenital schistosomiasis and soil-transmitted helminthiasis in schoolchildren on Unguja Island, Zanzibar. Trans R Soc Trop Med Hyg. 103: 1031–1044.
14. Njenga SM, Mwandawiro CS, Muniu E, Mwanje TM, Haji MF, et al (2011) Adult population as potential reservoir of NTD infections in rural villages of Kwale district, Coastal Kenya: implications for preventive chemotherapy interventions policy. Parasit Vectors, 4:175: 3–4.
15. Makau JK, Muhoho N, Awazawa T, Njomo D, Mukoko DA, et al (2004) Integrated parasite control: Effects or DEC-Albendazole antifilarial regimen on soil-transmitted helminths infection in Kwale District, coastal Kenya. In 25th African Health Sciences Congress; Nairobi. Abstract B/022/04.
16. Pullan RL, Gething PW, Smith JL, Mwandawiro CS, Sturrock HJW, et al (2011) Spatial Modelling of Soil-Transmitted Helminth Infections in Kenya: A Disease Control Planning Tool. PLoS Negl Trop Dis 5(2): 4–9.
17. Kenya National Bureau of Statistics (2010) 2009 Kenyan Population and Housing Census Report. Nairobi: KNBS.
18. World Health Organization. (2006) Preventive chemotherapy in human helminthiasis: coordinated use of anthelminthic drugs in control interventions: a manual for health professionals and programme managers.
19. World Health Organization. (2011) Assuring safety of preventive chemotherapy interventions for the control of neglected tropical diseases, 1–54.
20. Adoubryn KD, Kouadio-Yapo CG, Ouhon J, Aka NA, Bintto F, et al (2012) Intestinal parasites in children in Biankouma, Ivory Coast (mountaineous western region): efficacy and safety of praziquantel and albendazole. Med Sante Trop. 22(2): 170–6.
21. N'Goran EK, Gnaka HN, Tanner M, Utzinger J (2003) Efficacy and side-effects of two praziquantel treatments against *Schistosoma haematobium* infection, among schoolchildren from Côte d'Ivoire. Ann Trop Med Parasitol. 97: 37–51.
22. Raso G, N'Goran KE, Toty A, Luginbühl A, Adjoua AC, et al (2004) Efficacy and side effects of praziquantel against *Schistosoma mansoni* in a community of western Côte d'Ivoire. T Roy Soc Trop Med H. 98(1): 18–27.
23. Erko B, Degarege A, Tadesse K, Mathiwos A, Legesse M. (2012) Efficacy and side effects of praziquantel in the treatment of *Schistosoma mansoni* in schoolchildren in Shesha Kekele Elementary School, Wondo Genet, Southern Ethiopia. Asian Pac J Trop Biomed. 2(3): 235–9.
24. Horton J (2000) Albendazole: a review of anthelmintic efficacy and safety in humans. Parasitology. 121: S113–S132.
25. Berhe N, Gundersen SG, Abebe F, Birrie H, Medhin G, et al (1999) Praziquantel side effects and efficacy related to *Schistosoma mansoni* egg loads and morbidity in primary school children in north-east Ethiopia. Acta Trop. 72: 53–63.
26. Jaoko WG, Muchemi G, Oguya FO (1996) Praziquantel side effects during treatment of *Schistosoma mansoni* infected pupils in Kibwezi, Kenya. East Afr Med J. 73: p. 499–501.
27. Njomo DW, Tomono N, Muhoho N, Mitsui Y, Josyline CK, et al (2010) The adverse effects of albendazole and praziquantel in mass drug administration by trained schoolteachers. African Journal of Health Sciences. 17: 3–4.
28. Olds GR, King C, Hewlett J, Olveda R, Wu G, et al (1999) Double-blind placebo-controlled study of concurrent administration of albendazole and praziquantel in schoolchildren w with schistosomiasis and geohelminths. J Infect Dis 179(4): 996–1003.
29. Mohammed KA, Haji HJ, Gabrielli AF, Mubila L, Biswas G, et al (2008) Triple Co-Administration of Ivermectin, Albendazole and Praziquantel in Zanzibar: A Safety Study. PLoS Negl Trop Dis. 2(1): 4–5.

27

The Impact of Sexual Abuse in Patients Undergoing Colonoscopy

Melianthe P. J. Nicolai[1]*, Josbert J. Keller[2], Lieke de Vries[3], Andrea E. van der Meulen-de Jong[4], Jan J. Nicolai[2], James C. H. Hardwick[4], Hein Putter[5], Rob C. M. Pelger[1], Henk W. Elzevier[1]

1 Department of Urology, Leiden University Medical Center, Leiden, the Netherlands, **2** Department of Gastroenterology, HAGA Teaching Hospital, The Hague, the Netherlands, **3** Department of Urology, Westeinde Hospital, The Hague, the Netherlands, **4** Department of Gastroenterology, Leiden University Medical Center, Leiden, the Netherlands, **5** Department of Medical Statistics, Leiden University Medical Center, Leiden, the Netherlands

Abstract

Background: Sexual abuse has been linked to strong effects on gastrointestinal health. Colonoscopy can provoke intense emotional reactions in patients with a sexual abuse history and may lead to avoidance of endoscopic procedures.

Objective: To determine whether care around colonoscopy needs adjustment for patients with sexual abuse experience, thereby exploring targets for the improvement of care around colonoscopic procedures.

Methods: Questionnaires were mailed to patients (n = 1419) from two centers within 11 months after colonoscopy. Differences in experience of the colonoscopy between patients with and without a sexual abuse history were assessed and patients' views regarding physicians' inquiry about sexual abuse and care around endoscopic procedures were obtained.

Results: A total of 768 questionnaires were analyzed. The prevalence of sexual abuse was 3.9% in male and 9.5% in female patients. Patients born in a non-western country reported more sexual abuse (14.9%) than those born in a western country (6.3%; $p = 0.008$). Discomfort during colonoscopy was indicated on a scale from 0 to 10, mean distress score of patients with sexual abuse was 4.8($\pm$3.47) compared to 3.5($\pm$3.11) in patients without a sexual abuse history ($p = 0.007$). Abdominal pain was a predictor for higher distress during colonoscopy ($\beta = -0.019$ (SE = 0.008); $p = 0.02$, as well as the number of complaints indicated as reason for colonoscopy ($\beta = 0.738$ (SE = 0.276); $p = 0.008$). Of patients with sexual abuse experience, 53.8% believed gastroenterologists should ask about it, 43.4% said deeper sedation during colonoscopy would diminish the distress.

Conclusions: Sexual abuse is prevalent in patients presenting for colonoscopy. Patients with a sexual abuse history experience more distress during the procedure and indicate that extra attention around and during colonoscopy may diminish this distress.

Editor: Yong-hui Dang, Xi'an Jiaotong Univesity School of Medicine, China

Funding: These authors have no support or funding to report.

Competing Interests: The authors have declared that no competing interests exist.

* E-mail: melianthenicolai@gmail.com

Introduction

The prevalence of sexual abuse (SA) in modern western societies is estimated to be 12% to 25% for females and 8% to 10% for males [1–3]. SA has been linked to abdominal pain and functional gastrointestinal disorders [4,5], more healthcare utilization and exacerbated (pelvic) pain perception [6–8]. In community samples, patients with an abuse history have a 1.5 to 2 times increased risk of reporting gastrointestinal (GI) complaints compared to non-abused individuals [9,10]. Furthermore, SA has been linked to discomfort and traumatic reactions during pelvic examinations [11,12] and has been reported to make patients feel vulnerable when undergoing invasive endoscopic procedures [13–15]. Disclosure of abuse in the gastroenterological setting may allow for earlier consultation with mental health professionals [6].

In a recent survey among gastroenterologists, the majority stated to be aware of the importance of inquiring about SA. Nevertheless many indicated a lack of training in dealing with abuse-related problems [16]. Patients' beliefs regarding routine direct inquiry about SA in gastroenterology practice have never been assessed and it is unknown whether colonoscopy is experienced differently by patients with a history of SA. Hypothesizing attention for SA in gastroenterology practice is limited; we were interested in patients' beliefs and attitudes regarding care for SA. We aimed to assess if patients with a SA history experience colonoscopic procedures differently and to identify whether care around colonoscopy needs adjustment for patients with SA experience, exploring targets for the improvement of patient-centered care around colonoscopic procedures.

Materials and Methods

Ethics statement

Written informed consent was obtained from all participants. The study was approved by the Medical Ethical Testing Committee of Southwest Holland.

Patients and procedure

All patients ≥18 years old who had undergone colonoscopy in the selected timeframe were included. Patients were excluded if the procedure was performed under general anesthesia. Patients from the LUMC with inflammatory bowel disease (IBD) were excluded because participation in a study addressing sexuality in IBD was offered to those patients in the same period. IBD-patients from the HAGA teaching hospital were not excluded.

Within 11 months after the colonoscopy took place, the selected patients (n = 2348) received an introduction letter containing information about the study, a consent form and a freepost return envelope. Those returning the consent form with an affirmative answer received the questionnaire (in Dutch or English) within one month. The consent form contained an opt-out section in which reason for opting out was not asked for, as required by the medical ethical testing committee (MEC). One reminder letter was sent to non-respondents and one reminder letter was sent to respondents that agreed to participate but did not return a (completed) questionnaire.

Colonoscopy

Colonoscopies were performed according to the routine protocols of both centers. Each endoscopy team consisted of an endoscopist (gastroenterologist, resident in gastroenterology or specialized nurse endoscopist) and one or more specialized endoscopy nurses. Conscious sedation with intravenous midazolam and fentanyl was used in all patients undergoing colonoscopy. Rarely, flumazenil or naloxone were given to counteract the sedative action of midazolam or fentanyl, and in some patients butylscopalamine was given, based upon the judgment of the performing endoscopist.

Questionnaire

The questionnaire (appendix) was developed by the researchers. It was designed for both men and women. An expert panel with experience with the development of questionnaires checked its comprehensiveness and quality. A pilot study among 5 gastroenterologists, 3 residents in gastroenterology and 10 patients visiting one of the participating gastroenterology clinics was performed to assess the suitability, validity and comprehensiveness of the questionnaire.

The questionnaire included questions about sociodemographic data (age, gender, country of origin, way of referral and indication for colonoscopy), sexual function, micturition, SA history and the patient experience at colonoscopy. Furthermore, questions were included regarding patients' views on conversations about sexual function and SA with the gastroenterologist/physician. Several questions used were from The Pelvic Floor Inventories Leiden (PeLFIs), which is a validated tool to assess complaints of the pelvic floor and about SA [17,18]. For respondents that confirmed a history of SA, additional questions were posed regarding desired forms of healthcare. No distinction was made between adult and childhood SA. Questionnaires were processed by independent researchers (M.P.N. and L. de V.), and could not be traced back to patient records. Data were strictly anonymous as prerequisite by the MEC. In order to process the data correctly the questionnaires were numbered and the corresponding address data were saved and handled separately. Because answering the questionnaire was potentially distressing for subjects, an independent sexologist/psychologist was available in case support was needed.

Statistical analysis

Results were summarized by reporting responses on all surveyed items. Frequencies of demographic characteristics and answers to the questions were all presented. Numerical demographic values were summarized as mean (SD). Differences in numerical data between demographic groups were analyzed with independent sample t-tests. χ^2 Tests were used to assess association between categorical respondents' characteristics and categorical responses. Linear regression analysis was used to identify predictors of distress caused by colonoscopy and to correct for these factors. Statistical significance was defined as $p<0.05$, all tests were two-sided. Confidence intervals were defined as 95%. Analyses were conducted using SPSS release 20 (SPSS Inc., Chicago, IL, USA), GraphPath Prism 5 was used to design the figures.

Results

Subjects

From the 2348 patients who received the information letter and consent form, 1419 forms were returned (60.4%). Of these respondents, 610 (43.1%) declined participation and 809 (57.0%) were willing to participate. Of the 809 patients that received the questionnaire, 13 did not return it and 10 were incomplete for more than 30% and therefore excluded. One respondent was excluded because she indicated not to remember anything about the colonoscopy. Seventeen respondents were excluded because they underwent sigmoidoscopy and should not have been invited in the first place. The above led to a total of 768 questionnaires available for analysis (Figure 1). Mean time span between colonoscopy and return of the competed questionnaires was 274.0 days (±70.3).

Mean age of participants was 61.2 years (±14.5 years), female participants were younger than male participants with a mean age of 59.9 (±15.3 years) compared to 62.8 (±13.2) years respectively (p = 0.02). There was no difference in age between patients that declined participation (mean age 61.4±15.9) and participants. Non-respondents were younger than participants with a mean age of 53.8 years (±16.4) (p<0.001). Of the included patients, 43.9% were male. The majority of respondents were born in the Netherlands (88.4%, n = 674), 3.4% was from an other western country (n = 26) and 8.2% from a non-western country (including Turkey, Morocco, Surinam, and the Dutch Antilles, n = 63) (Table 1). From the respondents included for analysis, 81.4% underwent colonoscopy in the general teaching hospital and 18.4% in the tertiary referral center (LUMC).

Indications for colonoscopy were listed in Table 1. The most common indications were abdominal pain (not specified) (30.4%) and rectal blood loss (28.4%).

Almost three quarter of respondents indicated one complaint to be the reason for colonoscopy (73.3%; n = 563), 20.2% (n = 155) indicated two complaints, 5.2% (n = 40) three and 1.0% (n = 8) indicated four different reasons for the colonoscopy.

The majority was referred for colonoscopy by the general practitioner (48.8%). Almost a third (27.3%) was indicated for colonoscopy by the gastroenterologist him/herself and 11.1% by a physician in internal medicine (otherwise), 3.7% was referred by a surgeon.

Voiding complaints were present in 33.1% of respondents (n = 254): 52.5% of them mentioned frequency, 27.5% urgency and 24.3% urinary incontinence.

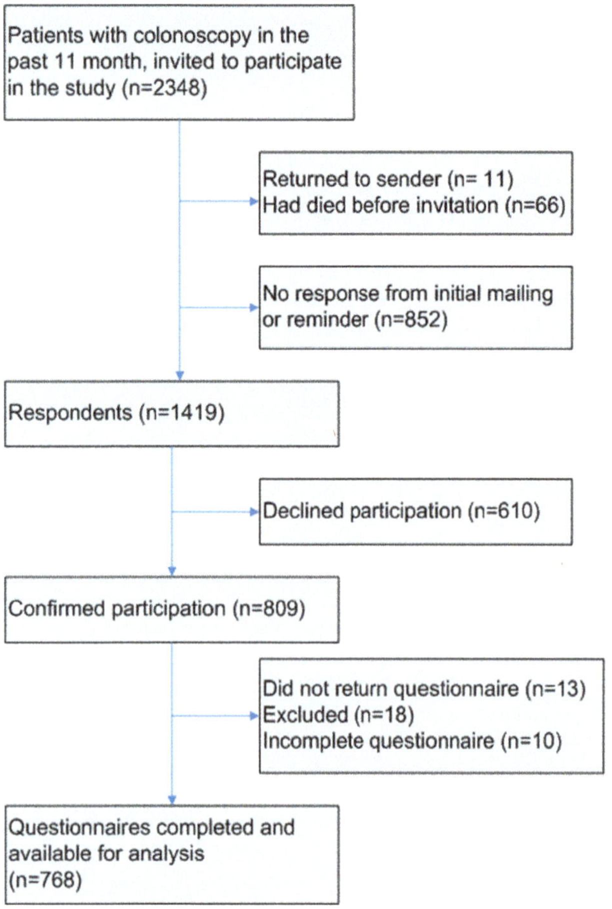

Figure 1. Study flow diagram.

A quarter of the patients (25.7%) reported sexual dysfunction (n = 197), this was more prevalent in male (34.5%) than in female patients (18.4%).

Sexual abuse

SA was reported by 53 (7.0%) of the 752 respondents that answered the question 'have you ever been a victim of sexual abuse?' Sexual abuse occurred in 40 (9.5%) of females (n = 421) and in 13 (3.9%) of males (n = 331). Patients born in a non-western country reported more SA compared to patients born in the Netherlands or another western country (14.9% versus 6.3%; p = 0.008). More details about the distribution of sexual abuse can be found in Table 2 and Figure 2.

Thirteen of 722 respondents indicated that a physician inquired about SA (1.8%), six were asked by the GP (0.8%) and three by the gastroenterologist (0.4%). Of the patients that reported SA (n = 53), 24.5% had professional help to deal with the experience and 64.1% said to have found a way to cope with it. More than half of patients with SA believed the gastroenterologist should ask about it (53.8%). Of them (n = 28), 35.7% said they would benefit from advice about dealing with the past, this option was marked significantly more often in male (80.0%) than in female patients (26.0%; p = 0.023). To the question "Do you think gastroenterologists need to have more training on the subject sexual health?" 46.7% said 'yes', 25.1% said 'no' and the remaining 21.6% answered with "I do not know".

Of patients with SA, 24 (45.3%) indicated gastroenterologists should not ask about SA (n = 24). One of the most common reasons for this answer was: "I am unable to talk about it". Female patients gave this answer significantly more often than male patients (29.2% vs. 0% respectively, p = 0.05), see Table 3.

Patients without SA experience (n = 715) were asked to answer the question: "Do you think gastroenterologists should ask their patients about sexual abuse?" 36% said "Yes" and 64% said "No". However, of all respondents (n = 768), only 23.7% believed a question about SA in an intake questionnaire would be peculiar (n = 182). No significant difference was seen between patients with and without a SA history concerning this question (22.4% resp. 24.7%; p = 0.723). Of the respondents stating that a question about SA in an intake questionnaire would be peculiar, the reason for this answer was mostly because they did not see the relationship (56.0%) or the relevance (31.1%) of SA in the context. No significant differences were seen between male and female respondents concerning their answers to the above questions.

Victims of SA noted significantly more sexual dysfunction (64.0%) compared to those without SA (24.4%; p<0.001), more micturition complaints (58.8% versus 30.9%; p<0.001) and a combination of both complaints (37.3 versus 11.4%; p<0.001).

Significantly more patients with SA history indicated a change in bowel habit as the reason for colonoscopy (p = 0.006) (Figure 2). Abdominal pain was significantly correlated to sexual abuse in men (r = 0.572, p = 0.031) and to a lesser extent in women (r = 0.291, p = 0.052). More than one GI-complaint was correlated with SA (r = 0.1, p = 0.006), as well as age under 60 years (r = −0.108, p = 0,003).

Discomfort during colonoscopy

Patients were asked to rate discomfort experienced during their last colonoscopy on a 10-point Likert scale in which 0 meant "no discomfort" and 10 meant "extreme discomfort". Patients with a sexual abuse history rated more discomfort (mean score 4.78±3.47) compared to non-abused subjects (mean score 3.54±3.11; p = 0.007) (Figure 3). Using linear regression, we controlled for age, gender, ethnicity, indication(s) for colonoscopy, and time between the colonoscopy and filling in the questionnaire. Several factors were found to influence the distress. Age and abdominal pain were influencing factors (β = −0.019 (SE = 0.008); p = 0.02 respectively β = 0.354 (SE = 0.156); p = 0.024) as well as the number of complaints presented (β = 0.738 (SE = 0.276); p = 0.008) and country of origin (Table 4). After controlling for these factor, sexual abuse was still a significant predictor for distress during colonoscopy (β = 0.991 (SE = 0.466); p = 0.034). Time between participation in the study and colonoscopy was not of influence (β = <0.001 (SE = 0.022); p = 0.914), see Table 4.

Patients with SA were asked to indicate which changes around and during colonoscopy would have made the procedure easier for them. Of 51 patients with a sexual abuse history that answered this question, a quarter (25.4%, n = 13) said the procedure went well, however 88.3% (n = 45) identified one or multiple options that would make the endoscopic procedure less uncomfortable, these options can be found in Figure 4.

Discussion

This cohort showed a SA prevalence of 3.9% in men and 9.5% in women. Many of the patients which experienced SA were born in a non-western country. Importantly, a SA history was associated with more discomfort during the colonoscopic procedure. Abdominal pain, multiple gastrointestinal complaints at presentation for colonoscopy and sexual dysfunction were associated with

Table 1. Characteristics of study sample.

Gender n(%)	**Female: 429 (56.1)[a]**	**Male: 336 (43.9)[a]**	**Difference *p*-value**
Age, mean (SD), years	59.9 (15.3)	62.8(13.2)	0.02
Age, ≤39 years, n(%)	41 (9.6)	25 (7.4)	0.08
Age, 40–49 years, n(%)	63 (14.7)	25 (7.4)	0.19
Age, 50–59 years, n(%)	84 (19.6)	60 (17.9)	0.07
Age, 60–69 years, n(%)	127 (29.6)	124 (36.9)	0.04
Age, 70–79 years, n(%)	74 (17.2)	72 (21.4)	0.34
Age, 80–89 years, n(%)	38 (8.9)	29 (8.6)	0.004
Age ≥90 years, n(%)	2 (0.5)	1 (0.3)	n/a
Country of origin n (%)	**Female n = 428[a]**	**Male n = 335[a]**	**Difference *p*-value**
The Netherlands	378 (88.3)	296 (88.4)	0.98
Other West-European country	13 (3.0)	9 (2.7)	0.78
Morocco	2 (0.5)	2 (0.6)	0.80
Turkey	3 (0.7)	4 (1.2)	0.48
Surinam	12 (2.8)	10 (3.0)	0.89
Dutch Antilles	3 (0.7)	4 (1.2)	0.48
Elsewhere western	2 (0.5)	2 (0.6)	0.80
Elsewhere non-western	15 (3.5)	8 (2.4)	0.38
Reason for colonoscopy[b] n (%)	**Female n = 428[b]**	**Male n = 336[b]**	**Difference *p*-value**
Abdominal pain	150 (35.0)	81 (24.1)	0.001
Rectal blood loss	110 (25.6)	108 (32.1)	0.05
Surveillance (hereditary) colon carcinoma/polyposis/polyps[c]	111 (25.9)	97 (28.9)	0.37
Changes defecation pattern	104 (24.3)	68 (20.2)	0.18
Chronic diarrhea, constipation or mucus in stool	37 (8.6)	15 (4.5)	0.02
Inflammatory Bowel Disease	18 (4.2)	22 (6.5)	0.15
Pain anal region	18 (4.2)	20 (6.0)	0.27
Anemia	9 (2.1)	14 (4.2)	0.10
Other[d]	38 (8.9)	31 (9.2)	0.51

n/a = not applicable.
a. Based on data from n = 768 respondents of which 429 women and 336 men (due to missing values), columns do not necessarily add to 768.
b. Multiple answers were possible.
c. Significantly more patients with the indication 'surveillance for colonoscopy for hereditary colon carcinoma/polyposis/polyps' were seen in the tertiary center (41.3%) compared to the general teaching hospital (23.6%; $p<0.001$).
d. Under which: loss of weight, diarrhea, eating disorders etc.

SA and more discomfort during the procedure. Most sexually abused patients indicated that gastroenterologists should ask about it before performing colonoscopy. Several minor adjustments where indicated as options to diminish distress during and beforehand of the procedure.

The prevalence rates of SA in our population were comparable with those obtained in a survey among patients visiting a general urology practice in the Netherlands [19]. In studies assessing SA in selected samples of patients with (functional) gastrointestinal illness from referral gastroenterology clinics, up to 44% of women and 11% of men reported sexual abuse [20–23]. However, when the same questions about sexual abuse were posed in community samples, the reported prevalence rates of SA with physical contact (touching and penetration) were comparable to the rates found in present study [24,25]. Because we were restricted by the MEC the specific form of abuse experience could not be asked about, therefore the demarcated question: 'Have you ever been a victim of sexual abuse?' was used. Because this question implicates sexual abuse with contact, patients with less explicit forms of abuse such as exposure to exhibitionists or (verbal) sexual intimidation will not have felt addressed. This will have led to an underestimation of sexual abuse in our sample, together with the effects of selection and non response bias.

To minimize potential biases we provided detailed assurances of confidentiality, pilot tested and refined the instrument and used balanced keying. Still, traumatized patients may have elected not to participate in the study to avoid reliving painful memories and nonrespondents may have had no affinity with the subject or may have considered their participation irrelevant for the study. Some patients with SA may have refused colonoscopy and therefore did not receive the invitation to participate in the study. The initial response rate was no higher than 32.7% (768/2348), but in the first mailing (2348 patients) only the letter with study information was sent out. Patients were requested to send back the consent form in order to obtain a questionnaire or opt out of the study. This step must therefore be regarded as study recruitment; a part of this initial sample was not eligible due to changes in address, illness, memory loss or death. Therefore the eligible response rate

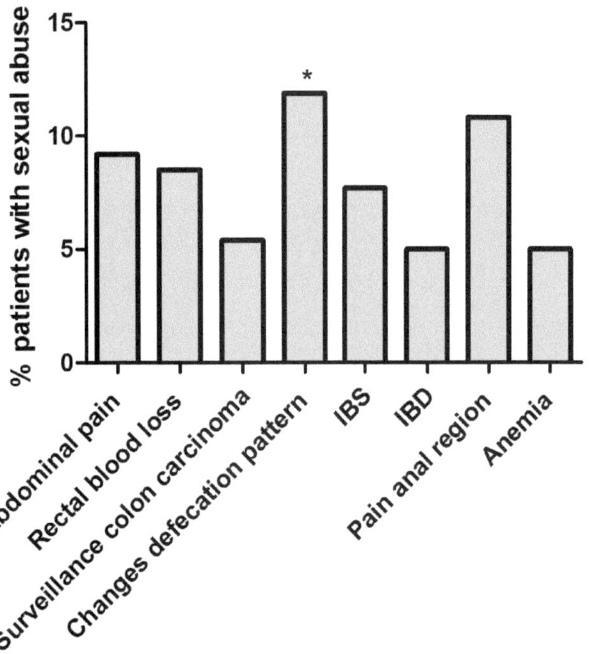

Figure 2. Indication for colonoscopy in patients with sexual abuse. * p = 0.006. Based on results for 53 patients, multiple answers were possible

Table 3. Should gastroenterologists ask about sexual abuse? Answered by patients with a sexual abuse history.

"No, the GE should not ask about SA", n(%)	**24 (45.3)[a]**
If not, what is the reason you do not want to talk about it?[b]	
I am ashamed of it	6 (25.0)
I do not believe the GE can help me with this problem	7 (29.1)
I am not able to talk about it	7 (29.1)
I am afraid to tell	5 (20.8)
It is not important for me anymore	7 (29.1)
It is too intimate to discuss	6 (25.0)
"Yes, the GE should ask about SA", n(%)	**28 (52.8)[a]**
If yes, 'what should the GE do after you told him about the SA?'[b]	
Just listen to me	7 (25.0)
Give me some advise about dealing with it	10 (35.7)
Refer me to psychologist	6 (21.4)
Refer me to a sexologist	6 (21.4)
Refer me to a pelvic floor physiotherapist	3 (10.7)
Refrain from performing a colonoscopy	2 (7.1)
Give me some information to read about it	10 (35.7)

GE = gastroenterologist, SA = sexual abuse.
a. Columns do not add to 53 because one patient with SA did not answer these questions.
b. Multiple answers were possible.

Table 2. Distribution of sexual abuse prevalence.

Patients Characteristics	Female n(%)	Male n(%)	Difference *p*-value
Total sexual abuse: 53 (7.0)	**40 (9.5)**	**13 (3.9)**	**0.003**
Age			
≤39 years	9 (22.5)	1 (1.5)	0.05
40–49 years	9 (22.5)	2 (2.3)	0.42
50–59 years	7 (17.5)	0	0.02
60–69 years	9 (22.5)	4 (1.6)	0.18
70–79 years	3 (7.5)	5 (3.5)	0.45
80–89 years	3 (7.5)	1 (1.6)	0.39
Age ≥90 years	0	0	n/a
Country of origin	**Female n(%)[a]**	**Male n(%)[a]**	**Difference *p*-value**
The Netherlands	32 (80)	10 (77.0)	0.93
Other West-European country	1 (2.5)	0	0.57
Turkey	0	0	n/a
Morocco	0	0	n/a
Surinam	2 (5.0)	0	0.42
Dutch Antilles	0	2 (15.4)	0.019
Elsewhere western	1 (2.5)	0	0.57
Elsewhere non-western[c]	4 (10.0)	1 (7.7)	0.82
Total Western country	33 (82.5)	10 (76.9)	0.004
Total Non-Western country [d]	7 (17.5)	3 (23.1)	0.412

Based on data from n = 752 respondents of which 421 women and 331 men (due to missing values).
Percentage of the total respondents with sexual abuse, by gender.
Total exceeds 100% because multiple answers where possible.
Namely: Brazil, Colombia, Egypt (male victim), Indonesia, Iran and Russia.
Included: Morocco, Surinam, Dutch Antilles, elsewhere non-western.

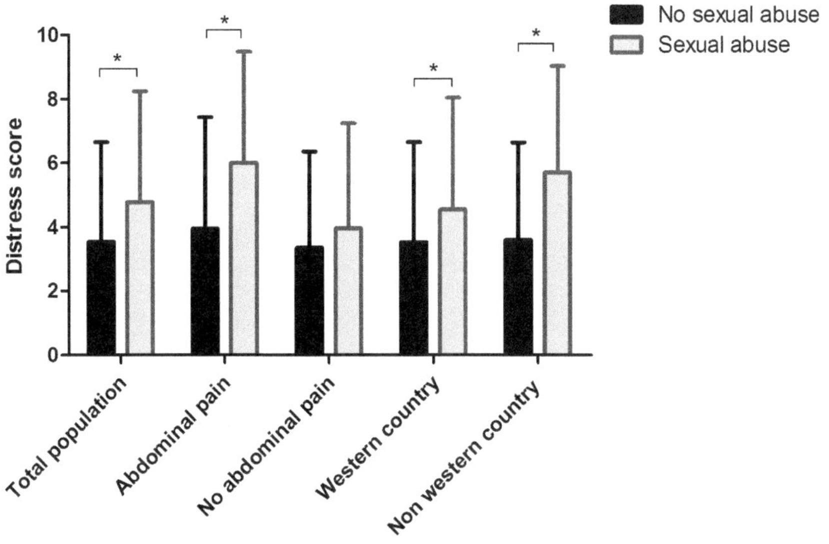

Figure 3. Distress during colonoscopy in patient with and without sexual abuse. * = significant difference.

of 54.1% (768/1419 respondents) should be used and considered representative [26].

An obvious limitation regarding the interpretation of discomfort experienced during colonoscopy is the absence of control for confounding variables such as length of the procedure and the amount of additional sedation used. Due to restrictions imposed by the MEC, we could not link questionnaires with patient files and therefore were unable to obtain these data.

Furthermore, recall bias may have occurred. The validity of retrospective reports by adults of their own adverse experiences in childhood has been extensively studied; so called infantile amnesia, the effect of mood and false or recovered memory may all influence retrospective recall of traumatic experiences [27,28]. In response, methods for addressing the issues of reporting unreliability and recall bias in retrospective reports of child sexual abuse were explored. The influence of recall bias was found to be small, accounting for less than 1% of the reporting variance [29]. Moreover, longitudinal data have to rely on retrospective recall for measures of experiences since the last interview as well, which will often involve reporting over a period of several years. And because longitudinal data are very expensive to collect, the discussion about methodology ended with the conclusion that retrospective reports about childhood abuse have a worthwhile place in research until better methods are found [30].

In spite of these limitations, this was the first study obtaining an inventory of SA in colonoscopy patients, identifying their needs regarding the colonoscopic procedure and comparing experienced discomfort during colonoscopy between patients with and without SA. Our results were consistent with prior research showing that

Table 4. Distress experienced during colonoscopy.

	Sexual abuse		No sexual abuse		
	Mean (±SD)	**Total (n)**	**Mean (±SD)**	**Total (n)**	***p*-value**
Total	4.8(±3.47)	50[a]	3.5(±3.11)	684	0.007
Male	5.0(±3.82)	11	3.2(±2.93)	311	0.052
Female	4.7(±3.47)	39	3.8(±3.23)	371	0.102
Age≤60 years	4.8(±3.55)	32	3.8(±3.06)	288	0.082
Age> 60years	4.7(±3.41)	18	3.4(±3.13)	396	0.071
With abdominal pain	6.0(±3.48)	20	4.0(±3.48)	204	0.009
No abdominal pain	4.0(±3.26)	30	3.4 (±2.99)	480	0.289
Western country	4.6(±3.50)	40	3.5 (±3.12)	631	0.048
Non-western country	5.7(±3.34)	10	3.6(±3.03)	53	0.053
Sexual complaints	5.3(±3.38)	31	3.7(±3.18)	153	0.011

Of the respondents with SA three did not fill in the distress-score.
Based on answers of 734 respondents, 34 respondents did not indicate distress during colonoscopy.

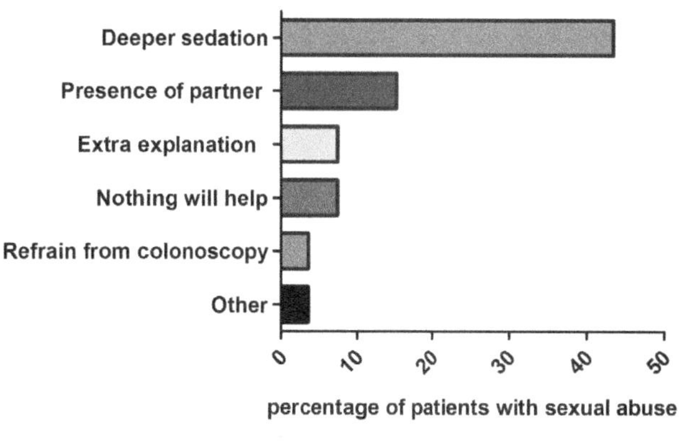

Figure 4. Possible options to diminish distress during and around colonoscopy, answers of patients with a history of sexual abuse[a]. a. Answers to the multiple choice/open question: "The colonoscopy experience would have been easier/more comfortable for me if..." Based on answers of 51 patients with sexual abuse experience. b. In the free space provided, one patient said: only start about sexual abuse if it has to do with the complaints, and one said 'not declare you as depressed'.

female patients with a history of SA reported more discomfort and anxiety during gynecological examination [12,31–33]. And confirmed the link between sexual abuse, abdominal pain and multiple GI-complaints already found in the early nineties by Drossman et al. which has been verified in many studies afterwards [6,34,35].

The reason a history of SA results in more pain during pelvic examinations may be explained by a variety of neural and humoral pathways that link brain, pelvic floor and gut [36]. Alterations in psychopathological and cortico-limbic pain modulatory systems have been described as mediating mechanisms for the association between SA and gastrointestinal disorders [7]. In addition, anxiety and trauma, especially SA, are significantly associated with dysfunction of the pelvic floor [37], leading to FGID [37,38], dyspareunia [39], dysfunctional voiding [40] and chronic pelvic pain [41]. In patients with IBS and a history of SA significantly more pain was reported to aversive rectal distention (similar to colonoscopy) compared with patients with IBS or abuse alone. Patients with IBS and SA reported higher pain scores and greater anterior mid cingulate activation with rectal distention than patients with either IBS or SA [42]. It is therefore remarkable that, however significant, the differences in mean distress scores found between patients with and without SA where rather mild (3.5 versus 4.8). This could be due to the fact that anxiety, depression and post-traumatic stress disorders play a major part in both perception of pain and symptoms as well [43]. A recent study using in-person interviews among gastroenterologists and endoscopy nurses to obtain information regarding development of psychological and/or physical symptoms after gastrointestinal endoscopy, fourteen of the 29 gastroenterologists (48%, 95% CI = 30.7–66.2%) reported encountering patients with new onset psychological symptoms lasting for more than a month after upper endoscopy or colonoscopy. A history of psychiatric illness was noted in 11 of 19 patients (58%) and a history of sexual abuse was noted in five of 19 patients (26%). Physicians reported that the endoscopic procedure was longer or more difficult than usual in six of 19 patients and that four of 19 patients had requested to prematurely terminate the procedure [44]. Our study specifically focused on SA in relation to distress experienced during colonoscopy. Patients with psychological problems, but without a SA history may have caused the diluted difference in discomfort between patients with and without SA.

Given the mounting evidence of the long-term detrimental effects of SA, especially as regards to gastrointestinal complaints [37], routine inquiry about SA in the gastroenterology practice might be expected. However, only 1.8% of the responding patients reported their gastroenterologist asked about 'negative sexual experiences' or abuse during consultation. Accordingly, a recent study among gastroenterologists showed that 2.5% of them asked female patients and 0.6% asked male patients about SA before performing colonoscopy. However, the majority of gastroenterologists' rated it as important to pay more attention to SA during their training [16].

From a patients' perspective, in the present study we found that three-quarters of the patients would not find it peculiar if a question about SA would be asked in an intake questionnaire beforehand of the colonoscopy. On the contrary, a third of respondents without SA believed the gastroenterologist should ask about it, and of the patients with SA experience, more than half believed so. More inquiry about SA may result in a better understanding between physician and patient, which is known to be the most important aspect of the pelvic examination experience for women [45]. If the endoscopist is informed about patients' traumas, compassionate and individualized care around and during the endoscopic procedure might diminish its impact. This study indicated that offering options such as use of a chaperone, deeper sedation and/or clear communication about the steps taken during the procedure may decrease discomfort, helping the patients to undergo the examination. Offering extra attention to patients with a history of sexual abuse may limit avoidance of transanal endoscopic procedures and may improve cooperation during procedures and therapy.

In conclusion, the results of this study have several implications for clinical practice. At least a tenth of women and up to four percent of men undergoing colonoscopy indicated experiencing SA. Colonoscopy was shown to be more distressing for patients with a history of SA. Consequently, especially in the gastroenterology practice this subject deserves attention. Discussing SA in medical practice seems difficult for both physician and patient. This study indicates that the use of a standardized intake questionnaire including questions about SA could be a solution to this problem.

Acknowledgments

We would like to thank Dr. M. Poelsma of the HAGA teaching hospital for her help, being available as physician/sexologist for respondents that indicated to need sexual health or psychological care after participating in this survey study. Furthermore we thank Ms. B. Breugelsdijk-Terveer for helping us with the processing of the databases and Ms. C. de Jong-Mom and Ir. W.D. Knijnenburg for their active assistance with mailing of the questionnaires.

Author Contributions

Conceived and designed the experiments: MPN JJK AEvdMdJ JJN HWE. Performed the experiments: MPN LdV. Analyzed the data: MPN LdV HP HWE. Contributed reagents/materials/analysis tools: JJK JJN AEvdMdJ. Wrote the paper: MPN. Revised the manuscript for important intellectual content: JJK AEvdMdJ JJN JCH RCP HWE. Final approval of the manuscript: RCP HWE.

References

1. Basile KC, Chen J, Black MC, Saltzman LE (2007) Prevalence and characteristics of sexual violence victimization among U.S. adults, 2001-2003. Violence Vict 22: 437–448.
2. Kellogg N (2005) The evaluation of sexual abuse in children. Pediatrics 116: 506-512. 116/2/506 [pii];10.1542/peds.2005-1336 [doi].
3. Stoltenborgh M, van Ijzendoorn MH, Euser EM, Bakermans-Kranenburg MJ (2011) A global perspective on child sexual abuse: meta-analysis of prevalence around the world. Child Maltreat 16: 79–101. 1077559511403920 [pii]; 10.1177/1077559511403920 [doi].
4. Walker E, Katon W, Harrop-Griffiths J, Holm L, Russo J, et al. (1988) Relationship of chronic pelvic pain to psychiatric diagnoses and childhood sexual abuse. American Journal of Psychiatry 145: 75–80.
5. Parris WC, Jamison RN (1985) Chronic pain in adults with a history of childhood sexual abuse. J Tenn Med Assoc 78: 493–495.
6. Drossman DA, Li Z, Leserman J, Toomey TC, Hu YJ (1996) Health status by gastrointestinal diagnosis and abuse history. Gastroenterology 110: 999–1007. S0016508596001874 [pii].
7. Leserman J, Drossman DA (2007) Relationship of abuse history to functional gastrointestinal disorders and symptoms: some possible mediating mechanisms. Trauma Violence Abuse 8: 331–343. 8/3/331 [pii];10.1177/1524838007303240 [doi].
8. Walker EA, Gelfand AN, Gelfand MD, Green C, Katon WJ (1996) Chronic pelvic pain and gynecological symptoms in women with irritable bowel syndrome. J Psychosom Obstet Gynaecol 17: 39–46.
9. McCauley J, Kern DE, Kolodner K, Dill L, Schroeder AF, et al. (1997) Clinical characteristics of women with a history of childhood abuse: unhealed wounds. JAMA 277: 1362–1368.

10. Talley NJ, Fett SL, Zinsmeister AR, Melton LJ III (1994) Gastrointestinal tract symptoms and self-reported abuse: a population-based study. Gastroenterology 107: 1040–1049.S0016508594002945 [pii].
11. Hilden M, Sidenius K, Langhoff-Roos J, Wijma B, Schei B (2003) Women's experiences of the gynecologic examination: factors associated with discomfort. Acta Obstet Gynecol Scand 82: 1030–1036.253 [pii].
12. Leeners B, Stiller R, Block E, Gorres G, Imthurn B, et al. (2007) Effect of childhood sexual abuse on gynecologic care as an adult. Psychosomatics 48: 385–393. 48/5/385 [pii];10.1176/appi.psy.48.5.385 [doi].
13. Davy E (2006) The endoscopy patient with a history of sexual abuse: strategies for compassionate care. Gastroenterol Nurs 29: 221–225.00001610-200605000-00003 [pii].
14. Borum ML, Igiehon E, Shafa S (2009) Sexual abuse history in patients... Davy (2006), "The endoscopy patient with a history of sexual abuse: strategies for compassionate care". Gastroenterol Nurs 32: 222–223.
15. Bal BS, Crowell MD, Kohli DR, Menendez J, Rashti F, et al. (2012) What factors are associated with the difficult-to-sedate endoscopy patient? Dig Dis Sci 57: 2527–2534. 10.1007/s10620-012-2188-2 [doi].
16. Nicolai MPJ, Fidder HH, Beck JJH, Bekker MD, Putter H, et al. (2012) Sexual abuse history in GI illness, how do gastroenterologists deal with it? Journal of Sexual Medicine 9: 1277–1284.
17. Voorham-van der Zalm PJ, Stiggelbout AM, Aardoom I, Deckers S, Greve IG, et al. (2008) Development and validation of the pelvic floor inventories Leiden (PelFIs). Neurourol Urodyn 27: 301–305. 10.1002/nau.20514 [doi].
18. Voorham-van der Zalm PJ, Berzuk K, Shelly B, Kamin B, Putter H, et al. (2011) Validation of the Pelvic Floor Inventories Leiden (PelFIs) in English. Neurourol Urodyn 30: 536–540. 10.1002/nau.21053 [doi].
19. Beck JJ, Bekker MD, van Driel MF, Roshani H, Putter H, et al. (2011) Prevalence of sexual abuse among patients seeking general urological care. J Sex Med 8: 2733–2738. 10.1111/j.1743-6109.2011.02389.x [doi].
20. Baccini F, Pallotta N, Calabrese E, Pezzotti P, Corazziari E (2003) Prevalence of sexual and physical abuse and its relationship with symptom manifestations in patients with chronic organic and functional gastrointestinal disorders. Dig Liver Dis 35: 256–261.
21. Delvaux M, Denis P, Allemand H (1997) Sexual abuse is more frequently reported by IBS patients than by patients with organic digestive diseases or controls. Results of a multicentre inquiry. European Journal of Gastroenterology and Hepatology 9: 345–352.
22. Leserman J, Drossman DA, Li Z, Toomey TC, Nachman G, et al. (1996) Sexual and physical abuse history in gastroenterology practice: how types of abuse impact health status. Psychosom Med 58: 4–15.
23. Leroi AM, Bernier C, Watier A, Hemond M, Goupil G, et al. (1995) Prevalence of sexual abuse among patients with functional disorders of the lower gastrointestinal tract. Int J Colorectal Dis 10: 200–206.
24. Longstreth GF, Wolde-Tsadik G (1993) Irritable bowel-type symptoms in HMO examinees. Prevalence, demographics, and clinical correlates. Dig Dis Sci 38: 1581–1589.
25. Fleming JM (1997) Prevalence of childhood sexual abuse in a community sample of Australian women. Med J Aust 166: 65–68.
26. Sitzia J, Wood N (1998) Response rate in patient satisfaction research: an analysis of 210 published studies. Int J Qual Health Care 10: 311–317.
27. Koriat A, Goldsmith M, Pansky A (2000) Toward a psychology of memory accuracy. Annu Rev Psychol 51: 481–537. 10.1146/annurev.psych.51.1.481 [doi].
28. Loftus EF (1993) The reality of repressed memories. Am Psychol 48: 518–537.
29. Fergusson DM, Horwood LJ, Boden JM (2011) Structural equation modeling of repeated retrospective reports of childhood maltreatment. Int J Methods Psychiatr Res 20: 93–104. 10.1002/mpr.337 [doi].
30. Hardt J, Rutter M (2004) Validity of adult retrospective reports of adverse childhood experiences: review of the evidence. J Child Psychol Psychiatry 45: 260–273.
31. Weitlauf JC, Frayne SM, Finney JW, Moos RH, Jones S, et al. (2010) Sexual violence, posttraumatic stress disorder, and the pelvic examination: how do beliefs about the safety, necessity, and utility of the examination influence patient experiences? J Womens Health (Larchmt) 19: 1271–1280. 10.1089/jwh.2009.1673 [doi].
32. Huber JD, Pukall CF, Boyer SC, Reissing ED, Chamberlain SM (2009) "Just relax": physicians' experiences with women who are difficult or impossible to examine gynecologically. J Sex Med 6: 791–799. JSM1139 [pii];10.1111/j.1743-6109.2008.01139.x [doi].
33. Farley M, Golding JM, Minkoff JR (2002) Is a history of trauma associated with a reduced likelihood of cervical cancer screening? J Fam Pract 51: 827–831.jfp_1002_00827 [pii].
34. Drossman DA, Talley NJ, Leserman J, Olden KW, Barreiro MA (1995) Sexual and physical abuse and gastrointestinal illness. Review and recommendations. Ann Intern Med 123: 782–794.
35. Drossman DA (2011) Abuse, trauma, and GI illness: is there a link? Am J Gastroenterol 106: 14–25. ajg2010453 [pii];10.1038/ajg.2010.453 [doi].
36. Drossman DA, Leserman J, Li Z, Keefe F, Hu YJ, et al. (2000) Effects of coping on health outcome among women with gastrointestinal disorders. Psychosom Med 62: 309–317.
37. Paras ML, Murad MH, Chen LP, Goranson EN, Sattler AL, et al. (2009) Sexual abuse and lifetime diagnosis of somatic disorders: a systematic review and meta-analysis. JAMA 302: 550–561. 302/5/550 [pii];10.1001/jama.2009.1091 [doi].
38. Imhoff LR, Liwanag L, Varma M (2012) Exacerbation of symptom severity of pelvic floor disorders in women who report a history of sexual abuse. Arch Surg 147: 1123–1129. 1485770 [pii];10.1001/archsurg.2012.1144 [doi].
39. Both S, van LR, Weijenborg P, Laan E (2012) A new device for simultaneous measurement of pelvic floor muscle activity and vaginal blood flow: a test in a nonclinical sample. J Sex Med 9: 2888–2902. 10.1111/j.1743-6109.2012.02910.x [doi].
40. Klingele CJ, Lightner DJ, Fletcher JG, Gebhart JB, Bharucha AE (2010) Dysfunctional urinary voiding in women with functional defecatory disorders. Neurogastroenterol Motil 22: 1094-e284. NMO1539 [pii];10.1111/j.1365-2982.2010.01539.x [doi].
41. Faubion SS, Shuster LT, Bharucha AE (2012) Recognition and management of nonrelaxing pelvic floor dysfunction. Mayo Clin Proc 87: 187–193. S0025-6196(11)00024-3 [pii];10.1016/j.mayocp.2011.09.004 [doi].
42. Ringel Y, Drossman DA, Leserman JL, Suyenobu BY, Wilber K, et al. (2008) Effect of abuse history on pain reports and brain responses to aversive visceral stimulation: an FMRI study. Gastroenterology 134: 396–404. S0016-5085(07)02024-0 [pii];10.1053/j.gastro.2007.11.011 [doi].
43. Bouchoucha M, Hejnar M, Devroede G, Babba T, Bon C, et al. (2012) Anxiety and depression as markers of multiplicity of sites of functional gastrointestinal disorders: A gender issue? Clin Res Hepatol Gastroenterol. S2210-7401(12)00330-0 [pii];10.1016/j.clinre.2012.10.011 [doi].
44. Berzin TM, Blanco PG, Lamont JT, Sawhney MS (2010) Persistent psychological or physical symptoms following endoscopic procedures: an unrecognized post-endoscopy adverse event. Dig Dis Sci 55: 2869–2873. 10.1007/s10620-010-1197-2 [doi].
45. Swahnberg K, Wijma B, Siwe K (2011) Strong discomfort during vaginal examination: why consider a history of abuse? Eur J Obstet Gynecol Reprod Biol 157: 200–205. S0301-2115(11)00137-0 [pii];10.1016/j.ejogrb.2011.02.025 [doi].

Typhoid Outbreak in Songkhla, Thailand 2009–2011: Clinical Outcomes, Susceptibility Patterns, and Reliability of Serology Tests

Wannee Limpitikul[1], Narong Henpraserttae[2], Rachanee Saksawad[3], Kamolwish Laoprasopwattana[4]*

1 Department of Pediatrics, Songkhla Hospital, Songkhla, Thailand, **2** Bureau of Epidemiology, Department of Disease Control, Ministry of Public Health in Songkhla, Songkhla, Thailand, **3** Department of Pediatrics, Hat Yai Education Center, Hat Yai Hospital, Hat Yai, Songkhla, Thailand, **4** Department of Pediatrics, Faculty of Medicine, Prince of Songkla University, Hat Yai, Songkhla, Thailand

Abstract

Objective: To determine the clinical manifestations and outcomes, the reliability of *Salmonella enterica* serotype Typhi (*S* ser. Typhi) IgM and IgG rapid tests, and the susceptibility patterns and the response to treatment during the 2009–2011 typhoid outbreak in Songkhla province in Thailand.

Method: The medical records of children aged <15 years with *S* ser. Typhi bacteremia were analysed. The efficacy of the typhoid IgM and IgG rapid tests and susceptibility of the *S* ser. Typhi to the current main antibiotics used for typhoid (amoxicillin, ampicillin, cefotaxime, ceftriaxone, co-trimoxazole, and ciprofloxacin), were evaluated.

Results: *S* ser. Typhi bacteremia was found in 368 patients, and all isolated strains were susceptible to all 6 antimicrobials tested. Most of the patients were treated with ciprofloxacin for 7–14 days. The median time (IQR) of fever before treatment and duration of fever after treatment were 5 (4, 7) days and 4 (3, 5) days, respectively. Complications of ascites, lower respiratory symptoms, anemia (Hct <30%), and ileal perforation were found in 7, 7, 22, and 1 patients, respectively. None of the patients had recurrent infection or died. The sensitivities of the typhoid IgM and IgG tests were 58.3% and 25.6% respectively, and specificities were 74.1% and 50.5%, respectively.

Conclusion: Most of the patients were diagnosed at an early stage and treated with a good outcome. All *S* ser. Typhi strains were susceptible to standard first line antibiotic typhoid treatment. The typhoid IgM and IgG rapid tests had low sensitivity and moderate specificity.

Editor: Alex Friedrich, University Medical Center Groningen, Netherlands

Funding: The only funding received for this manuscript was grant no. 56-210-01-1-3 from the Faculty of Medicine, Prince of Songkla University. The funder had no role in study design, data collection and analysis, decision to publish, or preparation of the manuscript.

Competing Interests: The authors have declared that no competing interests exist.

* Email: kamolwish@gmail.com

Introduction

Enteric fever (typhoid or paratyphoid fever) is an important cause of morbidity in developing countries, particularly among children and adolescents in Africa and South and Southeast Asia. The incidence in some counties is as high as 800/100,000 people/year. In 2000, the estimated number of enteric fever cases worldwide was 26.9 million, with 200,000 deaths [1].

The mortality rate in any particular country or area varies according to several factors, such as early diagnosis or available treatment. In patients treated prior to developing a serious complication such as bowel perforation the mortality rate is lower than 1%, but in patients treated only after developing a serious complication the mortality rate is as high as 15% [2–4].

In Thailand, where enteric fever is endemic, the incidence varies according to region (central, northern, north-eastern, and southern), and whether or not there is a current outbreak. For example, in 2013 the incidence among the different regions of Thailand varied from 0.9 to 83.6/100,000 people [5], while during 2009–2011, during a typhoid fever outbreak in Songkhla province in the south of Thailand, the estimated incidence increased from 1.8 (the average incidence in the 5 years before the outbreak) to 25.2/100,000 people [6].

Blood culture is the standard method for confirming a typhoid diagnosis; however this method is problematic for resource limited areas, and there is also a time problem, as cultures need at least 1–2 days to report the results, and effective treatment must begin as soon as possible, so a 2-day delay while waiting for a positive diagnosis is not good for the patients. In addition, the sensitivity of blood culture varies in its reliability - if performed during the first seven days of fever it is 60–80%, but if blood is cultured after the 7th day of fever the sensitivity drops to 20–30% [7,8]. Also, blood cultures can be influenced by previously received antibiotics and/or the volume of blood which need blood to broth ratio of 1:5 to

1:10 [9]. The currently most commonly used serology test, the Widal test, has low specificity to diagnose typhoid fever and reports on other recently developed rapid tests for enteric fever have found varying results for the sensitivity and specificity of these tests [10–21].

A developing problem in dealing with various diseases including typhoid fever is that in recent years multidrug-resistant bacteria have been increasingly encountered. In South and Southeast Asia, *Salmonella enterica* serotype Typhi (*S* ser. Typhi) resistance to the current first-line treatment, fluoroquinolones, is increasing [22–26]. Close monitoring of *S* ser. Typhi resistance to first line antibiotics, and knowing the resistance profile of *S* ser. Typhi, is important in helping the physician to choose the appropriate antibiotic when an outbreak occurs.

This study aimed to determine the clinical manifestations and outcomes, the reliability of *S* ser. Typhi IgM and IgG rapid tests, and the susceptibility patterns and the response to treatment during the 2009–2011 typhoid outbreak in Songkhla province in Thailand.

Materials and Methods

Permission from the institutional review board of Prince of Songkla University was obtained prior to conducting the study. We retrospectively reviewed the medical records of all children ($<$ 15 years of age) from 3 major hospitals in Songkhla province, Thailand (Songkhla Hospital, Songklanagarind Hospital and Hat Yai Hospital) treated during the October 2009–July 2011 typhoid outbreak in this area. Our study involved the use of patient medical data, from which any information that could specifically identify any patient was removed before the analysis was performed. All patients were diagnosed for typhoid fever through a blood culture positive for *S* ser. Typhi, using a BD Phoenix Automated Microbiology System (Becton Dickinson, Sparks, MD). Blood cultures were performed by technicians in the hospitals where the patients first presented.

Demographic characteristics, clinical profiles, treatments and complications, and typhoid immunochromatographic assays for IgM and IgG (SD Bioline *S* ser. Typhi IgG/IgM Test, South Korea) performed on the same day as the blood cultures, were recorded. The *S* ser. Typhi IgG/IgM rapid tests (available only in patients who visited Songkhla Hospital) were immediately performed after the blood samples were collected and the results were interpreted within 15–30 minutes by one of the technicians in Songkhla Hospital. Blood cultures were used as the gold standard to determine the sensitivity, specificity, negative predictive value (NPV), and positive predictive value (PPV) of the SD Bioline *S* ser. Typhi IgG/IgM tests in patients suspected of typhoid fever who lived in the outbreak area with febrile illness without another cause identified. Antimicrobial susceptibility testing (BBL Sensi-Disc; Becton Dickinson, USA) was performed using the Clinical and Laboratory Standards Institute (CLSI) standard disk diffusion method [27]. Six commonly used antimicrobial agents were evaluated: amoxicillin, ampicillin, cefotaxime, ceftriaxone, co-trimoxazole, and ciprofloxacin. Pulsed field gel electrophoresis (PFGE) was performed using the method of Ward et al. [28].

Statistical analysis

Data were evaluated using descriptive statistics (mean and standard deviation, median and interquartile range (IQR), or frequency and percentage, as appropriate). Comparisons between groups of patients were made using the Student's *t*-test or Mann-Whitney *U*-test for normally distributed and non-normally distributed continuous variables, respectively. Chi-square or Fisher's exact test was used for comparisons of categorical data. R 3.0.2 for Windows was used for statistical analysis.

Results

Outbreak periods and patients

S ser. Typhi bacteremia was found in 333, 27, and 8 patients from Songkhla Hospital, Songklanagarind Hospital and Hat Yai Hospital, respectively, for a total of 368 cases. Most of the patients were students from at least 10 primary schools in Songkhla province. The mean age of all patients was 7.5±3.0 years, and 44.8% were male. There were 2 separate outbreaks during the Songkhla epidemic, the 1st from October 2009 to March 2010 and the 2nd from September 2010 to July 2011 (Figure 1), with 137 (37.2%) and 231 (62.8%) patients in the two periods, respectively. The clinical characteristics, mean day of fever when initial treatment was begun (5.1±2.7 vs 5.5±2.9 days, $p = 0.18$) and outcomes were not different between the 1st and 2nd periods of the outbreak. However, the mean age of the patients in the1st period was greater than in the 2nd period (8.0±2.8 vs 7.2±3.0 years, $p = 0.01$). All of the *S* ser. typhi strains isolated in both periods were susceptible to all six of the tested antibiotics.

During the peak of the 1st outbreak (December 2009–January 2010), the Songkhla branch of the Bureau of Epidemiology, Department of Disease Control, Thailand Ministry of Public Health found that residual chlorine in the water supply from the schools with the highest numbers of typhoid cases schools was 0.1 parts per million (ppm), with no *S* ser. Typhi strains isolated from the tap water in either school, and only non-Typhi *Salmonella* strains found from rectal swabs in 16/88 (18%) of food handlers (4/7, 1/19, and 11/62 food handlers from schools A and B and street venders in front of schools A and B). All 28 food and water samples from these schools were organism-free. However, in market A, non-Typhi *Salmonella* was found in raw pork and raw chicken and *Aeromonas caviae* was found in coconut milk being sold. After 14 days of ciprofloxacin, these 4 and 18 food handlers form schools A and B had a repeat rectal swab, and no growths were found. PFGE from 52 samples (different schools and month of outbreak) had the same pattern of 92–100%. During the second outbreak, the Ministry of Public Health in Songkhla tried to find the source of *S* ser. Typhi as in the first outbreak, but none of samples collected form the environment or food handlers rectal swabs found *S* ser. Typhi.

Clinical characteristics and outcomes of typhoid patients treated before and after 5 days of fever

All of the 368 confirmed typhoid patients initially presented with high grade fever. Non-mucus bloody diarrhea, vomiting, abdominal pain, and headache were found in 48.4%, 36.7%, 22.8%, and 21.2% of the patients, respectively. The hospitalization rate was 70.7% and the mean duration of hospitalization was 4.7±2.8 days. Most of the hospitalized patients were initially treated with intravenous ceftriaxone or ciprofloxacin, and then continued with oral ciprofloxacin when their clinical status improved and they could tolerate oral intake for the treatment duration of 10–14 days. Most of the out-patients were treated with oral ciprofloxacin for 7–14 days. Sixteen patients were treated with other antibiotics - oral amoxicillin/clavulanate, co-trimoxazole, or azithromycin were given to those who could not tolerate ciprofloxacin (7, 5 and 4 patients, respectively). None of the patients had recurrent infection and all survived.

Of the 357 patients who self-reported the first date of fever, all except 3 were treated within 14 days of the onset of fever. The median day (IQR) of fever before treatment was 5 (4, 7) days and

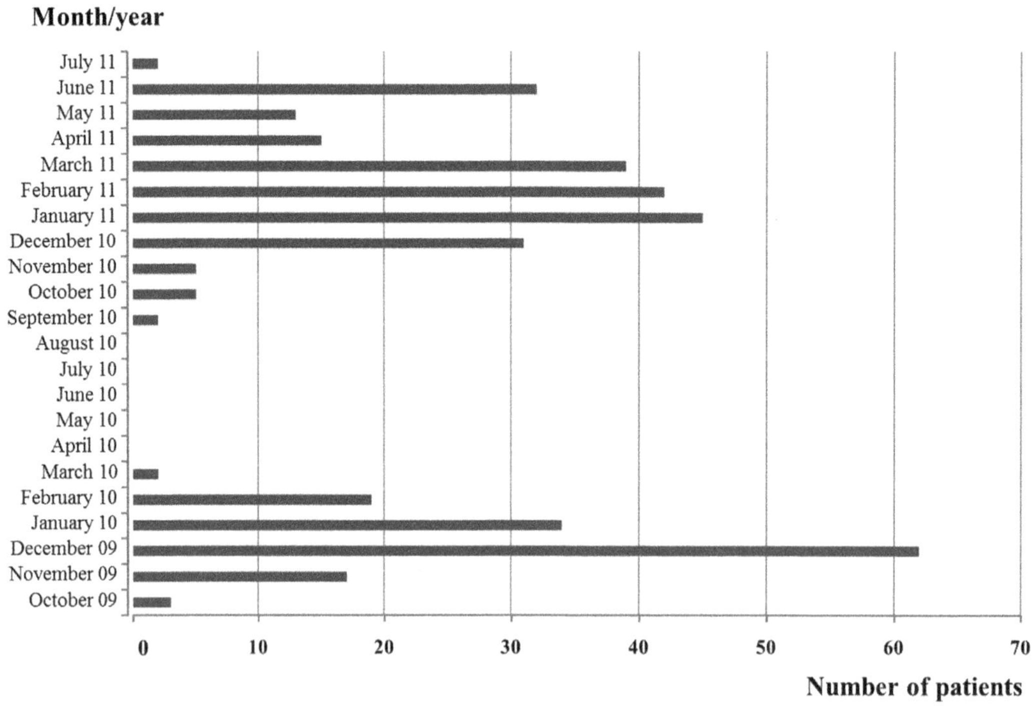

Figure 1. The first and second periods of the 2009–2011 typhoid fever outbreak, showing cases by month and hospital.

duration of fever after treatment was 4 (3, 5) days (267 patients had available last date of fever data). Patients whose treatment began after day 5 of their fever were more likely to have mucus bloody diarrhea, hepatomegaly, hospitalization, and anemia than those who were treated on or before the 5th day (Table 1, 2).

Complications, mainly moderate to severe gastrointestinal (GI) symptoms, lower respiratory symptoms, anemia (Hct <30%), thrombocytopenia (<100,000 platelets/mm^3), seizure, and acute kidney injury, were found in 49/368 (13.3%) patients; 5 patients had 2 complications and none died. Complications associated with moderate to severe GI symptoms were found in 8 patients; ascites with abdominal pain (confirmed by abdominal ultrasonography) was found in 7 patients and 1 patient who had fever 28 days prior to treatment had a terminal ileal perforation. None of the patients

Table 1. Clinical characteristics and outcomes of typhoid patients treated before and after the 5th day of fever.

Clinical factors and outcomes	Stage of fever when treatment begun		P
	≤5 days N = 208	>5 days N = 149	
Clinical characteristics			
BT, °C, mean ± SD	40.2±0.7, n = 138	40.0±0.7, n = 116	0.35
Pulse rate/minute, mean ± SD	126±11, n = 133	122±15, n = 111	0.04
Diarrhea, no. (%)	94 (45.2)	83 (55.7)	0.06
Mucus bloody, no. (%)	0	5 (3.4)	0.01
Abdominal pain, no. (%)	52 (25.0)	32 (21.5)	0.52
Vomiting, no. (%)	86 (41.3)	49 (32.9)	0.13
Cough, no. (%)	68 (32.7)	57 (38.3)	0.33
Hepatomegaly, no. (%)	10 (4.8)	20 (13.4)	<0.01
Splenomegaly, no. (%)	0	3 (2.0)	0.07
Outcomes			
Hospitalization, no. (%)	141 (67.8)	119 (79.9)	0.01
Complication, total, no. (%)	23 (11.1)	25 (16.8)	0.12
GI complication, no. (%)	0	8	<0.01
Non-GI complication, no. (%)	23	17	0.91

BT, body temperature; GI, gastrointestinal tract.

Table 2. Comparison of complete blood counts results tested before and after the 5th day of fever.

Laboratory investigation	Period of fever when tested		p
	≤5 days	>5days	
	N = 221	N = 128	
Hematocrit, %, median (IQR)	35.7±3.8	34.3±4.0	<0.01
Hematocrit <35%, n, (%)	79 (35.7)	63 (49.2)	0.01
Hematocrit <30%, n, (%)	11 (5.0)	13 (10.2)	0.07
White blood cells, cells/mm^3, median (IQR)	6,800	6,800	0.53
	(5,400–8,710)	(5,300–8,075)	
Neutrophils, %, mean ± SD	60.7±13.0	58.4±12.2, n = 127	0.10
Lymphocytes, %, mean ± SD	29.4±11.9, n = 158	33.3±11.2, n = 104	<0.01
Platelets x 10^3/mm^3, median (IQR)	198 (159–245)	200 (160–253)	0.61
	n = 212	n = 115	
<100,000 platelets/mm^3, n, (%)	11 (5.2)	4 (3.5)	0.59

who were treated prior to the 5th day of fever had GI complications (Tables 1 and 2). Of the 7 patients who had abdominal pain with ascites, 6 developed the symptom on day 6 of fever and one on day 8, and all responded well to antibiotic treatment, although one had a seizure. Lower respiratory symptoms were found in 7 patients, of whom one had underlying asthma; all had infection-induced wheezing and 5/7 patients developed the symptom before the 5th day of fever. Anemia (Hct <30%) was the most common complication, found in 25/354 (6.8%) patients. Three patients developed hemolytic anemia, two of whom had an underlying disease, one with glucose-6-phosphate dehydrogenase (G-6 PD) deficiency and the other with hemoglobin H disease, with the lowest hematocrits of 16% and 18%, respectively. The patient who had an unknown cause of hemolytic anemia also had acute kidney injury (AKI) with an initial blood urea nitrogen (BUN)/creatinine (Cr) level of 33/2.3 mg/dL; his BUN/Cr level decreased to 14/1.1 mg/dL on day 4 after beginning treatment. Fifteen patients had thrombocytopenia, 4 with <50,000 platelets/mm^3 but none with active bleeding.

Sensitivity, specificity, negative predictive value and positive predictive value of serology tests for typhoid fever

The mean day of fever when blood was drawn for the serology tests was 6.0±4.0 days. Of the 368 blood-culture confirmed patients, Typhi IgM and IgG tests were performed in 199 and 135 patients, respectively. The positive rate of both Typhi IgM and IgG tests did not increase when compared among the 3 periods of fever, before day 5, days 6–10, and after day 10; the three positive rates for the three periods were *S* ser. Typhi IgM (51.4%, 66.7%, 41.7%) and *S* ser. Typhi IgG (28.2%, 40.0%, 42.9%), respectively. The sensitivity, specificity, PPV, and NPV of the *S* ser. Typhi IgM tests were 56.3%, 74.1%, 31.4%, and 88.9%, respectively, and of the *S* ser. Typhi IgG tests were 33.3%, 50.5%, 7.7%, and 85.9%, respectively. Of the 126 cases who had both *S* ser. Typhi IgM and IgG rapid tests, 82 (65.1%) and 20 (15.9%) cases were positive to one of or both IgM and IgG, respectively (Table 3).

Discussion

We found good clinical outcomes of most typhoid fever cases during the 2009–11 outbreak in Songkhla, Thailand, as most of the patients were treated within 2 weeks of the first appearance of fever and all of the *S* ser. Typhi strains isolated were susceptible to our standard first line antibiotics.

We found that both of the *S* ser. Typhi IgM/IgG tests had low sensitivity for diagnosing typhoid fever, with IgM only 56.3% and IgG only 33.3%. A previous study found higher sensitivity of both IgM (69.0%) and IgG (70.7%) [29]. The specificity of IgM in our study was similar to this same study (74.1% vs 79.3%), but we found a lower specificity of IgG (50.5% vs 76.9%) [29]. However, both our study and this previous study found a high NPV for both *S* ser. Typhi IgM and IgG tests, suggesting that it is safe for the physician to wait for blood culture results if the rapid test is negative.

The first outbreak lasted for 6 months and entered a period of remission between April and August 2010, which could be explained by the April to May summer school break in Thailand, along with the implementation of various measures to improve sanitation at the affected schools, including providing health education messages for communities and in schools, promoting hand washing for food handlers and students, avoiding foods and beverages from street vendors, cleaning and renovating the kitchens and toilets in the outbreak schools and nearby markets, closing the schools for 7 days during school renovation, encouraging the students to eat homemade lunches/beverages using their own plates and spoons, providing ciprofloxacin to all school food handlers for 14 days, and adding chlorine to the tap water to increase chlorine levels from 0.1 ppm to 0.5 ppm. After these measures were implemented, the number of typhoid cases decreased, and the epidemic seemed to go into remission in April; however, 3–4 months later, after the schools reopened, a second outbreak was underway, which had a greater number of cases than the first outbreak, and lasted for 11 months, after which the overall outbreak ended as typhoid levels returned to historical norms. During the second outbreak, the Ministry of Public Health in Songkhla expected that after control measures were implemented in the schools and in local markets, the outbreak would go into remission as in the first outbreak, so vaccinations were not given to the students, as the current typhoid vaccines are only moderately effective for short periods of time, are costly, and multiple doses are required [30,31]. However, without accurate source identification as in our situation, typhoid vaccine implementation would be an important tool to help control the outbreak [32]. We found

Table 3. Sensitivity, specificity, negative predictive value, and positive predictive value of *S* ser. Typhi IgM/IgG rapid test.

Test	Results				Sensitivity (%)	Specificity (%)	PPV(%)	NPV (%)
	TP	FN	FP	TN				
IgM rapid test	112	87	244	697	56.3	74.1	31.4	88.9
Typhoid IgG	45	90	536	548	33.3	50.0	7.7	85.9

TP, true positive; FN, false negative; FP, false positive; FN, false negative.

that PFGE profiles from the 52 tested samples had the same pattern, indicating that the *S* ser. Typhi strains isolated from the patients from different schools were likely to have come from the same source. A large outbreak in Nepal lasted only 8 weeks after the source of the outbreak was found in the water supply, which suggests that isolating the source of *S* ser. Typhi quickly is an important factor in controlling such outbreaks [23].

We found that all of the *S* ser. Typhi strains isolated were susceptible to all first line antibiotics, including ciprofloxacin and ceftriaxone, as all of our patients responded well to these antibiotics and none had treatment failure or relapse [22,33]. According to the Thai health policy which requires patients to access services in their local health district, there were no patients who suffered a second episode of typhoid fever during the outbreak, which indicates that there were no typhoid relapses or treatment failures, although a few patients might have moved to another province.

Although ciprofloxacin is recommended as the first line antibiotic for the treatment of typhoid and was successfully used in our situation, other studies have noted a high resistance rate to first line antibiotics; for example, studies from the United States, Cambodia and Vietnam found multidrug resistant *S* ser. Typhi in 13%, 58%, and 85% of cases, respectively [24–26]. Monitoring the current resistance in typhoid endemic areas of *S* ser. Typhi susceptibility is important to ensure an appropriate antibiotic is used when an outbreak occurs.

We found, as in previous studies, that cough or wheezing was common in typhoid fever patients [10,34]. Acute hemolysis can occur in patients who have thalassemia or G-6PD deficiency [34]. We found that one-third of our patients had a dry cough without rhinorrhea, similar to a previous study which found cough in 39% of the typhoid fever cases [10]. In general, typhoid complications such as abdominal pain or pneumonitis will develop in the second week in patients who do not receive an appropriate antibiotic [2,35]. However, most of patients in our study who had abdominal pain with ascites developed symptoms by the end of the first week of illness. In addition, most of patients who had dyspnea developed the symptom within the first week of illness, but all responded well to antibiotics and bronchodilator.

In summary, there were 2 related outbreaks of typhoid fever in Songkhla during 2009–2011, with a 5-month gap between them. Most of the patients were diagnosed at an early stage and treated with a good outcome. Patients who were treated within the first five days of fever had no typhoid-related GI complications. The *S* ser. Typhi IgM and IgG tests (SD Bioline) had low sensitivity for diagnosing typhoid fever in Thai children.

Supporting Information

Data S1 Typhoid Outbreak in Songkhla, Thailand 2009-2011.

Acknowledgments

The authors wish to thank Miss Walailuk Jitpiboon for assistance with data analysis, and David Patterson for help with the English, both of whom work with the Faculty of Medicine, Prince of Songkla University.

Author Contributions

Conceived and designed the experiments: WL NH KL. Performed the experiments: WL NH RS. Analyzed the data: KL. Contributed reagents/materials/analysis tools: WL. Wrote the paper: KL.

References

1. Buckle GC, Walker CL, Black RE (2012) Typhoid fever and paratyphoid fever: Systematic review to estimate global morbidity and mortality for 2010. J Glob Health 2: 10401.
2. Parry CM, Hien TT, Dougan G, White NJ, Farrar JJ (2002) Typhoid fever. N Engl J Med 347: 1770–1782.
3. Saxe JM, Cropsey R (2005) Is operative management effective in treatment of perforated typhoid? Am J Surg 189: 342–344.
4. Ugwu BT, Yiltok SJ, Kidmas AT, Opaluwa AS (2005) Typhoid intestinal perforation in north central Nigeria. West Afr J Med 24: 1–6.
5. Thailand Bureau of Epidemiology, Department of Disease Control, Ministry of Public Health Typhoid surveillances. Available at: http://www.boe.moph.go.th/boedb/surdata/506wk/y56/d08_4256.pdf. Accessed 4 October 2013.
6. Henpraserttae N (2010) Typhoid outbreak in Songkhla Province, Thailand, October 2009–April 2010. Available at: http://203.157.15.4/wesr/file/y54/F5474.pdf. Accessed 4 October 2013.
7. Farooqui BJ, Khurshid M, Ashfaq MK, Khan MA (1991) Comparative yield of Salmonella typhi from blood and bone marrow cultures in patients with fever of unknown origin. J Clin Pathol 44: 258–259.
8. Vallenas C, Hernandez H, Kay B, Black R, Gotuzzo E (1985) Efficacy of bone marrow, blood, stool and duodenal contents cultures for bacteriologic confirmation of typhoid fever in children. Pediatr Infect Dis 4: 496–498.
9. Wain J, Pham VB, Ha V, Nguyen NM, To SD, et al. (2001) Quantitation of bacteria in bone marrow from patients with typhoid fever: relationship between counts and clinical features. J Clin Microbiol 39: 1571–1576.
10. Thriemer K, Ley BB, Ame SS, Deen JL, Pak GD, et al. (2013) Clinical and epidemiological features of typhoid fever in Pemba, Zanzibar: assessment of the performance of the WHO case definitions. PLoS One 7: e51823.
11. Das S, Rajendran K, Dutta P, Saha TK, Dutta S (2013) Validation of a new serology-based dipstick test for rapid diagnosis of typhoid fever. Diagn Microbiol Infect Dis 76: 5–9.
12. Choo KE, Razif AR, Oppenheimer SJ, Ariffin WA, Lau J, et al. (1993) Usefulness of the Widal test in diagnosing childhood typhoid fever in endemic areas. J Paediatr Child Health 29: 36–39.
13. Keddy KH, Sooka A, Letsoalo ME, Hoyland G, Chaignat CL, et al. (2011) Sensitivity and specificity of typhoid fever rapid antibody tests for laboratory diagnosis at two sub-Saharan African sites. Bull World Health Organ 89: 640–647.
14. Begum Z, Hossain MA, Musa AK, Shamsuzzaman AK, Mahmud MC, et al. (2009) Comparison between DOT EIA IgM and Widal Test as early diagnosis of typhoid fever. Mymensingh Med J 18: 13–17.
15. Bhutta ZA, Mansurali N (1999) Rapid serologic diagnosis of pediatric typhoid fever in an endemic area: a prospective comparative evaluation of two dot-enzyme immunoassays and the Widal test. Am J Trop Med Hyg 61: 654–657.
16. Dutta S, Sur D, Manna B, Sen B, Deb AK, et al. (2006) Evaluation of new-generation serologic tests for the diagnosis of typhoid fever: data from a community-based surveillance in Calcutta, India. Diagn Microbiol Infect Dis 56: 359–365.
17. Gasem MH, Smits HL, Goris MG, Dolmans WM (2002) Evaluation of a simple and rapid dipstick assay for the diagnosis of typhoid fever in Indonesia. J Med Microbiol 51: 173–177.
18. Hatta M, Goris MG, Heerkens E, Gooskens J, Smits HL (2002) Simple dipstick assay for the detection of Salmonella typhi-specific IgM antibodies and the evolution of the immune response in patients with typhoid fever. Am J Trop Med Hyg 66: 416–421.
19. House D, Wain J, Ho VA, Diep TS, Chinh NT, et al. (2001) Serology of typhoid fever in an area of endemicity and its relevance to diagnosis. J Clin Microbiol 39: 1002–1007.
20. Naheed A, Ram PK, Brooks WA, Mintz ED, Hossain MA, et al. (2008) Clinical value of Tubex and Typhidot rapid diagnostic tests for typhoid fever in an urban community clinic in Bangladesh. Diagn Microbiol Infect Dis 61: 381–386.
21. Khanam F, Sheikh A, Sayeed MA, Bhuiyan MS, Choudhury FK, et al. (2013) Evaluation of a typhoid/paratyphoid diagnostic assay (TPTest) detecting anti-Salmonella IgA in secretions of peripheral blood lymphocytes in patients in Dhaka, Bangladesh. PLoS Negl Trop Dis 7: e2316.
22. Thaver D, Zaidi AK, Critchley J, Azmatullah A, Madni SA, et al. (2009) A comparison of fluoroquinolones versus other antibiotics for treating enteric fever: meta-analysis. BMJ 338: b1865.
23. Lewis MD, Serichantalergs O, Pitarangsi C, Chuanak N, Mason CJ, et al. (2005) Typhoid fever: a massive, single-point source, multidrug-resistant outbreak in Nepal. Clin Infect Dis 40: 554–561.
24. Lynch MF, Blanton EM, Bulens S, Polyak C, Vojdani J, et al. (2009) Typhoid fever in the United States, 1999-2006. JAMA 302: 859–865.
25. Dolecek C, Tran TP, Nguyen NR, Le TP, Ha V, et al. (2008) A multi-center randomised controlled trial of gatifloxacin versus azithromycin for the treatment of uncomplicated typhoid fever in children and adults in Vietnam. PLoS One 3: e2188.
26. Emary K, Moore CE, Chanpheaktra N, An KP, Chheng K, et al. (2012) Enteric fever in Cambodian children is dominated by multidrug-resistant H58 Salmonella enterica serovar Typhi with intermediate susceptibility to ciprofloxacin. Trans R Soc Trop Med Hyg 106: 718–724.
27. Clinical and Laboratory Standards Institute (2009) Performance standards for antimicrobial susceptibility testing: 19th informational supplement. CLSI document M100-S19. 19th ed. Clinical and Laboratory Standards Institute, Wayne, PA.
28. Ward LR, de Sa JD, Rowe B (1987) A phage-typing scheme for Salmonella enteritidis. Epidemiol Infect 99: 291–294.
29. Kawano RL, Leano SA, Agdamag DM (2007) Comparison of serological test kits for diagnosis of typhoid fever in the Philippines. J Clin Microbiol 45: 246–247.
30. Martin LB (2012) Vaccines for typhoid fever and other salmonelloses. Curr Opin Infect Dis 25: 489–499.
31. Simanjuntak CH, Paleologo FP, Punjabi NH, Darmowigoto R, Soeprawoto, et al. (1991) Oral immunisation against typhoid fever in Indonesia with Ty21a vaccine. Lancet 338: 1055–1059.
32. Yang HH, Kilgore PE, Yang LH, Park JK, Pan YF, et al. (2001) An outbreak of typhoid fever, Xing-An County, People's Republic of China, 1999: estimation of the field effectiveness of Vi polysaccharide typhoid vaccine. J Infect Dis 183: 1775–1780.
33. Effa EE, Lassi ZS, Critchley JA, Garner P, Sinclair D, et al. (2011) Fluoroquinolones for treating typhoid and paratyphoid fever (enteric fever). Cochrane Database Syst Rev: CD004530.
34. Thisyakorn U, Mansuwan P, Taylor DN (1987) Typhoid and paratyphoid fever in 192 hospitalized children in Thailand. Am J Dis Child 141: 862–865.
35. Connor BA, Schwartz E (2005) Typhoid and paratyphoid fever in travellers. Lancet Infect Dis 5: 623–628.

29

Revisiting Russell's Viper (*Daboia russelii*) Bite in Sri Lanka: Is Abdominal Pain an Early Feature of Systemic Envenoming?

Senanayake A. M. Kularatne[1]*, Anjana Silva[2], Kosala Weerakoon[2], Kalana Maduwage[3], Chamara Walathara[4], Ranjith Paranagama[4], Suresh Mendis[4]

1 Department of Medicine, Faculty of Medicine, University of Peradeniya, Peradeniya, Sri Lanka, **2** Department of Parasitology, Faculty of Medicine and Allied Sciences, Rajarata University of Sri Lanka, Anuradhapura, Sri Lanka, **3** School of Medicine and Public Health, University of Newcastle, Callaghan, New South Wales, Australia, **4** Teaching Hospital, Anuradhapura, Sri Lanka

Abstract

The Russell's viper (*Daboia russelii*) is responsible for 30–40% of all snakebites and the most number of life-threatening bites of any snake in Sri Lanka. The clinical profile of Russell's viper bite includes local swelling, coagulopathy, renal dysfunction and neuromuscular paralysis, based on which the syndromic diagnostic tools have been developed. The currently available Indian polyvalent antivenom is not very effective in treating Russell's viper bite patients in Sri Lanka and the decision regarding antivenom therapy is primarily driven by clinical and laboratory evidence of envenoming. The non-availability of early predictors of Russell's viper systemic envenoming is responsible for considerable delay in commencing antivenom. The objective of this study is to evaluate abdominal pain as an early feature of systemic envenoming following Russell's viper bites. We evaluated the clinical profile of Russell's viper bite patients admitted to a tertiary care centre in Sri Lanka. Fifty-five patients were proven Russell's viper bite victims who produced the biting snake, while one hundred and fifty-four were suspected to have been bitten by the same snake species. Coagulopathy (159, 76.1%), renal dysfunction (39, 18.7%), neuromuscular paralysis (146, 69.9%) and local envenoming (192, 91.9%) were seen in the victims, ranging from mono-systemic involvement to various combinations. Abdominal pain was present in 79.5% of these patients, appearing 5 minutes to 4 hours after the bite. The severity of the abdominal pain, assessed using a scoring system, correlated well with the severity of the coagulopathy ($p<0.001$) and the neurotoxicity ($p<0.001$). Its diagnostic validity to predict systemic envenoming is – Sensitivity 81.6%, Specificity 82.4%, Positive predictive value 91.2%. Thus, abdominal pain is an early clinical feature of systemic Russell's viper bite envenoming in Sri Lanka. However, it is best to judge abdominal pain together with other clinical manifestations on decision making.

Editor: Edgardo Moreno, National University, Costa Rica

Funding: The authors have no support or funding to report.

Competing Interests: The authors have declared that no competing interests exist.

* E-mail: samkul@sltnet.lk

Introduction

The Russell's viper is considered a highly venomous snake throughout its range in Asia [1]. Based on the morphology and molecular evidence, the western and the eastern forms of this snake are now considered two separate species. The western form, *Daboia russelii* (Shaw and Nodder, 1797) is distributed throughout South Asia, west of the bay of Bengal, whereas the eastern form *Daboia siamensis* (Smith, 1917) is distributed in South-East Asia, east of the bay of Bengal [2]. Three sub species of the Russell's viper, *D. r. pulchella* (from Sri Lanka and southern India), *D. r. nordicus* (from northern India) and *D. r. russelii* (other areas) have been described from the regions to the west of the Bay of Bengal, based on morphology. Although these sub species have been placed under *Daboia russelii*, the taxonomic validity of this separation remains doubtful [2,3].

There are 37,000 snakebite admissions to Sri Lankan hospitals every year [4,5]. The Russell's viper (Figure 1) is responsible for 30–40% of the snake bites, and to the most number of severe envenoming and fatalities compared to other snakes in Sri Lanka [5,6]. Sri Lankans have been well aware of the aggressive nature and the lethality of the Russell's viper over many generations. In 1910, Abercromby [7] noted "...they [native Sri Lankans] consider the Russell's viper (Tic Polonga) as a personification of the devil." Bites by Russell's vipers commonly occur in paddy (rice) fields and on footpaths at dusk and at dawn, affecting a large number of agricultural workers and so considered an occupational hazard in Sri Lanka [8].

The clinical profile of Russell's viper bites in Sri Lanka was first studied in detail by Jeyarajah in 1984 based on 22 cases [9], followed by a study of 23 cases by Phillips et al., in 1988 [10]. Kularatne [8] studied the epidemiology and clinical profile of Russell's viper bites in Sri Lanka based on 336 cases. Coagulopathy and acute kidney injury had been the major life threatening systemic manifestations of bites by this snake in Sri Lanka [8,10]. Neuro-muscular paralysis, characterized by opthalmoplegia and ptosis, has been commonly observed in these with rare occurrence of respiratory muscle paralysis [8,9]. Rhabdomyolysis [10],

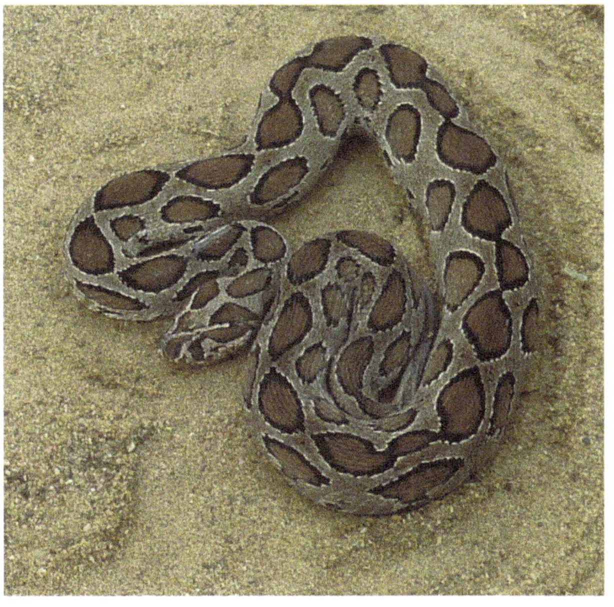

Figure 1. Russell's viper (*Daboia russelii*) adult specimen from Sri Lanka. Russell's vipers are distributed throughout Sri Lanka except at higher elevations (>1500 m) and are abundant in agricultural lands in the rural areas of the island's dry zone.

chronic renal failure [11], myocardial infarction [12] and secondary hypopituitarism [13] have also been reported in Russell's viper bite patients in Sri Lanka. Although generally not severe, local swelling has been a common feature seen in this country [8,10].

Differences in venom composition between Sri Lankan and northern Indian Russell's vipers have been used to support separation into two subspecies [14]. An attempt at developing a monospecifc antivenom against the venom of the Sri Lankan Russell's viper was successful, but it did not go beyond clinical trials [15]. The only antivenom available for Russell's viper bites in Sri Lanka is Indian-made polyvalent antivenom which has been raised against the venoms of four Indian snakes including Russell's vipers. This Indian polyvalent antivenom has been shown to be poorly effective in treating Sri Lankan Russell's viper bites [10]. It is noteworthy that this clinico-epidemiological information which lays the foundation for further clinical research as well as affecting clinical management, relies heavily on a few studies only, the latest being published ten years ago [8,10]. Based on the observation that the clinical profile of Russell's viper bites in Sri Lanka presented as unique clinical syndromes, epidemiological tools for the syndromic identification of Russell's viper bite envenoming have been developed [16,17]. The availability of offending snake specimens in snakebite instances has been less than 30% [8], therefore this method has been useful in making a presumptive diagnosis of Russell's viper bite envenoming. The incidence of recognised clinical features of Russell's viper envenoming are local envenoming 92%, coagulopathy 77%, neurotoxicity 78% and renal failure 18%, either in various combinations or as isolated manifestations [8]. When the combinations of clinical features do not follow a described pattern, the application of the syndromic diagnosis method to identify the offending snake could lead to an erroneous conclusion. To overcome this possibility more precise clinical evidence should be established by prospective clinical studies looking for variations of clinical manifestations.

In Russell's viper bite, the reported incidence of dry bite has been low, with most bites resulting in significant envenoming [8]. At the same time there were situations where, in proven cases of Russell's viper bite, acute renal failure was the sole manifestation of envenoming developing many hours after the bite [18]. From the clinicians' perspective, early recognition of significant systemic envenoming is of great importance as it would enable taking an early decision regarding antivenom therapy. At present there is no early sign or symptom that has been identified in Russell's viper bite that could be considered a clinical predictor of significant systemic envenoming. Abdominal pain has been documented as a clinical feature in some studies of Russell's viper envenoming [19,20]. But abdominal pain is also a known clinical feature of envenoming by other snakes, particularly by the common krait [21]. However, epidemiology of common krait bite is unique that it happens exclusively at night when victims are in sleep causing neuromuscular paralysis. Nevertheless, many practicing clinicians believe that abdominal pain is a feature of systemic envenoming in Russell's viper bite (personal communication, Dr. W P Dissanayake, consultant physician). This observation is strengthened by the fact that in a comparative study of the patients of Russell's viper and Hump-nosed pit viper (*Hypnale* spp.) bites, abdominal pain was present only among the Russell's viper bite patients [20].

These issues indicated that there was justification for revisiting the clinico-epidemiology of Russell's viper bites in Sri Lanka, using a well designed prospective clinical study in order to broaden the present understanding of the clinical profile and analysing the place of abdominal pain as an early feature of significant envenoming. The objectives of the present study therefore are to re-evaluate the clinico-epidemiology of Russell's viper envenoming in Sri Lanka and to examine the place of abdominal pain as a possible early clinical feature of significant envenoming.

Materials and Methods

Ethical background

Ethical clearance for this study was obtained from the Ethics Review Committee of the Faculty of Medicine, University of Peradeniya, Sri Lanka. Written informed consent was obtained from the participants in this study prior to data collection. Proxy consent was obtained from the relatives of those who were unconscious and of those below the age of 18 years.

Study setting

The study was carried out in the Emergency Treatment Unit (ETU) of the Teaching Hospital, Anuradhapura (THA), from January to December 2010.

THA is a tertiary care centre and the largest hospital in the North Central Province and indeed, in the entire dry zone of Sri Lanka, from where the highest number of snakebites is reported annually [4]. The hospital receives patients from a large catchment that consists mostly of rural paddy (rice) and *chena* (slash and burn) farming areas.

Data collection

Patients who were admitted to the hospital with a history of snakebite were screened and those with confirmed Russell's viper bites authenticated with the positive identification of the offending snake and suspected Russell's viper bite patients were enrolled in the study. Data collection was prospective using investigator administered questionnaires. Information regarding patients with altered consciousness and about children was obtained from relatives, parents or those in attendance. IBM SPSS version 20.0 was used for the data analysis.

Table 1. The scoring system adopted to grade the severity of envenoming and the severity of abdominal pain.

Description of the clinical manifestation category	Severity score
Abdominal pain	
Occurs within 6 hours of bite	1
Onset within 30 minutes of bite	0.5
Lasting more than 1 hour	0.5
Bearable with difficulty/Unbearable	0.5
Local envenoming	
Presence of local swelling	1
Swelling involving more than half the limb	1
Necrosis/Gangrene/Compartment syndrome	1
Coagulopathy	
On admission 20WBCT prolonged (>20 min)	1
Subsequent 20WBCTs prolonged (repeated 6 hourly, if any)	1
Spontaneous bleeding (local bleeding/gum bleeding/epistaxis/subconjunctival haemorrhage	1
Severe bleeding (gasterointestinal bleeding/haematuria)	1
Neuromuscular paralysis	
Ptosis/Opthalmoplegia	1
Neck/limb muscle weakness	1
Respiratory paralysis	1
Renal dysfunction	
Blood urea >13 mmol/l	1
Oliguria with high blood urea nitrogen/high serum K^+	1
Renal failure requiring renal replacement therapy	1
Cardiovascular dysfunction	
Systolic blood pressure <90 mmHg and signs of early circulatory collapse	1
Severe circulatory collapse (shock)/arrhythmias	1
Acute myocardial infarction/heart failure	1

Snake identification

The Department of Wildlife Conservation, Sri Lanka, permitted (by permit letter no: WL/3/2/1/7) the retention of the killed snakes brought along with snakebite victims that were then taken to the University of Peradeniya where the identification was done using identification keys in De Silva, 1980. In addition, whenever the assailant snake specimen is not available for identification, preserved specimens and photographs of Russell's vipers were shown to the patients for the tentative establishment of the identity of the assailant snake. However these cases were considered as suspected cases of Russell's viper bite.

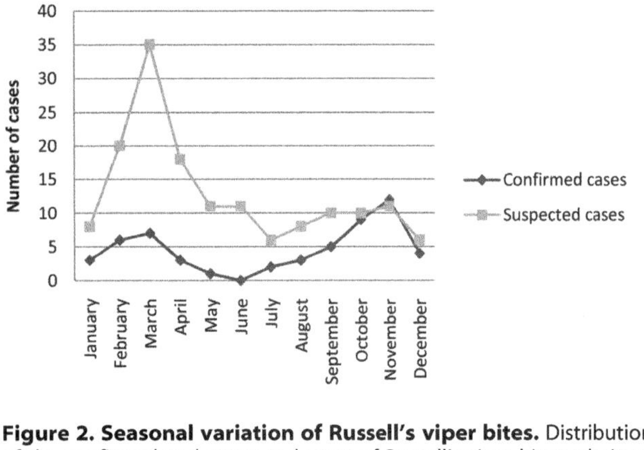

Figure 2. Seasonal variation of Russell's viper bites. Distribution of the confirmed and suspected cases of Russell's viper bites admitted to the Teaching Hospital, Anuradhapura from January to December, 2010. Note the high rate of admissions during February – April and September – November representing paddy harvesting and chena cultivation seasons.

Clinical assessment

The severity of envenoming was assessed using the scoring system described in table 1 where each manifestation, namely local envenoming, coagulopathy, neuromuscular paralysis, renal dysfunction, cardiovascular dysfunction and abdominal pain was given a score on a cumulative scale. Each manifestation could score a minimum of 1 point with additional points depending on increasing severity of involvement. Severity of antivenom reactions were assessed retrospectively as mild, moderate or severe based on clinical parameters: normal blood pressure with cutaneous manifestation was categorized as a mild reaction; dropping of systolic blood pressure below 90 mm Hg was considered a moderate reaction; and patients who had cardiovascular collapse with unrecordable blood pressure and thready pulse were considered to have a severe reaction.

Table 2. Clinical findings of the 55 proven and 154 suspected Russell's viper bite patients. (percentages within parenthesis).

Clinical findings	Proven cases (n, 55)	Probable cases (n,154)
Local envenoming at the site of bite		
Total	49 (89)	143 (93)
Swelling	49 (89)	143 (93)
Pain	53 (96)	150 (97)
Blistering	1 (2)	0
Necrosis	1 (2)	0
Coagulopathy		
Total	38 (69)	121 (79)
Incoagulable blood (20 WBCT)	38 (69)	121 (79)
Spontaneous bleeding		
Gum bleeding	2 (4)	1 (0.65)
Epistaxis	0	2 (1)
Gastrointestinal bleeding	1 (2)	5 (3)
Haematuria	1 (2)	23 (15)
Time duration from bite to coagulopathy (Minutes, range within parenthesis)	167.5 (35–960)	165 (55–1050)
Renal dysfunction		
Total	5 (9)	34 (22)
Mild	3 (5)	18 (12)
Moderate	2 (4)	11 (7)
Severe (requiring renal replacement therapy)	0	5 (3)
Neuromuscular paralysis		
Total	30 (55)	116 (75)
Ptosis	30 (55)	109 (71)
Ophthalmoplegia	30 (55)	111 (72)
Neck muscle weakness	14 (25)	50 (32)
Respiratory paralysis	0	2 (1)
Cardiovascular dysfunction		
Total	1 (2)	11 (7)
Mild		10 (6.5)
Moderate		1 (0.65)

Results

Demographic and epidemiological data

Of the study group, 92.7% patients directly came to the THA. During the study period, 55 specimen-authenticated (proven) and 154 suspected Russell's viper bite patients were treated in the study setting and were thus included in the study. The majority of victims were in the 20–50 year age group: 72.7% and 76.6% in the proven and suspected Russell's viper bite groups respectively. Most affected were males (81% and 84%) and farmers (45% and 67%) in both groups. However, a range of other occupations, including security personnel, school teachers, businessmen and school children were seen among the participants of this study. The vast majority (88% and 93%) of the Russell's viper bite patients in the two groups had received school education only up to grade 11 or age 16. Figure 2 shows the seasonal distribution of

Table 3. Systemic involvement of the proven Russell's viper bite patients (n = 55) (percentages within parenthesis).

Description of the systemic involvement	Number of patients
Coagulopathy alone	7 (13)
Coagulopathy and Neuromuscular paralysis	27 (49)
Coagulopathy and Renal dysfunction	2 (4)
Coagulopathy, Neuromuscular paralysis and Renal dysfunction	2 (4)
Neuromuscular paralysis and Renal dysfunction	1 (2)

Table 4. Correlations between length of the snake versus different clinical parameters of 48 from the 55 confirmed Russell's viper bite patients.

Description	Correlation Coefficient	P value
Length of the snake	1.000	-
Envenoming severity	−0.084	0.572
Coagulopathy	−0.016	0.916
Neuromuscular paralysis	−0.006	0.966
Local envenomation	−0.189	0.199
Renal dysfunction	.005	0.971

(Statistical test -Spearman's rho.).

these patients. There are high rates of Russell's viper bites during February to May and September to December, the paddy (rice) harvesting and chena cultivating seasons in the dry-zone of Sri Lanka. Bites had occurred in chenas (53% and 66%), paddy fields (5.5% and 13%), in and around residential compounds (20% and 11%) and by the roadside (20% and 9%) among the proven and suspected Russell's viper bite patients. In the above two groups, 67% and 61% of all bites had occurred during the period 12.00–21.00 hours, respectively.

First aid treatment

Washing the bite site (62%, 51%) and application of a tourniquet proximal to the bite site (42%, 57%) were the commonest first aid measures practiced prior to hospital admission in proven bites and suspected Russell's viper bites respectively. No first aid had been administered to 22% of the proven Russell's viper bite victims and 0.65% of the others. The median time interval between the snakebite and hospital admission was 28 and 30 minutes (range 10–180 minutes) in proven and suspected Russell's viper bite victims respectively.

Table 6. Correlations between abdominal pain severity versus different clinical parameters of the 55 proven Russell's viper bite patients.

Severity score	Number of	Correlation Coefficient	P value
Abdominal pain			
1	14	1.000	-
1.5	11		
2	5		
2.5	1		
Local envenoming			
1	47	0.167	0.224
2	2		
3	0		
Coagulopathy			
1	24	0.461	<0.001
2	12		
3	2		
4	0		
Neuromuscular paralysis			
1	16	0.553	<0.001
2	13		
3	0		
Renal dysfunction			
1	3	0.018	0.894
2	2		
3	0		

(Statistical test -Spearman's rho.).

Table 5. The numbers of antivenom vials and antivenom cycles received by the proven and probable Russell's viper bite patients.

	Proven cases (n, 55)	Probable cases (n, 154)
Number of vials		
10	2 (6)	4 (3)
15	0	2 (2)
20	22 (63)	64 (55)
25	0	1(1)
30	9 (26)	17 (15)
40	2 (6)	24 (21)
50	0	3 (3)
60	0	1 (1)
Number of antivenom cycles		
1	22 (63)	65 (56)
2	13 (37)	41 (35)
3	0	8 (7)
4	0	2(2)

(Percentages within parenthesis.).

Table 7. Validation of abdominal pain against systemic envenoming*.

	No. of Patients with systemic envenoming	No. of Patients without systemic envenoming	Total
No. of patients with abdominal pain	31	3	34
No. of patients without abdominal pain	7	14	21
Total	38	17	55

* [Sensitivity -81.6%, Specificity -82.4%, Positive predictive value -91.2%, Negative predictive value -66.7%, False positives 3 (17.6%), False negatives 7 (18.4%)].

Clinical features

The clinical findings of the study participants are described in table 2. Fifty-three (96%) of the proven Russell's viper bite patients had local or systemic envenoming, giving a dry bite rate of 4%, with 38 (69%) having systemic envenoming. All those with systemic envenoming also had local envenoming. Coagulopathy, characterized by prolonged clotting time (as determined by the twenty minute whole blood clotting test or 20WBCT) and spontaneous bleeding, was the commonest clinical manifestation of systemic envenoming among both groups. Neuro-muscular paralysis, renal toxicity and cardiovascular dysfunction were also seen in the study participants at varying degrees of severity and in various proportions (see table 2). These clinical manifestations occurred in isolation or in various combinations as described in table 3. The Spearman's rho test showed that the severity of each clinical manifestation did not correlate with the length of the snake (median =461 mm, range: 235–1320 mm) (table 4).

Antivenom therapy

Antivenom therapy was administered to 64% and 75% of study participants with proven and suspected Russell's viper bites respectively. The first dose of antivenom had been administered at the THA in 94% and 90% respectively. The median time interval from bite to first dose of antivenom was 332 (range: 105–1090) and 287 (range: 105–1225) minutes in the proven and suspected groups respectively. The ranges of total antivenom vials and antivenom cycles required for proven and suspected Russell's viper bite are described in table 5. The median time taken for the whole blood clotting time to become normal was 778 minutes (range: 125–2070) and 589 minutes (range: 105–1200) among proven and suspected patient groups respectively. A mild reaction at least was observed in all those who received antivenom in both groups. Moderate or severe reactions were observed among 31% and 6% of proven and among 14% and 5% of suspected Russell's viper bite patients respectively.

Abdominal pain

Abdominal pain was observed in 31 (79.5%) of the proven Russell's viper bite victims with systemic envenoming and in only 3 (25%) of those who had only local envenoming. The pain had developed 5 to 240 minutes (mean 71 minutes) after the bite and lasted up to the 2nd (40.7%) or 3rd day (18.2%), post bite. It was generalized in 52% of the patients, or localized to the umbilical (21%), epigastric (13%), supra-pubic (9%), right inguinal fossa (2.6%) or right lumbar (1.3%) region in others. The pain was described as colicky (60%), aching (32%), or burning (8%) in nature.

Abdominal pain co-existed with coagulopathy, neuromuscular paralysis and renal dysfunction in 78.9%, 80% and 60% of patients respectively. The Spearman's rank correlation coefficients between the abdominal pain scores and the respective severity scores of coagulopathy and neuromuscular paralysis (table 6) were highly significant. However, there were no statistically significant correlations between the abdominal pain scores and renal dysfunction or local envenoming. The analysis in terms of diagnostic validity of abdominal pain (table 7) found Sensitivity -81.6%, Specificity -82.4%, Positive predictive value -91.2%, False positives 3 (17.6%) and False negatives 7 (18.4%).

Discussion

This study shows that Russell's viper bites are common among young and middle aged male farmers in Sri Lanka. The bite rates are high during the chena cultivation and paddy harvesting seasons, with the vast majority of these bites occurring in agricultural lands. These factors together make Russell's viper bites a definite occupational health hazard of farmers in Sri Lanka. However, the large number of patients representing a range of occupations other than farming highlights the burden of Russell's viper bites on Sri Lanka. Involvement of the lower limbs in nearly 90% of the patients emphasizes the preventability of these bites by wearing protective footwear during agricultural work and when walking on foot paths. Very high antivenom reaction rates observed in these patients highlights the vexed question of the safety of Indian polyvalent antivenom for use in Sri Lankan Russell's viper bite patients and the desperate, urgent need of safe and effective antivenom for use in Sri Lanka.

This study demonstrates that Russell's viper envenoming in Sri Lanka affects multiple systems in various combinations as well as mono-systemic involvement, leading to a variety of clinical syndromes. It also shows that abdominal pain is a common clinical feature of Russell's viper envenoming and its severity has a significant correlation to the severity of systemic envenoming with coagulopathy and neurotoxicity.

Syndromes of Sri Lankan Russell's viper envenoming consist of local swelling, incoagulable blood and spontaneous bleeding, acute renal failure and neurotoxicity in various combinations [8,19]. Based on this observation, Ariaratnam et al. [17] developed an algorithm for identification of Russell's viper envenoming when the offending snake was not available. The signs included in the algorithm were combinations of neurotoxicity, incoagulable blood and renal failure. However, in our study, only 2 (4%) of the proven Russell's viper bite patients had all three systems involvement, raising a concern about the validity of the algorithmic approach as described above. Systemic involvement in Russell's viper envenoming seen in our study in rank order of frequency was as follows: coagulopathy and neurotoxicity; coagulopathy alone; coagulopathy and nephropathy; coagulopathy, neurotoxicity and nephropathy; neurotoxicity and nephropathy. Based on the results of our study, we emphasize the necessity of anticipating mono-systemic and possible combinations of multiple systemic effects in Russell's viper bite patients and it should be taken into consideration when making a clinical decision using syndromic approach.

The patient catchment of THA includes very remote areas, despite which 92.7% of all participants of this study were direct admissions. The median time interval from the incident to initiation of medical care was around 30 minutes, all the study participants having arrived within 3 hours, indicating that snakebite patients generally arrive quickly at a medical facility in Sri Lanka. The participants of this study received antivenom generally around 5 hours after the bite. The delay in commencing antivenom treatment following arrival in hospital, generally 4 ½ hours, was because of the time taken to confirm systemic envenoming by awaiting the appearance of specific clinical signs or the demonstration of coagulopathy by the 20WBCT.

Recently, the reliability of the 20WBCT performed in Sri Lankan hospitals for detecting Russell's viper bite induced coagulopathy has been questioned and reliance on clinical diagnosis of envenoming or the use of more accurate clotting studies over the 20WBCT suggested [22]. Prompt administration of antivenom following a bite resulting in systemic envenoming has the best chance of neutralising free venom and preventing the development of life-threatening situations. Delay in administration of antivenom, for example because the overt manifestation of clinical signs of systemic envenoming is delayed, reduces the chances of rapid venom elimination. In this situation the identification of early clinical features of severe Russell's viper envenoming would enable the early identification of the need for antivenom therapy. Abdominal pain, at present considered a non-specific symptom, is a likely candidate. It has long been neglected as a useful clinical sign of envenoming in Russell's viper bite patients in Sri Lanka. In developing the scoring system for syndromic identification of Russell's viper bite envenoming, abdominal pain has been taken as an unlikely clinical feature [16]. However, the results of the present study suggest the need of recognizing abdominal pain as an indicator of systemic envenoming due to Russell's viper bites, and an important observation on which to base the clinical decision regarding antivenom administration.

Russell's vipers and Hump-nosed pit vipers are responsible for most number of venomous snakebites in Sri Lanka [5]. Hump-nosed pit vipers commonly cause only local envenoming, less commonly, coagulopathy and renal failure [23] sometimes leading to a clinical picture somewhat similar to that of Russell's viper bites [20]. In about three-fourths of all snakebite instances in Sri Lanka, the offending snakes are not available for identification [7,23]. The Indian polyvalent antivenom is not indicated for hump-nosed pit viper bites in Sri Lanka, therefore the ability to distinguish one clinically from an actual Russell's viper bite in such instances becomes important. The availability of the snake specimen also does not guarantee the accurate distinction between the two vipers in routine hospital practice in Sri Lanka [17]. In the circumstances the results of this study suggests that abdominal pain in a snake bite victim where the identity of the biting snake is unknown should weigh heavily in favour of antivenom administration or prompt transfer to a hospital where that can be done. This will minimise unnecessary delay in antivenom therapy when that is indicated as well as prevent the unnecessary administration of antivenom when it is not. However, it is prudent to take abdominal pain together with other clinical manifestations such as local pathology, non specific symptoms and early features of specific systemic manifestation to avoid risk of using a single parameter to judge the onset and severity of envenoming.

Conclusion

Sri Lankan Russell's viper bites manifest as different combinations of system involvement as well as mono-system involvement, commonly isolated coagulopathy. It is felt that existing paradigms of syndromic approaches towards identifying Russell's viper envenoming needs careful re-assessment. Abdominal pain is a common, yet neglected early clinical feature in Russell's viper envenoming. Presence of abdominal pain and its severity is well correlated with the severity of coagulopathy, neurotoxicity and the severity of overall systemic envenoming, suggesting its use as a potential early clinical feature in Russell's viper bite envenoming in Sri Lanka.

Acknowledgments

Dr. Ishani Ratnayake (for data recording), Dr Chanaka Rathnayake (for data entry), and Dr. Malik Fernando (for editing the manuscript) are acknowledged.

Author Contributions

Conceived and designed the experiments: SAMK. Performed the experiments: KM CW RP SM. Analyzed the data: SAMK AS KW. Contributed reagents/materials/analysis tools: SAMK KM AS KW. Wrote the paper: AS SAMK KW. Managed the study patients: CW RP SM.

References

1. Warrell DA (1989) Snake venoms in science and clinical medicine. 1. Russell's viper: biology, venom and treatment of bites. Trans R Soc Trop Med Hyg 83: 732–40.
2. Thorpe RS, Pook CE, Malhotra A (2007) Phylogeography of the Russell's viper (*Daboia russelii*) complex in relation to variation in the colour pattern and symptoms of envenoming. Herpetol J 17: 209–18.
3. Wüster W (1998) The genus *Daboia* (Serpentes: Viperidae): Russell's viper. Hamadryad 23, 33–40.
4. Anonymous (2007) Annual Health Bulletin, Colombo: Ministry of Health, Sri Lanka.
5. Kasturiratne A, Pathmeswaran A, Fonseka MMD, Lalloo DG, Brooker S, et al. (2005) Estimates of disease burden due to land-snake bite in Sri Lankan hospitals. Southeast Asian J Trop Med Public Health 36: 733–740.
6. De Silva A, Ranasinghe L (1983) Epidemiology of snake-bite in Sri Lanka: a review. Ceylon Med J 28: 144–54.
7. Abercromby AF (1910) The snakes of Ceylon. London: Murray and Co.
8. Kularatne SA (2003) Epidemiology and clinical picture of the Russell's viper (*Daboia russelii russelii*) bite in Anuradhapura, Sri Lanka: a prospective study of 336 cases. Southeast Asian J Trop Med Public Health 34: 855–62.
9. Jeyarajah R (1984) Russell's viper bite in Sri Lanka. A study of 22 cases. Am J Trop Med Hyg 33: 506–510.
10. Phillips RE, Theakston RD, Warrell DA, Galigedara Y, Abeysekera DT, et al. (1988) Paralysis, rhabdomyolysis and haemolysis caused by bites of Russell's viper (*Vipera russelii pulchella*) in Sri Lanka: failure of Indian (Haffkine) antivenom. Q J Med 68: 691–715.
11. Herath HM, Wazil AW, Abeysekara DT, Jeewani ND, Weerakoon KG, et al. (2012) Chronic kidney disease in snake envenomed with acute kidney injury in Sri Lanka: a descriptive study. Postgrad Med J 88: 138–42.
12. Silva A, Pilapitiya S, Siribaddana S (2012) Acute myocardial infarction following a possible direct intravenous bite of Russell's viper (Daboia russelii). BMC Res Notes 5: 500.
13. Antonypillai CN, Wass JA, Warrell DA, Rajaratnam HN (2011) Hypopituitarism following envenoming by Russell's vipers (*Daboia siamensis* and *D. russelii*) resembling Sheehan's syndrome: first case report from Sri Lanka, a review of the literature and recommendations for endocrine management. Q J Med 104: 97–108.
14. Suzuki M, Itoh T, Anuruddhe BM, Bandaranayake IK, Shirani Ranasinghe JG, et al. (2010) Molecular diversity in venom proteins of the Russell's viper (*Daboia russelii russelii*) and the Indian cobra (*Naja naja*) in Sri Lanka. Biomed Res 31: 71–81.
15. Ariaratnam CA, Meyer WP, Perera G, Eddleston M, Kularatne SA, et al. (1999) A new monospecific ovine Fab fragment antivenom for treatment of envenoming by the Sri Lankan Russell's viper (*Daboia russelii russelii*): a preliminary dose-finding and pharmacokinetic study. Am J Trop Med Hyg 61: 259–65.

16. Pathmeswaran A, Kasturiratne A, Fonseka M, Nandasena S, Lalloo DG, et al. (2006) Identifying the biting species in snakebite by clinical features: an epidemiological tool for community surveys. Trans R Soc Trop Med Hyg 100: 874–8.
17. Ariaratnam CA, Sheriff MH, Arambepola C, Theakston RD, Warrell DA (2009) Syndromic approach to treatment of snake bite in Sri Lanka based on results of a prospective national hospital-based survey of envenomed by identified snakes. Am J Trop Med Hyg 81: 725–31.
18. Kularatne SAM, Gawarammana IB (2001) Monosystemic effects of Russell's viper envenoming in Sri Lanka: isolated neurotoxicity, nephrotoxicity and haematotoxicity. Abstracts of the Fourth World Congress of Herpetology: 58.
19. Ariaratnam CA, Sjöström L, Raziek Z, Kularatne SA, Arachchi RW, et al. (2001) An open, randomized comparative trial of two antivenoms for the treatment of envenoming by Sri Lankan Russell's viper (*Daboia russelii russelii*). Trans R Soc Trop Med Hyg 95: 74–80.
20. Kularatne K, Budagoda S, Maduwage K, Naser K, Kumarasiri R, et al. (2011) Parallels between Russell's viper (Daboia russelii) and hump-nosed viper (Hypnale species) bites in the central hills of Sri Lanka amidst the heavy burden of unidentified snake bites. Asian Pac J Trop Med 4: 564–7.
21. Kularatne SA (2002) Common krait (*Bungarus caeruleus*) bite in Anuradhapura, Sri Lanka: a prospective clinical study, 1996–98. Postgrad Med J 78: 276–80.
22. Isbister GK, Maduwage K, Shahmy S, Mohamed F, Abeysinghe C, et al. (2013) Diagnostic 20-min whole blood clotting test in Russell's viper envenoming delays antivenom administration. Q J Med 106: 925–32.
23. Ariyaratnam CA, Thuraisingam V, Kularatne SAM, Sheriff MHR, Theakston RDG, et al. (2008) Frequent and potentially fatal envenoming by hump – nosed pit vipers (*Hypnale hypnale* and *H. nepa*) in Sri Lanka: lack of effective antivenom. Trans R Soc Trop Med Hyg 102: 1120–26.

30

Perceptions of Malaria in Pregnancy and Acceptability of Preventive Interventions among Mozambican Pregnant Women: Implications for Effectiveness of Malaria Control in Pregnancy

Helena Boene[1], Raquel González[1,2], Anifa Valá[1], Maria Rupérez[1,2], César Velasco[2], Sónia Machevo[1,4], Charfudin Sacoor[1], Esperança Sevene[1,4], Eusébio Macete[1,3], Clara Menéndez[1,2]❡, Khátia Munguambe[1,4]*❡

1 Centro de Investigação em Saúde da Manhiça, Manhiça, Mozambique, 2 Barcelona Centre for International Health Research, Hospital Clinic - Universitat de Barcelona, Barcelona, Spain, 3 Direcção Nacional de Saúde Pública, Ministério da Saúde, Maputo, Mozambique, 4 Universidade Eduardo Mondlane, Faculdade de Medicina, Maputo, Mozambique

Abstract

Background: Intermittent Preventive Treatment (IPTp) and insecticide treated nets (ITNs) are recommended malaria in pregnancy preventive interventions in sub-Saharan Africa. Despite their cost-effectiveness and seemingly straight-forward delivery mechanism, their uptake remains low. We aimed at describing perceptions of pregnant women regarding malaria and the recommended prevention interventions to understand barriers to uptake and help to improve their effectiveness.

Methods and findings: We used mixed methods to collect data among 85 pregnant women from a rural area of Southern Mozambique. Information was obtained through observations, in-depth interviews, and focused ethnographic exercises (Free-listing and Pairwise comparisons). Thematic analysis was performed on qualitative data. Data from focused ethnographic exercises were summarized into frequency distribution tables and matrices. Malaria was not viewed as a threat to pregnancy. Participants were not fully aware of malaria- associated adverse maternal and birth outcomes. ITNs were the most preferred and used malaria preventive intervention, while IPTp fell between second and third. Indoor Residual Spraying (IRS) was the least preferred intervention.

Conclusions: Low awareness of the risks and adverse consequences of malaria in pregnancy did not seem to affect acceptability or uptake to the different malaria preventive interventions in the same manner. Perceived convenience, the delivery approach, and type of provider were the key factors. Pregnant women, through antenatal care (ANC) services, can be the vehicles of ITN distribution in the communities to maximise overall ITN coverage. There is a need to improve knowledge about neonatal health and malaria to improve uptake of interventions delivered through channels other than the health facility.

Editor: Thomas Eisele, Tulane University School of Public Health and Tropical Medicine, United States of America

Funding: This work was supported by a grant from the European and Developing Countries Clinical Trials Partnership (EDCTP–IP.07.31080.002). Helena Boene is supported by a grant by EDCTP (EDCTP–CT.2006.33111.001). Maria Ruperez is supported by a grant by Rio Hortega (CM11/00278). The Manhiça Health Research Center receives core funding from the Spanish Agency for International Cooperation and Development. The funders had no role in study design, data collection and analysis, decision to publish, or preparation of the manuscript.

Competing Interests: The authors have declared that no competing interests exist.

* E-mail: khatia.munguambe@manhica.net

❡ These authors contributed equally to this work.

Introduction

Pregnant women are the main adult group at risk of malaria in sub-Saharan Africa, where approximately 25 million pregnancies are exposed to the infection and an estimated 10,000 maternal deaths attributable to malaria occur every year [1]. To control malaria in pregnancy the World Health Organisation (WHO) recommends IPTP with sulfadoxine-pyrimetamine (SP), use of insecticide treated nets (ITNs), and effective treatment of malaria episodes [2]. Despite the fact that both IPTp with SP and ITNs are highly cost-effective in improving maternal and infant health [3], and have been rolled out for many years in several malaria endemic countries, their coverage is still unacceptably low in sub-Saharan Africa [4].

Several factors may explain the low uptake, and hence low effectiveness of preventive interventions for malaria in pregnancy, such as, limited access to ANC services, health system factors which include drugs and ITN stock outs, health professionals' attitudes and practices, low patient adherence, or community attitudes towards one intervention among others [5,6].

Anthropological studies have suggested variations in individual and community's malaria-related beliefs according to their socio-cultural, educational, economic, and environmental contexts and backgrounds, which in turn affect malaria prevention outcomes [7,8]. For example, in Malawi it has been reported that local taboos prohibiting the ingestion of bitter substances during pregnancy posed limitations on the acceptability of potential anti-malarial drugs for IPTp [7]. In addition, the belief that drugs lead to miscarriage or to difficult labour due to large-sized babies have also been suggested to be related to the low uptake of preventive drugs for malaria in pregnancy [5].

It is recognized that there has been more focus on quantitative data collection approaches on perceptions of malaria in pregnancy and acceptability of preventive interventions compared to qualitative or mixed methods [8]. Moreover, studies on acceptability of malaria preventive interventions often examine them in isolation from other interventions. Therefore there is a need to better understand women's perceptions, acceptability and adherence to these interventions when they are integrated with other health services offered to them, such as ANC services [5,9].

In Mozambique, since 2006 IPTp is administered under directly observed therapy, and ITNs are delivered to pregnant women free of charge through ANC [10]. However, the average country uptake of at least two IPTp doses is still only 23% and the proportion of households with pregnant women who have at least one ITN is about 19% [11]. There is a lack of information about the acceptability of specific malaria preventive interventions among Mozambican pregnant women. A context-specific analysis might provide insights as to what extent factors such as perceptions and beliefs, may be related to the low uptake of malaria preventive interventions.

This study aimed at describing the perceptions and behaviours of pregnant women in relation to malaria and the acceptability of currently recommended malaria preventive interventions. This information may serve to understand the barriers that affect the uptake of malaria preventive interventions in pregnancy and help to improve their effectiveness.

Materials and Methods

Study site and population

The study was conducted in Manhiça, southern Mozambique, located 80 Km north of Maputo city. The district covers an area of 2,360 Km2 and its population in 2007 was around 160,000 inhabitants, of which 23% comprised women of reproductive age [12]. Malaria transmission is perennial, with moderate seasonality that peaks during the rainy season (from November to March), and mainly due to Plasmodium falciparum [13]. The prevalence of HIV in women attending the ANC clinic was 29.4% in 2010 [14].

The population of Manhiça belongs mainly to the Changana ethnic group. They are mostly subsistence farmers, informal traders, employees of two local sugar estates, and migrant labours in South Africa [15]. Adult illiteracy rate is 71%, being more prevalent among women [15].

Around 92.000 inhabitants are under continuous follow-up through a Demographic Surveillance System (DSS), which covers an area of around 500 Km^2 (also known as the Demographic Surveillance Area) and routinely registers pregnancies, births, deaths, and migrations. During 2009, the DSS registered 2,539 new pregnancies (unpublished data, Manhiça DSS 2009), and around 2,000 women attended ANC visits (unpublished data, MDH 2009).

The ANC clinic at the Manhiça District Hospital (MDH) offers maternal and child health treatment and preventive services that include screening and treatment of syphilis, anaemia, and urinary tract infections, IPTp with SP (administered 3 times during pregnancy), ITNs distribution, antihelmintic, ferrous sulphate and folate tablets, tetanus toxoid vaccination, and prevention of mother to child transmission (PMTCT) of HIV with administration of antiretrovirals [16].

For malaria prevention, in addition, indoor residual spraying (IRS) is carried out in yearly rounds in the community.

Study design and data collection

This was a mixed method study, generating qualitative and quantitative data. Specifically, standard qualitative data collection approaches namely observation of ANC clinic activities and in-depth interviews (IDIs) with pregnant women were combined with focused ethnographic study (FES) data collection approaches [17,18]. Focused ethnographic studies address some of the limitations of the classic ethnographic design, by making use of a package of exercises that can be applied during the course of individual or group interviews [18,19]. The exercises used in this study were Free-listing and Pairwise comparison. The exercises help to swiftly generate, organize and categorize insights regarding local perceptions and behaviours and how these are shaped by cultural norms.

Data was collected by a trained female Mozambican social scientist with experience in conducting qualitative studies (HB) assisted by a local female interviewer (RP), who was specifically trained for this study. Both of them are fluent in Portuguese and Changana languages. The majority of interviews and FES exercises were conducted in Changana and very few were conducted in Portuguese. Choice of language was determined by participants' convenience.

Through in-depth interviews (Form S1), perceptions about malaria in pregnancy, and the use and acceptability of conventional and traditional malaria preventive interventions were explored. The interviews targeted both women attending ANC and women who had not attended any ANC visit during their current pregnancy. Participants not attending ANC were involved in a single interview at home, while ANC attendants were expected to be involved in three interviews. The first interview with ANC attendants was conducted at the health facility immediately after the administration of the first IPTp dose. For the second and third interviews women were followed up at home, up to two weeks after administration of the second IPTp dose, and up to 24 weeks after the end of the pregnancy respectively. While the first and second interviews focused on aspects related to pregnant women's perceptions and experiences with the different interventions offered to them during ANC, the third interview dealt, in addition, with their overall degree of satisfaction with regards to such interventions in the light of the pregnancy outcome, and any other issues that the interviewer had not managed to address during the previous interviews. Interviewing the participants several times and outside the health facility environment allowed rapport building between the interviewer and the participant.

During the IDIs with ANC attendants, Free-listing and Pairwise comparison exercises were conducted as part of the Focused Ethnographic Study component. Through the Free-listing exercise (Form S2), a list of perceived and experienced health problems and complaints during pregnancy was generated, through an open-ended question, at the start of each IDI. The interviewer then probed about perceived causes and consequences of each of the identified health problems both for the mother and the foetus. The exercise ended by the interviewer revisiting each of the mentioned complaints and discussing the perceived severity and the perceived risk of contracting the illness.

Pairwise comparison consisted in the use of pictorial vignettes representing malaria preventive interventions and other interventions delivered through ANC. First, the vignettes were presented to the participants all at once, and an agreement was reached between the participant and the interviewer as to which intervention each vignette represented. The participant was asked to organize the vignettes from the most preferred to the least preferred intervention. The interviewer used a data extraction form to register the preferences (Form S3). Secondly, the vignettes were presented to the participant in pairs, i.e., each vignette was matched one-on-one with another vignette at a time, encouraging the participant to think about the relative advantages and disadvantages of each of the presented interventions. For each pair, the participant was asked to elect the favourite one, and a discussion followed regarding the reasons for the choice.

Lastly, observations were carried out at the ANC clinics, both in the waiting and consultation rooms. The latter generated information about the participants' interaction with health care providers, as well as on their reactions to the procedures offered to them. It also provided insights about the possible contextual factors impeding or facilitating the implementation and acceptability of the interventions.

Recruitment

This study took place from September 2010 to November 2011. Two groups of participants were recruited. One group comprised pregnant women attending the first ANC visit and willing to participate in the qualitative study. Every day, the ANC nurse recruited the first two patients who fulfilled the inclusion criteria. The social scientist then asked for consent and arranged for the appropriate time and place for an initial interview.

To capture the views and opinions of those who had not had access to ANC services, a second group of participants was recruited, consisting of randomly selected pregnant women identified through the DSS. Every day, two women were recruited by the DSS fieldworker who annotated the directions of the household and possible dates for an initial interview.

A minimum sample size of 20 per group was foreseen in order to fulfil the study objectives. A final sample size of 85 women was obtained based on the saturation point, which is reached when the inclusion of new participants is suspended due to redundancy in the data being generated [20].

The number of observations was also determined by saturation, giving a total of 30 observations conducted at the ANC clinic over a period of six months.

Ethics statement

Ethical approval for this study was granted by the National Health Bioethics Committee in Mozambique (IRB nr. 00002657).

Written informed consent was sought from all participants. Among the participants of this study we included a subgroup of 11 pregnant women between the ages of 15 and 18, reflecting the range of ages of pregnant women at risk of malaria in the study area. Regarding participation of these women in the study, a waiver for parental consent was given by the IRB because they are considered to be *mature minors* who make autonomous decisions regarding their pregnancy and foetus. In fact, the majority of them were either married or not living with their parents. Moreover, culturally, the likelihood of an undisclosed pregnancy in the first trimester is high, therefore parental permission, which implied disclosure of pregnancy status, would pose more social harm to the participants than the participation in the study without parental permission. Participation of this group of women was crucial because they are the group most at risk of malaria-related pregnancy adverse consequences. Exclusion of this group from studies like this may deny benefits to this group on the long run.

Data management and analysis

All data analysis was performed using MS Excel [21] and Paired Comparison Worksheet [22].

For the data generated through the Free-listing exercise, all the illnesses that were identified by the participants were sorted in decreasing order of frequency of being mentioned. Further, for each illness, the perceived symptoms, preventive measures, and known treatment options were tabulated according to the frequency of being mentioned [17,18,23].

Analysis of Pairwise comparisons was performed in two steps. First, for the component of the Pairwise comparison whereby each participant was asked to rank their preference among the seven interventions presented to them all at once, the interventions were tabulated according to the frequency in which these interventions were elected as 1st, 2nd, ...nth choice ($n = 7$). Secondly, for the component of the Pairwise comparison whereby participants were asked to choose their preference between interventions that were presented in pairs, each intervention obtained one to three points according to the difference in the frequency mentioned compared to the alternative, and zero points for a tie. Interventions were then ranked according to the total number of points obtained after the scores of all possible comparison pairs were added [24].

The in-depth interviews and the discussions held during the FES exercises were digitally recorded and transcribed *verbatim* and field notes were taken during observations. Transcriptions and field notes were read and data were extracted and tabulated according to three key themes: (i) perceptions and knowledge of malaria in pregnancy; (ii) knowledge and acceptability of ANC services; (iii) acceptability and use of malaria preventive interventions in general and IPTp in particular.

Results

Characteristics of respondents

A total of 85 pregnant women participated in the study, of which 21 were recruited at the community and 64 at the ANC. Women recruited at the community participated in only one interview because as they were not ANC service users, there were no anticipated further issues to discuss with them after the first interview. Of the 64 women recruited at the ANC, all participated in the first interview (immediately after the 1st IPTp dose), 36 participated in the second (four to six weeks after the 1st dose, assuming that the 2nd dose would have been given four weeks after the 1st dose and adding a window period of two weeks to allow for tracking of participants at home), and 54 in the third (up to 24 weeks after the end of the pregnancy). The reasons for lower participation in the second and third interviews are presented in Table 1. The majority of losses to follow-up in the second round of interviews were because their first dose was administered very close to the due date, which implied that they had delivered when they were visited at home for the second round of interviews and therefore had to skip to the final interview, ending up with only two interviews.

The participants were between 15 and 40 years of age. Most women had primary education level (65%), 21% had secondary education level, and the majority were housewives (69%). Sixty percent of the respondents were in a marital union. Detailed socio-demographic characteristics are presented in Table 2.

Table 1. Reasons for non-participation in rounds 2 and 3 of interviews (n = 64).

Interview round	Number not interviewed	Reasons for not being interviewed	
2	28	Unavailable	1
		Had given birth	27
3	10	Unavailable	3
		Refused	3
		Internal migration	4

Perceptions of malaria in pregnancy

When responding to the open-ended question about perceived illnesses in pregnancy, malaria (locally referred as *Dzedzedze*) was the most frequently mentioned health problem in pregnancy, followed by abdominal, back and body pains. Headache, fever, chills, and joint pains were mentioned as the main symptoms of malaria in pregnancy (Table 3). The majority of pregnant women (74%), perceived the mosquito bite as the main mode of malaria transmission. Other ways of transmission were mentioned, such as unhygienic backyards and heat.

Table 2. Socio-demographic characteristics of respondents.

Characteristic	Frequency (%)
Age	
15–24	52 (61)
25–34	26 (31)
35–44	7 (8)
Education level	
No formal education	11 (13)
Primary	56 (66)
Secondary	18 (21)
Marital Status	
Married/Union	51 (60)
Casual relationship	9 (11)
Separated/Divorced	25 (29)
Occupation	
Housewife	59 (70)
Student	12 (14)
Vendor	5 (6)
Subsistence Farmer	4 (5)
Formally employed	5 (5)
Parity	
0 Children	31 (36)
1–2 Children	33 (38)
≥3 Children	22 (26)
Gestational age at recruitment	
≤3 months	7 (8)
4 to 6 months	58 (68)
7 to 9 months	20 (24)
Total	85 (100)

More than half (65%) of the participants reported that pregnant women and children were the groups most at risk for the infection.

> *"Pregnant women are those who catch malaria more easily. Even among those who are not pregnant, there are those who catch malaria more easily. But it happens more often to us, pregnant women, because we can catch any type of disease easily, because of our state [being pregnant]".* 24 year old pregnant women, IDI2

In the view of the participants, the increased risk of malaria in pregnant women resulted from sharing their protection with the unborn child, and therefore, being more fragile and susceptible to malaria.

In contrast to their knowledge about pregnant women's vulnerability to malaria, 58% of participants did not consider themselves at risk or ignored the risk of malaria because they felt protected by ITNs and IPTp.

> *"No, [I don't feel at risk of getting malaria] because every day I sleep under a net, and I take the tablets in the hospital, the ones they said are to treat malaria".* - 24 years old pregnant women, IDI1

Fifty-four women believed that malaria in pregnancy had adverse consequences. When asked through an open-ended question about the specific deleterious effects of malaria, the majority only referred to the consequences for the pregnant woman (maternal death, and hallucinations), very few mentioned consequences for the foetus or the baby (miscarriage, stillbirth, congenital malaria, prematurity) having only one respondent indicated low birth weight.

Preferences of malaria preventive interventions in the context of ANC routine activities

Regarding pregnant women's preferences of the different interventions against all others, Table 4 presents the frequency distribution of interventions among those elected as first, second, and subsequently up to seventh choice. Of note, 62.5% of the first choices were ITNs, followed by IPTp which amounted to 12.5% of the first choices. Nine percent of the first choices were iron supplements and HIV PMTCT. The interventions which were least elected as the first choice were tetanus toxoid vaccine (TT vaccine), antihelmintics, and IRS. The top second choices were IPTp and iron supplements and the bottom three choices were antihelmintics, IRS and HIV PMTCT.

Table 5 shows, for each intervention, the proportion of times elected as favourite, second choice and subsequently until the last choice. In terms of malaria interventions, ITNs were by far mostly mentioned as first choice (69%). IPTp was mostly mentioned as second choice (28%), but also and less frequently, elected as first

Table 3. Perceived symptoms of illnesses during pregnancy.

Illness	Symptoms*
Malaria	**Headache, fever, chills, joint pains**, abdominal pain, lack of appetite, nausea, palpitations, asthenia, dizziness, flu symptoms, hot flushes
Abdominal pain	**Pain**
Swollen feet	#
Joint pain	#
Vomiting	#
Womb pain	#
Vaginal discharge	#
Back and body pains	Pain
Cough	Pain
Weakness	#

*Perceived principal symptoms in bold type.
#No description of symptoms because according to the respondents the illness name was self explanatory of the symptoms.

and third choice (15% and 14% respectively). IRS was mostly mentioned between the third and the last three choices and hardly elected as the first choice (1.2%). In terms of other interventions, iron supplements were mostly elected between the second, third and fourth choices, and tetanus vaccine was more skewed towards the third, fourth and fifth choices. Both antihelmintics and HIV PMTCT were mostly elected among the last three choices.

Table 6 shows the comparison of each intervention against one alternative at a time. This comparison revealed that ITNs (with a total score of 14 points) were relatively more important than all other interventions except for HIV PMTCT. IPTp (with 5 points) was only more important than IRS and antihelmintics, which had been revealed to be the two least favourite interventions in the first step of the Pairwise comparison exercise (Tables 4 and 5). IRS (0 points) was consistently less preferred than all other interventions. Among the other interventions delivered through ANC, HIV PMTCT (8 points) and tetanus toxoid vaccine (7 points) were the relatively most important ones compared to each of the other interventions.

Perceptions of IPTp

According to the IDIs, women perceived that the different drugs given at the ANC were to prevent diseases in general, but most (70%) could not distinguish them apart (neither by name nor by description) nor could mention the single health problem targeted by such drug. They used the term *comprimidos* (Portuguese term for "tablet") to refer to those drugs and were aware that one of the tablets was given to prevent malaria, although very few could specify which tablet. Very few referred to it as *Fansidar* (Commercial name for SP in Mozambique). Therefore, after the initial open-ended question about the purpose of the different tablets given at ANC was answered, and in order to further explore the topic of IPTp, the interviewer referred to it as "the white tablets given to pregnant women at the ANC to prevent malaria and normally taken in front of the nurse".

All participants attending ANC reported to have accepted to take the tablets given by the nurse. In terms of perceived side effects of such tablets, some reported dizziness, vomiting, malaise and nausea. The majority (59%) of the women who reported side effects attributed them to taking the tablets too early in the morning and on an empty stomach.

> *"I felt normal after taking those tablets, but, because I left my house without taking matabicho (breakfast), I felt very weak".* – 18 years old pregnant women, IDI1

Table 4. Distribution of malaria preventive interventions and other interventions delivered through ANC among each choice.

	Percentage distribution of interventions among each choice						
Prevention interventions	**1st choice**	**2nd choice**	**3rd choice**	**4th choice**	**5th choice**	**6th choice**	**7th choice**
ITN	62.5	10.5	7.6	7.6	3.8	1.3	0.0
IPTp	12.5	25.6	15.2	10.1	10.3	11.4	10.7
IRS	1.1	11.6	17.7	13.9	16.7	19.0	22.7
Iron supplements	9.1	23.3	21.5	25.3	9.0	13.9	4.0
Tetanus vaccine	3.4	15.1	25.3	24.1	23.1	6.3	5.3
HIV PMTCT	9.1	9.3	7.6	10.1	19.2	20.3	21.3
Antihelmintic	2.3	4.7	5.1	8.9	17.9	27.8	36.0
Total	100	100	100	100	100	100	100

Table 5. Distribution of the choices made for each malaria preventive interventions and other interventions delivered through ANC.

	Percentage distribution of the choices among each intervention							
Prevention interventions	**1st choice**	**2nd choice**	**3rd choice**	**4th choice**	**5th choice**	**6th choice**	**7th choice**	**Total**
ITN	68.8	11.3	7.5	7.5	3.8	1.3	0.0	100
IPTp	14.1	28.2	15.4	10.3	10.3	11.5	10.3	100
IRS	1.2	12.3	17.3	13.6	16.0	18.5	21.0	100
Iron supplements	9.3	23.3	19.8	23.3	8.1	12.8	3.5	100
Tetanus vaccine	3.7	15.9	24.4	23.2	22.0	6.1	4.9	100
HIV PMTCT	10.4	10.4	7.8	10.4	19.5	20.8	20.8	100
Antihelmintic	2.5	5.0	5.0	8.8	17.5	27.5	33.8	100

For the majority of women (76%), the fact that the tablets were provided at the health facility made IPTp trustworthy. Other sources of tablets (such as informal vendors) were seen as dangerous for pregnant women.

Reported use of malaria preventive strategies at home

When discussing home-based malaria preventive strategies, again the majority of the women (75%) reported sleeping under an ITN (Table 7), and those who did not use it claimed that it was due to difficulties in hanging the net. According to the women, ITNs were preferred because they provide protection against mosquitoes to more than one person at once, and that, unlike insecticides this protection is long-lasting.

All participants were aware that because they were pregnant they had priority in receiving and using ITNs. Small children and their mothers were also perceived as priority groups.

> *"If the decision depended on me, I would have priority in the use of mosquito net because I'm pregnant and I need to protect myself".* 20 years old pregnant woman, IDI2

When probed about other methods they frequently used to protect against mosquitoes and malaria at home, including traditional ones, insecticide sprays, coils, and traditional smoke repellents were mentioned although much less frequently than ITNs. IRS was the least frequently mentioned malaria-preventive strategy adopted at home. Participants did not believe in the effectiveness of IRS, alleging that the chemical used "increased the burden of insects in the house, apart from not killing mosquitoes and others bugs".

Discussion

There is very limited information on what perceptions pregnant women exposed to malaria have about the infection, and what their acceptability to the recommended malaria preventive interventions is. With very few exceptions [25], specific studies on the acceptability of malaria preventive interventions tend to look at them in the context of clinical trials or examine such interventions in isolation from other interventions delivered through the same mechanism [26], for example ANC. This study adds to the body of evidence regarding prevention of malaria in pregnancy as an integral component of maternal and newborn health services.

The results of this study indicate that although the majority of pregnant women from this rural area in Mozambique recognize malaria infection as a health problem in pregnancy, in general they do not perceive it as dangerous for the pregnancy and the foetus. In this setting, where the high ANC attendance rate and the favourable delivery mechanisms for ITNs and IPTp offer potential to achieve the required coverage and use, there is a risk of the unwanted consequence of leaving pregnant women feeling not-at-risk. This finding calls for increased awareness raising about pregnant women's risk of malaria infection and its consequences in endemic areas where malaria continues to be an important health problem for pregnant women and children [27,28,29].

The observed limited awareness in this study regarding the adverse consequences of malaria in pregnancy, especially in

Table 6. Pairwise comparison matrix with scores of each intervention matched against all others.

	A: ITNs	**B: IPTp**	**C: IRS**	**D: Iron**	**E: TT vaccine**	**F: HIV PMTCT**	**G: Anti-Helmintic**
A: ITNs		A (2)	A (3)	A (3)	A (3)	A (0)/F (0)	A (3)
B: IPTp			B (3)	D (2)	E (1)	B (0)/F (0)	B (2)
C: IRS				D (2)	E (3)	F (3)	G (2)
D: Iron					D (0)/E (0)	F (1)	D (1)
E: TT vaccine						F (1)	E (3)
F: HIV PMTCT							F (3)
G: Anti-helmintic							
Total score per intervention	**A: 14**	**B: 5**	**C: 0**	**D: 5**	**E: 7**	**F: 8**	**G: 2**

Table 7. Reported use of malaria preventive measures among the interviewed women (n = 85)*.

Preventive tools at the household	Frequency mentioned (%)**
ITN	65 (77)
Insecticides (sprays or coils)	7 (8)
Burning of biomaterials *(Sule)*	6 (7)
Domestic hygiene (sweeping the backyard, cutting the grass, pruning the trees)	2 (2)
Insect repellent	2 (2)
IRS	1 (1)
None	2 (2)

*Responses from 1st round of interviews.
**Participants were allowed to mention more than one strategy.

relation to the foetus and the newborn, might contribute to low acceptability which in turn can negatively influence adherence, regarding malaria preventive interventions. For example, the low preference for IRS among pregnant women was evident in this study. A possible reason could be that the inconveniences and perceived ineffectiveness of the intervention could be superseding the perceived advantages of preventing malaria during pregnancy. This is in agreement with previously reported results from the same setting [30,31]. This should be taken into account when defining malaria prevention recommendations for pregnant women in particular and the population as a whole.

ITNs were the highest ranked malaria preventive intervention by the pregnant women in this study. This finding offers an opportunity to improve the current coverage of ITNs in the households, which is still inadequately low in Mozambique (28%) [4,32], by reinforcing ITN distribution through ANC services. This must be coupled with the provision, during the ANC health education sessions, of clear instructions and demonstrations on how to hang the ITN.

IPTp did not strongly feature as first choice by the women, and dominated the second and third choices compared to the other interventions. One-on-one Pairwise comparisons showed that among malaria preventive interventions, IPTp is preferable compared to IRS but neither prevails over ITNs, nor over most of the other ANC interventions. Provided that both IPTp and ITNs were rolled out to serve the same purpose of preventing malaria in pregnancy, the factors underlying preference of ITNs over IPTp should be critically examined. Again, convenience factors offered by ITNs, i.e., providing a physical barrier against the high burden mosquito bites [33,34], may be playing a more important role in influencing acceptability and use, compared to the recognition of the threat of malaria in pregnancy.

Even though IPTp was not amongst the most preferred ANC intervention, there seemed to be adherence to it, as reported by study participants. In accordance, data from the DSS indicates that nearly 80% of women who delivered at the health facilities within the Manhiça Demographic Surveillance Area (DSA) had taken at least one dose of IPTp (unpublished data, Manhiça DSS 2010). In contrast to previous studies in Africa, which identified perceived adverse reactions to the drugs as a negative factor for adherence [8], there were no indications from this study that perceived adverse reactions could be negatively influencing adherence, since the participants who mentioned adverse reactions reported to still take the tablets. The administration of IPTp through the directly observed therapy may have favoured the reported adherence to this intervention. However, this is only applicable in settings like Manhiça District, where ANC attendance is high.

It has been shown that the nature of the provider does influence adherence to a given health intervention [8,26,35,36]. In this setting, the hospital was viewed by the respondents as a "well-intentioned" entity, and their trust and obedience towards the health system, expressed by the term "the rule of hospital", is consistent with findings from previous studies in the same setting [30,37]. Interestingly, despite the presence of informal drug vendors and other sources of anti-malarial drugs in the study area, the study participants only trusted the formal health system for prescribing drugs to pregnant women. This positive behaviour should be reinforced and the existing awareness of the dangers posed by informally prescribed drugs should be transferred to other population groups.

A limitation of the study however, was the fact that part of the recruitment of participants as well as the first interviews with ANC attendants, took place at the health facility. This could have limited the level of comfort to openly discuss interventions provided by the health system. Involvement of pregnant women who had not attended ANC and conducting follow-up interviews at home contributed to the minimization of this social desirability bias [38]. However, community-based studies in similar settings are needed in order to provide supporting evidence regarding patients' judgement of the interventions.

A second limitation of the study rises from the assumption that preferences and ranking of interventions serve as proxies for acceptability. We acknowledge that these indicators cannot capture all dimensions of acceptability, but can be used as predictors of adherence to an intervention, taking into account its perceived relative importance over other interventions delivered through the same scheme. Future studies are recommended to explore further dimensions of acceptability of preventive interventions for malaria in pregnancy.

Conclusion

In this malaria endemic area, low awareness among pregnant women of the risks and adverse consequences of malaria for pregnant women and neonates did not seem to affect acceptability or adherence to all of the recommended malaria preventive interventions in the same manner. Acceptability seemed to be intervention-specific and dependent on perceived convenience and other immediate benefits. The approach used for delivery, and the nature of the provider also played an influential role on adherence to the intervention. In the efforts to maximize overall coverage, pregnant women, through ANC services, can be the vehicles for ITN distribution in the community.

Malaria preventive interventions requiring community-based delivery mechanisms, such as IRS or drugs requiring self-administration, are expected to have a reduced adherence, unless the risks averted by the interventions are clearly understood by the target population. Therefore, improving the knowledge about the effects of malaria on maternal and neonatal health may help increase the acceptability and adherence to malaria preventive interventions, especially if delivered through channels other than the health facility.

Supporting Information

Form S1 In-depth Interview guide.

Form S2 Free-listing data extraction form.

Form S3 Pairwise comparison data extraction form.

Acknowledgments

The authors would like to thank the pregnant women participating in the study. They are also grateful to Rosa Pires, Francisco Gomes, Guilhermina Dinis, and the health staff of Manhiça District Hospital, in particular the ANC clinic.

Author Contributions

Conceived and designed the experiments: KM HB CM ES RG EM. Performed the experiments: HB. Analyzed the data: HB KM CV. Contributed reagents/materials/analysis tools: CS KM RG AV MR SM CV. Wrote the paper: HB KM CM CV EM. Interpreted the results: KM CM RG HB ES CV.

References

1. Dellicour S, Tatem AJ, Guerra CA, Snow RW, Kuile FOt (2010) Quantifying the number of pregnancies at risk of malaria in 2007: a demographic study. Plos Med 7: e1000221. doi 1000210.1001371/Journal.Pmed.1000221.
2. WHO, UNICEF (2005) Protecting vulnerable groups in malaria-endemic areas in Africa through accelareted deployment of insecticide-treated nets WHO/HTM/RBM 57.
3. Sicuri E, Bardaji A, Nhampossa T, Maixenchs M, Nhacolo A, et al. (2010) Cost-effectiveness of intermittent preventive treatment of malaria in pregnancy in southern Mozambique. PLoS One 5.
4. van Eijk AM, Hill J, Alegana VA, Kirui V, Gething PW, et al. (2011) Coverage of malaria protection in pregnant women in sub-Saharan Africa: a synthesis and analysis of national survey data. Lancet Infect Dis 11: 190–207.
5. Mbonye AK, Neema S, Magnussen P (2006) Perceptions on use of Sulfadoxine-pyrimethamine in pregnancy and the policy implication form malaria control in Uganda. Health Policy 77: 279–289.
6. Ribera JM, Muela SH, D'Alessandro U, Grietens KP (2007) Malaria in Pregnancy: What can the Social Sciences contribute? PLos Medicine. 2007 ed. pp. 0631–0635.
7. Heggenhougen HK (2003) The behavioural and social aspects of malaria and its control. UNDP/World Bank/WHO. Special Programme for Research and Training in Tropical Diseases (TDR) 03: 1–228.
8. Pell C, Straus L, Andrew EV, Menaca A, Pool R (2011) Social and cultural factors affecting uptake of interventions for malaria in pregnancy in Africa: a systematic review of the qualitative research. PLoS One 6: e22452.
9. Brentlinger PE, Montoya P, Rojas AJ, Correia MA, Dgedge M, et al. (2007) Prevalence and predictors of maternal peripheral malaria parasitemia in central Mozambique. Am J Trop Med Hyg 77: 228–234.
10. MISAU (2006) Normas de manejo de casos de malária em Moçambique. Programa Nacional de Controlo da Malária.
11. MISAU (2012) Plano Estratégico da Malária 2012–2016. Direção Nacional de Saúde Pública. Programa Nacional de Controlo da Malária. Maputo: Ministério da Saúde.
12. INE (2007) III Recenseamento Geral da População e Habitação. Maputo: Instituto Nacional de Estatística.
13. Saute F, Aponte J, Almeda J, Ascaso C, Abellana R, et al. (2003) Malaria in southern Mozambique: malariometric indicators and malaria case definition in Manhica district. Trans R Soc Trop Med Hyg 97: 661–666.
14. Gonzalez R, Munguambe K, Aponte J, Bavo C, Nhalungo D, et al. (2012) High HIV prevalence in a southern semi-rural area of Mozambique: a community-based survey. HIV Med.
15. INE (2012) Estatisticas do Distrito da Manhica. Maputo.
16. Direcção Nacional de Saúde (2006) Política Nacional de Saúde Neonatal e Infantil em Moçambique. In: Departamento de Saúde da Comunidade, editor. Maputo: MISAU.
17. Pelto GH, Gove S (1992) Developing a focused ethonographic study for the WHO acute respiratory infection (ARI) control programme. In RAP: Rapid Assesment Procedures Qualitative Methodologies for planning and evaluation of health related programmes Edited by: Scrimshaw N, Gleason G Boston, Massachusetts: International Nutrition Foundation for Developing Countries: 215–255.
18. Gove S, Pelto GH (1994) Focused ethonographic studies in the WHO programmes for the control of acute respiratory infection. Medical anthropology 15: 409–424.
19. Green J, Thorogood N (2004) Qualitative methods for health research London. Sage.
20. Fontanella BJB, Ricas j, Turato ER (2008) Amostragem por saturação em pesquisas qualitativas em saúde: contribuições teóricas. Cadernos de Saúde Pública 24.
21. Microsoft Corporation (2007) Microsoft Excel 2007.
22. MindTools (1996–2013) Paired Comparison Analysis: Working Out Relative Importances.
23. Borgatti S (1998) Elicitation Techniques for Cultural Domain Analysis. In: Schensul J, editor. Ethnographer's Toolkit. Newbury Park: SAGE.
24. MindTools Ltd (206–2012) Paired Comparison Worksheet London.
25. Brentlinger PE, Dgedge M, Correia MA, Rojas AJ, Saute F, et al. (2007) Intermittent preventive treatment of malaria during pregnancy in central Mozambique. Bull World Health Organ 85: 873–879.
26. Smith LA, Jones C, Adjei RO, Antwi GD, Afrah NA, et al. (2010) Intermittent screening and treatment versus intermittent preventive treatment of malaria in pregnancy: user acceptability. Malar J 9.
27. Bardaji A, Sigauque B, Bruni L, Romagosa C, Sanz S, et al. (2008) Clinical malaria in African pregnant women. Malar J 7: 27.
28. Saute F, Menendez C, Mayor A, Aponte J, Gomez-Olive X, et al. (2002) Malaria in pregnancy in rural Mozambique: the role of parity, submicroscopic and multiple Plasmodium falciparum infections. Trop Med Int Health 7: 19–28.
29. Menendez C, Bardaji A, Sigauque B, Sanz S, Aponte JJ, et al. (2010) Malaria prevention with IPTp during pregnancy reduces neonatal mortality. PLoS One 5: e9438.
30. Montgomery CM, Munguambe K, Pool R (2010) Group-based citizenship in the acceptance of indor Residual Spraying (IRS). Social Science Medicine 70: 1648–1655.
31. Munguambe K, Pool R, Montgomery C, Bavo C, Nhacolo A, et al. (2011) What drives community adherence to indoor residual spraying (IRS) against malaria in Manhica district, rural Mozambique: a qualitative study. Malaria Journal 10.
32. INE (2012) Moçambique - Inquérito Demográfico e de Saúde 2011 - Relatório Preliminar. Maputo: Instituto Nacional de Estatística, Ministério da Saúde.
33. Munguambe K (2006) Patterns and factors associated with household environmental health practices in Manhiça, Mozambique. London: University of London.
34. Enato E, Okhamafe A, Okpere E (2007) A survey of knowledge, attitudes and practice of malaria management among pregnant women from two health facilities in Nigeria. Acta Obstet Gynocol Scand 86: 33–36.
35. Mbonye AK, Byqbjerg I, Magnussen P (2007) Intermittent preventive treatment of malaria in pregnancy: evaluation of a new delivery approach and the policy implicatios for malaria control in Uganda Health Policy 81: 228–241.
36. Brabin L, Stokes E, Dumbaya I, Owens S (2009) Gambian womens reliance on health workers to deliver sulphadoxine-pyrimethamine as recommended intermittent preventive treatment for malaria in pregnancy. Malar J 8.
37. Strauss L, Munguambe K, Bassat Q, Machevo S, Pell C, et al. (2011) Inherent ilnesses and attacks: an ethographic study of interpretations of childhood Acute Respiratory Infections (ARI's) in Manhica, southern Mozambique. BMC Public Health 11.
38. Lewis-Beck MS, Bryman l, Liao TF (2004) The SAGE Encyclopedia of Social Science Research Methods: SAGE.

Permissions

All chapters in this book were first published in PLOS ONE, by The Public Library of Science; hereby published with permission under the Creative Commons Attribution License or equivalent. Every chapter published in this book has been scrutinized by our experts. Their significance has been extensively debated. The topics covered herein carry significant findings which will fuel the growth of the discipline. They may even be implemented as practical applications or may be referred to as a beginning point for another development.

The contributors of this book come from diverse backgrounds, making this book a truly international effort. This book will bring forth new frontiers with its revolutionizing research information and detailed analysis of the nascent developments around the world.

We would like to thank all the contributing authors for lending their expertise to make the book truly unique. They have played a crucial role in the development of this book. Without their invaluable contributions this book wouldn't have been possible. They have made vital efforts to compile up to date information on the varied aspects of this subject to make this book a valuable addition to the collection of many professionals and students.

This book was conceptualized with the vision of imparting up-to-date information and advanced data in this field. To ensure the same, a matchless editorial board was set up. Every individual on the board went through rigorous rounds of assessment to prove their worth. After which they invested a large part of their time researching and compiling the most relevant data for our readers.

The editorial board has been involved in producing this book since its inception. They have spent rigorous hours researching and exploring the diverse topics which have resulted in the successful publishing of this book. They have passed on their knowledge of decades through this book. To expedite this challenging task, the publisher supported the team at every step. A small team of assistant editors was also appointed to further simplify the editing procedure and attain best results for the readers.

Apart from the editorial board, the designing team has also invested a significant amount of their time in understanding the subject and creating the most relevant covers. They scrutinized every image to scout for the most suitable representation of the subject and create an appropriate cover for the book.

The publishing team has been an ardent support to the editorial, designing and production team. Their endless efforts to recruit the best for this project, has resulted in the accomplishment of this book. They are a veteran in the field of academics and their pool of knowledge is as vast as their experience in printing. Their expertise and guidance has proved useful at every step. Their uncompromising quality standards have made this book an exceptional effort. Their encouragement from time to time has been an inspiration for everyone.

The publisher and the editorial board hope that this book will prove to be a valuable piece of knowledge for researchers, students, practitioners and scholars across the globe.

List of Contributors

Joerg Latus, Daniel Kitterer and M. Dominik Alscher
Department of Internal Medicine, Division of Nephrology, Robert-Bosch Hospital, Auerbachstrasse 110, Stuttgart, Germany

Klara Tenner-Racz, Paul Racz and Daniel Cadar
Bernhard Nocht Institute for Tropical Medicine, WHO Collaborating Centre for Arbovirus and Haemmorrhagic Fever Reference and Research, Bernhard-Nocht-Strasse 74, Hamburg, Germany

German Ott
Department of Diagnostic Medicine, Division of Pathology, Robert-Bosch Hospital, Auerbachstrasse 110, Stuttgart, Germany

Jonas Schmidt-Chanasit
Bernhard Nocht Institute for Tropical Medicine, WHO Collaborating Centre for Arbovirus and Haemmorrhagic Fever Reference and Research, Bernhard-Nocht-Strasse 74, Hamburg, Germany
German Centre for Infection Research (DZIF), partner site Hamburg-Luebeck-Borstel, Hamburg, Germany

Yan-Yan Dong
Department of Gastroenterology, Qilu Hospital, Shandong University, Jinan, Shandong, People's Republic of China
The Key Laboratory of Cardiovascular Remodeling and Function Research, Chinese Ministry of Education and Chinese Ministry of Health, Qilu Hospital, Shandong University, Jinan, Shandong, People's Republic of China

Fei-Xue Chen, Yan-Bo Yu, Chao Du, Qing-Qing Qi, Han Liu and Yan-Qing Li
Department of Gastroenterology, Qilu Hospital, Shandong University, Jinan, Shandong, People's Republic of China

Winfried Häuser and Eva Jung
Department Internal Medicine I, Klinikum Saarbrücken, Saarbrücken, Germany
Department of Psychosomatic Medicine and Psychotherapy, Technische Universität München, München, Germany

Brigitte Erbslöh-Möller
Rheumatology Medical Practice, Neunkirchen, Germany

Mechthild Gesmann
Psychosomatic Medicine and Pain Therapy Medical Practice, Herford, Germany

Hedi Kühn-Becker
Psychosomatic Medicine and Pain Therapy Medical Practice, Zweibrücken, Germany

Franz Petermann
Centre of Clinical Psychology and Rehabilitation, Universität Bremen, Bremen, Germany

Jost Langhorst
Department Internal Medicine V (Intergrative Medicine), Kliniken Essen-Mitte, Essen, Germany

Thomas Weiss
Outpatient Clinic Mannheim, Mannheim, Germany

Andreas Winkelmann
Department of Physical Medicine and Rehabilitation, Klinikum der Universität München, München, Germany

Frederick Wolfe
National Data Bank for Rheumatic Diseases, Wichita, Kansas, United States of America
University of Kansas School of Medicine, Wichita, Kansas, United States of America

Stefan A. W. Bouwense
Pain and Nociception Neuroscience Research Group, Department of Surgery, Radboud University Nijmegen Medical Center, Nijmegen, The Netherlands

Søren S. Olesen
Mech-Sense, Department of Gastroenterology and Hepatology, Aalborg Hospital, Aarhus University Hospital, Aalborg, Denmark

Asbjørn M. Drewes
Mech-Sense, Department of Gastroenterology and Hepatology, Aalborg Hospital, Aarhus University Hospital, Aalborg, Denmark

Center for Sensory-Motor Interaction (SMI), Department of Health Science and Technology, Aalborg University, Aalborg, Denmark

Jan-Werner Poley
Department of Gastroenterology and Hepatology, Erasmus MC, University Medical Center, Rotterdam, The Netherlands

Oliver H. G. Wilder-Smith
Pain and Nociception Neuroscience Research Group, Department of Anaesthesiology, Pain and Palliative Care, Radboud University Nijmegen Medical Center, Nijmegen, The Netherlands

Gilaad G. Kaplan
Division of Gastroenterology, University of Calgary, Calgary, Alberta, Canada
Departments of Medicine, University of Calgary, Calgary, Alberta, Canada
Community Health Sciences, University of Calgary, Calgary, Alberta, Canada

Mieczyslaw Szyszkowicz, Eugeniusz Porada and Renaud Vincent
Environmental Health Sciences and Research Bureau, Health Canada, Ottawa, Ontario, Canada

Jakub Fichna
Department of Biomolecular Chemistry, Medical University of Lodz, Lodz, Poland

Brian H. Rowe
Department of Emergency Medicine and School of Public Health, University of Alberta, Edmonton, Alberta, Canada

Karen Madsen
Department of Medicine, Division of Gastroenterology, University of Alberta, Edmonton, Alberta, Canada

Subrata Ghosh
Division of Gastroenterology, University of Calgary, Calgary, Alberta, Canada
Departments of Medicine, University of Calgary, Calgary, Alberta, Canada

Martin Storr
Division of Gastroenterology, University of Calgary, Calgary, Alberta, Canada
Departments of Medicine, University of Calgary, Calgary, Alberta, Canada
Department of Medicine, Ludwigs-Maximilians University, Munich, Germany

Junya Yokobe, Masaki Kitahara and Shoichi Uezono
Department of Anesthesiology, The Jikei University School of Medicine, Minato, Tokyo, Japan

Masato Matsushima
Division of Clinical Epidemiology, The Jikei University School of Medicine, Minato, Tokyo, Japan

Rocchina Colucci, Narcisa Ghisu, Marco Tuccori, Matteo Fornai, Luca Antonioli and Corrado Blandizzi
Division of Pharmacology and Chemotherapy, Department of Clinical and Experimental Medicine, University of Pisa, Pisa, Italy

Dario Gambaccini, Francesco Costa, Nicola De Bortoli, Angelo Ricchiuti, Maria Gloria Mumolo, Santino Marchi and Massimo Bellini
Unit of Gastroenterology, Department of Translational Medicine, University of Pisa, Pisa, Italy

Giuseppe Rossi
Unit of Epidemiology and Biostatistics, Institute of Clinical Physiology, National Research Council, Pisa, Italy

James Sejvar and Stephan Monroe
Division of High-Consequence Pathogens and Pathology, National Center for Emerging and Zoonotic Infectious Diseases (NCEZID), Centers for Disease Control and Prevention (CDC), Atlanta, Georgia, United States of America

Emily Lutterloh
Scientific Education and Professional Development Program Office, Epidemic Intelligence Service, CDC, Atlanta, Georgia, United States of America
Current Position, New York State Department of Health, Albany, New York, United States of America

Jeremias Naiene
Ministry of Health, Maputo, Mozambique

Andrew Likaka, Robert Manda and Tadala Khaila
Ministry of Health, Lilongwe, Malawi

Benjamin Nygren, Michael Humphrys, Deborah Talkington and Eric Mintz
Division of Foodborne, Waterborne, and Environmental Infectious Diseases, NCEZID, CDC, Atlanta, Georgia, United States of America

Sara A. Lowther, Linda Capewell, Kashmira Date, David Townes and Yanique Redwood
Scientific Education and Professional Development Program Office, Epidemic Intelligence Service, CDC, Atlanta, Georgia, United States of America

Joshua Schier and Ben Blount
Division of Environmental Hazards and Health Effects, National Center for Environmental Health (NCEH), CDC, Atlanta, Georgia, United States of America

Beth Tippett Barr and Austin Demby
Global AIDS Program, CDC, Lilongwe, Malawi

Macpherson Mallewa and Sam Kampondeni
Malawi-Liverpool-Wellcome Trust, College of Medicine, Blantyre, Malawi

Gregory L. Armstrong
Division of Viral Diseases, National Center for Immunization and Respiratory Diseases, CDC, Atlanta, Georgia, United States of America

Yafang Hu, Haishan Jiang, Qun Wang, Zuoshan Xie and Suyue Pan
Department of Neurology, Nanfang Hospital, Southern Medical University, Guangzhou, People's Republic of China

Vincent A. Mukkada
Department of Pediatrics, Hasbro Children's Hospital, Providence, Rhode Island, United States of America

Shaolei Lu, Shamlal Mangray, Kelly Cleveland, Nick Shillingford and Murray B. Resnick
Department of Pathology and Laboratory Medicine, Rhode Island Hospital, the Alpert School of Medicine, Brown University, Providence, Rhode Island, United States of America

Christoph Schorl and Alexander S. Brodsky
Department of Molecular Biology, Cell Biology and Biochemistry, Brown University, Providence, Rhode Island, United States of America

Wen-Ling Lin, Chen-June Seak and Yi-Ming Weng
Department of Emergency Medicine, Chang Gung Memorial Hospital, Taoyuan, Taiwan, and Chang Gung University College of Medicine, Taoyuan, Taiwan

Jiunn-Yih Wu and Hang-Cheng Chen
Department of Emergency Medicine, Chang Gung Memorial Hospital, Keelung, Taiwan, and Chang Gung University College of Medicine, Taoyuan, Taiwan

Liesbeth Knaepen, Maarten van Kleef, Jacob Patijn and Elbert A. Joosten
University Pain Center Maastricht, Department of Anesthesiology/Pain Management, Maastricht University Medical Center, Maastricht, The Netherlands

Ine Rayen
School for Mental Health and Neuroscience, Maastricht University, Maastricht, The Netherlands

Thierry D. Charlier and Dick Tibboel
University of Liege, GIGA-Neurosciences, Liège, Belgium

Marianne Fillet and Virginie Houbart
Laboratory of Analytical Pharmaceutical Chemistry, Department of Pharmacy, CIRM, University of Liège, Liège, Belgium

Harry W. Steinbusch
School for Mental Health and Neuroscience, Maastricht University, Maastricht, The Netherlands

Jodi L. Pawluski
School for Mental Health and Neuroscience, Maastricht University, Maastricht, The Netherlands
University of Liege, GIGA-Neurosciences, Liège, Belgium

Anthony G. Doufas
Department of Anesthesia, Stanford University School of Medicine, Stanford, California, United States of America
Outcomes Research Consortium, Cleveland, Ohio, United States of America

Orestis A. Panagiotou
Department of Hygiene and Epidemiology, University of Ioannina School of Medicine, Ioannina, Greece

John P. A. Ioannidis
Stanford Prevention Research Center, Department of Medicine, Stanford University School of Medicine, Stanford, California, United States of America,
Department of Health Research and Policy, Stanford University School of Medicine, Stanford, California, United States of America,

Department of Statistics, Stanford University School of Humanities and Sciences, Stanford, California, United States of America

Shizuka Seino, Satoshi Watanabe, Namiko Ito, Motoyori Kanazawa and Shin Fukudo
Department of Behavioral Medicine, Tohoku University Graduate School of Medicine, Sendai, Japan

Konosuke Sasaki and Kaori Shoji
Health Science, Tohoku University Graduate School of Medicine, Sendai, Japan

Shoko Miura and Kanoko Kozawa
Department of Clinical Physiology, Tohoku University Hospital, Sendai, Japan

Kunihiko Nakai and Hiroshi Sato
Department of Environmental Health Science, Tohoku University Graduate School of Medicine, Sendai, Japan

Kathryn T. Hall and Ted J. Kaptchuk
Division of General Medicine and Primary Care, Beth Israel Deaconess Medical Center and Harvard Medical School, Boston, Massachusetts, United States of America
Program in Placebo Studies, Beth Israel Deaconess Medical Center and Harvard Medical School, Boston, Massachusetts, United States of America

Anthony J. Lembo and Efi Kokkotou
Program in Placebo Studies, Beth Israel Deaconess Medical Center and Harvard Medical School, Boston, Massachusetts, United States of America
Department of Gastroenterology, Beth Israel Deaconess Medical Center and Harvard Medical School, Boston, Massachusetts, United States of America

Dimitrios C. Ziogas
Department of Internal Medicine, University of Athens, Athens, Greece

Irving Kirsch
Program in Placebo Studies, Beth Israel Deaconess Medical Center and Harvard Medical School, Boston, Massachusetts, United States of America
School of Psychology, University of Plymouth, Devon, United Kingdom

Jeffrey Douaiher
Department of Surgery, Johns Hopkins, Baltimore, Maryland, United States of America

Karin B. Jensen
Program in Placebo Studies, Beth Israel Deaconess Medical Center and Harvard Medical School, Boston, Massachusetts, United States of America
Department of Psychiatry, Massachusetts General Hospital, Harvard Medical School, Boston, Massachusetts, United States of America

Lisa A. Conboy
Program in Placebo Studies, Beth Israel Deaconess Medical Center and Harvard Medical School, Boston, Massachusetts, United States of America

John M. Kelley
Program in Placebo Studies, Beth Israel Deaconess Medical Center and Harvard Medical School, Boston, Massachusetts, United States of America
Department of Psychiatry, Massachusetts General Hospital, Harvard Medical School, Boston, Massachusetts, United States of America
Endicott College, Beverly, Massachusetts, United States of America

Alison L. Drake
Department of Global Health, University of Washington, Seattle, Washington, United States of America

Alison C. Roxby
Department of Medicine, University of Washington, Seattle, Washington, United States of America

James Kiarie
Department of Obstetrics and Gynaecology, University of Nairobi, Nairobi, Kenya

Barbra A. Richardson
Department of Global Health, University of Washington, Seattle, Washington, United States of America
Department of Biostatistics, University of Washington, Seattle, Washington, United States of America
8 Divisions of Vaccine and Infectious Diseases, Fred Hutchinson Cancer Research Center, Seattle, Washington, United States of America

Anna Wald
Department of Medicine, University of Washington, Seattle, Washington, United States of America
Department of Epidemiology, University of Washington, Seattle, Washington, United States of America

Department of Laboratory Medicine, University of Washington, Seattle, Washington, United States of America
Divisions of Vaccine and Infectious Diseases, Fred Hutchinson Cancer Research Center, Seattle, Washington, United States of America

Grace John-Stewart
Department of Global Health, University of Washington, Seattle, Washington, United States of America
Department of Medicine, University of Washington, Seattle, Washington, United States of America
Department of Epidemiology, University of Washington, Seattle, Washington, United States of America
Department of Pediatrics, University of Washington, Seattle, Washington, United States of America

Carey Farquhar
Department of Global Health, University of Washington, Seattle, Washington, United States of America
Department of Medicine, University of Washington, Seattle, Washington, United States of America
Department of Epidemiology, University of Washington, Seattle, Washington, United States of America

Jui-Yang Hong
Gail and Gerald Oppenheimer Family Center for Neurobiology of Stress, University of California Los Angeles, Los Angeles, California, United States of America
Department of Medicine, University of California Los Angeles, Los Angeles, California, United States of America
Division of Digestive Diseases, University of California Los Angeles, Los Angeles, California, United States of America
Department of Bioengineering, University of California Los Angeles, Los Angeles, California, United States of America

Zhiguo Jiang
Department of Biomedical Engineering, New Jersey Institute of Technology, Newark, New Jersey, United States of America
Human Performance and Engineering Laboratory, Kessler Foundation Research Center, West Orange, New Jersey, United States of America

Jennifer S. Labus
Gail and Gerald Oppenheimer Family Center for Neurobiology of Stress, University of California Los Angeles, Los Angeles, California, United States of America
Pain and Interoception Imaging Network (PAIN), University of California Los Angeles, Los Angeles, California, United States of America
Department of Medicine, University of California Los Angeles, Los Angeles, California, United States of America
Brain Research Institute, University of California Los Angeles, Los Angeles, California, United States of America
Division of Digestive Diseases, University of California Los Angeles, Los Angeles, California, United States of America

Cody Ashe-Mcnalley, Arpana Gupta and Tillisch
Gail and Gerald Oppenheimer Family Center for Neurobiology of Stress, University of California Los Angeles, Los Angeles, California, United States of America
Pain and Interoception Imaging Network (PAIN), University of California Los Angeles, Los Angeles, California, United States of America
Department of Medicine, University of California Los Angeles, Los Angeles, California, United States of America
Division of Digestive Diseases, University of California Los Angeles, Los Angeles, California, United States of America

Ivo Dino
University of Michigan School of Nursing, Ann Arbor, Michigan, United States of America

Yonggang Shi
Laboratory of Neuro-Imaging, University of Southern California, Los Angeles, California United States of America

Jean Stains, Nuwanthi Heendeniya and Suzanne R. Smith
Gail and Gerald Oppenheimer Family Center for Neurobiology of Stress, University of California Los Angeles, Los Angeles, California, United States of America
Department of Medicine, University of California Los Angeles, Los Angeles, California, United States of America

Division of Digestive Diseases, University of California Los Angeles, Los Angeles, California, United States of America

Kirsten Emeran A. ayer
Gail and Gerald Oppenheimer Family Center for Neurobiology of Stress, University of California Los Angeles, Los Angeles, California, United States of America
Pain and Interoception Imaging Network (PAIN), University of California Los Angeles, Los Angeles, California, United States of America
Department of Medicine, University of California Los Angeles, Los Angeles, California, United States of America
Department of Psychiatry, University of California Los Angeles, Los Angeles, California, United States of America
Ahmanson Lovelace Brain Mapping Center, David Geffen School of Medicine, University of California, Los Angeles, California

Joshua G. X. Wong, Victor C. Gan and Ee-Ling Ng
Institute of Infectious Disease and Epidemiology, Tan Tock Seng Hospital, Singapore, Singapore

Yee-Sin Leo
Institute of Infectious Disease and Epidemiology, Tan Tock Seng Hospital, Singapore, Singapore
Saw Swee Hock School of Public Health, National University of Singapore, Singapore, Singapore
Lee Kong Chian School of Medicine, Nanyang Technologicial University, Singapore, Singapore
Yong Loo Lin School of Medicine, National University of Singapore, Singapore, Singapore

Siew-Pang Chan
Institute of Infectious Disease and Epidemiology, Tan Tock Seng Hospital, Singapore, Singapore
Stata Users Group, Singapore, Singapore
Department of Mathematics and Science, La Trobe University, Melbourne, Victoria, Australia

Robin Choo
Stata Users Group, Singapore, Singapore
Singapore Institute for Clinical Sciences, Brenner Centre for Molecular Medicine, Singapore, Singapore

David C. Lye
Institute of Infectious Disease and Epidemiology, Tan Tock Seng Hospital, Singapore, Singapore
Yong Loo Lin School of Medicine, National University of Singapore, Singapore, Singapore

Liping Yang, Yu Chen, Bingling Zhang, Chunxiao Chen, Min Yue, Juan Du, Chaohui Yu and Youming Li
Department of Gastroenterology, the First Affiliated Hospital, College of Medicine, Zhejiang University, Hangzhou, China

Zhang Fangbin, Hao Weiwei, Zheng Cong, Chu Yanjun and Xu Feng
Department of Gastroenterology, The First Affiliated Hospital of Zhengzhou University, Zhengzhou, People's Republic of China

Zhao Wugan
Department of Pathology, The First Affiliated Hospital of Zhengzhou University, Zhengzhou, People's Republic of China

Xinxue Liu, Angela Wong, Sudarshan R. Kadri, Andrej Corovic, Pierre Lao-Sirieix and Rebecca C. Fitzgerald
MRC Cancer Unit, University of Cambridge, Cambridge, United Kingdom

Maria O'Donovan
Department of Histopathology, Addenbrooke's Hospital, Cambridge, United Kingdom

Rodney W. Burnham
Queen's Hospital, Romford, Essex, United Kingdom

Laurence B. Lovat
University College London Hospital (UCLH), London, United Kingdom

Janne Laine
Tampere University Hospital, Department of Internal Medicine, Tampere, Finland
National Institute of Health and Welfare, Epidemiologic Surveillance and Response Unit, Helsinki, Finland

Jukka Lumio
University of Tampere, School of Medicine, Tampere, Finland

Salla Toikkanen, Mikko J. Virtanen and Markku Kuusi
National Institute of Health and Welfare, Epidemiologic Surveillance and Response Unit, Helsinki, Finland

Terhi Uotila
Tampere University Hospital, Department of Internal Medicine, Tampere, Finland

Markku Korpela
Tampere University Hospital, Department of Internal Medicine, Tampere, Finland
University of Tampere, School of Medicine, Tampere, Finland

Eila Kujansuu
Nokia Health Centre, Nokia, Finland

Giuseppe Lanza and Raffaele Ferri
Department of Neurology I.C., Oasi Institute for Research on Mental Retardation and Brain Aging (I.R.C.C.S.), Troina (Enna), Italy

Mariagiovanna Cantone and Manuela Pennisi
Department of Chemistry, University of Catania, Catania, Italy

Carmela Cinzia D'Agate, Pietro Naso and Giuseppe Aprile
Gastroenterology and Endoscopy Unit, University of Catania, Catania, Italy

Giulia Malaguarnera
Department of Biomedical Sciences, University of Catania, Catania, Italy

Giovanni Pennisi, Salvatore Giuffrida, Luisa Vinciguerra, Valentina Puglisi and Rita Bella
Department "G.F. Ingrassia", Section of Neurosciences, University of Catania, Catania, Italy

Ignasi Puig
Digestive Diseases Department, Althaia Xarxa Assistencial Universitària de Manresa, Barcelona, Spain
Universitat Internacional de Catalunya, Barcelona, Spain
Departament de Medicina, Universitat Autònoma de Barcelona, Barcelona, Spain

Xavier Calvet
Departament de Medicina, Universitat Autònoma de Barcelona, Barcelona, Spain
Digestive Diseases Department, Corporació Sanitària Parc Taulí, Sabadell, Barcelona, Spain
Centro de Investigación Biomédica en Red de enfermedades hepáticas y digestivas (CIBERehd), Madrid, Spain

Mireia Baylina
Departament de Medicina, Universitat Autònoma de Barcelona, Barcelona, Spain
Internal Medicine Department, Corporació Sanitària Parc Taulí, Sabadell, Barcelona, Spain

Álvaro Isava, Pau Sort, Jordina Llaó, Francesc Porta and Francesc Vida
Digestive Diseases Department, Althaia Xarxa Assistencial Universitària de Manresa, Barcelona, Spain
Universitat Internacional de Catalunya, Barcelona, Spain

Mujahed Shraim
Arthritis Research UK Primary Care Centre, Keele University, Keele, United Kingdom
Work Environment Department, University of Massachusetts Lowell, Lowell, Massachusetts, United States of America
Center for Disability Research, Liberty Mutual Research Institute for Safety, Hopkinton, Massachusetts, United States of America

Milisa Blagojevic-Bucknall, Christian D. Mallen and Kate M. Dunn
Arthritis Research UK Primary Care Centre, Keele University, Keele, United Kingdom

Sammy M. Njenga
Eastern and Southern Africa Centre of International Parasite Control (ESACIPAC), Kenya Medical Research Institute (KEMRI), Mbagathi Road, Nairobi, Kenya

Paul M. Ng'ang'a and Mariam T. Mwanje
Division of Vector-Borne Diseases & Neglected Tropical Diseases (DVBD-NTD), Ministry of Health, Nairobi, Kenya

Fatuma S. Bendera
Environmental Health Department, Kwale County, Kenya

Moses J. Bockarie
Centre for Neglected Tropical Diseases, Liverpool School of Tropical Medicine, Liverpool, United Kingdom

Melianthe P. J. Nicolai, Rob C. M. Pelger and Henk W. Elzevier
Department of Urology, Leiden University Medical Center, Leiden, the Netherlands

Josbert J. Keller and Jan J. Nicolai
Department of Gastroenterology, HAGA Teaching Hospital, The Hague, the Netherlands

Lieke de Vries
Department of Urology, Westeinde Hospital, The Hague, the Netherlands

Andrea E. van der Meulen-de Jong and James C. H. Hardwick
Department of Gastroenterology, Leiden University Medical Center, Leiden, the Netherlands

Hein Putter
Department of Medical Statistics, Leiden University Medical Center, Leiden, the Netherlands

Wannee Limpitikul
Department of Pediatrics, Songkhla Hospital, Songkhla, Thailand

Narong Henpraserttae
Bureau of Epidemiology, Department of Disease Control, Ministry of Public Health in Songkhla, Songkhla, Thailand

Rachanee Saksawad
Department of Pediatrics, Hat Yai Education Center, Hat Yai Hospital, Hat Yai, Songkhla, Thailand

Kamolwish Laoprasopwattana
Department of Pediatrics, Faculty of Medicine, Prince of Songkla University, Hat Yai, Songkhla, Thailand

Senanayake A. M. Kularatne
Department of Medicine, Faculty of Medicine, University of Peradeniya, Peradeniya, Sri Lanka

Anjana Silva and Kosala Weerakoon
Department of Parasitology, Faculty of Medicine and Allied Sciences, Rajarata University of Sri Lanka, Anuradhapura, Sri Lanka

Kalana Maduwage
School of Medicine and Public Health, University of Newcastle, Callaghan, New South Wales, Australia

Chamara Walathara, Ranjith Paranagama and Suresh Mendis
Teaching Hospital, Anuradhapura, Sri Lanka

Helena Boene, Anifa Valá and Charfudin Sacoor
Centro de Investigação em Saúde da Manhiça, Manhiça, Mozambique

Raquel González, Maria Rupérez and Clara Menéndez
Centro de Investigação em Saúde da Manhiça, Manhiça, Mozambique
Barcelona Centre for International Health Research, Hospital Clinic - Universitat de Barcelona, Barcelona, Spain

César Velasco
Barcelona Centre for International Health Research, Hospital Clinic - Universitat de Barcelona, Barcelona, Spain

Sónia Machevo, Esperança Sevene and Khátia Munguambe
Centro de Investigação em Saúde da Manhiça, Manhiça, Mozambique
Universidade Eduardo Mondlane, Faculdade de Medicina, Maputo, Mozambique

Eusébio Macete
Centro de Investigação em Saúde da Manhiça, Manhiça, Mozambique
Direcção Nacional de Saúde Pública, Ministério da Saú de, Maputo, Mozambique

Index

A

Abdominal Pain, 1-5, 9, 20, 30-37, 45-48, 51, 56-57, 60-63, 66, 76-79, 89, 92, 94-95, 97-98, 100-101, 105-107, 109-111, 117, 119-120, 123-125, 127, 130-132, 134-135, 137-146, 148, 150-153, 156-159, 163, 170, 172, 177, 179, 181-186, 188-190, 192-195, 197-198, 201-204, 206-208, 210-212, 218

Allergic Disorder, 65

Allergic Inflammation, 65, 73

Anchor Descriptors, 38-43

Anchor Label, 39, 42

Antiretrovirals, 114, 215

Appendicitis, 7, 31, 36-37

B

Back Pain, 5, 42-43, 56, 77, 80, 95, 97-99, 119-120, 128-129, 172, 179, 181, 184-185

Baep Peak Latency, 102

Biopsies, 1-3, 6-7, 65-69, 74, 124, 146

Brainstem Auditory Evoked Potential, 100-102

Breastfeeding, 92, 114, 121

C

Capsule Endoscopy, 137-138, 140

Catechol-o-methyltransferase, 108, 113

Central Nervous System, 24-26, 28, 52, 101, 106, 118, 162-163, 167

Chi-square Test, 39-40, 78, 81, 164

Children's Somatization Inventory, 100-101, 178

Chronic Kidney Disease, 76, 79, 81-82, 212

Chronic Pain, 20-21, 24-25, 27-28, 38-39, 41-43, 84, 93, 97-99, 108, 113, 124, 127-130, 135, 198

Chronic Pancreatitis, 20-21, 23-25, 28-29, 129, 176

Chronic Pancreatitis Patients, 20-21, 23-25, 28

Colonoscopy, 1-3, 46, 106, 138, 140-143, 145-147, 154, 192-198

Computed Tomography, 76, 137-138, 140, 162, 164

Corticosterone Levels, 86, 88, 90-92

E

Electroencephalogram, 63, 100-101, 164

Electrophysiological, 100, 163, 165-166

Emergency Department, 30-37, 43, 76-77

Encephalopathy, 51, 53-54, 56-57, 59, 118

Eosinophilic Esophagitis, 65, 67, 75

Episodic Ataxia, 60-61, 63-64

F

Fibromyalgia Syndrome, 14, 18-19, 99, 186

Fluoxetine Exposure, 84, 88-92

Fms Patients, 14

Functional Constipation, 8-10, 13, 143

Functional Dyspepsia, 8-10, 12

Functional Gastrointestinal Disorders, 8, 12-13, 49, 106-107, 129, 199

G

Gastrointestinal, 1, 3, 8-9, 11-13, 30-31, 33, 36-37, 45, 49-50, 52, 57, 97, 100, 106-107, 109, 113, 118-120, 129, 137, 139-142, 146, 149, 156-161, 169, 173, 176-177, 179, 181-185, 190, 192, 194-195, 198-199, 202, 209

Gastrointestinal Health, 192

Genotyping, 46, 50, 109, 112

Gi Symptoms, 2, 100-103, 105-106, 125, 202

H

Hantavirus Infection, 1, 3, 7

Hantavirus Species, 1

Headaches, 62, 93, 97, 99, 106, 185-186, 189-190

Hpa System, 84-85, 88-89, 91-92

Hyperalgesia, 20-21, 23-29, 37, 50, 92, 106

I

Immunohistochemical, 1-4, 7, 54

Infant Safety, 114-116

Inflammatory Bowel Diseases, 31, 37, 123, 146

Insomnia, 93-94, 97-99

Intestinal Biopsies, 1, 3

Irritable Bowel Syndrome, 8-13, 21, 26, 28, 30, 37, 45, 49-50, 100, 106-109, 113, 123, 129-130, 142, 146, 156, 158, 161, 182

J

Joint Symptoms, 156-158, 160-161

L

Lamina Propria, 1-4, 146

M

Maternal Safety, 117, 119, 121

Mental State Examination, 39, 162, 164-165

Mirnas, 65-75
Monoclonal Antibody, 2, 4, 92
Mrna Transcriptome, 65

N
Nephropathia Epidemica, 1, 7
Neurologic Illness, 51-58
Neuroplastic Changes, 123
Nociception Behavioral, 85, 87
Non-specific Abdominal Pain, 30-37
Norovirus, 156-157, 159-161
Nucleocapsid Antigen, 1, 3-6

P
Pain Catastrophizing, 39-40, 44
Pain Detection Threshold, 20, 23, 25
Pain Intensity, 38-43, 128, 131-132, 135
Pain Outcomes, 93-95, 97-98
Parental Bonding, 100-102, 104-106
Parental Bonding Instrument, 100, 102, 104, 106
Patient Selection, 76
Placebo Responders, 108, 111-113
Placebo Responses, 109, 111
Polymerase Chain Reaction, 45-46
Polymorphism, 45-47, 49-50, 63, 108-109, 111-113, 146
Pressure Pain Thresholds, 21, 23-24, 27
Pro-nociceptive Pain, 21, 23
Psychological Factors, 8, 11-12, 39, 159
Puumala Virus, 1, 7

Q
Quantitative Sensory Testing, 20-21, 23-24, 29

R
Renal Infarction, 76-79, 81-82

S
Schistosomiasis, 187-188, 190-191
Selective Serotonin Reuptake Inhibitor, 84
Serotonin Transporter, 45, 48-50, 111
Sexual Abuse, 192, 194-199
Signed-rank Test, 39-40, 42
Sleep Disorders, 93, 99
Sleep Disturbance, 93-99
Sleep-related Outcomes, 94, 98
Soil-transmitted Helminths, 187-188, 191
Somatic Symptom, 14-15, 18, 46, 48
Somatization, 13, 100-103, 106, 178, 185-186

T
Temporomandibular Joint, 93, 97, 99
Terminal Ileal Lesions, 141, 144
Thrombocytopenia, 1, 58, 202-203
Treatment, 2, 6-7, 12-13, 18, 20-21, 23-29, 31-33, 36, 46, 50, 57-58, 60-61, 63-70, 73-77, 82, 84-85, 87-97, 99, 101, 106, 108-115, 119, 128-131, 135, 140, 142-143, 145, 161, 168, 171-172, 186-191, 200-205, 207, 210, 212-216, 221
Typhoid Fever, 51-55, 57-58, 200-205

V
Valacyclovir, 114-122
Visceral Pain Syndromes, 123, 128

W
Widespread Pain Index, 14-15, 17